Contents

FUNDAMENTAL PRINCIPLES OF PATIENT MANAGEMENT

COMMON COMPLAINTS

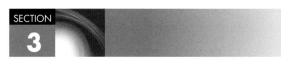

CANCER AND POTENTIALLY MALIGNANT DISORDERS

COMMON AND IMPORTANT OROFACIAL CONDITIONS

SECTION 5

RELEVANT SYSTEMIC DISORDERS

SECTION 6

EPONYMOUS AND OTHER CONDITIONS

THIRD EDITION

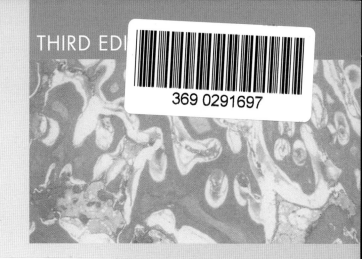

Oral and Maxillofacial Medicine

THE BASIS OF DIAGNOSIS AND TREATMENT

Commissioning Editor: Alison Taylor
Development Editor: Lynn Watt
Project Manager: Louisa Talbott
Designer/Design Direction: Miles Hitchen
Illustration Manager: Jennifer Rose
Illustrator: Dartmouth Inc./Antbits Ltd.

THIRD EDITION

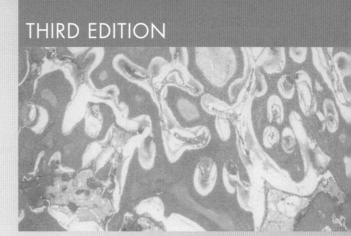

Oral and Maxillofacial Medicine

THE BASIS OF DIAGNOSIS AND TREATMENT

Crispian Scully CBE

MD PhD MDS MRCS BSc FDSRCS FDSRCPS FFDRCSI FDSRCSE FRCPath FMedSci FHEA FUCL DSc DChD DMed[HC] DrHC

Emeritus Professor, University College London, London, UK

Honorary Consultant University College London Hospitals NHS Foundation Trust, HCA International Hospitals and Great Ormond Street Hospital for Children, London, UK

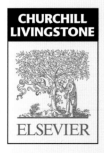

CHURCHILL LIVINGSTONE

ELSEVIER

Edinburgh   London   New York   Oxford   Philadelphia   St Louis   Sydney   Toronto   2013

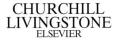

First edition 2004
Second edition 2008
Third edition 2013

ISBN 978-0-7020-4948-4

British Library Cataloguing in Publication Data
A catalogue record for this book is available from the British Library

Library of Congress Cataloging in Publication Data
A catalog record for this book is available from the Library of Congress

Notices
Knowledge and best practice in this field are constantly changing. As new research and experience broaden our understanding, changes in research methods, professional practices, or medical treatment may become necessary.

Practitioners and researchers must always rely on their own experience and knowledge in evaluating and using any information, methods, compounds, or experiments described herein. In using such information or methods they should be mindful of their own safety and the safety of others, including parties for whom they have a professional responsibility.

With respect to any drug or pharmaceutical products identified, readers are advised to check the most current information provided (i) on procedures featured or (ii) by the manufacturer of each product to be administered, to verify the recommended dose or formula, the method and duration of administration, and contraindications. It is the responsibility of practitioners, relying on their own experience and knowledge of their patients, to make diagnoses, to determine dosages and the best treatment for each individual patient, and to take all appropriate safety precautions.

To the fullest extent of the law, neither the Publisher nor the authors, contributors, or editors, assume any liability for any injury and/or damage to persons or property as a matter of products liability, negligence or otherwise, or from any use or operation of any methods, products, instructions, or ideas contained in the material herein.

 your source for books,
journals and multimedia
in the health sciences

www.elsevierhealth.com

Working together to grow
libraries in developing countries

www.elsevier.com | www.bookaid.org | www.sabre.org

ELSEVIER   BOOK AID International   Sabre Foundation

The
Publisher's
policy is to use
**paper manufactured
from sustainable forests**

Printed in China

Preface to third edition

I am pleased to say that the first two editions were so well received and popular, that there have been multiple reprints. The first edition was awarded the First Prize of the Royal Society of Medicine and Society of Authors for a new authored book and the second edition was Highly Commended in the British Medical Association Book Awards.

In the preface to the first edition I noted I would be delighted to receive any comments about the text, but received no suggested improvements. Therefore, to reassure myself, the publishers have had the book peer-reviewed blindly, and I have incorporated suggestions received. Further, to ensure the book continues to be up-to-date, I have again taken the opportunity to refine and restructure; to thoroughly revise, clarify and update the text and the Further reading and Useful websites.

I have also added new material and clinical pictures, tables, boxes and algorithms. Advisers have requested more information on drug interactions and contraindications, but dissuaded me from adding too many additional clinical pictures, suggesting that Atlases were most suitable for these.

I have also increased the content in terms of expansion and rearrangement of the section dealing with potentially malignant disorders and cancer; added new material on the genetic influences in many conditions; and added some fairly recently recognised relevant conditions including various adverse drug reactions, autonomic neuropathies, drug-induced hypersensitivity syndrome, hypereosinophilic syndrome, immune reconstitution inflammatory syndrome (IRIS), IgG4 syndrome, lichenoid and granulomatous stomatitis, trigeminal autonomic cephalgias (TACs), TUGSE (traumatic ulcerative granuloma with stromal eosinophilia), and a new oral mucosal condition similar to orofacial granulomatosis described in solid organ-transplanted children.

Finally, I have also expanded therapeutics – including emergent therapies. Few of the agents used in oral medicine have been produced specifically for orofacial diseases, many also being employed in other fields such as dermatology, rheumatology and gastroenterology and their use in orofacial disease is often 'off label'. Some complementary medicine products are also increasingly in use, with an even weaker evidence base. Few agents have thus been tested in randomized controlled double blind clinical trials but, nevertheless, I have endeavoured to highlight the level of evidence for the various therapies most commonly used and introduced a 'likely benefit' scheme similar to that used in *Clinical Evidence* – the British Medical Journal publication. There will always be some controversy between the categories 'likely to be beneficial' and 'unproven effectiveness'. The evidence base is often sparse and changing but patients must be offered some help and hope.

Drug doses quoted are for healthy adults only and must be reduced in children and older and/or ill patients. Contraindications to drug use are often relative and not absolute, and drug interactions can range from potentially lethal to theoretical only. Doses, contraindications and possible interactions should always be checked with an authoritative source.

In any book there is always a potential conflict between the need for basic and more advanced knowledge: I have endeavoured to address this by including some boxes on the basic causes of conditions, along with expanded versions including more advanced lists.

My additional thanks also are again to Prof Mervyn Shear and Dr David Wiesenfeld for advice; to Dr Aubrey Craig of Medical and Dental Defence Union of Scotland for occasional guidance; to Drs Rachel Cowie, Rachael Hampton and Yazan Hassona for clinical assistance, to Dr Mo El-Maaytah for figure 56.2, to Dr Tony Brooke for figure 53.9 and also to Drs Andrew Robinson, Eleni Georgakopoulou and Dimitris Malamos for constructive comments on the previous edition.

CS
2013

No-one who achieves success does so without acknowledging the help of others.

Alfred North Whitehead

Preface to second edition

I am pleased to say that the first edition was very well received and proved popular. Indeed, the book was awarded the First Prize of the Royal Society of Medicine and Society of Authors, for a new authored book.

Nevertheless, I have taken the opportunity to restructure; to thoroughly revise and update the text; to reformat where this could enhance clarity; to add new material and clinical pictures and some basic histopathology, tables, boxes and algorithms; to add new chapters on sialorrhoea and drooling, other conditions, and adverse drug reactions; and to update Further reading.

My additional thanks are to John Huw Evans for his technical assistance, to Dr Stefano Fedele for his comments overall, to Dr Mohamed El-Maaytah and Dr Navdeep Kumar for providing a few figures, to Professor John Eveson for kind permission to use histopathology from our book Eveson, J.W. and Scully, C. *Colour Atlas of Oral Pathology* (1995). Mosby-Wolfe (London) and to Peter Reichart, David Sidransky and Dr L. Barnes for permission to reproduce their WHO Classifications from *Pathology and Genetics of Tumours of the Head and Neck* (2005) and to Professor Mervyn Shear for commenting on the Chapter on Odontogenic Cysts and Tumours.

CS
2007

The wise should consider that health is the greatest of human blessings.

Hippocrates

Preface to first edition

Oral medicine is that area of special competence in dentistry concerned mainly with diseases involving the oral and perioral structures, especially the oral mucosa, and the oral manifestations of systemic diseases. The specialty, in some countries termed 'stomatology', deals not only with oral disease but also with perioral lesions, and is increasingly known as 'oral and maxillofacial medicine'. Furthermore, apart from the obvious close relationships with oral pathology (oral and maxillofacial pathology) and with oral surgery (oral and maxillofacial surgery), there is a close relationship with special care dentistry and hospital dentistry.

This book attempts to present for those interested in oral medicine and hospital dentistry, the basics of the specialty of oral medicine in a useful and digestible format; by offering the information in a range of modes and levels of detail and offering practical guidance to diagnosis, therapy and sources of information for patient and clinician, both on the Internet and elsewhere.

The first section reviews the fundamental principles of the history, examination and investigations and principles of management. In the absence of randomized controlled trials, many of the therapies suggested are unable to be thoroughly evidence based. Hopefully, future multicentre studies will rectify this deficiency. The second section discusses the more common symptoms and signs in oral medicine.

The third section covers in some detail the most common and important conditions seen in oral medicine. This section also includes synopses of a number of eponymous and other conditions relevant to oral medicine; if a specific condition is not found there, the reader is referred to the index, since it may well be located elsewhere in the book.

The fourth section is a discussion of the important areas of HIV infection and iatrogenic diseases.

The other relevant oral manifestations of systemic disorders are tabulated in Appendix 1: further detail can be found in *Medical Problems in Dentistry* (Scully and Cawson: Elsevier, Edinburgh, 2004).

Agents used in the treatment of patients with oral diseases are outlined in Appendix 2. Only a limited number of these are prescribed by dental practitioners, but practitioners may have to cope with questions from patients about their treatment, or to recognize or deal with treatment complications. Further details can be found in textbooks such as *Basic Pharmacology and Clinical Drug Use in Dentistry* (Cawson, Spector and Skelly: Churchill Livingstone, Edinburgh, 1995).

An attempt has been made to present the material in such a way as to highlight the more important conditions – important because of frequency or seriousness – and to guide the reader through didactic and problem-oriented approaches. However, it is impossible to position every subject in a perfect location, not least because few conditions affect only one site (e.g. even erythema migrans can have lesions in sites other than on the tongue), some affect even more than one tissue (e.g. ectodermal dysplasia affects skin, salivary glands and teeth) and several have a range of clinical presentations (e.g. lichen planus and cancer can both present with white, red or ulcerative lesions, and can be symptomless or cause extreme discomfort). Cross-referring between sections will help the user get full value from the content.

The book is not intended to give all the details of the various investigative and therapeutic modalities, since these are covered in other texts by the author, or in pharmacopoeias. The book offers illustrative examples of the more common and important conditions, but cannot provide the more comprehensive selection of illustrations such as can be found in atlases such as *Oral Diseases* (Scully, Flint, Porter and Moos: Dunitz, London, 2004).

I thank my patients and nurses who have taught me so much over the years, and continue so to do, and all those students and colleagues with whom I have worked and interacted, who may have shared the clinical care of some patients, and/or may have knowingly or otherwise contributed ideas or content.

In this respect I thank especially Professors Oslei Almeida (Brazil), Jose-Vicente Sebastian-Bagan (Spain), Johann Beck-Managetta (Austria), Roman Carlos (Guatemala), Marco Carrozzo (Italy), Roderick Cawson (UK), Pedro Diz Dios (Spain), Drore Eisen (USA), Joel Epstein (Canada), Sergio Gandolfo (Italy), George Laskaris (Greece), Jens Pindborg (Denmark; deceased), Stephen Porter (UK), Peter Reichart (Germany), Pierre-Luigi Sapelli (Italy), Sol 'Bud' Silverman (USA) and Isaac Van der Waal (The Netherlands).

Thanks are also due to: Alan Drinnan (USA) for his innovative introduction of the Bulletin Board in Oral Pathology (BBOP), a useful world forum for oral medicine and pathology; to Miguel Lucas-Tomas (Spain), who founded the European Association for Oral Medicine – a major European forum; and to Dean Millard (USA) and David Mason (UK), who had the foresight to institute the World Workshops in Oral Medicine; to John Greenspan (USA) who had the foresight to organize the Oral AIDS workshops; and to Newell Johnson with whom I founded and co-edit Oral Diseases. These giants have helped the progression of oral medicine to the high level at which it now stands.

Much of my work could not be done without the support of my family (Zoe and Frances) and my work colleagues who help with information collection, particularly John Evans, Avril Gardner, Lesley Garlick and Karen Widdowson, to whom thanks are due. I thank Jose-Vicente Sebastian Bagan and Isaac van der Waal, and also my nephew, Dr Athanassios Kalantzis, for their helpful, friendly and constructive comments on the text.

Finally, I would be delighted to receive any comments about this text, in the hope that I can improve further in the future.

CS
2003

Learning aims and objectives

- Describe oral and maxillofacial diseases and their relevance to prevention, diagnosis and treatment
- Explain general and systemic disease of particular relevance to oral health
- Explain the aetiology and pathogenesis of orofacial disease
- Obtain, record, and interpret a comprehensive and contemporaneous patient history
- Undertake an appropriate systematic intra and extra-oral clinical examination
- Manage appropriate clinical and laboratory investigations
- Undertake appropriate special tests and diagnostic procedures
- Assess patients' levels of anxiety, experience and expectations in respect of dental care
- Generate a differential diagnosis
- Formulate an appropriate treatment plan based on the patient assessment and diagnosis
- Describe the range of orthodox complementary and alternative therapies that may impact on patient management
- Refer patients for treatment or advice when and where appropriate
- Explain and manage the impact of medical and psychological conditions in the patient
- Discuss the need for and make arrangements for appropriate follow-up care
- Recognise the responsibilities of a dentist as an access point to and from wider healthcare
- Provide patients with comprehensive and accurate preventive education and instruction in a manner which encourages self-care and motivation
- Describe the principles of preventive care and incorporate as part of a comprehensive treatment plan
- Underpin all patient care with a preventive approach that contributes to the patient's long-term oral and general health
- Describe in appropriate detail the health risks of diet, drugs and substance misuse, and substances such as tobacco, alcohol and betel on oral and general health and provide appropriate advice and support
- Assess and manage the health of soft tissues taking into account risk and lifestyle factors
- Manage oral disease and refer when and where appropriate
- Describe, take account of and explain to the patient the impact of the patient's health on the overall treatment plan and outcomes
- Evaluate, for individual patients, the need for more complex treatment and refer appropriately
- Recognise all stages of malignancy, the aetiology and development of tumours and the importance of early referral for investigation and biopsy
- Identify and explain appropriately to patients the risks, benefits, complications and contra-indications to medical and surgical interventions
- Communicate appropriately, effectively and sensitively at all times with and about patients, their representatives and the general public and in relation to difficult circumstances, such as when breaking bad news, and when discussing issues, such as alcohol consumption, tobacco smoking or diet.

Intended learning outcomes

This text will deal with oral and maxillofacial diseases and their medical management, and it is intended that, having read this text, the reader will be able to:

- Adopt a systematic approach to medical history taking that extends routine questions into certain relevant areas of enquiry that involve the body in general.
- Examine patients and their oral lesions systematically and use the findings of specific features of the lesion and associated signs and symptoms, to start formulating differential diagnoses.
- Identify which sites may be affected by the presenting condition and what to look for at those sites.
- Identify relevant follow-up questions that may further clarify the findings of the clinical examination and refocus the history.
- Understand when clinical investigations are indicated, which are appropriate, and how to perform these investigations.
- Interpret the findings of routine clinical investigations (e.g. blood test results) and develop a sense of the potential implications for the patient.

- Recognize the scope of oral and maxillofacial diseases and the importance of medical management in addition to the traditional dental focus of the discipline.
- Advise the patient about the aetiology of oral lesions, and predisposing factors.
- Identify lesions and interpret the findings and develop a sense of the potential implications for the patient.
- Understand how prevention may impact positively upon the condition.
- Identify a range of therapeutic options for the patient and understand the need for regular review and re-appraisal of the condition.
- Understand how treatment may impact, positively or negatively, upon the condition.
- Identify the need to refer for advice, investigations or treatment by dental, medical or surgical specialists.
- Recognize the importance of close liaison with colleagues in other disciplines, particularly imaging, medicine, pathology and surgery.

Education is not filling a bucket but lighting a fire
William Butler Yeates

FUNDAMENTAL PRINCIPLES OF PATIENT MANAGEMENT

It is better to know what kind of patient has the disease than what kind of disease the patient has.
Sir William Osler

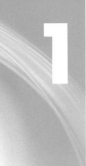

Diagnosis: history

INTRODUCTION

Diagnosis means 'through knowledge' and entails acquisition of data about the patient and their complaint using the senses (HOTS):

- hearing
- observing
- touching
- sometimes smelling (**Fig. 1.1**).

The purpose of making a diagnosis is to be able to offer the most:

- effective and safe treatment
- accurate prognostication.

Diagnosis is made by the clinical examination, which comprises the:

- history (anamnesis) – this offers the diagnosis in about 80% of cases
- physical examination
- supplemented in some cases by investigations.

Each is based on a thorough, methodical routine. Diagnosis most importantly involves a careful history; the patient will often deliver the diagnosis from the history, though the findings from examination and investigations can be helpful, as can reference to the literature and Internet. To state the obvious, it is difficult to diagnose a condition that is unknown to the diagnostician; thus extensive reading of recent literature, clinical experience and discussion with colleagues is continually needed, as well as an enquiring mind. Continuing education is essential.

There are many types of diagnosis, including:

- Clinical diagnosis: made from the history and examination.
- Pathological diagnosis: provided from the pathology results.
- Direct diagnosis: made by observing pathognomonic features. This is occasionally possible, for example in dentinogenesis imperfecta where the abnormally translucent brownish teeth are characteristic.
- Provisional (working) diagnosis: the more usually made diagnosis. This is an initial diagnosis from which further investigations can be planned.
- Deductive diagnosis: made after due consideration of all facts from the history, examination and investigations.
- Differential diagnosis: the process of making a diagnosis by considering the similarities and differences between similar conditions.
- Diagnosis by exclusion: identification of a disease by excluding all other possible causes.

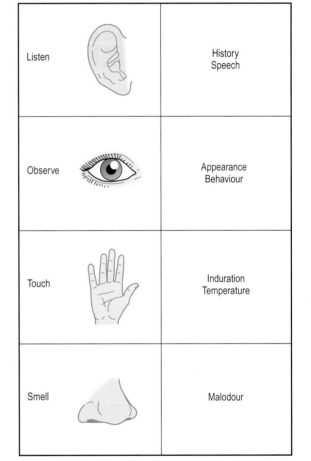

Listen	History Speech
Observe	Appearance Behaviour
Touch	Induration Temperature
Smell	Malodour

Fig. 1.1 The senses in diagnosis

- Diagnosis ex-juvantibus: made on the results of response to treatment. For example, the pain of trigeminal neuralgia may be atypical, and the diagnosis can sometimes be confirmed only by a positive response to the drug carbamazepine.
- Provocative diagnosis: the induction of a condition in order to establish a diagnosis. This is rarely needed, except in possible drug reactions or allergies, when the patient may need to be re-exposed to the potentially culpable substance, but this should always be carried out where appropriate medical support and resuscitation are available.

PROGNOSIS

Prognosis (from the Greek – literally fore-knowing, foreseeing) is a medical term to describe the likely outcome of an illness. A number of conditions and lesions seen in oral medicine, especially cancer and pemphigus, can have potentially serious prognoses (**Table 1.1**).

In any event, the crucial point is communicating clearly with the patient.

COMMUNICATING WITH THE PATIENT

Patients' attitudes to healthcare, the benefits and risks from examination, investigations and treatment, and the extent to which they find adverse effects tolerable, can differ markedly from assumptions of the clinicians. Effective healthcare communication incorporates not only medical and dental information, but also sensitive discussion of the patients' emotional and social wellbeing, always being culturally sensitive and tailoring to the patient's ability to understand.

Patients have personal wishes, needs and concerns that demand the understanding and respect of the clinician. Involving patients as full partners in decisions about treatment leads to better health outcomes. Healthcare should:

- provide respectful care
- meet the patient's personal, cultural and religious needs
- educate and inform on relevant health issues
- facilitate patients making their own choices
- respect those choices.

Communicating requires time and patience and expertise: language can be a huge barrier. One of the most obvious ways to assist communication is to have material available in relevant different languages and easily readable and understood.

Patient interviews are an opportunity to listen and ascertain the patient's feelings and concerns about healthcare and to explore what beliefs and practices are important to them. The clinician should use 'LEAPS':

- **L**isten
- **E**mpathize
- **A**sk
- **P**araphrase
- **S**ummarize.

The clinician should thereby endeavour to:

- Elicit the:
  - patient's main problems
  - patient's perceptions of their problems
  - physical, emotional and social impact of problems.
- Tailor information to what the patient wants to know, always checking understanding.
- Elicit the patient's reaction to information given.
- Determine how much the patient wants to participate in decision-making.
- Discuss management options.

Greetings can 'make' or 'break' the professional relationship, especially as is often the case, if the patient is older and/or from a different culture. Key points to remember include to:

- smile
- speak clearly and directly, making eye contact as appropriate
- greet using 'Good morning' or 'Good afternoon', or the greeting appropriate to their culture
- never use the first name alone, except when requested. Ask the patient what they prefer to be called but as a default and at the initial greeting use their title and surname
- be careful about touching
- explain who you are and what you do, what is happening and what will happen
- sensitively check whether the patient understands the conversation
- say a few words to put the patient at ease.
- encourage the patient to establish a professional relationship.

For many people from non-Anglo-Saxon cultures, the customary greeting is a gesture other than the handshake. In addition, some may be uncomfortable shaking hands with a person of the opposite gender. Unless you are certain of their culture or religion, it is better to greet a patient with a handshake, seeing first if the person offers their hand, and then say 'Good morning/afternoon' and use their title followed by their last name.

Communication can thus be achieved through:

- active listening
- empathy
- appropriately using open questions
- frequently summarizing
- clarifying where needed
- clearly explaining concepts
- checking patient's understanding
- checking patient's compliance with management recommendations.

Specific skills such as questioning styles, active listening, providing information and avoiding negative communication behaviours (e.g. inappropriate affect, the inappropriate use of closed questions, or offering premature advice/reassurance), are crucial to success.

Avoid also the use of:

- technical terms and expressions
- abbreviations
- professional jargon
- abstract concepts
- colloquialisms
- idiomatic expressions
- slang
- metaphors
- euphemisms
- stereotype figures or symbols.

Give any bad or unpleasant news tactfully and slowly, maintain confidentiality and check with the patient exactly who can be told about their condition, when, and what they can be told.

A key healthcare professional (HCP) should be identified who the patient can contact for further information and act as an advocate. Most important is verbal interaction, but alternative information sources (e.g. written leaflets, computer systems, DVDs, etc.) can help.

Table 1.1 Clinical situations with potentially serious or life-threatening connotations

Features	Comments
Abnormal blood vessels supplying a lump	May be malignancy
Actinic cheilitis (solar elastosis)	Potentially malignant
Angioedema	Potentially lethal through airway obstruction
Behçet syndrome	May cause thromboses of dural sinuses or vena cavae
Cancer	Potentially lethal
Dysphagia	May be malignancy
Erythema multiforme	Potentially lethal if Stevens–Johnson syndrome or toxic epidermal necrolysis (TEN)
Facial palsy	May be malignancy or cerebrovascular event
Extraction socket not healing	May be malignancy
Headache	Any patient older than 50 years who develops headaches for the first time or who has a change in a chronic headache pattern should be taken very seriously. Raised intracranial pressure is also serious, since it may be caused by malignant hypertension, a tumour, abscess or haematoma. Meningeal irritation may indicate meningitis, metastases or subarachnoid haemorrhage and may present with severe headache with nausea, vomiting, neck pain or stiffness (with inability to kiss the knees) or pain on raising the straightened legs (Kernig sign). Subdural haematomas, malignancies and trigeminal neuralgia can be serious. Giant cell arteritis needs to be treated promptly to avoid loss of vision
HIV infection	Potentially lethal
Indurated lesion	Firm infiltration beneath the mucosa may be malignant
Lesion fixed to deeper tissues	To deeper tissues or to overlying skin or mucosa may be malignant
Leukoplakia	Potentially malignant
Lichen planus	Potentially malignant
Lump	Especially if hard may be malignant
Lymph node enlargement	Especially if there is hardness in a lymph node or fixation. Enlarged cervical nodes in a patient with oral carcinoma may be caused by infection, reactive hyperplasia secondary to the tumour, or metastatic disease. Occasionally, a 'positive' lymph node is detected in the absence of any obvious primary tumour
Lymphoma	Potentially lethal
Numbness	May be malignancy
Pain	May be malignancy
Pemphigus	Potentially lethal
Red lesion	Erythroplasia or erythroplakia may be malignant or potentially malignant
Red/white mixed lesion	Erythroleukoplakia may be malignant or potentially malignant
Submucous fibrosis	Potentially malignant
Syphilis	Potentially lethal
Tooth mobility	May be malignancy
Tuberculosis	Potentially lethal
Ulcer	If persistent, with fissuring or raised exophytic margins may be malignant or chronic infection
Weight loss	May be malignancy or infection such as HIV or TB
White lesion, especially if irregular surface	Verrucous leukoplakia may be malignant or potentially malignant

HISTORY TAKING

The first contact with the patient is crucial to success and there should be a courteous approach to the patient with a professional introduction and every effort to establish communication, rapport and trust, and make the patient feel the focus of the clinician's interest. History taking is part of the initial communication between the dentist and patient. It is important to adopt a professional appearance and manner, and introduce oneself clearly and courteously. The clinician should enquire early on as to the main complaint and relevant social aspects such as occupation. The patient will know if you care, well before they care if you know.

The clinician should encourage the patient to tell the story in their own words, and use methodical questioning to elucidate further details.

Perhaps not surprisingly, many patients are apprehensive when confronted by a clinician, and therefore they may be easily disturbed if, for example, the clinician appears indifferent or unsympathetic. This can result in barriers to effective communication, which will simply hinder the clinician.

Due cognizance must also always be taken of the age, cultural background, understanding and intelligence of the patient when taking the history. It is the clinician's responsibility to elicit an accurate history; if that necessitates finding an interpreter, for example, then the clinician must arrange this.

The history is best given in the patient's own words, though the clinician often needs to guide the patient, and may use protocols to ensure collection of all relevant points.

It is important to cover the following areas:

- general information (name, date of birth, gender, ethnic origin, place of residence, occupation)
- presenting complaint(s)
- history of each of the present complaints
- past medical history
- dental history
- family history
- social and cultural history including lifestyle habits (e.g. use of tobacco, alcohol, betel)
- patient expectations.

By the end of the history, the clinician should have an idea of the patient's concerns, have assessed the patient's current problems and also have drawn up a provisional or differential diagnosis.

PRESENTING COMPLAINT

The history taking commences by identifying the current complaint(s), e.g. 'sore mouth'. The 'history of the present complaint' is then taken.

HISTORY OF THE PRESENT COMPLAINT

This should cover aspects relevant to the particular main complaint, such as:

- date of onset
- duration
- location(s)
- aggravating and relieving factors
- investigations thus far
- treatment already received.

'Leading questions' (i.e. those which suggest the answer) should be avoided. 'Open questions', which do not suggest an answer, are preferred. The history should be directed by the complaint and in most oral medicine patients it is important to establish whether there are cutaneous, gastrointestinal, genital, ocular or joint problems or a history of fever. Some patients bring descriptions or diagrams (**Fig. 1.2**). Then a series of relevant questions should elicit the 'past or relevant medical history'.

PAST OR RELEVANT MEDICAL HISTORY

The medical history should be taken to elicit all matters relevant to the:

- diagnosis
- treatment
- prognosis.

As a double check on the verbal history, the use of preprinted, standardized, self-administered questionnaires is helpful, and may encourage more truthful responses to sensitive questions (**Table 1.1**).

The history should uncover, for example, medical history relevant to:

- Previous episodes of similar or related complaints.
- Other complaints that may be relevant. For example, in patients with mucosal disorders, it is important to ascertain whether there have been lesions affecting other mucosae (ocular or anogenital) or skin, hair or nails, gastrointestinal complaints, or fever.
- Important to include are:
  - General symptoms, such as fever or weight loss.
  - Relevant symptoms related to body systems, such as:
    - nervous system (e.g. sensory loss)
    - respiratory system (e.g. cough)
    - gastrointestinal disorders that may be associated with oral ulcers and other lesions
    - skin lesions (solitary or rashes), itch or discolourations, which are common symptoms of skin disease, and there are sometimes oral lesions
    - ocular problems or visual disturbance
    - anogenital lesions, such as ulcers or warts
    - psychiatric disorders, such as anxiety, depression and eating disorders, and drug abuse are relevant to orofacial conditions.
  - Medical or surgical consultations, investigations and treatments, including radiotherapy.
- Current prescribed drugs (including self-medications and alternative medicines), since these may cause oral complaints or influence management. *The British National Formulary (BNF)* or equivalent is often indispensable, since patients commonly misspell or do not know the names of, drugs they are taking.
- Complementary medicine.
- Previous illnesses.
- Hospitalizations and previous consultations.
- Operations.
- General anaesthetics.
- Specific medical problems that may influence operative procedures, particularly:
  - allergies.
  - bleeding tendency
  - cardiorespiratory problems.

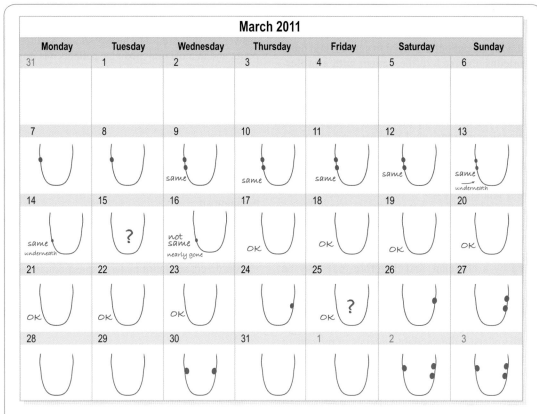

Fig. 1.2 Diary provided by patient showing recurrent tongue lesions

- drug therapy such as anticoagulants or corticosteroids
- endocrine disorders – especially diabetes
- infectious diseases.

Patients may also carry formal warnings of certain conditions relevant to dental care. These may be written cards, smart cards (there are two kinds – memory cards and microprocessor cards), or MedicAlert type bracelets or necklaces. These types of MedicAlert warning devices are recommended to be carried by anyone with:

- allergies to any drug or agent with the potential for causing a serious reaction
- chronic health problems, which might necessitate emergency treatment of a specific nature, such as: diabetes, epilepsy, glaucoma, or malignant hyperthermia
- the need to take regular medication, prosthesis, implants, and conditions which might lead to difficulty in diagnosis during emergency care, e.g. long-term anticoagulants, or long-term systemic corticosteroids.

Some patients bring quite precise written information which can be helpful (**Fig. 1.3**).

ABC

The medical history of dental patients should be directed to elicit any relevant systemic disease. For example, this may be achieved by an ABC:

- **Allergies or anaemia;** allergies can be a contraindication to use of materials such as latex. Anaemia: a reduction in haemoglobin level below the normal for age and gender can:

- be a contraindication to general anaesthesia
- cause oral complications (i.e. candidosis, sore mouth, burning tongue, glossitis, ulcers, angular stomatitis).
- **Bleeding tendency:** a hazard to any surgical procedure, including some injections, and a contraindication to aspirin and some other nonsteroidal antiinflammatory drugs (NSAIDs).
- **Cardiorespiratory disease:** this may be a contraindication to general anaesthesia. Patients with various cardiac lesions are predisposed to develop endocarditis, which may be precipitated as a consequence of the bacteraemia associated with some forms of dental treatment. Cardiac patients may have a bleeding tendency because of anticoagulants. Oral lesions may be seen – such as calcium channel blocker-induced gingival swelling, or oral ulceration with nicorandil. NSAIDs and itraconazole are contraindicated in severe cardiac failure.
- **Drug use, allergies and abuse:** these may cause orofacial lesions or give an indication about underlying pathology, or may influence dental procedures or drug use. Drug allergies are a contraindication to the use of the responsible or related drugs. Drug abuse may give rise to behavioural problems and a risk of cross-infection. Corticosteroids absorbed systemically produce adrenocortical suppression. Such patients may not respond adequately to the stress of trauma, operation or infection, and stress may produce adrenal crisis and collapse.
- **Endocrine disease.**
  - Diabetes may cause:
    - the danger of hypoglycaemia if meals are interfered with
    - oral complications such as sialosis, dry mouth and periodontal breakdown.

PRINCESS GRACE HOSPL. Harley Street London	Repair of right direct inguinal hernia using an open mesh technique. OPERATION .BFV3627- 13-11-01
Wimpole Street London W1G 8YF	Re Blood Pressure & Heart. Myocardial Perfusion Scan – 18-10-01
The London Clinic	Haemorrhoidectomy H5100 & Sigmoidoscopy OPERATION 17-05-2000
King Edward V11 Hospital	Cystoscopy (GA) M4510 OPERATION 29-06-1999
THE LONDON CLINIC	Laparoscopic cholecystectomy OPERATION 31-08-1996
King Edward V11 Hospital	Cystoscopy OPERATION 07-03-96
The Harley Street Clinic	Cystourethroscopy Bladder Biopsy & Cystodiathermy Urethral dilation. Ligation left Varicocoele. Excision left epididymal Cyst. OPERATION 16-05-1995
NORTHWICK PARK HOSPITAL	Lithotripsy (ESWL) ureteric calculus. 10-03-1994
CLEMENTINE CHURCHILL HOSPITAL	Cystoscopy, ureteroscopic Manipulation of calculus, instertion of Ureteric JJ stent M3000 & M2920 OPERATION 22-02-1994 Removal of JJ ureteric stent 04-03-1994
Harley Street Clinic	Cystourethroscopy & Transurethral Prostatectomy OPERATION 08-02-1990

Fig. 1.3 Part of medical history provided by patient

- Hyperparathyroidism may cause:
  - jaw radiolucencies/rarefaction
  - loss of lamina dura
  - giant cell granulomas (central)
  - hypercalcaemia and hyposalivation.
- **Fits and faints:** epilepsy and other causes of unconsciousness should be elicited before embarking on any procedures.

Oral lesions may be seen, such as phenytoin-induced gingival swelling.

- **Gastrointestinal disorders:** are relevant mainly because of possible vomiting with general anaesthesia, and possible oral manifestations.
- **Hospital admissions, attendances and operations:** this information often helps fill in gaps in the medical history, and may be relevant if, for example, the patient has had a previous halothane anaesthetic or has had radiotherapy. Successful prior surgery in the absence of any serious postoperative haemorrhage also suggests the absence of any inherited bleeding tendency.
- **Infections:** the possibility of transmission of infection to patients or staff is ever present:
  - blood-borne infections: hepatitis viruses B and C, and HIV are the main agents of concern
  - respiratory infections: current or very recent respiratory infections, particularly tuberculosis, may be transmissible and a contraindication to general anaesthesia
  - sexually shared infections: imprecise diagnosis or empirical treatment serves only to spread these infections, as contact tracing is normally undertaken only on proven cases of sexually transmitted (venereal) disease.
- **Jaundice and liver disease:** these are important because of the associated bleeding tendency, drug intolerance and possible viral hepatitis and oral carcinoma.
- **Kidney disease:** this may cause a bleeding tendency and impaired drug excretion. The other main problems are in relation to the immunosuppression created following a kidney transplant, liability to neoplasia, and gingival swelling from ciclosporin.
- **Likelihood of pregnancy:** because of the danger of abortion or teratogenicity, it is important during pregnancy, particularly the first trimester, to avoid or minimize exposure to drugs, radiography and infections. Pregnancy can influence some conditions such as aphthae, pyogenic granulomas and Behçet syndrome, and may produce gingivitis or epulides.
- **Malignant disease,** including those on radiotherapy or chemotherapy (where oral lesions may occur): malignant disease may underlie some oral complaints, such as pain or sensory changes and can result in significant morbidity and even mortality. Oral complications are very common after cancer therapies.
- **Neuropsychiatric conditions:**
  - Down syndrome: there are many oral problems and cervical spine involvement may predispose to spinal cord damage during general anaesthesia
  - mental health: there are many oral problems and drug therapy may produce oral conditions, such as dry mouth.
- **Other relevant conditions:** every condition which is elicited from the medical history should be checked for relevance, but the following can be highly relevant:
  - glucose-6-phosphate dehydrogenase deficiency is a contraindication to some drugs
  - hereditary angioedema: any dental trauma may result in oedema and a hazard to the airway
  - malignant hyperthermia (malignant hyperpyrexia): various general anaesthetics and other agents may be contraindicated

- porphyria: intravenous barbiturates, metronidazole and other agents may be contraindicated
- rheumatoid arthritis: cervical spine involvement may predispose to spinal cord damage if the neck is flexed during general anaesthesia; Sjögren syndrome is a common complication
- suxamethonium sensitivity: suxamethonium is contraindicated.
- **Prosthesis and transplant patients:** patients after transplants may be at risk from infection, neoplasms and iatrogenic problems, such as bleeding, gingival swelling or graft-versus-host disease (Ch. 54). Patients with transplants are also liable to present a number of complications to dental treatment – in particular the need for a corticosteroid cover, a liability to infection and a bleeding tendency.

There is no good evidence for infection of prosthetic joints arising from oral sepsis. However, if the orthopaedic surgeon wishes an antimicrobial cover, the dentist must consider the medicolegal implications.

The complications of infection of ventriculo-atrial valves are so serious that, although there is little evidence for an oral source, it may be reasonable to give an antimicrobial cover, if the responsible neurosurgeon so advises.

Patients with cardiac pacemakers and similar devices may be in danger in relation to the use of equipment which can interfere, such as MRI, diathermy and electrosurgery.

DENTAL HISTORY

The dental history will give an idea of the:

- regularity of attendance for dental care
- attitude to dental professionals and to treatment
- recent relevant dental problems
- recent restorative treatment.

FAMILY HISTORY

This may reveal familial outbreaks of diseases such as contagious infections (e.g. herpangina; tuberculosis) and hereditary problems, such as amelogenesis imperfecta, haemophilia or hereditary angioedema, and familial conditions, such as recurrent aphthous stomatitis or diabetes. Some diseases are more prevalent in certain ethnic groups, e.g. pemphigus in Jews and Asians; Behçet syndrome in people from Asia or the Mediterranean area.

SOCIAL AND CULTURAL HISTORY

The social history may reveal:

- whether the patient has a family or a partner – and the degree of support that can be anticipated
- information about the patient's attitudes to treatment (e.g. some patients may refuse operation, others may decline medication)
- information about the patient's residence, which can suggest the socioeconomic circumstances of the patient

Table 1.2 Systematic recording of relevant medical history

System	Specific problems	No	Yes
CVS	Heart disease, hypertension, angina, syncope Cardiac surgery, endocarditis Bleeding disorder, anticoagulants, anaemia		
RS	Asthma, bronchitis, TB, other chest disease, smoker		
GU	Renal, urinary tract or sexually shared disease Pregnancy, menstrual problems		
GI/Liver	Coeliac disease, Crohn disease Hepatitis, other liver disease, jaundice		
CNS	CVE, multiple (disseminated) sclerosis, other neurological disease Psychiatric problems, drug or alcohol abuse Sight or hearing problems		
LMS	Bone, muscle or joint disease		
Endocrine	Diabetes, thyroid, other endocrine disease		
Allergy	Allergies – e.g. latex, aspirin, penicillin, plaster (band-aids)		
Drugs	Recent or current drugs/medical treatment Corticosteroids, anticoagulants		
Others	Previous operations, GA or serious illness Other conditions (including congenital anomalies) Family medical history Born, residence or travel abroad Pets Infections e.g. HIV		

CVS, cardiovascular system; RS, respiratory system; GU, genitourinary system; GI, gastrointestinal system; CNS, central nervous system; LMS, locomotor system.

- information about contacts with pets and other animals, which may be relevant to some infectious diseases, such as cat-scratch disease or toxoplasmosis
- whether the patient has travelled overseas, which may be relevant to some infectious diseases, such as tuberculosis, tropical diseases such as Leishmaniasis and deep mycoses such as histoplasmosis
- the patient's sexual history, which may be relevant to some infectious diseases, such as human immunodeficiency virus (HIV), herpes simplex virus (HSV), papillomavirus (HPV) and hepatitis viruses A (HAV), B (HBV) and C (HCV)
- any occupational problems, which may be relevant to some disease, and access to care
- relevant habits (tobacco, alcohol, betel and recreational drug use) – for example, tobacco use underlies several oral diseases, including periodontal disease and cancer
- relevant hobbies, such as swimming in pools that may cause tooth erosion or scuba diving that may underlie temporomandibular pain
- information about the patient's culture and diet – may lead, for example, to vitamin deficiencies and glossitis or angular cheilitis (as in vitamin B_{12} deficiency in vegans)
- information about stress; several orofacial complaints are stress-related or modulated by stress.

Standardized forms will help with the recording of data, the relevance of which can sometimes be surprising (**Table 1.2**).

Patient expectations can only be assessed by polite enquiry. Each patient is an individual with their own specific thoughts and beliefs. Some cultures have medical understanding quite separate from that of westernised medicine.

FURTHER READING

Abraham-Inpijn, L., 2000. Local anesthesia and patients presenting with medical pathologies; the use of anamnesis in the prevention of medical complications in the dental office. Rev. Belge Med. Dent. 55 (1), 72–79.

Abraham-Inpijn, L., Abraham, E.A., Backman, N., et al., 2000. Is het nog wel veilig in de tandartsstoel? Ned. Tandartsenbl. 55, 14–15.

Ferlito, A., Boccato, P., Shaha, A.R., et al., 2001. The art of diagnosis in head and neck tumors. Acta Otolaryngol. 121, 324–328.

Maguire, P., Pitceathly, C., 2002. Key communication skills and how to acquire them. BMJ 325, 697–700.

Ragonesi, M., Ivaldi, C., 2005. Anaesthesiological risk assessment in young/adult and older dental patients. Gerodontology 22 (2), 109–111.

Scully, C., Kalantzis, A., 2005. Oxford handbook of dental patient care, second ed. Oxford University Press, Oxford.

Scully, C., Wilson, N., 2006. Culturally sensitive oral health care. Quintessence Publishers, London.

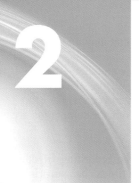

Diagnosis: examination

The patient will know if you care, well before they care if you know.

Anonymous

INTRODUCTION

The clinical examination of the patient should start as the patient enters the clinic and is greeted by the clinician. The history and clinical examination are designed to put the clinician in a position to make a provisional diagnosis, or a differential diagnosis. Special tests or investigations may be required to confirm or refine this diagnosis or elicit other conditions. Physical disabilities, such as those affecting gait, and learning disability are often immediately evident as the patient is first seen, and blindness, deafness or speech and language disorders may be obvious. You should also be able to assess the patient's mood and general wellbeing but, if in any doubt, ask for advice. Other disorders, such as mental problems, may become apparent at any stage. The patient should be carefully observed and listened to during history taking and examination; speech and language can offer a great deal of information about the medical and mental state. Some patients bring written material that can be helpful (e.g. an accurate list of their illnesses and/or medications) and increasingly patients use the internet and come with print-outs. Others may bring less meaningful drawings or histories, which have led some to coin the phrase – la maladie du petits papiers – the illness of small pieces of paper. All these factors can help build a picture of the patient and their condition. As a general rule, if you think a patient looks ill, they probably are.

Always remember that the patient has the right to refuse all or part of the examination, investigations or treatment. A patient has the right under common law to give or withhold consent to medical examination or treatment. This is one of the basic principles of healthcare. Patients are entitled to receive sufficient information in a way they can understand about the proposed investigations or treatments, the possible alternatives and any substantial risk or risks, which may be special in kind or magnitude or special to the patient, so that they can make a balanced judgment (UK Health Department, 19.2.99. HSC 1999/031).

There may be cultural sensitivities but, in any case, no examination should be carried out in the absence of a chaperone – preferably of the opposite sex to the practitioner.

GENERAL EXAMINATION

Medical problems may manifest in the fully clothed patient with abnormal appearance or behaviour, pupil size, conscious level, movements, posture, breathing, speech, facial colour, sweating or wasting. General examination may sometimes include the recording of body weight and the 'vital signs' of conscious state, temperature, pulse, blood pressure and respiration. The dentist must be prepared to interpret the more common and significant changes evident in the clothed patient.

VITAL SIGNS

Vital signs include conscious state, temperature, pulse, blood pressure and respiration:

- The conscious state: any decrease in this must be taken seriously, causes ranging from drug use to head injury.
- The temperature: the temperature is traditionally taken with a thermometer, but temperature-sensitive strips and sensors are available. Leave the thermometer in place for at least 3 min. The normal body temperatures are: oral 36.6°C; rectal or ear (tympanic membrane) 37.4°C; and axillary 36.5°C. Body temperature is usually slightly higher in the evenings. In most adults, an oral temperature above 37.8°C or a rectal or ear temperature above 38.3°C is considered a fever (pyrexia). A child has a fever when ear temperature is 38°C or higher.
- The pulse: this can be measured manually or automatically (**Fig. 2.1**). The pulse can be recorded from any artery, but in particular from the following sites:
  - the radial artery, on the thumb side of the flexor surface of the wrist
  - the carotid artery, just anterior to the mid-third of the sternomastoid muscle
  - the superficial temporal artery, just in front of the ear.

Pulse rates at rest in health are approximately as follows:

- infants, 140 beats/min
- adults, 60–80 beats/min.

Pulse rate is increased in:

- exercise
- anxiety or fear
- fever
- some cardiac disorders
- hyperthyroidism and other disorders.

The rhythm should be regular; if not, ask a physician for advice. The character and volume vary in certain disease states and require a physician's advice.

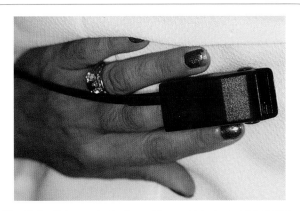

Fig. 2.1 Pulse meter (nail varnish must be removed from the finger tested)

- The blood pressure: this can be measured with a sphygmomanometer (**Fig. 2.2**), or one of a variety of machines. With a sphygmomanometer the procedure is as follows: seat the patient; place the sphygmomanometer cuff on the right upper arm, with about 3 cm of skin visible at the antecubital fossa; palpate the radial pulse; inflate the cuff to about 200–250 mmHg or until the radial pulse is no longer palpable; deflate the cuff slowly while listening with the stethoscope over the brachial artery on the skin of the inside arm below the cuff; record the systolic pressure as the pressure when the first tapping sounds appear; deflate the cuff further until the tapping sounds become muffled (diastolic pressure); repeat; record the blood pressure as systolic/diastolic pressures (normal values about 120/80 mmHg, but these increase with age).

RESPIRATION

The normal reference range for respiration in an adult is 12–20 breaths/min.

OTHER SIGNS

- Weight: weight loss is seen mainly in starvation, malnutrition, eating disorders, cancer (termed cachexia), HIV disease (termed 'slim disease'), malabsorption and tuberculosis and may be extreme as in emaciation. Obesity is usually due to excessive food intake and insufficient exercise.

- Hands: conditions such as arthritis (mainly rheumatoid or osteoarthritis) (**Figs 2.3** and **2.4**) and Raynaud phenomenon (Ch. 56; **Fig. 2.3**), which is seen in many connective tissue diseases, may be obvious. Disability, such as in cerebral palsy, may be obvious (**Fig. 2.5**).
- Skin: lesions, such as rashes – particularly blisters (seen mainly in skin diseases, infections and drug reactions), pigmentation (seen in various ethnic groups, Addison disease and as a result of some drug therapy).
- Skin appendages: nail changes, such as koilonychia (spoon-shaped nails) – seen in iron deficiency anaemia, hair changes, such as alopecia, and finger clubbing (**Fig. 2.6**), seen mainly in cardiac or respiratory disorders. Nail beds may reveal the anxious nature of the nail-biting person (**Fig. 2.7**).

Extraoral head and neck examination

The face should be examined for lesions (**Table 2.1**) and features such as:

- swellings, seen in inflammatory and neoplastic disorders in particular
- pallor, seen mainly in the conjunctivae or skin creases in anaemia
- rash, such as the malar rash in systemic lupus erythematosus. Malar erythema may indicate mitral valve stenosis.
- erythema, seen mainly on the face in an embarrassed or angry patient, or fever (sweating or warm hands), and then usually indicative of infection.

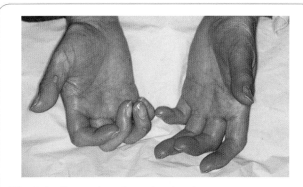

Fig. 2.3 Raynaud syndrome in scleroderma

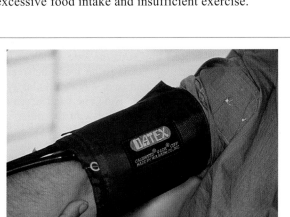

Fig. 2.2 Sphygmomanometer

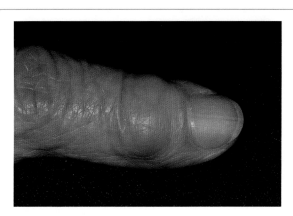

Fig. 2.4 Heberden nodes of osteoarthritis

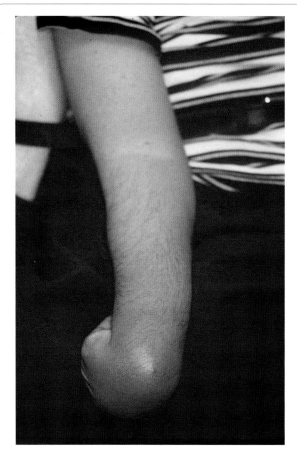

Fig. 2.5 Cerebral palsy

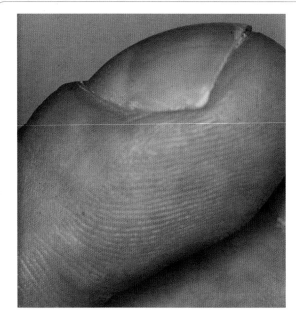

Fig. 2.6 Clubbing

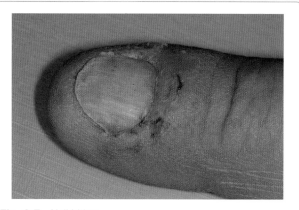

Fig. 2.7 Nail biting

Eyes should be assessed for visual acuity and examined for features such as:

- corneal arcus which may be seen in hypercholesterolaemia
- exophthalmos (prominent eyes), seen mainly in Graves thyrotoxicosis
- jaundice, seen mainly in the sclerae in liver disease
- redness, seen in trauma, eye diseases, or Sjögren syndrome
- scarring, seen in trauma, infection or pemphigoid.

Inspection of the neck, looking particularly for swellings or sinuses, should be followed by careful palpation of all cervical lymph nodes and salivary and thyroid glands, searching for swelling or tenderness. The neck is best examined by observing the patient from the front, noting any obvious asymmetry or swelling, then standing behind the seated patient to palpate the lymph nodes (**Fig. 2.8**). Systematically, each region needs to be examined lightly with the pulps of the fingers, trying to roll the lymph nodes against harder underlying structures:

- Lymph from the superficial tissue of the head and neck generally drains first to groups of superficially placed lymph nodes, then to the deep cervical lymph nodes (**Figs 2.9–2.12 and Table 2.2**).
- Parotid, mastoid and occipital lymph nodes can be palpated simultaneously using both hands.
- Superficial cervical lymph nodes are examined with lighter fingers as they can only be compressed against the softer sternomastoid muscle.
- Submental lymph nodes are examined by tipping the patient's head forward and rolling the lymph nodes against the inner aspect of the mandible.
- Submandibular lymph nodes are examined in the same way, with the patient's head tipped to the side which is being examined. Differentiation needs to be made between the submandibular salivary gland and submandibular lymph glands. Bimanual examination using one hand beneath the mandible to palpate extraorally and with the other index finger in the floor of the mouth may help.
- The deep cervical lymph nodes which project anterior or posterior to the sternomastoid muscle can be palpated. The jugulodigastric lymph node in particular should be specifically examined, as this is the most common lymph node involved in tonsillar infections and oral cancer.
- The supraclavicular region should be examined at the same time as the rest of the neck; lymph nodes here may extend up into the posterior triangle of the neck on the scalene muscles, behind the sternomastoid.

Table 2.1 The commoner descriptive terms applied to lesions

Term	Meaning
Atrophy	Loss of tissue with increased translucency, unless sclerosis is associated
Bullae	Visible accumulations of fluid within or beneath the epithelium, >0.5 cm in diameter (i.e. a blister)
Cyst	Closed cavity or sac (normal or abnormal) with an epithelial, endothelial or membranous lining and containing fluid or semisolid material
Ecchymosis	Macular area of haemorrhage >2 cm in diameter (bruise)
Erosion	Loss of epithelium which usually heals without scarring; it commonly follows a blister
Erythema	Redness of the mucosa produced by atrophy, inflammation, vascular congestion or increased perfusion
Exfoliation	The splitting off of the epithelial keratin in scales or sheets
Fibrosis	The formation of excessive fibrous tissue
Fissure	Any linear gap or slit in the skin or mucosa
Gangrene	Death of tissue, usually due to loss of blood supply
Haematoma	A localized tumour-like collection of blood
Keloid	A tough heaped-up scar that rises above the rest of the skin, is irregularly shaped and tends to enlarge progressively
Macule	A circumscribed alteration in colour or texture of the mucosa
Nodule	A solid mass in the mucosa or skin which can be observed as an elevation or can be palpated; it is >0.5 cm in diameter
Papule	A circumscribed palpable elevation <0.5 cm in diameter
Petechia (pl. petechiae)	A punctate haemorrhagic spot approximately 1–2 mm in diameter
Plaque	An elevated area of mucosa >0.5 cm in diameter
Pustule	A visible accumulation of free pus
Scar	Replacement by fibrous tissue of another tissue that has been destroyed by injury or disease An *atrophic* scar is thin and wrinkled A *hypertrophic* scar is elevated with excessive growth of fibrous tissue A *cribriform* scar is perforated with multiple small pits
Sclerosis	Diffuse or circumscribed induration of the submucosal and/or subcutaneous tissues
Tumour	Literally a swelling The term is used to imply enlargement of the tissues by normal or pathological material or cells that form a mass The term should be used with care, as many patients believe it implies a malignancy with a poor prognosis
Ulcer	A loss of epithelium, often with loss of underlying tissues, produced by sloughing of necrotic tissue
Vegetation	A growth of pathological tissue consisting of multiple closely set papillary masses
Vesicle	Small (<0.5 cm in diameter) visible accumulation of fluid within or beneath the epithelium (i.e. small blister)
Wheal	A transient area of mucosal or skin oedema, white, compressible and usually evanescent (AKA urticaria)

- Parapharyngeal and tracheal lymph nodes can be compressed lightly against the trachea.
- Some information can be gained by the texture and nature of the lymphadenopathy.
- Tenderness and swelling should be documented. Lymph nodes that are tender may be inflammatory (lymphadenitis). Consistency should be noted. Nodes that are increasing in size and are hard, or fixed to adjacent tissues may be malignant.
- Both anterior and posterior cervical nodes should be examined as well as other nodes, liver and spleen if systemic disease is a possibility. Generalized lymphadenopathy with or without enlargement of other lymphoid tissue, such as liver and spleen (hepatosplenomegaly), suggests a systemic cause.

The temporomandibular joints (TMJ) and muscles of mastication should be examined and palpated. Although disorders that affect the TMJ often appear to be unilateral, the joint should not be viewed in isolation, but always considered along with its opposite joint, as part of the stomatognathic system. Some practitioners palpate using a pressure

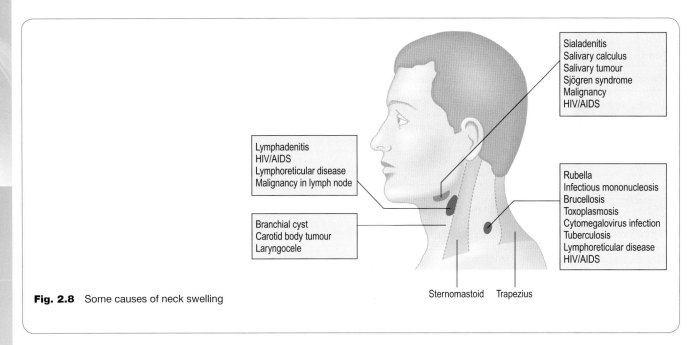

Sialadenitis
Salivary calculus
Salivary tumour
Sjögren syndrome
Malignancy
HIV/AIDS

Lymphadenitis
HIV/AIDS
Lymphoreticular disease
Malignancy in lymph node

Branchial cyst
Carotid body tumour
Laryngocele

Rubella
Infectious mononucleosis
Brucellosis
Toxoplasmosis
Cytomegalovirus infection
Tuberculosis
Lymphoreticular disease
HIV/AIDS

Sternomastoid   Trapezius

Fig. 2.8 Some causes of neck swelling

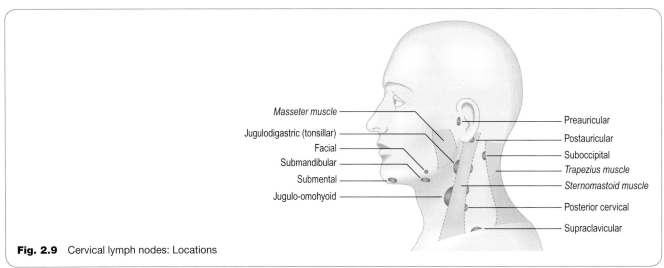

Masseter muscle
Jugulodigastric (tonsillar)
Facial
Submandibular
Submental
Jugulo-omohyoid

Preauricular
Postauricular
Suboccipital
Trapezius muscle
Sternomastoid muscle
Posterior cervical
Supraclavicular

Fig. 2.9 Cervical lymph nodes: Locations

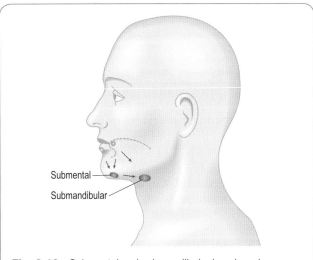

Submental
Submandibular

Fig. 2.10 Submental and submandibular lymph node drainage

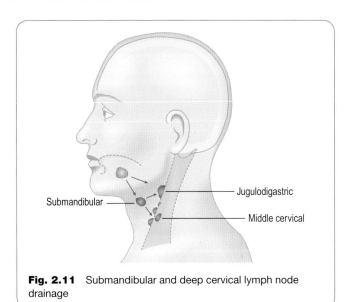

Submandibular

Jugulodigastric
Middle cervical

Fig. 2.11 Submandibular and deep cervical lymph node drainage

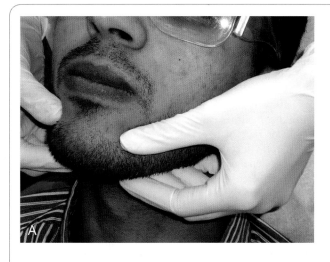
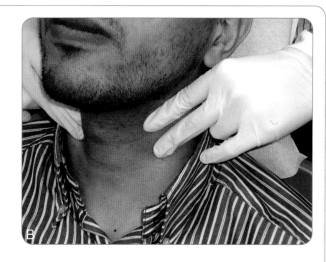
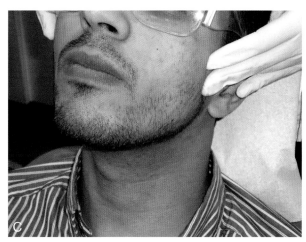
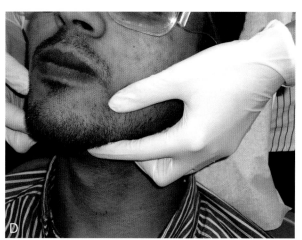

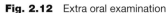

Fig. 2.12 Extra oral examination

algometer to standardize the force used, and undertake range-of-movement (ROM) measurements. The area should be examined by inspecting:

- Facial symmetry, for evidence of enlarged masseter muscles (masseteric hypertrophy) suggestive of clenching or bruxism. A bruxchecker can help confirm bruxism.
- Mandibular opening and closing paths, noting any noises or deviations.
- Mandibular opening extent, measuring the inter-incisal distance at maximum mouth opening.
- Lateral excursions, measuring the amount achievable.
- Joint noises, by listening (a stethoscope placed over the joint can help).
- Both condyles, by palpating them, via the external auditory meatus, to detect tenderness posteriorly, and by using a single finger placed over the joints in front of the ears, to detect pain, abnormal movements or clicking within the joint.
- Masticatory muscles on both sides, noting tenderness or hypertrophy:
  - Masseters, by intraoral–extraoral compression between finger and thumb. Palpate the masseter bimanually by placing a finger of one hand intraorally and the index and middle fingers of the other hand on the cheek over the masseter over the lower mandibular ramus.

- Temporalis, by direct palpation of the temporal region and by asking the patient to clench the teeth. Palpate the insertion of the temporalis tendon intraorally along the anterior border of the ascending mandibular ramus.
  - Lateral pterygoid (lower head), by placing a little finger up behind the maxillary tuberosity (tenderness is the 'pterygoid sign'). Examine it indirectly by asking the patient to open the jaw against resistance and to move the jaw to one side while applying a gentle resistance force.
  - Medial pterygoid muscle, intraorally lingually to the mandibular ramus.
- The dentition and occlusion. This may require monitoring of study models on a semi or fully adjustable articulator. Note particularly missing premolars or molars, and attrition.
- The mucosa. Note particularly occlusal lines and scalloping of the tongue margins, which may indicate bruxism and tongue pressure.

Examine the jaws. There is a wide normal individual variation in morphology of the face. Most individuals have facial asymmetry but of a degree that cannot be regarded as abnormal. Maxillary, mandibular or zygomatic deformities or lumps may be more reliably confirmed by inspection from above (maxillae/zygomas) or behind (mandible). The jaws should be palpated to detect swelling or tenderness. Maxillary air sinuses

Table 2.2 The cervical lymph nodes and their main drainage areas

Area	Draining lymph nodes
Scalp, temporal region	Superficial parotid (pre-auricular)
Scalp, posterior region	Occipital
Scalp, parietal region	Mastoid
Ear, external	Superficial cervical over upper part of sternomastoid muscle
Ear, middle	Parotid
Over angle of mandible	Superficial cervical over upper part of sternomastoid muscle
Medial part of frontal region, medial eyelids, skin of nose	Submandibular
Lateral part of frontal region, lateral part of eyelids	Parotid
Cheek	Submandibular
Upper lip	Submandibular
Lower lip	Submental
Lower lip, lateral part	Submandibular
Mandibular gingivae	Submandibular
Maxillary teeth	Deep cervical
Maxillary gingivae	Deep cervical
Tongue tip	Submental
Tongue, anterior two-thirds	Submandibular, some midline cross-over of lymphatic drainage
Tongue, posterior third	Deep cervical
Tongue ventrum	Deep cervical
Floor of mouth	Submandibular
Palate, hard	Deep cervical
Palate, soft	Retropharyngeal and deep cervical
Tonsil	Jugulodigastric

can be examined by palpation for tenderness over the maxillary antrum, which may indicate sinus infection. Transillumination or endoscopy can be helpful. The major salivary glands should be inspected and palpated (parotids and submandibulars) for:

- symmetry
- evidence of enlargement
- evidence of salivary flow from salivary ducts
- evidence of the normal salivary pooling in the floor of mouth
- saliva appearance
- evidence of oral dryness (food residues; lipstick on teeth, scarce saliva, mirror sticks to mucosa), sialometry (salivary flow rate) shows hyposalivation.

Salivary glands are palpated in the following way:

- Parotid glands are palpated by using fingers placed over the glands in front of the ears, to detect pain or swelling. Early enlargement of the parotid gland is characterized by outward deflection of the lower part of the ear lobe, which is best observed by looking at the patient from behind. This sign may allow distinction from simple obesity. Swelling of the parotid sometimes causes trismus. Swellings may affect the whole or part of a gland, or tenderness may be elicited. The parotid duct (Stensen duct) is most readily palpated with the jaws clenched firmly, since it runs horizontally across the upper masseter where it can be gently rolled; the duct opens at a papilla on the buccal mucosa opposite the upper molars.
- The submandibular gland is best palpated bimanually with a finger of one hand in the floor of the mouth lingual to the lower molar teeth, and a finger of the other hand placed over the submandibular triangle. The submandibular duct (Wharton duct) runs anteromedially across the floor of the mouth to open at the side of the lingual fraenum.

Examine the cranial nerves (**Table 2.3**). In particular, facial movement should be tested and facial sensation determined. Facial symmetry is best seen as the patient is talking. Movement of the mouth as the patient speaks is important, especially when they allow themselves the luxury of some emotional expression. Examination of the upper face (around the eyes and forehead) is carried out in the following way:

- If the patient is asked to close their eyes any paralysis (palsy) may become obvious, with the affected eyelid failing to close and the globe turning up so that only the white of the eye is showing (Bell sign).
- Weakness of orbicularis oculi muscles with sufficient strength to close the eye can be compared with the normal side by asking the patient to close the eyes tight and observing the degree of force required to part the eyelids.
- If the patient is asked to wrinkle the forehead, weakness can be detected by the difference between the two sides.

The lower face (around the mouth) is best examined by asking the patient to:

- smile
- bare the teeth or purse the lips
- blow out the cheeks or whistle.

The cranial nerves can be examined further:

- Facial sensation: progressive lesions affecting the sensory part of the trigeminal nerve initially result in a diminishing response to light touch (cotton wool or air spray) and pin-prick (gently pricking the skin with a sterile pin or needle without drawing blood), and later there is complete anaesthesia.
- The corneal reflex: this depends on the integrity of the trigeminal and facial nerves, either of which if defective will give a negative response. This is tested by gently touching the cornea with a wisp of cotton wool twisted to a point. Normally, this procedure causes a blink but, if the cornea is anaesthetic (or if there is facial palsy), no blink follows, provided that the patient does not actually see the cotton wool. If the patient complains of complete facial or hemifacial anaesthesia, but the corneal reflex is retained or there is apparent anaesthesia over the angle of the mandible (an area not innervated by the trigeminal nerve), then the symptoms are probably functional (non-organic).

Table 2.3 Cranial nerve nomenclature and examination

Cranial nerve		Findings in lesions
I	Olfactory	Impaired sense of smell for common odours (do not use ammonia)
II	Optic	Visual acuity reduced using Snellen types ± ophthalmoscopy: nystagmus Visual fields by confrontation impaired Pupil responses may be impaired
III	Oculomotor	Diplopia; strabismus; eye looks down and laterally ('down and out') Eye movements impaired Ptosis (drooping eyelid) Pupil dilated Pupil reactions: direct reflex impaired, but consensual reflex intact
IV	Trochlear	Diplopia, particularly on looking down Strabismus (squint) No ptosis Pupil normal and normal reactivity
V	Trigeminal	Reduced sensation over face ± corneal reflex impaired ± taste sensation impaired Motor power of masticatory muscles reduced, with weakness on opening jaw; jaw jerk impaired Muscle wasting
VI	Abducens	Diplopia (double vision) Strabismus Lateral eye movements impaired to affected side
VII	Facial	Impaired motor power of facial muscles on smiling, blowing out cheeks, showing teeth, etc. Corneal reflex reduced ± taste sensation impaired
VIII	Vestibulocochlear	Impaired hearing (tuning fork at 256 Hz) Impaired balance ± nystagmus ± tinnitus
IX	Glossopharyngeal	Reduced gag reflex Deviation of uvula Reduced taste sensation Voice may have nasal tone
X	Vagus	Reduced gag reflex Voice may be impaired
XI	Accessory	Motor power of trapezius and sternomastoid reduced
XII	Hypoglossal	Motor power of tongue impaired, with abnormal speech ± fasciculation, wasting, ipsilateral deviation on protrusion

Intraoral examination

Most oral diseases have a local cause and can be recognized fairly readily. Even those that are life-threatening, such as oral cancer in particular, can be detected at an exceedingly early stage. However, even now, oral cancer is sometimes overlooked at examination, and the delay between the onset of symptoms of oral cancer and the institution of definitive treatment still often exceeds 6 months. The same story applies to pemphigus – another potentially lethal disease that presents in the mouth. Any lesion persisting over 3 weeks should be taken seriously.

Many systemic diseases, particularly infections and diseases of the blood, gastrointestinal tract and skin, also cause oral signs or symptoms that may constitute the main complaint, particularly, for example, in some patients with HIV, leukopenia or leukaemia.

The examination, therefore, should be conducted in a systematic fashion to ensure that all areas are included. If the patient wears any removable prostheses or appliances, these should be removed in the first instance, although it may be necessary later to replace the appliance to assess its fit, function and relationship to any lesion.

Complete visualization with a good source of light is essential (**Fig. 2.13**); magnifying loupes or microscope help

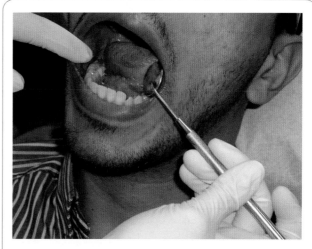

Fig. 2.13 Mouth examination

enormously. All mucosal surfaces should be examined, starting away from the location of any known lesions or the focus of complaint, and lesions recorded on a diagram (**Fig. 2.14**).

Attempts to improve the visualization of mucosal lesions include the use of toluidine blue vital dye, and fluorescence visualization, where a light source is used to enhance the visualization or to identify the optimal site for biopsy have not proven superior to conventional visual examination in terms of specificity or sensitivity. A review of currently available products showed insufficient evidence (**Table 2.4**):

■ that commercial devices based on autofluorescence enhance visual detection beyond a conventional visual and tactile examination
■ that commercially available devices based on tissue reflectance enhance visual detection beyond a conventional visual and tactile examination.

Although these aids may have their limitations, developments in this field such as narrow band imaging (NBI) and others must surely offer hope for the future. Until then, conventional oral examination remains the gold standard.

The lips should first be inspected. The labial mucosa, buccal mucosa, floor of the mouth and ventrum of the tongue, dorsal surface of the tongue, hard and soft palates, gingivae and teeth should then be examined in sequence (**Box 2.1**):

■ Lips: features, such as cyanosis, are seen mainly in the lips in cardiac or respiratory disease; angular cheilitis is seen mainly in oral candidosis or iron or vitamin deficiencies. Many adults have a few yellowish pinhead-sized papules in the vermilion border (particularly of the upper lip) and at the commissures; these are usually ectopic sebaceous glands (Fordyce spots), and may be numerous, especially as age advances.
■ Labial mucosa normally appears moist with a fairly prominent vascular arcade. Examination is facilitated if the mouth is gently closed at this stage, so that the lips can then be everted to examine the mucosa. In the lower lip, the many minor salivary glands, which are often exuding mucus, are easily visible. The lips, therefore, feel slightly nodular and the labial arteries are readily felt.

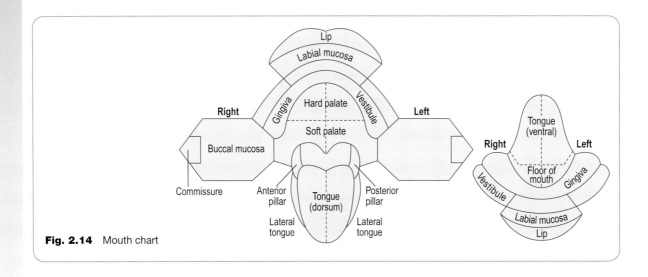

Fig. 2.14 Mouth chart

Table 2.4   Attempts at aids for earlier detection of sinister lesions

Basis	Product	Sensitivity/specificity	Comment
Vital dye	Toluidine blue (TB) (tolonium chloride)	High sensitivity 93–97% for identifying oral squamous cell carcinomas and specificity 73–92%	Many studies had methodological flaws
Light-based detection systems	Chemiluminescence (Vizilite®. Zila Pharmaceuticals, Phoenix, Arizona, USA)	High sensitivity (100%), but low specificity (0–14.2%) and low positive predictive value Combination with TB (Vizilite Plus®) may have better specificity and positive predictive value	Few reliable studies have appeared
	Chemiluminescence (Microlux/DL®. AdDent Inc., Danbury, Connecticut, USA)	Sensitivity and specificity for the detection of oral cancer and precancer are 77% and 70% respectively	
	Tissue fluorescence imaging (VELscope® Visually Enhanced Lesion Scope. LED Dental Inc., White Rock, British Columbia, Canada)	Sensitivity 97–100% and specificity 94–100%	More studies awaited
Exfoliative cytology	Brush biopsy (OralCDx® Laboratories Inc., Suffern, New York, USA)	Sensitivity for detection of abnormal cells 52–100% and specificity 29–100%	Scalpel biopsy usually preferred

BOX 2.1   The more commonly used tooth notations

Palmer
Permanent dentition

Upper

87654321 | 12345678

Right   Left

87654321 | 12345678

Lower

Deciduous dentition (anonymous classification)

EDCBA | ABCDE

EDCBA | ABCDE

Haderup
Permanent dentition

(8+)(7+)(6+)(5+)(4+)(3+)(2+)(1+) | (+1)(+2)(+3)(+4)(+5)(+6)(+7)(+8)

(8-)(7-)(6-)(5-)(4-)(3-)(2-)(1-) | (-1)(-2)(-3)(-4)(-5)(-6)(-7)(-8)

Deciduous dentition

(50+)(40+)(30+)(20+)(10+) | (+01)(+02)(+03)(+04)(+05)

(50-)(40-)(30-)(20-)(10-) | (-01)(-02)(-03)(-04)(-05)

Universal
Permanent dentition

1 2 3 4 5 6 7 8 | 9 10 11 12 13 14 15 16

32 31 30 29 28 27 26 25 | 24 23 22 21 20 19 18 17

Deciduous dentition

A B C D E | F G H I J

T S R Q P | O N M L K

Fédération Dentaire Internationale (two-digit)
Permanent dentition

18 17 16 15 14 13 12 11 | 21 22 23 24 25 26 27 28

48 47 46 45 44 43 42 41 | 31 32 33 34 35 36 37 38

Deciduous dentition

55 54 53 52 51 | 61 62 63 64 65

85 84 83 82 81 | 71 72 73 74 75

one where lesions are most easily missed. During this part of the examination the quantity and consistency of saliva should be assessed. Examine for the pooling of saliva in the floor of the mouth; normally there is a pool of saliva.

- The dorsum of the tongue is best inspected by protrusion, when it can be held with gauze. The anterior two-thirds is embryologically and anatomically distinct from the posterior third, and separated by a dozen or so large circumvallate papillae. The anterior two-thirds is coated with many filiform, but relatively few fungiform papillae. Behind the circumvallate papillae, the tongue contains several large lymphoid masses (lingual tonsil) and the foliate papillae lie on the lateral borders posteriorly. These are often mistaken for tumours. The tongue may be fissured (scrotal), but this is a developmental anomaly. A healthy child's tongue is rarely coated, but a mild coating is not uncommon in healthy adults. The voluntary tongue movements and sense of taste should be formally tested (Ch. 22). Abnormalities of tongue movement (neurological or muscular disease) may be obvious from dysarthria (abnormal speech) or involuntary movements, and any fibrillation or wasting should be noted. Hypoglossal palsy may lead to deviation of the tongue towards the affected side on protrusion.

- The palate and fauces consist of an anterior hard palate and posterior soft palate, and the tonsillar area and oropharynx. The mucosa of the hard palate is firmly bound down as a mucoperiosteum (similar to the gingivae) and with no obvious vascular arcades. Ridges (rugae) are present anteriorly on either side of the incisive papilla that overlies the incisive foramen. Bony lumps in the posterior centre of the vault of the hard palate are usually tori (torus palatinus). Patients may complain of a lump distal to the upper molars that they think is an unerupted tooth, but the pterygoid hamulus or tuberosity is usually responsible for this complaint. The soft palate and fauces may show a faint vascular arcade. Just posterior to the junction with the hard palate is a conglomeration of minor salivary glands. This region is often also yellowish. The palate should be inspected and movements examined when the patient says 'Aah'. Using a mirror, this also permits inspection of the posterior tongue, tonsils, oropharynx, and can even offer a glimpse of the larynx. Glossopharyngeal palsy may lead to uvula deviation to the contralateral side. Bifid uvula may signify a submucous cleft palate.

- Gingivae in health are firm, pale pink, with a stippled surface, and have sharp gingival papillae reaching up between the adjacent teeth to the tooth contact point. Look for gingival deformity, redness, swelling, or bleeding on gently probing the gingival margin. The 'keratinized' attached gingivae (pale pink) is normally clearly demarcated from the non-keratinized alveolar mucosa (vascular) that runs into the vestibule or sulcus. A Basic Periodontal Examination (BPE) may be helpful. Bands of tissue, which may contain muscle attachments, run centrally from the labial mucosa onto the alveolar mucosa and from the buccal mucosa in the premolar region onto the alveolar mucosa (fraenae).

- Teeth: the dentition should be checked to make sure that the expected complement of teeth is present for the patient's age. Extra teeth (supernumerary teeth) or deficiency of teeth (partial loss – hypodontia or oligodontia – or

- Cheek (buccal) mucosa is readily inspected if the mouth is held half open. The vascular pattern and minor salivary glands so prominent in the labial mucosa are not obvious in the buccal mucosa, but Fordyce spots may be conspicuous, particularly near the commissures and retromolar regions in adults and there may be a faint horizontal white line where the teeth meet (linea alba). Place the surface of a dental mirror against the buccal mucosa; it should slide and lift off easily but, if it adheres to the mucosa, then there is probably hyposalivation.

- The floor of the mouth and the ventrum of the tongue are best examined by asking the patient to push the tongue first into the palate and then into each cheek in turn. This raises for inspection the floor of the mouth – an area where tumours may start (the coffin or graveyard area of the mouth). Its posterior part is the most difficult area to examine well and complete loss (anodontia)) can be features of many syndromes, but teeth are far more frequently missing because they are unerupted, impacted or lost as a result of caries or periodontal disease. The teeth should be fully examined for signs of disease, either malformations, such as hypoplasia or abnormal colour, or acquired disorders such as dental caries, staining, tooth surface loss

or fractures. The laser fluorescence device DIAGNOdent may help caries detection. Apex locators, such as Propex (third generation) and Raypex-4 (fourth generation), may help define root fractures. The occlusion of the teeth should also be checked; it may show attrition or may be disturbed, as in some jaw fractures or dislocation of the mandibular condyles.

FURTHER READING

al Kadi, H., Sykes, L.M., Vally, Z., 2006. Accuracy of the Raypex-4 and Propex apex locators in detecting horizontal and vertical root fractures: an in vitro study. SADJ 61 (6), 244–247.

D'Cruz, L., 2006. Off the record. Dent. Update 33 (7), 390–392, 395–396, 399–400.

Leisnert, L., Mattheos, N., 2006. The interactive examination in a comprehensive oral care clinic: a three-year follow up of students' self-assessment ability. Med. Teach. 28 (6), 544–548.

Olmez, A., Tuna, D., Oznurhan, F., 2006. Clinical evaluation of DIAGNOdent in detection of occlusal caries in children. J. Clin. Pediatr. Dent. 30 (4), 287–291.

Onodera, K., Kawagoe, T., Sasaguri, K., et al., 2006. The use of a bruxchecker in the evaluation of different grinding patterns during sleep bruxism. Cranio 24 (4), 292–299.

Rethman, M.P., Carpenter, W., Cohen, E.E.W., et al., 2010. Evidence-based clinical recommendations regarding screening for oral squamous cell carcinomas. J. Am. Dent. Assoc. 141 (5), 509–520.

Scully, C., Bagan, J.V., Hopper, C., Epstein, J.B., 2008. Oral cancer; current and future diagnostic techniques. Am. J. Dent. 21, 199–209.

Scully, C., Kalantzis, A., 2005. Oxford handbook of dental patient care. Oxford University Press, Oxford.

Scully, C., Wilson, N., 2005. Sensitive oral health care. Quintessence Publishers, London.

Shintaku, W., Enciso, R., Broussard, J., Clark, G.T., 2006. Diagnostic imaging for chronic orofacial pain, maxillofacial osseous and soft tissue pathology and temporomandibular disorders. J. Calif. Dent. Assoc. 34 (8), 633–644.

Tan, E.H., Batchelor, P., Sheiham, A., 2006. A reassessment of recall frequency intervals for screening in low caries incidence populations. Int. Dent. J. 56 (5), 277–282.

Trullenque-Eriksson, A., Muñoz-Corcuera, M., Campo-Trapero, J., et al., 2009. Analysis of new diagnostic methods in suspicious lesions of the oral mucosa. Med. Oral Patol. Oral Cir. Bucal. 1; 14 (5), E210–E216.

Diagnosis: investigations

3

Accurate diagnosis is the only true cornerstone on which rational treatment can be built.

C Noyek

INFORMED CONSENT

It is the duty of dental staff to ensure they try and help patients understand their condition. Patients commonly complain that they have been ill-informed about their diagnosis, investigations and the results of these. Patients should always be involved in the decision-making about their management. Patients are increasingly well-informed: some attend with specific questions and a few have detailed dossiers and seek special investigations. Careful discussion with the patient is the best approach. Other ways to help are by:

- Writing important points down for the patient.
- Using patient information sheets, examples of which are included in this book.
- Offering guidance to other sources of information, such as written material and the internet.
- Arranging contact with other patients with the same problems, either individually or through a patient self-help group. Patients with chronic serious conditions, such as cancer, pemphigus, trigeminal neuralgia, Behçet syndrome or Sjögren syndrome, particularly may benefit from this.
- Explaining the condition, diagnosis, investigations, management and prognosis to someone who can act as an advocate. This could be the patient's parent, partner, friend or relative. This should only be done if appropriate and only with the patient's express consent.

Consent is implied for taking a history and performing relevant clinical examinations. However, investigations are another matter; the clinician must clearly explain the:

- nature of investigation
- potential benefit
- possible adverse effects
- problems and advantages of not carrying out the investigations.

These points must be explained clearly to the patient, in a way that can be readily understood. Routine urinalysis, for example, is usually accepted as part of medical and insurance examinations though some patients question its use in dentistry. For other procedures, informed consent should always first be obtained. It is also important where there could be adverse effects, such as pain, bleeding, infection, scarring or loss of sensation after a biopsy.

Verbal informed consent is adequate for non-invasive procedures, but for invasive or risky procedures a signed, witnessed and written informed consent should be obtained. Remember that patients are free to decline any or all investigations should they so wish, but it is wise for the clinician to clearly record that decision in writing in the case records.

A patient has the right under common law to give or withhold consent to medical examination of treatment. This is one of the basic principles of healthcare. Patients are entitled to receive sufficient information in a way they can understand about the proposed treatments, the possible alternatives and any substantial risk or risks which may be special in kind or magnitude or special to the patient, so that they can make a balanced judgement.

(UK Health Department 19.2.99. HSC 1999/031).

Remember also that patients are entitled to change their minds and to withdraw consent.

INVESTIGATIONS

Following history taking and examination, investigations may be required to help make or confirm the diagnosis and prognosis, or sometimes simply to exclude some diagnoses in order to reassure the patient (and partner, family or clinician). Inadequate investigation could lead to a:

- misdiagnosis
- missed diagnosis
- complaint of bad practice
- legal action.

However, superfluous investigations may be:

- liable to engender undue anxiety on the part of the patient, partner or relatives
- time consuming
- expensive
- occasionally associated with adverse effects, or even dangerous.

The following points should be borne in mind with regard to any form of investigation:

- The first principle must be to do no harm.
- Informed consent is required.
- Only an operator adequately skilled in a procedure should perform it.
- Surgical procedures are invasive and this includes venepuncture and biopsy; an oral biopsy is rarely a pleasant procedure.

21

This chapter discusses a number of common investigations: others appear elsewhere in the book.

All body fluids and tissues are potentially infectious. Barrier precautions must, therefore, always be employed in order to prevent transmission of infection to patients or staff during investigations involving body fluids or tissues.

These procedures can often be carried out in general practice but, for a number of reasons, the dental professional may elect to refer to a specialist. The same applies to other investigations, particularly where there are issues when medical experience or a medical or specialist opinion could be helpful if not essential.

URINALYSIS

This is routinely performed with 'dip-sticks'. It may reveal:

- glycosuria: which may suggest diabetes mellitus

- ketonuria: which may be a sign of diabetic ketoacidosis or starvation
- bilirubin or urobilinogen: which may indicate hepatobiliary disorders
- proteinuria: which may be due to menstruation, or indicate renal, urinary tract or cardiac disease
- haematuria: which may be due to menstruation, or indicate renal or urinary tract disease.

BLOOD TESTING

Details of the various blood tests commonly used are shown in **Table 3.1**. During venepuncture, remember:

- The antecubital fossa is most commonly used since veins are usually large and easily seen. Veins at other sites, such as the dorsum of hand or the cephalic vein, can be difficult to identify and venepuncture can be painful there.

Table 3.1 Blood tests in common use

Test	Blood sample required	Comments
Full blood count (FBC)	5 mL anticoagulated with dry potassium edetate (EDTA) and received in the haematology laboratory within 24 h	One of the laboratory investigations most frequently requested because anaemia and changes in the white blood cell count occur so commonly in a wide variety of diseases Blood cells are usually counted and sized in automatic blood cell counters Folate can be assayed on this sample Blood film is prepared from the same sample if indicated by the history or by the blood count results, for visual inspection of blood cells
Erythrocyte Sedimentation Rate (ESR), C-reactive protein (CRP) or PV (plasma viscosity)	As above	Global rate (ESR) or plasma measurements of non-specific plasma protein changes in viscosity ('plasma viscosity'): principally, increases in the concentration of certain globulins, and a fall in the albumin level The ESR also increases with anaemia.
Coagulation screen	5 mL anticoagulated with liquid sodium citrate and received in the haematology laboratory within 4 h or within 24 h for warfarin control by the prothrombin time or International Normalized Ratio (INR)	Required to diagnose coagulation disorders
Ferritin, iron, transferrin, folate and vitamin B12 (cobalamin) levels	10 mL added to a plain tube, and received in the haematology laboratory within 24 h	Useful in the diagnosis of anaemias due to deficiencies
Blood grouping and cross-matching	10 mL added to a plain tube, and received in the haematology laboratory within 4 h	Required prior to blood cell transfusion or major surgery
Blood glucose	Special tube (sodium fluoride)	Used to diagnose hypoglycaemia or hyperglycaemia, which is often due to diabetes mellitus
Serum urea, creatinine and electrolyte levels	Plain tube (no anticoagulant)	Used to diagnose renal failure (raised urea and creatinine levels) and electrolyte disturbance
Serum liver function tests include bilirubin, aspartate aminotransferase, alanine aminotransferase, alkaline phosphatase, albumin and globulin	10 mL added to a plain tube	Useful in the diagnosis of jaundice, liver and biliary tract disorders
Serum calcium, phosphate and alkaline phosphatase	10 mL added to a plain tube	Useful in the diagnosis of metabolic bone disease in particular
Serology	10 mL added to a plain tube	Useful for assay of various antibodies

- Blood is withdrawn automatically into a vacutainer. If a syringe is used, withdraw slowly, making sure that there is no air in the syringe. Too rapid removal of blood may cause haemolysis.
- If the specimen tube contains anticoagulant, ensure mixing by gently rolling the tube.
- Carefully dispose of the needle in the sharps container.
- Label the blood collection tubes with the patient's name, hospital or clinic number, date and time, etc.
- Complete and sign the appropriate request forms and give date, relevant clinical data, patient's name and number, etc.

SKIN TESTING

Absorption of many substances through the intact skin is poor and variable, but direct application to the surface of the skin is used for patch testing. The epidermal barrier may be overcome either by removing it or by introducing the material directly with a needle into the dermis. A positive test is typically a weal and flare and may be taken as one, which is significantly different from the control. Assessment of what is significant is difficult and varies with the enthusiasm of the tester. Resuscitation equipment and 1 in 1000 epinephrine (adrenaline) must be at hand to cope with any untoward allergic reactions.

The following techniques for skin testing are most commonly used.

Patch tests

Patch tests are usually carried out on the forearm and are used to detect contact allergy of the delayed hypersensitivity type. A battery of test allergens (European Standard Contact Dermatitis Testing Series) is often used. Patch testing is usually carried out with Finn chambers on Scanpor, a non-woven adhesive skin friendly tape which contains no colophony. Results are usually read at 48–72 h and again up to 1 week, but can also be read at 0.5 h to detect contact urticaria. At times patch testing may usefully be combined with scratch testing (see below).

Intradermal injections

A test solution must always be compared with a control solution (e.g. sterile saline) injected in a comparable site at the same time. The back, and the flexor aspects of the forearms are most conveniently used. The injections are made into the superficial layer of the dermis through a fine-bore (26 G or 27 G) needle with its bevel pointing upwards. The quantity of which may be conveniently injected varies from 0.01–0.1 mL. Precise measurement of smaller quantities is difficult and requires syringes with especially well-fitting plungers and a micrometer screw gauge. For routine clinical purposes an approximation is sufficient, either 0.05 mL or the amount, which just causes a visible wheal (0.01–0.02 mL).

Prick test

This is a modification of the intradermal injection. A small quantity of the test solution is placed on the skin and a prick made through it with a sharp needle. This should be superficial and not sufficient to draw blood. The size of the weal and flare are measured after 15 min. This test gives reproducible results and is convenient for much routine allergy testing.

Because of the discrepancy in quantities injected, the testing solutions are made up at different strengths for prick testing and intradermal testing. The intradermal injections of prick test solutions may be dangerous.

Modified prick test

Here a drop of the test solution is placed on the skin. A needle is then inserted very superficially and almost horizontally into the skin and lifted to raise a tiny tent of epidermis. This test is slightly more sensitive than the ordinary prick test, but gives no more reproducible results.

Scratch test

The scratch test resembles the prick test. A linear scratch about 1 cm long, but not sufficient to draw blood, is made through the epidermis. This test gives less reproducible results than the prick test.

The optimal time for reading intradermal reactions varies with the pharmacological agent or the type of immunological reaction. Most such tests are read at either 15–20 min or at 48 h, but it may be important to read the tests at other times, e.g. at 4–12 h or after 4 days.

BIOPSY

Biopsy is the removal of a small piece of tissue from the living body for the purpose of diagnosis by microscopic examination. It is often indicated in order to confirm or make a precise diagnosis, especially in the case of mucosal lesions, when a specimen for immunostaining is often also called for.

Indications for biopsy include (**Table 3.2**):

- lesions that have neoplastic or premalignant features or are enlarging
- persistent lesions that are of uncertain aetiology
- persistent lesions that are failing to respond to treatment

Table 3.2 Main indications for biopsy

Indication	Examples
Lesions which have neoplastic or premalignant features or are enlarging	Actinic cheilitis Erythroplakia Leukoplakia Lichen planus Focal pigmented lesions Lumps
Persistent lesions of uncertain aetiology	Soft or hard tissue
Persistent lesions failing to respond to treatment	Ulcers or lesions, such as some radiolucent or radio-opaque bone lesions
Persistent focal lesions involving the gingival/periodontium	Lumps, ulcers or non-healing extraction sockets
Confirmation of clinical diagnosis	Labial salivary gland biopsy to confirm Sjögren syndrome
Lesions causing the patient extreme concern	Patients may prefer biopsy or excision biopsy of a persistent red, white or pigmented lesion or lump

- confirmation of the clinical diagnosis
- lesions that are causing the patient extreme concern.

Biopsy precautions

Ensure that comprehensive medical history is completed and if patient is on:

- anticoagulants: warfarin requires up-to-date INR within 36 h of biopsy
- corticosteroids: if 10 mg or above for >3 months, requires 100 mg hydrocortisone i.v. 30 min before procedure
- immunocompromised: if neutropenic (neutrophils <1.5) requires antibiotic prophylaxis.

Biopsy technique

Tissue may be obtained by two main methods: techniques not requiring anaesthesia (e.g. exfoliative cytology and brush biopsy) and techniques requiring local anaesthesia (analgesia). Those requiring local anaesthesia are largely employed, and include:

- scalpel or tissue punch – incisional biopsy
- scalpel, diathermy or laser cutting – excisional biopsy

- curettage
- needle biopsy, these include:
  - cutting biopsy using a 14 G Tru-Cut needle, which is wide bore
  - cutting biopsy using a 16 G Vim Silverman needle
  - fine-needle cutting biopsy (FNCB) using an 18 G TSK Surecut needle
  - fine-needle aspiration biopsy (FNA or FNAB) or cytology (FNAC) using a 22 G or 25 G standard disposable needle, sometimes as ultrasound-guided fine-needle aspiration cytology (US-FNAC).

Figures 3.1–3.3 show equipment required. In the case of suspected potentially malignant or malignant mucosal lesions it can be difficult to decide exactly which is the part of the lesion that is best biopsied. Most significant information can be gained from red mucosal areas (erythroplasia) rather than white areas (leukoplakia) and it can sometimes be helpful to stain the mucosa before biopsy with toluidine blue dye (vital staining), which is taken up by nuclei and stains pathological areas mainly, causing suspect mucosal areas to stain blue. The technique is of limited value in a primary-care setting, but may have a place in the hands of an experienced clinician, in

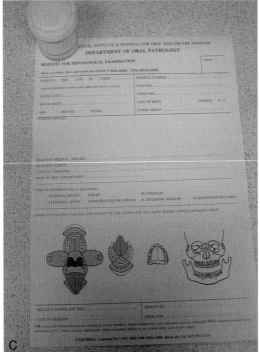
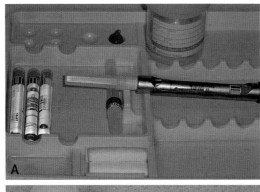
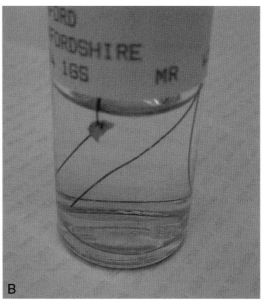

Fig. 3.1 (A) Biopsy tray, containing topical anaesthetic gel; local anaesthetic cartridges, needles and syringe; biopsy punch; pot with fixative; cotton wool rolls (B) pot and (C) form

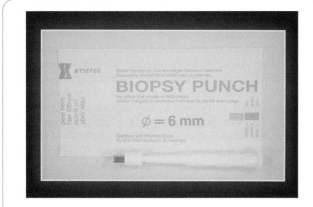

Fig. 3.2 Biopsy punch

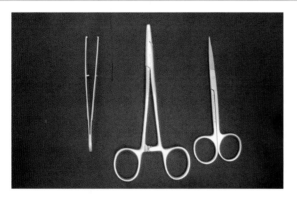

Fig. 3.3 Biopsy instruments: tissue forceps, suture forceps, scissors

patients at high risk of cancer (Ch. 31). The usual procedure is as follows: the patient is asked to rinse for 20 s with a solution of 1% acetic acid to cleanse the area of mucus, etc.; they then rinse for 20 s with plain water; they then rinse for 60 s with 1% aqueous toluidine blue solution; they then rinse for 20 s with a 1% solution of acetic acid; and, finally, they rinse for 20 s with water.

Usually a single biopsy is taken, but multiple biopsies may be indicated where:

- additional investigations, such as immunostaining, are required
- malignant disease is suspected
- there are widespread leukoplakic or erythroplakic field changes (such biopsies may be termed 'geographic' biopsies).

Biopsy procedure

Informed consent is mandatory for biopsy as for all operative procedures, particularly noting any possible adverse effects, such as postoperative pain, bleeding or loss of sensation. Care must be taken not to produce anxiety where it is not necessary; some patients equate biopsy with a diagnosis of cancer. Complete the request form with the:

- patient's full name
- patient's date of birth
- hospital number, if applicable

- date
- site of biopsy
- clinical résumé
- dates, and numbers, of all previous biopsies.

The container must be labelled clearly with:

- patient's full name
- patient's date of birth
- number
- date
- specimen site.

Mucosal biopsies

Mucosal biopsies are excisional (removal of the complete lesion) or incisional and taken with a scalpel or biopsy punch, or sometimes a diathermy or laser, usually under local analgesia. Excisional biopsy is preferred for small, isolated and probably benign lesions.

The biopsy should include lesional and normal tissue and should be large enough to handle, and to provide adequate information about the lesion. In the case of ulcerated mucosal lesions, most histopathological information is gleaned from the peri-lesional tissue, since by definition most epithelium is lost from the ulcer itself. Where there are similar lesions affecting several sites, which is often the case for example in lichen planus, then it is often better to biopsy buccal mucosal lesions than gingival, palatal or tongue lesions. Gingival biopsies may damage the gingival architecture, a protective pack such as Coe-pak must be worn for a week or so, and the lesions may be complicated to interpret histologically, since gingivitis is often superimposed. Palatal lesions similarly may need a dressing, and can be painful after biopsy. Tongue is a very sensitive, vascular and mobile organ, and biopsies can lead to discomfort, some interference with function, and the constant movement causes discomfort and may lead to sutures failing. In contrast, a biopsy from the buccal mucosa can be done virtually painlessly, with little post-operative swelling or discomfort, and sutures may not be needed – especially when a punch has been used. The punch has the advantages for incision biopsy that:

- the incision is controlled
- an adequate specimen is obtained (typically 4 mm or 6 mm in diameter)
- the patient is not disturbed by the sight of a scalpel
- suturing may not be required.

However, only a fairly small biopsy is obtained with the punch and, in some instances, epithelium may be sheared off – especially in vesiculobullous disorders. If a larger piece of tissue is needed, or the whole lesion is to be removed, the scalpel has advantages, particularly when the lesion is on the gingivae, especially lingually or other areas in which it is difficult to gain access with a punch or when mucosa is fragile (e.g. pemphigus). A number 15 blade is usually chosen.

To carry out a biopsy:

- A local anaesthetic should be given.
- Ensure tissue representative of the lesion is obtained. In mucosal lesions, include some normal tissue as well as the lesion (biopsies of ulcers alone are inadequate) (**Fig. 3.4**). When a vesiculobullous disorder is suspected, include perilesional tissue and use a scalpel rather than a punch (**Fig. 3.5**).

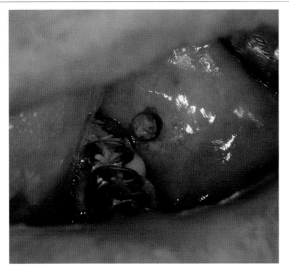

Fig. 3.4 Punch biopsy; the disc of tissue is removed with scissors or scalpel

- Do not squeeze with forceps as this can cause crush artefacts. Sutures may be used to hold the tissue and also to mark specific areas of biopsy.
- Place the biopsy specimen onto a small piece of paper before immersing in fixative, as this prevents curling. Put small specimens for histological examination immediately into buffered formalin or other fixative in at least its own volume of fixative, preferably 10-fold more, and leave at room temperature (20°C). A further biopsy specimen (or half of a larger biopsy) should also be immediately snap-frozen (−70°C) if immunostaining or a frozen section is required. If bacteriological examination is required, for example in suspected tuberculosis, send a separate specimen without fixative.
- Suture if necessary, preferably using a fine needle and resorbable suture such as Vicryl 3/0 or Vicryl Rapide 4/0, which will not require the patient to re-attend for removal (**Fig. 3.6**). Non-resorbable sutures, such as silk, are also available. For very small lesions suture may not be needed, or a silver nitrate stick can be used for haemostasis (**Fig. 3.5**).
- Use of an inverted suture technique means that there is no knot left in the mouth to irritate the patient.

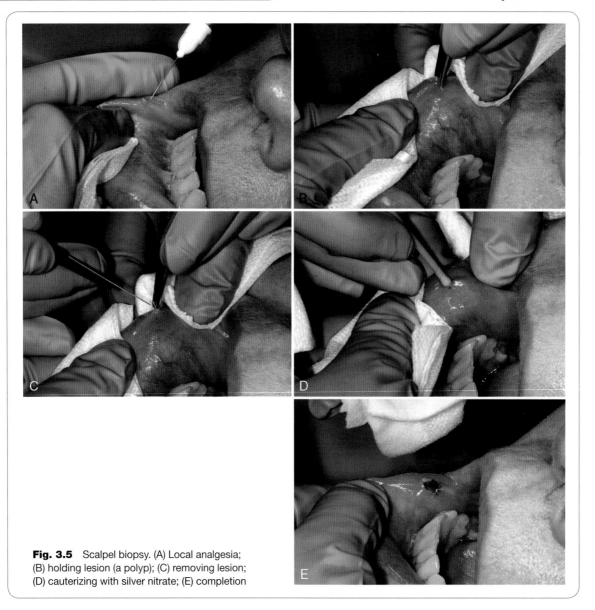

Fig. 3.5 Scalpel biopsy. (A) Local analgesia; (B) holding lesion (a polyp); (C) removing lesion; (D) cauterizing with silver nitrate; (E) completion

Immunostaining and immunofluorescence

Specimens for immunostaining should not be fixed in formalin, but must be handed immediately to laboratory staff for freezing, or immediately snap-frozen (on solid carbon dioxide or liquid nitrogen) and taken within an hour or so to the laboratory, or, occasionally put into Michel's solution if the specimen cannot be frozen:

- Direct immunofluorescence is a qualitative technique used to detect immune deposits (antibodies and/or complement) in the tissues. It is a one-stage technique, requiring patient lesional or perilesional tissue (**Fig. 3.7**). Immunostaining usually uses a fluorescein stain, which fluoresces apple green under ultraviolet light, and is termed 'immunofluorescence'. It is useful in the diagnosis particularly of vesiculobullous disorders, such as pemphigoid and pemphigus.
- Indirect immunofluorescence is a qualitative and quantitative technique used to detect immune deposits (circulating antibodies and/or complement) in the serum. It is a two or more stage technique requiring patient serum and animal tissue.

Oral smears for cytology

Cytology is rarely used but prepared in this way, smears will keep for up to 3 weeks:

- Take smears with a wooden or metal spatula, or dental plastic instrument.
- Spread smears evenly on the centres of two previously labelled glass slides.
- Fix smears immediately in industrial methylated spirit. Do not allow to dry in air, as cellular detail is rapidly lost and artefacts develop.
- After 20 min of fixation the smears can be left to dry in the air or left in fixative.

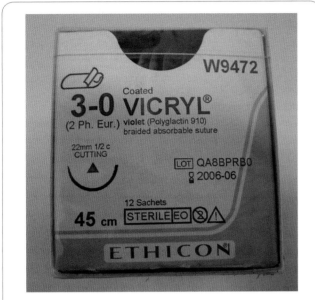

Fig. 3.6 Absorbable suture for biopsy closure if needed

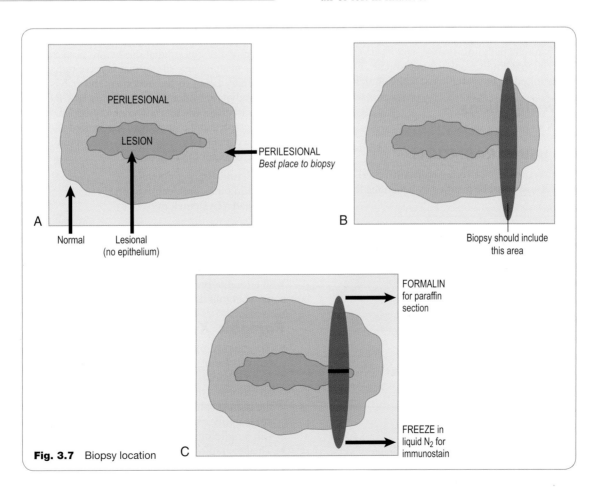

Fig. 3.7 Biopsy location

Lymph node biopsy

Lymph nodes should not be subjected to open biopsy if malignant disease is suspected: FNAB or FNAC are better, or the biopsy deferred until the time of operation. A sentinel lymph node is the first node(s) to which cancer is likely to spread from the primary cancer. To identify the sentinel lymph node (SLN), the surgeon injects in the area of the primary tumour, a radionuclide or dye. The substance is identified in the SLN by scanning (radionuclide) or visual inspection (dye). Once located the SLN is excised and examined histopathologically (this is SLN biopsy).

Labial salivary gland biopsy

- Warn the patient of possible postoperative mild hypoaesthesia.
- Give the patient local analgesia.
- Make a linear mucosal incision about 5–8 mm long (to one side of the midline in the lower labial mucosa) or an x-shaped incision over the swelling, which overlies the salivary gland (**Fig. 3.8**).
- Excise at least four lobules of salivary gland.
- Suture the wound if necessary.

Frozen sections for rapid diagnosis

This procedure, in which the section is examined whilst the patient is still under anaesthesia, is useful in cases where malignancy is suspect and in resections, to check the resection margin for tumour infiltration and to assess whether the margins are tumour-free.

Communicate with the pathologist at the latest by the day before the operation. Specimens should be immediately snap-frozen (on solid carbon dioxide or liquid nitrogen) and taken immediately to the laboratory, or collected by the pathology team. Telephone the laboratory when the specimen is on its way. Warn the pathologist about any tissue containing calcified material that could break the microtome. The results should be transmitted by the pathologist to the clinician direct.

Other investigations

Tables 3.3–3.8 summarize investigations of various sites.

IMAGING USING RADIATION

Because and the cumulative effect of radiation hazard, all investigations using X-rays must be justified by benefiting the patient.

The clinician requesting the examination or investigation must be satisfied that each investigation is necessary and that the benefit outweighs the risk.

In the UK, the Ionising Radiation Regulations (1988) required exposure of patients to be 'as low as reasonably achievable' (ALARA) and have been superseded by the Ionising Radiation Regulations (1999) (IRR99) and Ionising Radiation (Medical Exposure) Regulations (2000) (IR(ME)R2000).

Radiography

The request form for radiography should be completed and signed by the clinician or entered online and should include the following:

- Vital patient data: full name, address, date of birth, unit number, ward, clinic or outpatient department and specialist in charge.
- Details that facilitate correct investigations and accurate opinion:
  - investigations required (region to be examined and, where relevant, special investigation needed)
  - diagnostic problem
  - relevant clinical features
  - known diagnoses
  - previous relevant operations.
- Other information, for example, whether the patient is a walking or trolley case, whether there is an infectious risk, whether an urgent or routine report is required, the date, place and type of previous radiographs.

A protective lead apron having a lead equivalence of no less than 0.25 mm is worn by the patient only where the primary X-ray beam can strike the pelvis, such as in vertex-occlusal radiography, and a neck shield is indicated if the thyroid is to be exposed.

A particular problem arises during pregnancy, because of the hazard to the foetus. Enquiry as to pregnancy must always be made (risk of foetal irradiation) before performing radiography or other imaging procedures that involve radiation exposure by the primary beam to the abdomen and pelvis. Although most dental radiography does not constitute a risk, the clinician should always ascertain whether a woman is pregnant before requesting a radiograph and the investigation required should be discussed with the patient, who may wish to defer it until after pregnancy.

Note whether the patient:

- is of child-bearing potential
- is taking the contraceptive pill
- has had a hysterectomy
- has been sterilized.

Restricting X-ray investigations on women of child-bearing age to the 10 days following the start of a menstrual period (the 10-day rule) should be considered only for examinations with a relatively high gonad radiation risk, and has now fallen somewhat into disfavour.

Portable X-rays

- The quality of portable films is rarely as good as that of corresponding films taken using non-portable equipment.
- Examination should take place in the ward only if there is an absolute contraindication to the patient being brought to the radiography department. If there is any doubt about the advisability of bringing the patient to the department, consult a radiologist.
- Theatre radiography is done only when its results are needed during the operation.

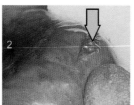
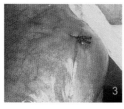
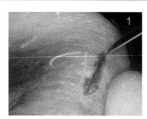

Fig. 3.8 Labial salivary gland biopsy (one method)

Table 3.3 Investigative procedures in diseases of the jaws and sinuses

Procedure	Advantages	Disadvantages	Remarks
Transillumination	Simple	–	Helpful to show a fluid level
Fibre-optic nasendoscopy	Simple; good visualization	Skill needed	Useful to examine nasal passages, pharynx and larynx
Radiography	Reveals much data not obvious on clinical examination	Specialized techniques may be difficult	Upper occlusal radiography is useful for detecting cysts Other radiographic views may fail to show cysts and diagnosis of a cyst can be very difficult if the antrum is large with outpouchings into the alveolar process and zygomatic bone, since these antral extensions may resemble cysts Occipitomental radiography (Waters) views of the skull are the best radiographs for viewing the antra These views can be taken at 15° and 30°, and can show an opaque antrum, a fluid level or fractures
Computed tomography (CAT, CT, CBCT), MRI	Reveal data often not seen on clinical or conventional radiographic examination Magnetic resonance imaging (MRI) uses no radiation	Expensive and not universally available Interpretation requires additional training	Demonstrate both hard and soft tissues and give spatial relationships Cone beam CT (CBCT) or coronal CAT of the antrum can be useful for showing the extent of a neoplasm, particularly in the posterior and superior maxilla CAT and MRI are useful particularly in detecting the extent of spread of a malignant neoplasm and have the great advantage of demonstrating the posterior maxilla, the intratemporal fossa, the floor of the orbit and the nasoethmoidal sinuses – sites not readily seen by other imaging
Aspiration	Simple	May introduce infection	May show the presence of haemangioma The protein content of cyst fluid may be of diagnostic value (protein levels lower than 4g/100mL in keratocysts)
Bone biopsy	Definitive	Invasive	Invasive
Bone scan	Surveys all skeleton	Those of any radionuclide procedure	May reveal pathology (e.g. metastases or osteomyelitis)

Table 3.4 Investigative procedures in temporomandibular joint disease

Procedure	Advantages	Disadvantages
Radiography	Simple Can reveal much pathology	Radiation exposure
CAT scan, CBCT	Can provide excellent information	Expensive Radiation exposure
Arthrography (double contrast)	Provides excellent information	Danger of introducing infection Painful
MRI	Provides excellent information without exposure to ionizing radiation	Non-invasive Expensive and not universally available
Arthroscopy	Minimally invasive Good visualization	Requires anaesthesia Technically demanding

Table 3.5 Investigative procedures in salivary gland disease

Procedure	Advantages	Disadvantages and comments
Sialometry* (salivary flow rates)	Simple rapid useful procedure which may confirm or refute hyposalivation	Somewhat imprecise Wide range of normal values Commonly used
Blood tests	Simple and useful to reveal systemic disease (e.g. rheumatoid arthritis or Sjögren syndrome)	Will not usually reflect local disease of salivary glands
MRI	Useful for investigating space-occupying lesions and suspect malignancy, or infections	Expensive, not universally available, but no irradiation
Ultrasound	Useful, inexpensive, non-invasive and often helpful diagnostically	Increasingly used
Plain radiography	Lower occlusal and oblique lateral or OPT may show submandibular calculi Soft PA film may show parotid calculi	Calculi may not be radio-opaque Sialography may be needed
CT, CBCT	Useful to investigate salivary duct obstruction, infections or abscesses	Not universally available; high radiation dose
Sialendoscopy	Useful to investigate salivary duct obstruction	Not universally available
Sialochemistry	Research investigation; rarely helpful clinically	Salivary composition varies with many factors Far less useful than blood and other tests Rarely used
Sialography	Useful to eliminate gross structural damage, calculi or stenoses	Time consuming and somewhat crude and insensitive May cause pain or, occasionally, sialadenitis† Uses X-rays Uncommonly used
Salivary gland biopsy	Labial gland (LSG) biopsy is simple and may reflect changes in other salivary (and exocrine) glands. Major gland biopsy and fine needle aspiration cytology (FNAC) may be useful	Biopsies are invasive Major gland biopsy may result in facial palsy or salivary fistula and thus uncommonly used
Scintigraphy and radiosialometry	Measures uptake of radionuclide‡ (radiosialometry more quantitative) High uptake (hotspots) may reveal tumours	Expensive and with hazards associated with use of radionuclides Taken up by thyroid gland; rare instances of thyroid damage Rarely used

*Unstimulated whole salivary flow rates are usually used; flow rates < 1.5 mL/15 min are low. Alternatively, stimulate parotid salivary flow with 1 mL 10% citric acid on to tongue; flow rates < 1 mL/min may signify reduced salivary function. Alternatively, pilocarpine 2.5 mg i.v. may be used, but is contraindicated in cardiac patients or those with hypertension.

†Combined sialography with CAT scanning may be useful in the diagnosis and localization of salivary gland lesions, particularly parotid neoplasms.

‡Usually technetium pertechnetate.

Plain radiography

This is useful in the diagnosis of fractures, dislocations, bone and tooth disorders, joint disease and foreign bodies.

Chest radiography

The chest radiograph is valuable in investigating chest disease, heart disease (e.g. heart failure) and general medical problems, such as malaise, fever or weight loss (e.g. bronchial carcinoma, tuberculosis and other chest infections). Spiral computed tomography is a major advance.

Abdominal radiography

Abdominal radiographs are valuable in the diagnosis of gastrointestinal obstruction or perforation, renal stones or gallstones.

Intra-oral radiography

- Periapical radiographs are useful for demonstrating pathology in the periapical region (abscess, granuloma, cyst, etc.) and in tooth root, periodontium and adjacent bone.
- Bitewing radiographs show both upper and lower premolar and molar teeth on one film, but do not show the tooth apex. They are useful for revealing approximal caries and demonstrating the alveolar crest.
- Occlusal films may be useful in assessing the facial and lingual cortices and adjacent areas such as floor of mouth and palate.

Dental panoramic tomography (DPT) (or orthopantomography (OPTG))

This is valuable as a general survey and typically shows the antra and temporomandibular joints well. The radiation dose

Table 3.6 Investigative procedures in oral mucosal disease

Procedure	Advantages	Disadvantages	Remarks
Biopsy	Gives definitive diagnosis in many instances	Invasive	Mucosal biopsies should be submitted for histopathological and often direct immunofluorescence examinations if a vesiculobullous disorder is suspected
Bacteriological smear and culture	Simple clinical procedure	Isolation of organisms does not necessarily imply causal relation with disease under investigation Some organisms are non-cultivable	Anaerobic techniques may be indicated especially in oral lesions in the immunocompromised host Nucleic acid studies increasingly used
Fungal smear	Simple clinical procedure	As above	Candida hyphae suggest Candida species are pathogenic Nucleic acid studies increasingly used
Viral culture	Simple sensitive clinical procedure Often gives diagnosis more rapidly than does serology	May require special facilities and may only give retrospective diagnosis	False-negative results possible Indicated in some acute ulcerative or bullous lesions Serology should also be undertaken Nucleic acid studies increasingly used
Microbial DNA studies	Polymerase chain reaction (PCR) or nucleic acid amplification tests (NAAT) now often used	May require special facilities	Rapid and specific results Increasingly used
Haematological screen, haemoglobin red cell and white cell indices	Simple clinical procedure	Detection rate may not be high	Essential to exclude systemic causes of oral disease, especially in ulcers, glossitis or angular stomatitis
Serology	Demonstration of a rise in titre-specific antibodies between acute and convalescent serum may be diagnostically useful Specific tests available, e.g. HIV antibodies	Serum autoantibodies may not mean disease Serum autoantibodies may be undetected in pemphigoid Diagnosis of viral infections is retrospective	Essential in suspected HIV and other infections, connective tissue disease, autoimmune or other immunological disorders

is considerably lower than a full mouth survey using periapical films, but it:

- lacks the detail obtained by other films, such as periapical radiography
- does not show detail in the anterior jaws
- does not show caries until this is advanced
- can result in ghost shadows and blurring
- examines only a slice of tissue.

Radiovisiography

Radiovisiography (RVG) is digital imaging, and is useful in reducing the radiation exposure, particularly where there is a need for repeated films, such as in endodontics.

Sialography

Sialography involves instillation of radio-opaque contrast media into the salivary duct followed by oblique lateral and postero-anterior (PA) or rotated PA radiographs. Use of a sialogogue, such as lemon juice, to empty the gland gives an 'emptying film'. Sialography is not commonly used nowadays but can occasionally help to:

- detect ductal obstruction
- detect the rare cases of salivary aplasia.

- assess patients with hyposalivation
- assess patients with salivary swelling.

Arthrography

Arthrography is rarely used. It involves injection of radio-opaque contrast media (usually iohexol or iopamidol) into the lower space of the temporomandibular joint. The main indication is in suspected internal joint derangements.

Angiography

Angiography involves injection of radio-opaque contrast media into arteries (arteriography) or veins (venography). The main indications include:

- diagnosis or delineation of vascular anomalies or tumours
- assessment of tumours in the deep lobe of the parotid gland
- assisting surgical procedures (e.g. microvascular surgery or embolization).

Computed axial tomography (CAT or CT)

CT integrates information from multiple radiographic 'slices' into images of internal tissues (e.g. brain, orbit, sinuses, neck, salivary glands, tongue). It has considerable advantages for visualizing complex head and neck anatomical

Table 3.7 Imaging available for lesions in different locations

Location of lesions	Plain radiography	Other imaging
Mandible	Rotational tomography Oblique lateral CT, CBCT	MRI Bone scan
Mandibular condyle	Reverse Towne Submentovertex CT, CBCT	MRI Bone scan
Temporomandibular joint	Rotational tomography Transcranial CT Transpharyngeal CT, CBCT	MRI Arthrography Bone scan
Maxilla	30 occipitomental CT, CBCT	MRI Bone scan
Paranasal sinuses	OM rotational tomography for maxillary antra Upper occlusal or lateral Submentovertex CT, CBCT	MRI Bone scan
Skull	PA skull rotational tomography 10 occipitomental Lateral skull CT	MRI Bone scan
Salivary glands	Oblique lateral Rotated PA CT	Ultrasound MRI Sialography Scintigraphy
Intra-oral	Rotational tomography CT, CBCT	Ultrasound MRI

Table 3.8 Significance of the more common serum autoantibodies

Autoantibody	Main significance*
DNA antibodies (ds-DNA (*Crithidia luciliae*))	Systemic lupus erythematosus
Anti-topoisomerase 1 (Sc1-70)	Scleroderma
Anticentromere antibodies (ACA)	Scleroderma
Rheumatoid factor (RF)	Rheumatoid arthritis (RA) (sometimes systemic lupus erythematosus)
Robert (Ro), also known as soluble substance A antigen (SS-A)	Sjögren syndrome
Lane (La), also known as soluble substance B antigen (SS-B)	Sjögren syndrome
Epithelial intercellular cement (desmoglein (dsg))	Pemphigus
Epithelial basement membrane zone (e.g. integrin)	Pemphigoid**
Parietal cell antibody; intrinsic factor antibodies	Pernicious anaemia

*The presence of autoantibodies does not always indicate disease.
**Or other immune-mediated subepithelial blistering diseases.

Scintiscanning (radionuclide scanning)

Radioactive pharmaceuticals with affinity for specific organs or tissues can be detected and measured by a gamma camera.

Salivary scintigraphy

Intravenous sodium pertechnetate is taken up by salivary (and thyroid) glands and secreted in saliva. Scintiscanning is not commonly used in salivary gland investigation but can sometimes help in the diagnosis of:

- Sjögren syndrome
- ductal obstruction
- salivary neoplasms
- salivary aplasia.

It may also help locate a lingual thyroid.

Bone scans

Intravenous technetium methylene diphosphonate is taken up by osteoblasts, and bone scans can be useful in:

- assessing condylar or coronoid hyperplasia
- detecting metastases
- detecting bone invasion
- determining activity of bone disease.

Positron emission tomography (PET)

PET can produces maps of tissue metabolic activity based either on blood flow or glucose utilization, and is increasingly used to detect second primary tumours and metastases (Ch. 31).

areas inaccessible to conventional radiographs and is good for visualizing hard tissue lesions especially. CT imaging of the head can provide images of bones, soft tissue, and blood vessels and is:

- particularly useful for determining tumour spread, to exclude cranial base or intracranial pathology and planning surgery and implant placement
- expensive
- a fairly high radiation exposure (CT of the head can give the equivalent exposure to about 100 chest radiographs).

Cone beam CT (CBCT) is a smaller, faster and safer modification of CT. Using a cone-shaped X-ray beam, the CBCT scanner size, scanning time and radiation dosage are all reduced; the time needed for a CBCT scan is typically under one minute and the radiation dosage is up to a hundred times less than that of a regular CT. CBCT is thus increasingly used to image jaws and related structures.

Functional CT using positron emission tomography (PET), four-dimensional computed tomography (4D-CT), and single photon emission computed tomography (SPECT) is increasingly used.

NON-RADIATION IMAGING
Magnetic resonance imaging (MRI)

MRI depends on the distribution of protons (hydrogen nuclei) in tissues and their effect on a magnetic field and does not involve ionizing radiation. The MRI signal has two components:

- T1, in which the proton is spinning under magnetic influence and radiofrequency to return to the original value (spin lattice or longitudinal relaxation time). T_1-weighted scans are a standard basic scan, in particular differentiating fat from water – with water darker and fat brighter. T_1-weighted images cause fat like the myelin in brain white matter to appear bright (light grey); grey matter appears grey, cerebrospinal fluid (CSF) appears black.
- T2, which depends on the gradual dephasing of the protons in the transverse or transaxial plane (spin-spin, or transverse relaxation times). T_2-weighted scans show fat darker, and water lighter. Brain white matter appears dark grey, grey matter appears grey and CSF appears white.

The advantages of MRI are that it is:

- especially good for visualizing soft tissues and lesions
- useful for imaging the temporomandibular joint
- good for revealing bone invasion.

The disadvantages of MRI are that it is:

- not good for imaging bone
- fraught with producing image artefacts where metal objects are present (dental metal restorations, implants, orthodontic and other metal-containing appliances, bone plates, metallic foreign bodies, joint prostheses, etc.)
- expensive.

Contraindications to the use of MRI include the presence of ferromagnetic implanted devices in brain or eye, such as nerve stimulators, cochlear implants, or intracranial vascular clips. Metal objects outside the brain and eye are not a contraindication: cardiac valves, inferior vena cava filters, IUDs and metallic prostheses are safe, unless there is doubt as to positional stability. However, cardiac pacemakers, insulin pumps, neurostimulators, cochlear implants, etc. may be de-programmed.

Thus, MRI gives sensitive images of the internal organs and tissues (e.g. brain or spine), but in the presence of metal there may be artefacts.

Ultrasound scanning (US)

- 'Ultrasound' is a term that applies to sound waves with a frequency above the audible range of human hearing.
- US (diagnostic sonography) is non-invasive, simple, inexpensive and very helpful in imaging soft tissues with virtually no contraindications and is thus increasingly used.
- US gives useful imaging of soft tissues (e.g. subcutaneous tissues, muscle, tendons, vessels) and internal organs (e.g. lymph nodes, thyroid or salivary glands) and foreign bodies. Ultrasound (Doppler) is also useful for investigating vascular disease. Colour Doppler ultrasound (CDUS) may be useful.
- US diagnostically uses high frequency sound waves (2–18 Hz) with wavelengths of 0.6–0.01 mm, and involves no ionizing radiation exposure. Sonographers use a hand-held probe (a transducer) placed directly on and moved over the area to be imaged. When the sound strikes the interface between media, the energy reflects as an echo, which may be displayed as a unidimensional wave image (an A scan) or, when a sweeping beam is used, as a two-dimensional monochrome image (a B scan). There is abrupt impedance with calcified lesions, or foreign bodies, such as glass or metal.

Endoscopy

Endoscopy is typically performed with flexible fibre-optic endoscopes, under local analgesia, sometimes with conscious sedation or general anaesthesia. Relevant endoscopic procedures include:

- nasendoscopy
- oesophagoscopy
- bronchoscopy
- panendoscopy usually refers to triple endoscopy (nasendoscopy, oesophagoscopy and bronchoscopy)
- gastroscopy (the oesophagus, stomach and duodenum)
- sialoendoscopy
- colonoscopy.

Risks from endoscopy include possible:

- infection
- bleeding
- punctured organs.

Bleeding may occur at the site of a biopsy or polyp removal. Typically minor, such bleeding may simply cease spontaneously or be controlled by cautery. Surgery is seldom necessary. Perforation, however, generally requires surgery, though some cases may be treated with antibiotics and intravenous fluids.

Thermography

An infrared camera detects areas of changed vascularity, but has the disadvantage of needing the patient to be 'precooled'.

Photography

This is exceedingly useful to record lesions, and the advent of digital photography has considerably improved the quality.

INVESTIGATIONS OF SPECIFIC MEDICAL PROBLEMS RELEVANT IN ORAL MEDICINE

ALLERGIES

Allergy is an abnormal immune response (usually a type I or type IV hypersensitivity response) to an antigen – a protein or allergen. Many allergies have a hereditary component but the prevalence of allergies appears to be increasing and people who suffer allergies to one type of substance are more likely to suffer allergies to others. Common allergens are pollen, dust mites, mould, pet dander, nuts, shellfish, milk and egg proteins and latex but, in many cases, the allergen cannot be reliably identified.

Diagnosis is based on clinical history and presentation including a family history of allergy; plus skin-prick or patch testing to identify contact allergens (see above); or an elimination diet to identify food allergens.

Assays of serum IgE levels (PRIST: paper radio-immunosorbent test) and serum specific IgE antibodies (RAST: radioallergosorbent test) may help.

ANAEMIA

Deficiency of any of the vitamins and minerals essential for normal erythropoiesis (haematinics), including iron. copper, cobalt. vitamins A, B_{12}, B_6, C, E, folic acid, riboflavin and nicotinic acid, may be associated with defective erythropoiesis and eventually, a fall in haemoglobin (anaemia). Iron. vitamin B_{12} and folate are the haematinics for which deficiency states manifest most often clinically, sometimes even when haemoglobin levels are normal. Haematinics may be lacking from dietary or gastrointestinal causes, or from increased losses (e.g. iron in chronic or severe haemorrhage).

Dietary sources of iron and B_{12} are largely animal, while folate is present in green vegetables. Vegans may lack B_{12}.

Normal gastric function is required for iron absorption (hydrochloric acid is needed) and for B_{12} absorption (intrinsic factor from gastric parietal cells is needed). These haematinics are absorbed in the small intestine, B_{12} mainly in the ileum. Diseases in those sites may cause deficiencies, as may some drugs.

Iron is stored in haemoglobin and B_{12} in the liver, but stores of folate are lacking. Thus deficiencies take some months or years to manifest in patients with iron or B_{12} deficiencies.

Anaemia is caused mainly by:

- reduced erythropoiesis
- haemolysis
- haemorrhage.

The most usual cause of anaemia in resource-rich groups is iron deficiency caused by chronic haemorrhage (commonly menorrhagia). After a thorough history and examination, the following are required for diagnosis of the extent and type of anaemia:

- haemoglobin concentration
- a full blood film (full blood count/full blood picture/complete blood count)
- red cell indices
- white cell count and differential
- levels of serum iron (ferritin), vitamin B_{12} and corrected whole blood folate.

Deficiency states and anaemias

Once the type of deficiency or anaemia has been established, the cause must be found and treated.

In iron deficiency, unless it is clear that menorrhagia is the cause, the site of blood loss should be sought, usually in the gastrointestinal, or sometimes genitourinary, tract:

- Iron deficiency anaemia is usually microcytic (red cell mean corpuscular volume (MCV) is reduced) and managed by treatment of the cause, and oral iron supplements. Only rarely is blood transfusion necessary, usually when the haemoglobin is <9 g/dL and surgery is required urgently. Packed red cells should then be used in preference to blood.
- Folate or vitamin B_{12} deficiencies may result in a macrocytic (megaloblastic) anaemia (MCV raised).
- Folate deficiency is commonly dietary in origin. Treatment of folate deficiency is by treatment of the cause and with oral folic acid.

- Vitamin B_{12} deficiency is seen in vegans but otherwise is rarely dietary in origin; more commonly, it is caused by a gastrointestinal lesion or pernicious anaemia. Treatment is by treatment of the cause if possible and with vitamin B_{12}, usually by injection for life.
- Deficiencies of multiple haematinic factors, e.g. iron, folate and vitamin B_{12}, may well be caused by disease of the small intestine, such as coeliac disease (gluten-sensitive enteropathy).

Sickle cell anaemia

Sickle cell anaemia is the homozygous form of a hereditary condition affecting haemoglobin composition (sickle haemoglobin (HbS)) resulting in red blood cells adopting a sickle shape, especially in hypoxia. It is:

- found mainly in patients of African heritage and some originating from the Mediterranean countries and Asia
- a risk for general anaesthesia.

It is therefore important to rule out sickle cell anaemia in all black patients and record results to prevent unnecessary re-testing:

- Check the medical history. In sickle cell anaemia, at low oxygen tensions (≈45 mmHg), the erythrocytes become inelastic and sickle shaped and then either 'sludge', blocking capillaries and causing infarcts (e.g. in bone and brain), or rupture, causing haemolytic anaemia.
- Do a full blood picture.
- Do a sickle screening blood test, such as a simple solubility test (e.g. the SickleDex test) which detects any HbS and is, therefore, positive both in patients with sickle cell anaemia and the sickle trait (see below).
- Further haematological examination, including haemoglobin electrophoresis, is theoretically required for confirmation. In practice, however, a positive solubility test with a low haemoglobin level can be taken as being diagnostic of sickle cell anaemia. A positive solubility test with a normal haemoglobin level may indicate the sickle cell trait (see below).

In the sickle trait, sickling occurs only at much lower oxygen tensions (<20 mmHg), which are unlikely to occur in normal clinical practice.

BLEEDING TENDENCIES

A bleeding tendency can be caused mainly by a blood platelet defect (thrombocytopenia) or blood coagulation defect (anticoagulant drugs, haemophilia, von Willebrand disease). Screening tests typically include:

- platelet count
- function tests
- APTT (activated partial thromboplastin time)
- PT (prothrombin time) and international normalized ratio (INR) – the ratio of the patient's PT to a control
- clotting factor assays.

Screening tests will eliminate two-thirds of suspected cases, and the remaining third will require more detailed tests to accurately define a diagnosis. Consult the haematologist immediately before undertaking other investigations; bleeding and clotting time assays are quite unsatisfactory, and special investigations may well be required, such as factor VIII clotting activity or related antigen assay.

ENDOCRINE DISORDERS
Adrenocortical function testing

- Blood pressure: is low in hypoadrenocorticism (Addison disease), high in hyperadrenocorticism (Cushing disease).
- Plasma cortisol levels: the diurnal rhythm of plasma cortisol is a sensitive index of adrenal function; cortisol values are normally highest between 6.00 a.m. and 10.00 a.m. and lowest between midnight and 4.00 a.m. Samples taken at 8.00 a.m. and 4.00 p.m. should differ by at least 5 mg/100 mL. The sample taken at 8.00 a.m. should be 5–25 mg/100 mL. Plasma cortisol at 8.00 a.m. to 9.00 a.m. is often <6 mg/100 mL in hypoadrenocorticism. Diurnal variation in cortisol is lost in hyperadrenocorticism.
- Synacthen test (ACTH stimulation test): this is performed in the following way. Take blood at 8.00 a.m. to 9.00 a.m. for the plasma cortisol level; give 0.25 mg synacthen subcutaneously or intramuscularly; after 30 min, take a further blood sample for the cortisol level. Normally, synacthen results in a rise in cortisol levels to >18 mg/100 mL. This rise is lost in hypoadrenocorticism (at an earlier stage in disease than the low cortisol level is found).
- Abdominal radiography: this may show calcified adrenals if tuberculosis is the cause of hypoadrenocorticism.
- Serum autoantibodies: patients with Addison disease may have various circulating autoantibodies.
- Electrolytes: plasma potassium is raised and sodium reduced in Addison disease.

Diabetes

Diabetes is often detected at routine urinalysis by detecting glycosuria (and ketonuria), but there are other causes of glycosuria and of ketonuria, and diabetics do not always have glycosuria. Diabetes is best diagnosed by testing for raised blood glucose above 11 mmol/L or fasting level over about 7 mmol/L usually establishes the diagnosis (plasma glucose levels are about 1 mmol/L higher). Glucose tolerance testing is indicated only if blood sugar values are borderline. A widely accepted simplified glucose tolerance test (GTT) is as follows: give the patient 75 g glucose orally; assay blood glucose levels 2 h later; a level >11.1 mmol/L is diagnostic of diabetes; a level <11.1 mmol/L excludes diabetes.

Diabetic control is best by serial measurements of blood glucose levels throughout the day with a glucometer. Glycosylated haemoglobin or fructosamine are usually monitored regularly to assess longer-term control. Non-diabetics have up to 7% glycosylated haemoglobin: 7–9% represents good control, over 13% shows poor control in diabetes.

A small amount of ketonuria, as shown by Acetest tablet test, is usually of no importance, but a strongly positive test, especially if confirmed by a positive ferric chloride reaction (Gerhardt's test), indicates a serious degree of ketosis. Confirmation is obtained by finding a low serum bicarbonate concentration.

Hyperparathyroidism

Blood for calcium levels should be collected early in the morning from a fasting patient and a tourniquet should not be used (venous stasis and a fall in pH alter calcium levels). The blood collection should be done along with serum for albumin assay (albumin levels influence calcium levels) and may need repeating several times to exclude hyperparathyroidism.

GRANULOMATOUS DISORDERS

Granulomatous disorders may present a difficult differential diagnosis, which can include Crohn disease, orofacial granulomatosis, sarcoidosis and tuberculosis. Investigations indicated may then include:

- lesional biopsy
- erythrocyte sedimentation rate (ESR) or plasma viscosity (PV) or C reactive protein (CRP)
- serum angiotensin converting enzyme (SACE), and a gallium scan.
- a tuberculin skin test
- chest imaging
- gastrointestinal endoscopy, radiography and biopsy.

IMMUNODEFICIENCY

Immune defects should be suspected if there are recurrent or persistent infections or other features such as neoplasms. Laboratory tests needed to confirm the diagnosis of immunodeficiency and to identify the type of disorder include:

- total white blood cell count, the percentages of each main type and CD4 count
- antibody levels
- red blood cell count
- platelet count.
- levels of complement proteins.

Skin tests using candida or other antigens may be done if the immunodeficiency is thought to be due to a T-cell abnormality.

SEXUALLY SHARED INFECTIONS
HIV

Diagnosis of acute HIV disease is from other causes of glandular fever syndromes (**Table 3.9**) and diagnosis of HIV infection in any event includes:

- clinical features (Ch. 53)
- lymphopenia
- a severe T-helper lymphocyte defect (reduced CD4$^+$ cells and CD4:CD8 ratio)
- ideally, HIV antibody *and* p24 antigen are tested simultaneously (after counselling) These fourth generation assays are advantageous in reducing the time between HIV infection and testing HIV positive to 1 month – which is 1–2 weeks earlier than with sensitive third generation (antibody only detection) assays. HIV-RNA quantitative assays (viral load tests) are NOT recommended as screening assays because of the possibility of false positive results, and also because they have only marginal advantage over fourth generation assays for detecting primary infection. Confirmatory assays are then required to confirm HIV antibody and antigen/RNA
- excluding other sexually shared infections.

Syphilis

Dark ground/darkfield (DGM) of a lesion may demonstrate *Treponema pallidum* in lesion exudate or lymph nodes but is not reliable for examining oral lesions where contamination with commensal treponemes is likely. Test material from oral lesions submitted on dry swabs using the polymerase chain reaction (PCR).

Table 3.9 Glandular fever syndromes

Syndrome	Causal agents	Investigations
Infectious mononucleosis (classic glandular fever)	Epstein–Barr virus (EBV)	Paul–Bunnell test (heterophile antibodies) EBV antibodies
EBV-negative glandular fever	Cytomegalovirus (CMV)	CMV antibodies
Acute HIV seroconversion	Human immune deficiency viruses (HIV)	HIV antibody and antigen T4 (CD4) cell depletion
Erythema subtilum	Human herpes 6 virus	HHV-6 antibodies
Toxoplasmosis	*Toxoplasma gondii*	Sabin–Feldman dye test – specific IgM antibodies

Serology is indicated; a *Treponema pallidum* enzyme immunoassay (EIA), which detects both IgG and IgM, is recommended. The *Treponema pallidum* particle assay (TPPA) is preferred to the *Treponema pallidum* haemagglutination assay (TPHA), and is used in combination with a cardiolipin antigen/reagin test such as VDRL (Venereal Disease Research Laboratory) or RPR (rapid plasma reagin) to maximize the detection of primary infections. An EIA IgM test should be performed in addition to these routine screening tests since IgM becomes detectable in the serum 2–3 weeks after infection and IgG 4–5 weeks after infection. An additional test, such as immunoblotting based on recombinant antigens or the fluorescent antibody absorbed (FTA-abs) test, can be used in the case of a discrepancy between the EIA and TPPA. An EIA for anti-treponemal IgM should be performed on all sera reactive in one or more of the screening tests. Quantitative VDRL/RPR tests should then be performed before therapy.

Always exclude other sexually shared infections.

Gonorrhoea

Gonococcal pharyngitis may be seen, particularly in men who have sex with men. Always exclude other sexually shared infections. Microscopy, a direct smear for Gram-staining (Gram-negative diplococci) while useful for other sites, is not suitable for oral or pharyngeal specimens where many other bacteria are present including Gram-negative cocci of other genera. Take a bacteriological swab from the area, for culture and sensitivities. Direct plating of the specimen and use of transport swabs both give acceptable results. Transport swabs should be stored in the refrigerator at 4°C and transported to the laboratory as soon as possible, preferably within 48h. Tests that probe or amplify specific nucleic acid sequences (nucleic acid amplification tests (NAATs)) have the ability to detect small amounts of nucleic acid and can detect non-viable organisms but have had limited evaluation on oropharyngeal samples and although they may have increased sensitivity (>90%) compared to cultures (<60%) are currently not recommended because they do not provide viable organisms for susceptibility testing.

Hepatitis viruses B and C

Seroconversion for virus antibody may take 3 months so antibody tests may give false negative results when a patient presents with acute hepatitis.

Hepatitis B virus (HBV) testing is for hepatitis B surface antigen (HB$_s$Ag) and IgM anti-HBc antibody. If HB$_s$Ag-positive, proceed to hepatitis B 'e' antigen (HB$_e$Ag) and antibody (HB$_e$Ab) testing. About one in five are HB$_e$Ag positive and at high risk of infectivity. Those who have HB$_s$Ag should later be screened again at 3 months, and again if still positive. Those positive at 9 months are 'chronic carriers'. Assays for anti-HBc and HB$_s$Ag in saliva samples have been used for surveillance and research but are not available for diagnostic use.

Hepatitis C virus (HCV) testing includes second or third generation ELISA for serum anti-HCV or other immunoassays (e.g. chemiluminescence). Tests to confirm a positive result include a recombinant immunoblot assay (RIBA), using another ELISA, or proceeding directly to an assay for HCV-RNA by reverse-transcriptase polymerase chain reaction (RT-PCR) or another genome amplification assay.

COMMUNICATING THE DIAGNOSIS

Communicating a diagnosis is the act of 'communicating to the individual or his/her personal representative a diagnosis identifying a disease or disorder as the cause of symptoms of the individual in circumstances in which it is reasonably foreseeable that the individual or his/her personal representative will rely on the diagnosis, including to decide whether to agree to any intervention recommended'.

Clinicians should reassure the patient where possible, and:

- Communicate assessment findings and ensure that the information is understood by the patient or appropriate substitute decision-maker.
- Communicate further information about their disease or diagnosis as appropriate, or if requested.
- Follow their ethical and professional responsibility to refer the patient to another appropriate HCP if this is likely to be in the patient's best interests.

COMMUNICATING RISK

People with high-risk behaviours such as tobacco, alcohol or recreational drug use should not only be encouraged to change these behaviours but also to understand the need for vigilance and follow-up. Personalized communications (especially when supported by written and visual materials) are the most effective in promoting screening uptake.

COMMUNICATING A DIAGNOSIS OF A POTENTIALLY LETHAL CONDITION

While a diagnosis of a potentially lethal condition may not be unexpected to the patient, it cannot fail to be distressing to them and their families. Patients tend to recall only a little of the information that they are given, and so at the initial diagnosis the focus should be on stating the news and dealing with the initial emotional responses. Breaking bad news is difficult both for the patient and also the clinician, and the key principles are:

- Preparing: provide a conducive environment, making sure there is sufficient time, privacy and confidentiality as these factors are important, so minimize non-essential people in the room unless the patient needs or wants family, friends or an interpreter present
- Communicating the news
- State the news
- Elicit the response of the patient or carer or family member
- Deal tactfully with emotional responses
- Communicating bad news, especially across a language and/or cultural barrier can be difficult, time-consuming and frustrating. At the very least most patients will feel intimidated. It is important, therefore, to (if relevant):
  - ask the patient about their preferred language
  - never assume agreement or fluency until you are sure from the patient feedback
  - remember that even those with a good grasp of the language may well not understand medical or dental terminology. Explain as you proceed
  - use direct eye contact, and speak slowly and clearly, using uncomplicated terminology, remembering also that some individuals have hearing impairment
  - remember that head-nodding and smiles do not necessarily indicate understanding or agreement. Ask questions to ascertain understanding, not just enquiries with a 'yes' or 'no' answer. Silence can have many meanings and sometimes indicates lack of agreement
  - establish if there is a spokesperson for the patient and the patient's confidence in that person, and what the patient wishes the clinician to impart.

ENSURING FOLLOW-UP

- Arrange a follow-up meeting or discussion by telephone within 1 or 2 days.
- Arrange to meet the patient and carer or family member again
- Discuss and review the situation with the healthcare team, both in terms of impact on them and whether communications could have been improved.

PATIENT INFORMATION SHEET

Post-biopsy care

- A biopsy is the taking of a small piece of tissue for microscopic examination.
- This is carried out usually after a local anaesthetic injection in the area, such as used for fillings.
- Biopsy is painless, though a little sore when the injection wears off after a couple of hours.
- Stitches may or may not be used.
- Stitches may be resorbable or need to be removed in the next week. It is usually not a problem if the stitches come out earlier than 1 week.
- Any interventive procedure may occasionally result in complications, such as a little:
  - bleeding: pressure for 5–10 min from a gauze swab will almost invariably stop the bleeding
  - soreness or pain: paracetamol will usually control any discomfort; aspirin should not be used as it can cause bleeding
  - swelling: this should subside spontaneously over 3–4 days
  - bruising: this should clear spontaneously over 4–5 days.

Rarely there may be:

- altered sensation
- restricted mouth opening
- reactions to drugs
- allergies
- infection.
  If you are at all concerned, for advice kindly telephone.........

However, there are usually no long-term consequences. The scar is usually almost invisible, any discomfort goes quickly and any slight numbness recovers.

USEFUL WEBSITES

British Association for Sexual Health and HIV: http://www.bashh.org/

FURTHER READING

Alexander, R.E., Wright, J.M., Thiebaud, S., 2001. Evaluating, documenting and following up oral pathological conditions. J. Am. Dent. Assoc. 132, 329–335.

Apsey, D.J., Kaciroti, N., Loesche, W.J., 2006. The diagnosis of periodontal disease in private practice. J. Periodontol. 77 (9), 1572–1581.

Farman, A.G., 2006. Reproducible precision does not necessarily mean validity. Oral Surg. Oral Med. Oral Pathol. Oral Radiol. Endod. 102 (2), 145–146; author reply 146–147.

Gawkrodger, D.J., 2005. Investigation of reactions to dental materials. Br. J. Dermatol. 153 (3), 479–485.

Kutsch, V.K., 2006. Digital radiography: improving image quality. Pract. Proced. Aesthet. Dent. 18 (5), 289–290.

Morgan, A., 2006. Implementing technology to its fullest advantage. Dent. Today 25 (9), 140–141.

NRPB, 2001. Guidance notes for dental practitioners on the safe use of X-ray equipment. Department of Health. London.

Peloro, T.M., Ramsey, M.L., Marks, V.J., 2001. Surgical pearl: X marks the spot for the salivary gland biopsy. J. Am. Acad. Dermatol. 45, 122–123.

Scully, C., Kalantzis, A., 2005. Oxford handbook of dental patient care. Oxford University Press, Oxford.

Spielmann, N., Wong, D., 2011. Saliva: diagnostics and therapeutic perspectives. Oral. Dis. 17, 345–354.

Strong, S., 2006. Improving the standard of care using digital radiography: part I – implants and the general practitioner. Pract. Proced. Aesthet. Dent. 18 (7), 423–424.

Wilder-Smith, P., Holtzman, J., Epstein, J., Le, A., 2010. Optical diagnostics in the oral cavity: an overview. Oral Dis. 16, 717–728.

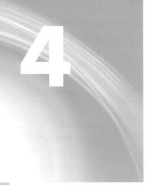

4 Treatment

Our universal aim should be to treat every patient as we would wish our families, or indeed ourselves, to be treated.

C Noyek

INTRODUCTION

Many of the conditions seen in oral and maxillofacial medicine practice have systemic manifestations, or they may be seen in patients with medical problems. It is crucial, therefore, always to collaborate closely with the medical and any other attendants in the care of the patient, as well as fully discussing issues with the patient. Clinical risk management concedes that there is an inherent risk in all health-care processes including treatments. This must be discussed with the patient, and informed consent obtained. Risk management should be considered before starting, during, and after treatment. Good communication skills are needed to allow clinicians to show empathy and to provide disclosure. Risk management after an adverse reaction includes skills in acknowledging bad outcomes or error and freedom to say 'sorry' as defined by 'apology laws'.

Some patients have conditions that are amenable to care in a primary care setting, or shared care with a specialist, but those patients who have severe disease, multisystem disease, or who require very sophisticated investigations, medications (see Ch. 5) or therapies are best managed by a specialist and often more than one medical/surgical specialist. Indeed, some orofacial conditions involve not only the mouth but also other mucosae (anogenital, ocular, pharyngeal, etc.), skin, other organs, mental health issues, or complex hospital-based therapies such as medical oncology, and so multi-disciplinary teams can often offer optimal healthcare.

QUALITY OF LIFE (QOL)

QoL is a concept encompassing many aspects, not only wealth, employment and housing, but also physical and mental health, recreation, leisure and social belonging and in healthcare, QoL is often seen in terms of how it is negatively affected, on an individual level, in a chronic debilitating illness such as cancer. Health related quality of life (HRQoL) is a subset of QoL, involving:

- physical functioning
- psychological functioning
- social interaction, and disease
- treatment related symptoms.

QoL can be assessed by interview or patient-completed 'instruments' (questionnaires) which include the:

- visual analogue scale (VAS)
- hospital anxiety and depression scale (HADS)
- short-form McGill pain questionnaire (SFMPQ)
- health related QoL questionnaire (HRQoL)
- oral health impact profile (OHIP-14)
- chronic oral mucosal diseases questionnaire (COMDQ).

EVIDENCE BASED MEDICINE AND TREATMENT

Few treatments available for patients with oral and maxillofacial medical problems have yet been rigorously studied in the disorders in question. The evidence base that guides the use of therapeutic agents in these conditions is therefore very limited. Ethically, this presents a complex challenge. It is difficult to decline care for a patient on the basis that there is no evidence-base. Rather it is essential to offer treatment to patients, and this is clearly the case even where the evidence base is limited, but clinicians must be aware of the danger of inappropriate or over-treatment.

PSYCHOLOGICAL AND SOCIOLOGICAL ASPECTS OF TREATMENT

Treatment is much more than the simple use of a drug or the performance of a procedure; an holistic approach involving the whole psychology of the patient is important. Remember always that patients know whether the clinician cares, well before they care whether the clinician knows all the answers.

Many orofacial conditions are chronic and have no cure, and for a few disorders the prognosis is poor or, fortunately rarely, the condition may even be lethal. Therefore, compassion and patient education and participation are important. Empowering patients allows them to take control of their lives and decisions affecting their wellbeing. Such education and reassurance is always helpful; a supportive and understanding clinician is invariably welcomed by the patient, their partner and family.

It is thus important to:

- do no harm
- manage the patient as a whole, in the context of their individual perceptions, aspirations, general health and social setting

- offer hope - not all conditions can be cured, but most can be controlled or at least ameliorated. General improvements in oral and systemic health also help control symptoms in several other orofacial disorders
- work with the patient and family, and involve the patient in all decisions. Discuss the condition, diagnosis and possible therapies with the patient (and possibly partner and family, provided the patient consents)
- warn of possible consequences (good and bad) of treatment or of no treatment
- obtain express informed consent before any invasive procedure
- offer advice on what patients themselves can do for their problems, including support from family, partners and friends, as well as care groups.

PROVIDING INFORMATION ABOUT TREATMENT

Information about financial issues and the impact of treatment on ability to work, function physically, relationships and quality of life, support from other bodies (e.g. alcohol, smoking or other drug support groups), disease support groups (e.g. cancer help groups or the pemphigus support groups, Sjögren Syndrome Society, etc.) or other information sources (e.g. patient information sheets, the internet) can be helpful. Many drugs used for oral conditions are used 'off-label' and this must be understood by, and agreed with, the patient (Ch. 5).

LIFESTYLE CHANGES

There is no doubt that certain lifestyle habits, such as the use of tobacco products, areca nut products, recreational drugs and alcoholic beverages, should be discouraged, especially in patients with oral mucosal diseases. Indeed, sometimes, the cessation of these habits may lead to resolution of the condition. Diet and/or oral hygiene may also benefit from improvement.

PREVENTIVE CARE

DENTAL BACTERIAL PLAQUE CONTROL

Dental staff should ensure the patient has appropriate oral health education, and maintains particularly good oral hygiene, since the limited evidence available suggests that good plaque control helps the resolution of some lesions as well as gingivitis.

The most important devices in oral hygiene are floss and a toothbrush; many are effective but:

- soft toothbrushes and silica-based toothpastes are least abrasive
- powered toothbrushes may assist oral hygiene especially in those with impaired manual dexterity
- interspace and other toothbrushes can access areas difficult to clean.

Toothpastes are available that offer tooth whitening, plaque control, desensitization, calculus (tartar) control, tooth remineralization and malodour control and some combine all facets (**Table 4.1**).

Antiplaque mouthwashes are commonly used to reduce infection and malodours, particularly if the patient is immunocompromised. Many mouthwashes have only a transient antiseptic activity (**Table 4.2**), but:

- Chlorhexidine digluconate is the most widely used antiplaque agent and is active, especially against Gramnegative rods, it helps control plaque and periodontal disease and has some anticaries and antifungal activity. It has good substantivity (ability to bind to hard and soft tissues and be released over a long period), but binds tannins and thus can cause dental staining if the patient drinks coffee, tea or red wine. Rarely, it causes other adverse effects, including:
  - overgrowth of enterobacteria (e.g. in leukaemic patients)
  - mucosal desquamation
  - hypersensitivity or anaphylaxis
  - salivary gland pain or swelling.
- Triclosan is a chlorinated bisphenol with some substantivity and a broad spectrum of antibacterial activity, and a significant antiplaque effect, without staining the teeth.
- Phenolics, such as Listerine, have some antiplaque effect and do not stain teeth, but have low substantivity.
- Oxygenating mouthwashes may have a place in the control of anaerobic infections, such as necrotizing gingivitis.
- Sanguinarine is marketed for activity against bacterial plaque and malodour, but with low activity in these respects. A toxic alkaloid extracted from some plants, including Bloodroot (*Sanguinaria canadensis*), Mexican Prickly Poppy (*Argemone mexicana*), *Chelidonium majus*, and *Macleaya cordata*, it has, however, also been incriminated in some oral white lesions.

CARIES PREVENTION

A low cariogenicity diet is important (see below). Fluoride is also helpful for anticariogenic activity, especially useful for patients with dry mouth (**Table 4.3**). Fluorides may be usefully applied in the dental office, and daily at home (1% sodium fluoride gels or 0.4% stannous fluoride gels). Young children may need fluoride supplements if their water supply has a low fluoride content. Amorphous calcium phosphate (ACP) may also help. Chewing gum may stimulate salivation and help caries prevention and reduce malodour.

DIET

A healthy balanced diet is indicated to help resolution of oral conditions. In particular:

- Many mucosal lesions are aggravated by irritants, such as tobacco and alcohol, and these also decrease salivary flow and should thus be avoided.
- A softish diet, avoiding toast and potato crisps, spices and acids, such as in tomatoes and citric fruits and drinks, may be indicated whilst a patient has a sore mouth. Foods that can be eaten, however, include:
  - milk and other dairy products, low-fat only
  - cooked, canned, or frozen vegetables
  - cooked or canned fruit with the skin and seeds removed, such as applesauce or canned peaches

Table 4.1 Active principles in toothpastes (dentifrices)

Anticaries	Antibacterials	Anti-hypersensitivity	Anti-tartar	Whiteners	Anti-malodour	Others
Amine fluorides	Chlorhexidine	Formaldehyde	Azocycloheptane diphosphonate	Benzalkonium chloride	Chlorhexidine	Enoxolone
Calcium phosphate	Fluorides	Potassium citrate	Gantrez acid (Polyvinyl methyl ether and maleic acid copolymer)	Calcium carbonate	Triclosan	Essential oils
Calcium pyrophosphate	Hexetidine	Potassium chloride		Calcium phosphates	Zinc chloride	Keratin
Calcium trimetaphosphate	Hydrogen peroxide	Potassium nitrate		Carboxymethyl cellulose	Zinc citrate	Panthenol
Nicomethanol fluorhydrate	Plant extracts	Sodium citrate	Potassium pyrophosphate	Citroxaine		Permethol
Potassium fluoride	Potassium peroxydiphosphate	Sodium fluoride	Zinc chloride	Pentasodium triphosphate		Provitamin B5
Sodium fluoride (NaF) 1450-1500 ppm (< 600 ppm in child paste)	Sanguinarine	Stannous fluoride	Zinc citrate	Potassium tetra pyrophosphate		Tocopherol
Sodium monofluorophosphate (NA$_2$ FPO$_3$)	Siliglycol	Strontium chloride hexahydrate		Sodium benzoate		Vitamin E
Stannous fluoride	Sodium bicarbonate	Strontium fluoride		Sodium bicarbonate		
Xylitol	Stannous pyrophosphate			Sodium tripolyphosphate		
	Triclosan					
	Urea peroxide					
	Xylitol					
	Zinc chloride					
	Zinc citrate					
	Zinc trihydrate					

Table 4.2 Some mouthwashes with significant antimicrobial activity

Agent	Dose	Comments*
Chlorhexidine gluconate	0.12–0.2% aqueous mouthwash, rinse for 1 min twice daily. Also 0.5–1.0% gel or spray	A cationic chlorinated bisbiguanide with significant antiplaque and antifungal activity and oral retention; traces can still be found in saliva after 24 h May stain teeth or tissues if patient drinks tea, coffee or red wine
Triclosan	0.03% mouthwash, rinse for 1 min twice daily	A non-ionic chlorinated bisphenolic antiseptic with moderate antiplaque and antifungal activity, but less retention in mouth than chlorhexidine More effective against plaque when with copolymer or zinc citrate
Cetylpyridinium chloride	0.05% mouthwash used twice daily	A quaternary ammonium compound with antiplaque activity, but less than chlorhexidine May stain teeth and cause oral burning sensation or ulceration

*All occasionally may cause mucosal irritation.

Table 4.3 Regime for caries prevention

Eliminate active caries	Restorative dental care
Preventive measures	Patient education Dietary modification Fluorides: 1.23% acidulated fluoride or 2% neutral fluoride gels in 4-min tray applications 4 times daily over 4 weeks; or home fluoride applications by gels or rinses Amorphous calcium phosphate (ACP) Xylitol chewing gum; chew for 5 min 5 times daily Chlorhexidine mouthwashes; 0.2% used twice daily for 1 min
Examine at 3 monthly recall appointments	Reinforce preventive message Monitor restorations Monitor cariogenic micro-organisms (*Streptococcus mutans* testing)

- breads, and pasta made with refined white flour
- refined hot cereals, such as oatmeal and cream of wheat
- lean, tender meats, such as poultry, whitefish, and shellfish that are steamed, baked, or grilled
- creamy peanut butter
- pudding and custard
- eggs
- tofu
- soup, especially broth
- tea.

In persons with dry mouth, pureed non-irritant foods and cool moist fruits, such as melon, are helpful, and patients should consider:

- Eating a soft, high protein moist diet.
- Substituting moist fish, eggs or cheese for red meat.
- Taking food and drinks lukewarm rather than hot.
- Soaking bread and/or rolls in milk or sauces.
- Eating moistened casseroles and meats with gravies, sauces, soups and stews.
- Using sour cream, and half cream as sauce bases (adds calories).
- Blending food and drink.
- Eating yogurt, fresh fruit, powdered milk.
- Eating fruit smoothies/slushies.
- Drinking milk shakes.
- Drinking soy or rice milk.
- Avoiding dry foods (bread, dry meat, pastries, toast and crackers, snack foods that are dry and salty).

- Avoiding citric foods, juices such as tomato, orange, grapefruit based products and sauces.
- Avoiding fizzy sodas and sparkling water.

Although vitamin and iron deficiencies are not common, supplements may be required if the diet is lacking.

SYMPTOMATIC CARE

Specific therapies are not available for all conditions, and the best that can then be offered is the control of symptoms; this is called symptomatic treatment. Attention should be directed to relieving the following (**Table 4.4**):

- Pain and discomfort: antipyretics/analgesics, such as paracetamol, help relieve pain and a soft diet may help. In mucositis, potent analgesics such as opioids or buprenorphin

Table 4.4 Topical agents that may help reduce pain from mucosal lesions

Agent	Use
Benzydamine hydrochloride	Rinse or spray every 1.5–3 h
Lidocaine	Topical solution or gel may ease pain
Carboxymethylcellulose	Paste or powder used after meals to protect area

may be indicated (see Chs 5 and 54). Erosive or ulcerative lesions can be protected with Orabase or Zilactin. Soft diet and topical agents, such as topical local anaesthetics (e.g. lidocaine) or 0.1% benzydamine mouth rinse or spray, may help symptomatically. Benzocaine should be avoided because of possible hypersensitivity and induction of methaemoglobinaemia. Methaemoglobin (MetHb) reduces the oxygen-carrying ability of erythrocytes and can lead to cyanosis with grey or blue-coloured skin, lips, or nail beds; dyspnoea; fatigue; confusion; headache; nausea; and change in pulse rate within minutes or 1–2 h after the first or several uses of benzocaine. In rare severe cases, methaemoglobinaemia can progress to coma and even to death.

- Fever: paracetamol helps relieve fever and adequate fluid intake is important.
- Malodour (Ch. 9).
- Anxiety: patient information is an important aspect in management and goes a long way to relieve anxiety, but there may need to be reassurance, and sometimes recourse to mild anxiolytics, such as diazepam 2.5 mg or temazepam 5 mg.

SURGERY

This can range from the simple excision of a lump such as a papilloma, to removal of a tooth, or to resection of a malignant neoplasm. Referral to a surgeon may be indicated.

- All surgery is invasive.
- Scalpel, laser or electrosurgery are widely available.
- Only an operator adequately skilled in a procedure should perform it.

OTHER LESS-INVASIVE OR NON-INVASIVE TREATMENTS

These include:

- cryotherapy
- soft laser therapy
- photodynamic therapy (PDT)
- appliances (e.g. splints, tissue conditioning).

DRUG TREATMENT

In UK, registered dentists are legally entitled to prescribe from the entirety of the *British National Formulary* (BNF) and *BNF for Children* (BNFC), but within the National Health Service (NHS) dental prescribing is restricted to those drugs contained within the 'List of Dental Preparations' in the *Dental Practitioners Formulary* (DPF). The National Prescriptions Centre offers guidance (www.npc.co.uk).

The BNF, published by the British Medical Association and the Royal Pharmaceutical Society of Great Britain, includes the DPF is a valuable source of information and advice on therapy. The BNF is revised twice yearly, and only the current issue should be consulted; it is available on the internet. Hand-held devices, such as PDAs can have software such as Epocrates, which holds comprehensive drug data.

Drugs do not necessarily have predictable effects: patients vary in their responses by virtue of various intrinsic or extrinsic factors (**Table 4.5**).

Table 4.5 Some factors influencing drug responses

Intrinsic	Extrinsic
Genetic	Alcohol
Absorption	Climate
Distribution	Culture
Metabolism	Diet
Excretion	Drug compliance
Body weight	Smoking
Enzyme polymorphisms	Stress
Height	Sunlight exposure
Race	
Gender	
Physiological	
Body weight	
Age	
Cardiovascular function	
Diseases	
Height	
Renal function	
Liver function	

Also, always remember the following:

- Avoid any drug if the patient is allergic to it.
- Use the safest drugs; virtually all drugs can have some adverse effects.
- Use only drugs with which you are totally familiar and use their generic (non-proprietary) drug names.
- Check that the prescription is legible, the drug doses, contraindications, interactions and adverse reactions.
- Warn the patient of, and discuss, possible adverse effects or interactions.
- Reduce drug doses for children, older patients and those suffering from liver or kidney disease.
- Consider the possibility of altered drug metabolism. For example:
  - Han Chinese or other Asians with the HLA allele *B*1502* may develop Stevens–Johnson syndrome (Ch. 56) and toxic epidermal necrolysis (Ch. 57) after exposure to carbamazepine or phenytoin
  - Thiopurine methyltransferase or thiopurine S-methyltransferase (TPMT) is an enzyme that metabolizes thiopurines such as azathioprine and 6-mercaptopurine (6MP). Patients who may need these drugs should first have their TMPT activity assayed as patients with low activity (10% prevalence) or absent activity (prevalence 0.3%) are at a heightened risk of drug-induced bone marrow failure.
  - The cytochrome P450 system of enzymes (CYP isoenzymes) in the gastrointestinal mucosa and liver metabolizes many drugs, and various isoenzymes metabolize drugs by oxidation, typically reducing their effect. CYP isoenzymes may have different activities between individuals and ethnic groups; this increases, for example, the activity of some anxiolytics such as diazepam (up to 6% of whites, but up to 23% of Asians are sensitive to diazepam). Antidepressants and analgesics may also be affected. Alcohol and smoking can affect CYP.

  Some drugs, for example erythromycin, inhibit CYP leading to the reduced ability to metabolize drugs, such as ciclosporin.

Grapefruit juice and Seville oranges contain flavenoids that can inhibit CYP and thus increase the activity of, for example, ciclosporin and some protease inhibitors.

Some over-the-counter (OTC) herbal preparations, such as St John's Wort, can induce CYP; they can thus reduce the effect of protease inhibitors, antidepressants, warfarin, anticonvulsants and the contraceptive pill:
- CYP2C9 influences phenytoin and warfarin effects
- CYP2C19 affects diazepam and citalopram
- CYP2D6 affects codeine.

- Avoid drug use in pregnancy and breast feeding, where possible.
- Avoid aspirin for children under 12 years of age, because of the risk of Reye syndrome (Ch. 56), patients with cardiac failure, those with peptic ulcers, or those with bleeding tendencies such as haemophilia or thrombocytopenia and in those taking anticoagulant drugs, since it exacerbates bleeding.
- Avoid NSAIDs in patients with cardiac failure, those with peptic ulcers, or those with bleeding tendencies such as haemophilia or thrombocytopenia and in those taking anticoagulant drugs, since they exacerbate bleeding.
- Avoid metronidazole, azole antifungals and some other antimicrobials in patients on warfarin, since they displace it from plasma proteins and increase bleeding.
- Avoid itraconazole in cardiac failure, as it can exacerbate it.
- Avoid tetracyclines in children under 8 years, pregnancy or breastfeeding, as they can cause tooth discolouration.
- Avoid macrolides (azithromycin, clarithromycin, erythromycin) in people with cardiac disease, as they can cause arrhythmias.
- Avoid intramuscular injections in patients with bleeding tendencies, such as haemophilia or thrombocytopenia, and in those taking anticoagulant drugs, as haematomas can result, and take care with surgery.
- Take care if surgery will involve bone in patients who have been on bisphosphonates, as osteochemonecrosis can result, or in patients who have been irradiated in the head and necks (osteoradionecrosis can arise).

PRESCRIBING FOR CHILDREN

- Doses of all drugs are much lower for children than for adults; always check against the recommended dose per unit body weight (**Table 4.6**).
- Some drugs are contraindicated (e.g. tetracyclines are contraindicated under the age of 7–8 years; also, aspirin is contraindicated in all children under 12 years old) (**Table 4.7**).
- Oral preparations are invariably preferable to injectable drugs.

Table 4.6 Rough guide for prescribing for children

Age of child (years)	Percentage of adult drug dose
1	25
6	50
12	75

Table 4.7 Drugs to avoid in children

Drug to avoid	Comments
Aspirin	May cause Reye syndrome in <12 year olds
Ciprofloxacin	Musculoskeletal damage
Diazepam	Paradoxical reactions
Ibuprofen	Gastrointestinal bleeding; cardiac damage
Nasal decongestants	Tachyphylaxis
Promethazine	Paradoxical reactions in <2 year olds
Sugar-containing medications	May cause caries/obesity
Tetracyclines	Tooth staining in <8 year olds

PRESCRIBING IN PREGNANCY AND DURING BREASTFEEDING

Because of the danger of damage to the foetus, all drugs should be avoided in pregnancy or where pregnancy is possible, unless their use is essential. In particular avoid tetracyclines, which stain teeth, and retinoids and thalidomide, which are teratogenic. The prescriber, patient and pharmacy must comply with regulations in terms of thalidomide: every prescription must be accompanied by a 'prescription authorization form'.

PRESCRIBING FOR THE OLDER PATIENT

- A number of drugs should be avoided for the older patient (**Box 4.1**), notably many drugs affecting the CNS and some NSAIDs.
- Lower drug doses are almost invariably indicated because even in apparently healthy older people, there are changes in body water:fat ratios, and reduced liver and kidney drug clearance, along with increased sensitivity to many drugs. Particular care should be taken when there is the possibility of renal or hepatic dysfunction; this will necessitate substantially reduced drug doses.
- Compliance may be poor.

DRUGS AND FOOD ABSORPTION

Most oral drugs are best given with or after food. However, oral drugs that should be given at least 30 min before food, since their absorption is otherwise delayed, include:

- aspirin
- erythromycin

BOX 4.1 Drugs to avoid in older patients (Beers criteria)

- Amitriptyline
- Benzodiazepines
- Chlorphenamine
- Doxepine
- Imipramine
- Indometacin
- Meperidine
- Naproxen
- Piroxicam
- Pentazocine
- Promethazine
- Propoxyphene

- paracetamol
- penicillins (including ampicillin and amoxicillin)
- rifampicin
- tetracyclines (except doxycycline).

Grapefruit juice disturbs the absorption and metabolism of some drugs and, therefore, should be avoided by persons taking:

- ciclosporin,
- calcium channel blockers (e.g. nifedipine)
- terfenadine.

PRESCRIBING IN DIFFERENT CULTURES

Some key concerns for different groups of patients are set out in **Table 4.8**.

Alcohol (ethanol) is used widely in pharmaceutical formulations as an antimicrobial preservative or as a solvent and may be unacceptable to Muslims and some other patients.

Gelatin is made of protein derived from animal bones, cartilage, tendons and other tissues, such as pigskin. The other most commonly used agents of animal derivation are insulin, heparin and haemostatic agents, such as blood coagulation factors and topical agents. Such products may be contraindicated for use on religious or cultural grounds.

Some artificial saliva preparations contain animal mucin, which may be unacceptable on religious grounds to some

Table 4.8 Main concerns about drugs and healthcare products for certain groups of patients

Groups	Main concerns
Buddhist	Animal and genetically modified (GM) products
Catholics	GM derivatives and those developed by foetal experimentation
Jehovah's witnesses	Not able to accept food and products that may contain blood or blood derivatives
Hindus	Gelatin-containing products, animal products and alcohol
Jains	Strict vegetarians, but will not eat root vegetables. Some patients, particularly those who follow vegan or vegetarian diets, may object to the use of animals to meet the needs of humans.
Muslims	Porcine and bovine derivatives, alcohol, non-Halal animal derivatives, E numbers derived from porcine products, and emulsifiers derived from animals
Jews	Products derived not only from pork, but also from any animal that had not been slaughtered according to Jewish law (Kosher). Devout Jews may wish to avoid alcohol
Sikhs	Beef and its derivatives

Use of healthcare products and consumables produced through exploitation of animal, if production has involved cruelty to animals or animal research, or exploitation of resource-poor or otherwise disadvantaged people may upset some people.
From Scully C, Wilson N 2005 Culturally sensitive oral healthcare. Quintessence Publications.

Muslims, Hindus, Jews and Rastafarians. Products containing carboxymethylcellulose may then be preferred.

Most oral healthcare products are licensed only as 'cosmetics', which are less rigorously tested than pharmacological products, although they must still be labelled with all active and inactive ingredients. Toothpastes fall into this category. Some oral healthcare products are licensed as pharmacological products and because they must be labelled with all ingredients – active and inactive – this readily affords the opportunity to avoid certain religious and ethnic group restrictions. Some mouthwashes contain colourants or excipients that may be animal derivatives and many contain alcohol, which may raise objections on religious grounds, although the objections are not always well-founded, when the religious rules are consulted. Some toothpastes may contain 'glycerin', manufactured synthetically or derived from animal fat, and this may not be included in the ingredients. Oral healthcare products that might contain animal derivatives could include some:

- analgesics
- antimicrobials
- bone fillers
- colourants
- drug capsules
- emulsifiers
- haemostatic materials
- polishing (bristle) brushes
- prophylaxis pastes
- toothpastes
- waxes.

ADVERSE REACTIONS TO DRUGS

No drug should be used unless there are good indications since almost any drug may produce unwanted or unexpected adverse reactions (side-effects). Some produce oral adverse reactions. The true incidence of adverse drug reactions is often not known, and many adverse reactions are probably not, at present, recognized as drug-related.

A full medical history should always be taken and questions should be asked specifically about drug use (including over-the-counter preparations) and adverse drug reactions, since the medical status may influence the choice of drugs used. G6PD deficiency must be excluded before using dapsone. TPMT must be assayed before azathioprine use. HLA-B1502 testing is necessary before carbamazepine use. Polypharmacy should be avoided and practitioners should use only drugs with which they are familiar.

Patients should be warned if serious adverse reactions are liable to occur (e.g. systemic corticosteroids), and provided with the appropriate warning card to carry.

After injections, there is always a small chance that anaphylactic shock or a vasovagal attack may occur.

ORAL USE OF DRUGS

The oral route is generally the preferred route for drug administration.

SUBCUTANEOUS INJECTION OF DRUGS

Subcutaneous injections can be given into a skin fold, pinched up over the anterior abdominal wall or anterior thigh, with vertical insertion of a 25 G (orange hub) needle and are used for injection of drugs such as:

- insulin
- heparin
- opiate analgesics.

INTRAMUSCULAR INJECTION OF DRUGS

This is used to obtain a more rapid effect than a subcutaneous injection, or where intravenous injection is impractical or carries a greater risk of anaphylactic or cardiac stimulant reaction. A 23 G (blue hub) needle is used. Intramuscular (i.m.) injection is used for:

- epinephrine (adrenaline) in the emergency treatment of anaphylactic shock or cardiac arrest
- glucagon, in the emergency treatment of hypoglycaemia
- antipsychotics (e.g. chlorpromazine, haloperidol) in the emergency treatment of acute psychoses
- midazolam or diazepam in the management of epileptic fit (buccal midazolam is superseding this)
- antimicrobials.

Adverse effects of intramuscular injections include the following:

- pain
- bruising, due to local haematoma formation. Intramuscular injections are contraindicated in patients with bleeding tendencies (e.g. haemophilia or induced by anticoagulant therapy)
- nerve damage, which may lead to paralysis, especially in bleeding disorders. This risk is minimized by using either the side of the thigh, or the upper, outer quadrant of the gluteus maximus muscle in the buttock or the deltoid muscle in the upper, outer arm
- collapse, usually due to a faint
- anaphylactic shock, especially after injections with antimicrobials, such as penicillins. The patient should be observed for 30 min after the injection, with facilities for resuscitation available.

INTRAVENOUS INJECTION OF DRUGS

Intravenous (i.v.) injection is used to achieve a rapid effect in emergencies, for example:

- epinephrine (adrenaline) in the management of cardiac arrest only
- diazepam in the management of status epilepticus
- heparin in the management of acute pulmonary embolism.

I.V. infusion through an indwelling catheter is used:

- when administration by other routes is not possible (e.g. blood transfusion, or fresh frozen plasma or coagulation factor concentrates)
- for hydration with intravenous fluids (e.g. saline or dextrose) when oral intake of fluids is not possible (e.g. unconsciousness or semiconsciousness, impaired swallowing (e.g. after stroke), vomiting, or fasting prior to surgery or other procedures)

- for antimicrobial treatment of severe infections or prophylaxis when using, for example, vancomycin.

Veins preferred for i.v. injections are those in the antecubital fossa, the preferred sites for infusions are the forearm or dorsal hand veins (which allow joint mobility). Note that:

- following insertion of the needle (usually 21 G (green hub) or 23 G (blue hub)) or catheter, the fact that the needle is in a vein and not elsewhere should be confirmed by aspiration of blood and by the absence of local pain or swelling on injection or infusion of a small amount of the material to be administered
- intravenous catheters should be taped in place, and sterile precautions (and rotation of catheter sites) observed to minimize the risk of local thrombosis and sepsis
- when prolonged IV access is required (e.g. in treatment of endocarditis or malnutrition), a central venous catheter can be inserted (under full sterile conditions) into the internal jugular or subclavian veins. Such Hickman lines (central catheters) are also useful in monitoring central venous pressure and fluid replacement in circulatory shock.
- The patient should be observed for 30 min after the injection, with facilities for resuscitation available.

REFERRAL TO A SPECIALIST

Referral may be indicated when the practitioner is faced with:

- a complicated or serious diagnosis (especially cancer, HIV infection, pemphigus, Behçet syndrome)
- a doubtful diagnosis
- a patient who has extraoral lesions or other indications of possible systemic disease
- a situation where investigations are required, but not possible or appropriate to carry out in general practice
- a situation where therapy may not be straightforward and may require potent agents
- a situation where drug use needs to be monitored with laboratory or other testing (e.g. for liver functional disturbances)
- a patient who needs access to an informed opinion or care outside normal working hours.

Should referral be required, it should always be in writing, giving a concise background to the referral (**Fig. 4.1**), including:

- patient's last name, first name(s), date of birth, full address and telephone, mobile phone, fax and e-mail where possible; primary care medical practitioner's name, address and telephone, fax and e-mail
- referring clinician's name, address, telephone, fax and e-mail
- referral urgency (real or perceived), reason, relevant history and findings
- provisional diagnosis
- treatment already offered
- relevant medical, dental and social history
- any special needs such as transport or translator.

PATIENT REFERRAL FORM (to be completed by referring CLINICIAN)

1.   PATIENT

LAST Name: ....   First Name(s) ....

Date of Birth: ....   Address: ....

Postcode: ....

Telephone: (Home) ....   (Work) ....

(Mobile) ....   (Fax) ....

Gender: M/F   Hospital No. (if known) ....

2.   REFERRING CLINICIAN

Name: ....   Telephone No.: ....

Address: ....

Postcode: ....

Fax: ....   E-mail: ....

3.   REFERRAL

Urgency with which you wish patient to be seen: if possible

Immediately ☐   within: 2 weeks ☐   within: 3 months ☐

Patient's main complaint ....

Purpose of referral: ....   for advice only ☐   for advice and care ☐

Comments ....

4.   HISTORY

Dental Specify ....   No ☐   Yes ☐

Medical: does the patient have

	No	Yes		No	Yes
Allergies			Bleeding tendency		
Heart problems			Diabetes		

Medication ....   No ☐   Yes ☐

Any other problem

Detail ....

Other (Specify) ....

Please enclose other relevant information such as medication, radiographs, study casts, lab results (if available)

Date: ....   Signature of Referer: ....

Fig. 4.1   Referral form

FURTHER READING

Alexander, R.E., Wright, J.M., Thiebaud, S., 2001. Evaluating, documenting and following up oral pathological conditions. J. Am. Dent. Assoc. 132, 329–335.

Allen, B.R., 2001. Thalidomide. Br. J. Dermatol 144, 225–228.

Baid, S.K., Nieman, L.K., 2006. Therapeutic doses of glucocorticoids: implications for oral medicine. Oral Dis. 12 (5), 436–442.

Eversole, L.R., 2006. Evidence-based practice of oral pathology and oral medicine. J. Calif. Dent. Assoc. 34 (6), 448–454.

Flaitz, C.M., Baker, K.A., 2000. Treatment approaches to common symptomatic oral lesions in children. Dent. Clin. North. Am. 44, 671–696.

Gonzalez-Moles, M., Scully, C., 2005. Vesiculo-erosive oral mucosal disease. management with topical corticosteroids: 1. Fundamental principles and specific agents available. J. Dent. Res. 84, 294–301.

Gonzalez-Moles, M., Scully, C., 2005. Vesiculo-erosive oral mucosal disease. management with topical corticosteroids: 2. Protocols, monitoring of effects and adverse reactions, and the future. J. Dent. Res. 84, 302–308.

Riordain, R.N., McCreary, C., 2010. The use of quality of life measures in oral medicine: a review of the literature. Oral Dis. 16, 419–430.

Riordain, R.N., McCreary, C., 2011. Validity and reliability of a newly developed quality of life questionnaire for patients with chronic oral mucosal diseases. J. Oral Pathol. Med. 40 (8), 604–609.

Scully, C., Kalantzis, A., 2005. Oxford handbook of dental patient care. Oxford University Press, Oxford.

Scully, C., Wilson, N., 2005. Culturally sensitive oral health health care. Quintessence Publisher, London.

Agents used in the treatment of patients with orofacial disease

It is a wise man's part, rather to avoid sickness, than to wish for medicines.

Thomas More

INTRODUCTION

Where specific therapies are available they should be used: for other conditions, the best that can be offered is symptomatic treatment – the control of symptoms (Ch. 4). Attention should first be directed to relieving pain, discomfort and anxiety.

However, clinicians and patients must understand that many orofacial conditions are chronic and although they can be ameliorated cannot be cured. Many mucosal conditions for example, can only be controlled with continued immunomodulatory therapy.

Many of the agents used for the treatment of oral diseases are used 'off label' – the practice of prescribing a drug for an unapproved indication or in an unapproved age group, unapproved dose or unapproved form of administration. Off-label use is very common in medicine and it is legal for a clinician to independently decide to prescribe a drug off-label, but it is illegal for the company to promote off-label uses to prescribers. However, according to the UK General Medical Council (GMC), off-label prescriptions must better serve patient needs than alternatives, and must be supported by evidence or experience to demonstrate safety and efficacy. GMC supports GMPs to prescribe off-label or unlicensed drugs if no appropriate licensed drug is available or they are satisfied it is as safe and effective as the licensed alternative. The European Medicines Agency (EMA) however, is dissatisfied with off-label use and has stated that for a European Union (EU) member state 'to encourage the use of a pharmaceutical for an indication for which it is not licensed would be a breach of EU legislation' and 'a medicine should be a treatment prescribed and dispensed with only the best interests of the patient in mind, and with the patient fully informed and involved in the decision-making process'.

In any event, patients must always be consulted and consent to off-label use of drugs.

See http://www.eaasm.eu and http://www.ema.europa.eu

ANALGESICS

Pain is the most important symptom suggestive of orofacial disease, but absence of pain does not exclude disease. There is considerable individual variation in response to pain, and the threshold is lowered by tiredness and psychogenic and other factors. It is important, therefore, where possible, to:

- identify and treat the cause of pain
- relieve factors that lower the pain threshold (fatigue, anxiety and depression)
- use analgesics (agents that relieve pain without causing loss of consciousness)
- try simple topical or oral analgesics, before embarking on more potent or injectable preparations or opioids. Nonopioid analgesics act primarily at the periphery, do not produce tolerance or dependence, and do not alter the patient's perception; they are used for mild to moderate pain. Opioid analgesics act on the CNS and alter the patient's perception; they are more often useful for severe pain
- avoid polypharmacy.

Pain control may require continued medication.

TOPICAL ANALGESICS

Topical analgesics are available as pain-relieving creams, lotions, rubs, gels, and sprays. The 3 main types of topical analgesics apart from benzydamine (which has an antihistamine action) include:

- local anaesthetics (mainly lidocaine, lidocaine-prilocaine cream (EMLA) and benzocaine): benzocaine however can cause methaemoglobinaemia. Topical analgesics such as lidocaine may ease mucosal discomfort or joint-related pain (Ch. 4).
- rubefacients or counter-irritants which act by counter-irritation: capsaicin, a preparation derived from peppers, and methylsalicylates, derived from willow bark and often combined with menthol; Capsaicin can, by depleting substance P in sensory nerve endings, and by blocking conduction in type-C nociceptive fibres, be helpful in oral dysaesthesia and post-herpetic neuralgia.
- nonsteroidal antiinflammatory agents which act by penetrating deep into tissues to inhibit cyclooxygenase (COX) enzymes responsible for development of inflammatory processes can be helpful in joint-related pain (Ch. 51).

SYSTEMIC ANALGESICS

Systemic analgesics (**Table 5.1**) can reduce pain, in some cases, such as NSAIDs, through an eicosanoid-depressing, antiinflammatory action. The term 'eicosanoids' is used as a collective name for molecules derived from 20-carbon

Table 5.1 Some analgesics

Agent	Adult dosage	Comments (see Tables 5.18 and 5.19)
Nonsteroidal antiinflammatory drugs (NSAIDS)		
Ibuprofen	400 mg up to 4 times daily	Caution in asthma, peptic ulcer, bleeding tendency, breastfeeding, cardiac, renal and liver disease, pregnancy, older patient, aspirin hypersensitivity. May cause arrhythmias and cardiac infarction
Mefenamic acid	250–500 mg up to 3 times daily	Caution in asthma, peptic ulcer, bleeding tendency, breastfeeding, cardiac, renal and liver disease, pregnancy, older patient, aspirin hypersensitivity
Non-NSAIDS		
Paracetamol	500–1000 mg up to 6 times daily (maximum 4 g/day)	Caution in liver or renal disease; those on zidovudine
Nefopam	30–60 mg up to 3 times daily	Contraindicated in convulsive disorders, pregnancy, older patient, renal, liver disease
Opioids		
Buprenorphine	5 µg/h slow release transdermal patches used for 7 days, or sublingual tablets 200 µg up to 4 times daily	Contraindicated in patients with head injury (interfere with pupillary responses and suppress respiration), liver disease, kidney disease, pregnancy, breastfeeding, taking MAOIs
Codeine phosphate	10–60 mg up to 6 times daily orally (or 30 mg i.m.)	Contraindicated in liver disease, late pregnancy
Dihydrocodeine	30 mg up to 4 times daily (or 50 mg i.m.)	Contraindicated in children, hypothyroidism, asthma, renal disease
Pentazocine	25–50 mg up to 4 times daily (or 30 mg i.m. or i.v.)	Contraindicated in pregnancy, children, hypertension, respiratory depression, head injuries or raised intracranial pressure
Methadone	5 mg tablets	Contraindicated in older or debilitated patients, since accumulation occurs
Oxycodone	5 mg capsules	Contraindicated in patients with head injury (interfere with pupillary responses and suppress respiration), liver disease, kidney disease, pregnancy, breastfeeding, taking MAOIs
Pethidine	50–100 mg i.m. or 5–10 mg subcutaneously or i.m.	Contraindicated in patients with head injury (interfere with pupillary responses and suppress respiration), liver disease, kidney disease, pregnancy, breastfeeding, taking MAOIs
Fentanyl	100–200 µg sublingual tablets or buccal lozenges, or transdermal patches releasing 12 µg/h used for 72 h	Contraindicated in patients with head injury (interfere with pupillary responses and suppress respiration), liver disease, kidney disease, pregnancy, breastfeeding, taking MAOIs

fatty acids – mainly the leukotrienes and prostanoids. Leukotrienes play an important role in inflammation, especially as part of the slow reacting substance of anaphylaxis. Prostanoids (prostaglandins (PGs), prostacyclin, thromboxanes) mediate local symptoms of inflammation such as vasoconstriction or vasodilatation, coagulation, pain and fever. All prostanoids originate from prostaglandin H catalyzed by the enzyme PGH2-synthase, which is a combination of a peroxidase and a cyclo-oxygenase (COX) (**Fig. 5.1**).

COX catalyzes the formation of prostaglandins and thromboxane from arachidonic acid (itself derived from cellular phospholipase A_2). Prostaglandins stimulate protective gastric mucin and bicarbonate but reduce gastric acid, renal excretion and blood platelet formation. Prostaglandins released via COX-2 act (among other things) as messenger molecules in inflammation.

NSAIDS

Most NSAIDs act as non-selective inhibitors of COX, inhibiting both the isoenzymes COX-1 and COX-2. NSAIDs, including aspirin, are useful analgesics, but can cause:

- further deterioration of cardiac function, if this is already impaired in cardiac failure
- peptic ulceration, especially in those over 75 years old or who have a history of peptic ulceration. Thus it is best to add a proton pump inhibitor, such as misoprostol. Ibuprofen appears to be the conventional NSAID with the lowest risk of gastrointestinal adverse effects but can produce thromboses, arrhythmias or myocardial infarction. COX-2 inhibitors, such as celecoxib, etoricoxib, valdecoxib and parecoxib, have fewer gastrointestinal effects, but may have serious cardiac adverse effects

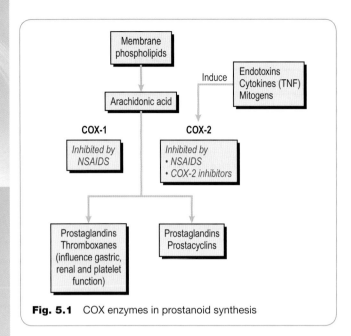

Fig. 5.1 COX enzymes in prostanoid synthesis

■ further deterioration of renal function, if this is already impaired

■ a bleeding tendency, by interfering with platelet activity

■ premature closure of the ductus arteriosus in pregnancy third trimester.

ASPIRIN

Aspirin has been in use longer than most other NSAIDs, and the efficacy and adverse effects are well recognized. Aspirin is a useful analgesic but it can also cause:

■ bleeding – irreversibly blocking the formation of thromboxane A_2 in platelets

■ asthma

■ fluid retention

■ nausea, diarrhoea or tinnitus

■ interference with a number of drugs, including antihypertensives, diuretics and methotrexate

■ allergies

■ Reye syndrome – a serious liver disease, in breastfeeding, by passing in milk to the child and in children under age 16 years (Ch. 56)

■ complications in mothers in late pregnancy.

PARACETAMOL

Paracetamol inhibits COX but, although it is sometimes grouped together with the NSAIDs, it lacks the adverse effects of NSAIDs, is not a true NSAID and lacks significant antiinflammatory properties. There is speculation that it acts through the inhibition of COX-3 isoform, or that it acts centrally. Generally speaking, paracetamol has few adverse effects, drug interactions or contraindications. Chronic pain requires regular analgesia (not just as 'required') however, and it is important not to overdose with paracetamol – which is hepatotoxic in high doses. In children, paracetamol can helpfully be given in sugar-free syrups.

OPIOIDS AND NARCOTICS

■ Opioids are analgesics used for moderate to severe pain such as that from cancer or mucositis.

■ Opioids are narcotics, controlled drugs and all are capable of causing addiction.

■ Opioids may cause constipation, respiratory depression, nausea, drowsiness and urinary retention.

NON-ANALGESIC AGENTS

Non-analgesic agents, which may be effective in some types of pain, include, for example, antidepressants and anticonvulsants.

OTHER CNS-ACTIVE DRUGS

ANTIDEPRESSANTS

Treatment of depression is by psychotherapy and medication. If there is any possibility of a suicide attempt, the patient must be seen by a psychiatrist as a matter of urgency. Antidepressants may, by altering brain neurotransmitters such as serotonin (5-hydroxytryptamine) and noradrenaline, control depression. Antidepressants (**Table 5.2**) can also be useful for the relief of some neuropathic pain, when they can have analgesic effect within 1–7 days (before they have any antidepressant effect) and at lower doses than needed for treatment of depression.

No antidepressant drugs is perfect and all suffer from at least one of the following drawbacks:

■ Delayed onset of action from 7–28 days. Although some improvements may be seen in the first few weeks, most antidepressant medications must be taken regularly for 3–4 weeks (in some cases, as many as 8 weeks) before the full therapeutic effect starts.

■ Anticholinergic effects.

■ Sedation.

■ Agitation.

■ Cardiotoxicity.

■ Weight gain.

Patients often are tempted to stop antidepressant medication too soon but they should continue for *at least* 4–9 months to prevent recurrence. The natural history of most depression is of remission after 3–12 months.

There are many different classes of antidepressants from which to choose therapies but the main ones are:

■ Tricyclic antidepressants (TCAs): often effective but frequently producing anticholinergic adverse effects such as dry mouth. TCAs with balanced effects on serotonin and noradrenaline re-uptake (e.g. amitriptyline, nortryptiline) may be more effective than those acting mainly on noradrenaline uptake (e.g. maprotiline).

■ Selective serotonin reuptake inhibitors (SSRIs): newer antidepressants, with the advantage over older antidepressants of less severe antimuscarinic activity, weight gain or cardiac conduction effects. SSRIs generally have fewer adverse effects than tricyclics and do not interact with alcohol and are thus often preferred by both patients and practitioners. However, gastrointestinal effects are common and they can produce dry mouth and arrhythmias.

Table 5.2 Some antidepressants

Drug	Dose	Comments (see Tables 5.18 and 5.19)
Amitriptyline	25–75 mg/day in divided doses	Contraindications: recent myocardial infarction, arrhythmias, liver disease
Clomipramine	25 mg 3 times daily or 75 mg at night	
Dosulepin (dothiepin)	25 mg 3 times daily or 75 mg at night	
Doxepin	10–100 mg/day in divided doses	
Fluoxetine	20 mg/day	Caution with: epilepsy, pregnancy, cardiac, liver or kidney disease, allergy, mania
Nortryptiline	75–100 mg/day	Contraindications: recent myocardial infarction, arrhythmias, liver disease
Venlafaxine	75 mg in morning	Contraindications: recent myocardial infarction, arrhythmias, liver disease

Antidepressants:

- Must be prescribed only in limited amounts, as there is a danger they may be used in a suicide attempt.
- May take up to 3–4 weeks before the antidepressant action takes place. Monitoring of plasma concentrations may be helpful in ensuring optimal dosage.
- Doses should be reduced for the older patient.
- Should not be withdrawn prematurely.
- Are usually contraindicated in patients with cardiac or liver disease.
- May have adverse effects, often via anticholinergic activity and thus cause:
  - dry mouth, but the complaint of dry mouth may also be a manifestation of depression
  - epileptogenic effects (tricyclics and fluoxetine)
  - drowsiness
  - visual impairment
  - constipation and urinary retention
- Antidepressants
  - may make it impossible for patients to drive vehicles, as they may suffer drowsiness and visual impairment
  - may interact with alcohol
- Tricyclic antidepressants interact with antiarrhythmics, antiepileptics, antihistamines, antihypertensives, antipsychotics, apraclonidine, beta blockers, brimonidine, diuretics, the contraceptive pill, nefopam, norepinephrine (noradrenaline) and tramadol. However, neither tricyclic (TCAs) nor monoamine oxidase inhibitor (MAOIs) antidepressants significantly interact with adrenaline in dental local anaesthetic solutions.

ANTICONVULSANTS

Anticonvulsants are the standard treatment of idiopathic trigeminal neuralgia (**Table 5.3**). As these agents may cause blood dyscrasias or hepatic dysfunction, it is important to monitor full blood counts and liver function (see Ch. 52).

HYPNOTICS

- Pain, anxiety or depression may cause insomnia.
- Hypnotics may help sleep, but should not be prescribed without forethought.

- Benzodiazepines such as temazepam 10 mg every night are, in general, the preferred hypnotics, but are contraindicated in severe respiratory disorders and are also addictive. Barbiturates and glutethimide should not be used; both are dangerous in overdose and barbiturates are addictive.
- Hypnotics often potentiate alcohol and other CNS depressants, and may impair judgement and dexterity.
- Hypnotics may be contraindicated in the older patient and in those with liver or respiratory disease.

ANXIOLYTICS

- Identify and treat the cause of the patient's anxiety wherever possible.
- It is important to differentiate between agitated depression and simple anxiety; the treatment is different.
- Reassurance is often remarkably effective at calming the anxious patient but there are times when a mild anxiolytic, such as a benzodiazepine like diazepam 1–10 mg, or a non-benzodiazepine, such as buspirone 5 mg orally three times daily, or zopiclone 3.75 mg orally up to three times daily can be helpful.
- Numerous benzodiazepines are now available as anxiolytics. All may produce dependence (especially lorazepam) and there is often little to choose in terms of anxiolytic effect between the different drugs. Most cause unsteadiness and some confusion.
- Buspirone (**Table 5.4**) probably acts by an effect on brain serotonin receptors and is not sedative. Buspirone may take up to 4 weeks at full dosage to have effect. Buspirone can interact with some antimicrobials, e.g. erythromycin, itraconazole and rifampicin, and should not be taken with MAOI antidepressants.
- Zopiclone, a benzodiazepine-like drug was introduced and initially promoted as having less dependence and withdrawal than benzodiazepines, but is now known to be addictive.
- Beta blockers (e.g. propranolol) may be more useful if anxiety is causing tremor/palpitations.
- Drowsiness (particularly when used together with alcohol) and impaired judgement are common in patients taking anxiolytics, so patients must be warned of the dangers of driving, operating machinery or making important decisions.
- Doses of anxiolytics should be reduced for the older patient, since adverse effects, particularly sedation, are common.

Table 5.3 Drugs for management of trigeminal neuralgia

Drug	Dose	Comments (see Tables 5.18 and 5.19 and Ch. 52)
Baclofen	5 mg three times daily	Contraindicated in peptic ulceration and pregnancy. Common adverse effect of sedation. Avoid abrupt withdrawal
Carbamazepine	Prophylactic for trigeminal neuralgia – not analgesic. Initially 100 mg once or twice daily. Many patients need about 200 mg 8-hourly. Do not exceed 1800 mg daily	Contraindicated in Han Chinese or other patients with HLA-B1502, cardiac, renal and liver disease, glaucoma and pregnancy. Occasional dizziness, diplopia, and blood dyscrasia, often with a rash and usually in the first 3 months of treatment. Interferes with contraceptive pill. Possible interactions with antimalarials, anticonvulsants, diltiazem, verapamil, gefitinib, diuretics, erythromycin, clarithromycin, dextropropoxyphene, fluconazole, miconazole, CNS depressants, cimetidine, isoniazid, lithium
Gabapentin	300 mg up to three times daily	Similar adverse effects to carbamazepine. Headache common. Contraindicated in psychiatric disease, renal disease, diabetes and pregnancy. Avoid sudden withdrawal
Phenytoin	150–300 mg daily	Contraindicated in Han Chinese or other patients with HLA-B1502, and in liver disease and pregnancy. Produces gingival swelling. Similar other adverse effects to carbamazepine. Avoid sudden withdrawal
Topiramate	25 mg daily	Contraindicated in glaucoma and breastfeeding. Avoid sudden withdrawal

Table 5.4 Anxiolytics

Drug	Dose	Comments (see Tables 5.18 and 5.19)
Buspirone	5 mg 2–3 times daily	Non-benzodiazepine. Avoid in epilepsy, liver disease, pregnancy, breastfeeding, care with alcohol, driving or operating machinery
Diazepam	2–30 mg/day in divided doses	Benzodiazepines. Avoid in glaucoma. Use with caution in the older patient, care with alcohol, driving or operating machinery
Temazepam	5–10 mg at night	
Zopiclone	3.75 mg 2–3 times daily	Non-benzodiazepine. Avoid in respiratory or neuromuscular disease, liver disease, renal disease, pregnancy, breastfeeding. Use with caution in the older patient, care with alcohol, driving or operating machinery

IMMUNOMODULATORY AGENTS

The aim of most immunomodulatory treatment is to suppress the damaging effects of inflammation. However, immuno-suppression can have a number of adverse effects (Ch. 54). Adverse effects are important mainly with systemic agents and thus the preference in the treatment of disease restricted to the oral cavity is usually for topical immunomodulatory agents, mainly the corticosteroids.

TOPICAL ANTIINFLAMMATORY AGENTS
Topical corticosteroids

Glucocorticoids are used for immunosuppression. They may have a wide range of antiinflammatory actions, including to inhibit:

- inflammatory cytokines
  - tumour necrosis factor alpha (TNF-α)
  - interleukins (IL-1, IL-3, IL-4, IL-5, IL-6 and IL-8)

- transcription of immune genes such as IL-2 gene. IL-2 is the main cytokine necessary for development of T cell immunologic memory (which depends upon the expansion of antigen-selected T cell clones)
- inflammatory cell (neutrophil, macrophage and mast cell) emigration, chemotaxis, phagocytosis, respiratory burst and the release of various inflammatory mediators (lyso-somal enzymes, cytokines, tissue plasminogen activator, chemokines, etc.) via lipocortin-1
- eicosanoid, prostaglandin and leukotriene production (via COX inhibition).

Topical corticosteroids (**Table 5.5**) are useful in the management of many oral ulcerative conditions where there is no systemic involvement, such as recurrent aphthous stomatitis:

- These corticosteroids are used locally on a lesion as a spray, gel or cream, or as a mouthwash if there are extensive lesions: many are used off-label and this must be discussed with the patient.
- Creams, gels and sprays are better than ointments, since the latter adhere poorly to the mucosa. However, creams can be bitter and gels can irritate.

Table 5.5 Examples of topical corticosteroids

Corticosteroid	Example	Use every 6h	Comments (see Tables 5.18 and 5.19)
Mild potency			
Hydrocortisone oromucosal 2.5 mg tablets (mucoadhesive buccal tablets)	Corlan	Dissolve in mouth close to ulcers	Use at an early stage of ulceration in recurrent aphthous stomatitis
Medium potency			
Betamethasone soluble phosphate 0.5 mg tablets	Betnesol	Use as mouthwash	Adrenal suppression unlikely
Betamethasone valerate 0.1% cream	Betnovate	Apply to lesion	Adrenal suppression unlikely
Flucinolone 0.025% cream	Synalar	Apply to lesion	Adrenal suppression unlikely
Mometasone furoate 0.1% cream	Elocon	Apply to lesion	Adrenal suppression unlikely
Triamcinolone acetonide 0.1% in carmellose gelatin paste	Adcortyl, Kenalog	Apply to lesion	Adheres best to dry mucosa; affords mechanical protection; of little benefit on tongue or palate. Unavailable in UK
High potency			
Beclometasone (beclomethasone) dipropionate spray	Beclometasone dipropionate	1 puff, 100 mL	Adrenal suppression possible
Budesonide spray	Budesonide	1 puff, 100 mL	Adrenal suppression possible
Fluocinonide 0.05% cream, gel or ointment	Metosyn	Apply to lesion	Adrenal suppression possible
Fluticasone propionate spray	Flixotide	1 puff	Adrenal suppression possible
Fluticasone propionate 0.05% cream	Cutivate	Apply to lesion	Adrenal suppression possible
Very high (super) potency			
Betamethasone dipropionate 0.05% cream	Diprosone	Apply to lesion	Adrenal suppression possible
Clobetasol propionate 0.05% cream	Dermovate	Apply to lesion	Adrenal suppression possible
Prednisolone sodium phosphate 5 mg suppositories	Predsol	Dissolve slowly in mouth	Adrenal suppression possible

- The corticosteroid needs to be in contact with the mucosa for some minutes for it to have any significant effect; patients should, therefore, time its use for at least 3 min on each occasion.
- Patients should not eat or drink for 30 min after using the corticosteroid, in order to prolong contact with the lesion.
- The corticosteroid can usefully be applied in a plastic splint worn overnight for treatment of desquamative gingivitis.

Topical corticosteroids are the primary therapeutic agents used to treat ulcerative mucosal lesions which have an immunologically-based aetiology (aphthae, erythema multiforme, lichen planus, pemphigoid). A mild potency agent such as hydrocortisone may be effective but more typically a medium potency corticosteroid such as betamethasone or a higher potency one such as fluocinonide or beclomethasone are required, moving to a super-potent topical corticosteroid, e.g. clobetasol, if the benefit is inadequate (**Table 5.5**).

With many topical corticosteroids there is little systemic absorption and thus no significant adrenocortical suppression but it is difficult to predict the absorption – especially through atrophic and/or inflamed and ulcerated mucosae. In patients using potent corticosteroids for more than a month it is prudent to add an antifungal, since candidosis may arise.

Drawbacks of the topical corticosteroids are that:

- there are few randomized controlled trials (RCTs)
- they are not uniformly effective
- occasionally candidosis is a complication
- they can damage collagen
- there is no evidence on possible oncogenicity
- they are often not licensed for use in the mouth so must be used 'off-label'.

INTRALESIONAL CORTICOSTEROIDS

These are occasionally useful in the management of intractable local lesions, such as erosive lichen planus and orofacial granulomatosis. Intra-articular corticosteroids are occasionally indicated where there is intractable pain from a noninfective arthropathy. Some examples include:

- prednisolone sodium phosphate, up to 22 mg
- methylprednisolone acetate, 4–80 mg
- triamcinolone acetonide, 2–3 mg
- triamcinolone hexacetonide, up to 5 mg.

TOPICAL CALCINEURIN INHIBITORS

These include (**Table 5.6**):

- Ciclosporin
- Tacrolimus
- Pimecrolimus.
- Calcineurin inhibitors act by binding to immunophilins (cyclophilin and macrophilin) and the resultant complexes inhibit calcineurin, which under normal circumstances induces the transcription of IL-2. Used off-label, they can be:
  - effective in oral ulcerative disorders
  - more effective if used along with topical corticosteroids
  - expensive.

Tacrolimus is:

- available as 0.1 and 0.03% creams
- liable to cause stinging for >15 min (decreases on continued use)
- only rarely associated with adverse effects, but the US Food and Drug Administration (FDA) in 2005, issued a public health advisory warning about possible carcinogenicity.

SYSTEMIC ANTIINFLAMMATORY AGENTS
Tetracyclines

Tetracyclines distinct from their non-antimicrobial actions have antiinflammatory actions, which include inhibition of:

- pro-inflammatory cytokines
- matrix metalloproteinases (MMPs), including collagenases MMP-1, MMP-8 and MMP-13
- prostaglandin synthesis
- nitric oxide release
- caspase activation (by minocycline).

Adverse effects of tetracyclines can include:

- hyperpigmentation of teeth and bones
- gastrointestinal discomfort
- nausea, anorexia
- photosensitivity
- hypersensitivity

- lupoid reactions
- serum sickness-type reactions.

Tetracyclines are therefore contraindicated in:

- children under 8 years and in pregnant/nursing mothers
- liver disease
- lupus erythematosus
- myasthenia gravis
- porphyria.

Tetracycline absorption is inhibited by zinc, iron and antacids.

SYSTEMIC IMMUNOSUPPRESSANTS

Systemic immunosuppressants are shown in **Table 5.7**. They are used especially in organ transplantation and in autoimmune disorders but their adverse effects can be serious and may include the following:

- infections, especially with viruses, fungi and mycobacteria, such as tuberculosis
- lymphoproliferative disorders
- malignancies, such as lip carcinoma
- teratogenicity.

SYSTEMIC CORTICOSTEROIDS
Indications

Systemic corticosteroids are often indicated for the management of:

- Bell palsy
- giant cell arteritis
- pemphigus
- multisystem diseases, such as some lichen planus, erythema multiforme or pemphigoid
- severe or resistant recurrent aphthae or aphthous-like ulceration.

Adverse effects

Systemic corticosteroids must always be used with caution because of potential adverse effects, which may include, apart from those noted above:

- Adrenocortical suppression: this may occur after a course of >3 weeks of systemic corticosteroids and may persist for 1 year or more. Adrenocortical suppression makes the patient liable to collapse if stressed, traumatized or having an infection, operation or general anaesthetic.
- Weight gain and mooning of the face: weight should be monitored. A diet low in salt, fats and calories helps control weight and prevent hypertension.

Table 5.6 Alternative topical immunosuppressants (calcineurin inhibitors)

Drug	Dose	Comments (see Tables 5.18 and 5.19)
Ciclosporin (Neoral or Sandimmun), used as mouthwashes or in an adhesive preparation	100–1500 mg/mL daily as a mouthwash; <50 mg/mL daily in an adhesive preparation	Adverse effects rare with topical applications
Tacrolimus (Protopic or Prograf)	0.1–0.03% ointment	Adverse effects rare with topical applications. Has 10- to 100-fold potency of ciclosporin FDA advisory caution: related to cancer arising in lichen planus

Table 5.7 Systemic immunomodulatory agents*

Agent	Dosage	Comments (see Tables 5.18 and 5.19)
Azathioprine	2–2.5 mg/kg daily (50–150 mg/day)	A 6-mercaptopurine pro-drug, which blocks nucleotides and DNA. Licenced for autoimmune bullous disorders, lupus, dermatomyositis. There is evidence to support the use of azathioprine outside its product licence for: ■ Atopic eczema ■ Maintenance therapy for Wegener granulomatosis ■ Behçet syndrome ■ Bullous pemphigoid. Assay TPMT (thio-purine methyl transferase) first; do not use azathioprine if level is low as there is myelotoxicity in low TPMT. TPMT testing only identifies a proportion of individuals at increased risk of haematological toxicity, hence the continued need for regular monitoring of blood counts irrespective of TPMT status. May take 2–3 months to have real effect. Regular checking of FBC is essential during long-term treatment. Macrocytosis is common. Leukopenia is the most common adverse event but anaemia, thrombocytopenia and, rarely, pancytopenia may be seen. May also cause nausea, hypersensitivity, susceptibility to infection, liver dysfunction, arrhythmias, hypotension, nephritis, carcinogenicity. Absolute contraindications are: hypersensitivity to azathioprine/6-MP; severe infections; severely impaired hepatic or bone marrow function; pancreatitis; live vaccines; pregnancy; and lactation. Interactions: allopurinol, cyclophosphamide, methotrexate, ciclosporin, co-trimoxazole, trimethoprim, clozapine, ribavirin and febuxostat (increase the myelotoxic effect), aspirin (bleeding), other immunosuppressants (increase the risk of infection), warfarin (reduced effect)
Ciclosporin (cyclosporin)	1–2 mg/kg daily	Nephrotoxic, hepatotoxic. May cause hypertension, blood dyscrasias, gingival swelling. Contraindicated in kidney disease, pregnancy and porphyria. Interactions: allopurinol, analgesics and antifungals (increase ciclosporin toxicity), anticonvulsants (reduced efficiency)
Colchicine	500 mg 3 times daily	An alkaloid, originally extracted from *Colchicum* (Autumn crocus – the 'meadow saffron'). Colchicine inhibits mitosis by binding to tubulin in microtubules, and thus depresses neutrophil motility and activity. Adverse effects include diarrhoea and myelotoxicity. Contraindicated in pregnancy, older patient, cardiac, renal or hepatic disease
Cyclophosphamide	1–2 mg/kg daily	Transformed by cytochrome p450 to active phosphoramide mustard and acrolein, which reacts with DNA. Leukopenia always – but reversible. Also causes cystitis. Small risk of cancer with prolonged use
Dapsone	1 mg/kg daily (usually 100–200 mg). Give also vitamin E 800 IU/day, and cimetidine	May take many months to have beneficial effect. Haemolysis, hypersensitivity Interactions: trimethoprim and methotrexate (both increase the risk of haematological complications). Protect from sun exposure
Hydroxychloroquine	200–400 mg/day	May take 3–6 months to have effect. May cause retinal damage and visual impairment. May cause myelotoxicity. Contraindicated in patients with renal or hepatic disease
Leflunomide	100 mg/day for 3 days, then 20 mg/day	A prodrug, completely converted to an active metabolite which blocks dihydro-orotate dehydrogenase, a key enzyme of pyrimidine synthesis. Teratogenic in both genders. Hepatotoxic (never use with methotrexate). Myelotoxic
Levamisole	50 mg 3 times daily for 3 days	Promotes leukocyte chemotaxis. May cause dizziness, taste disturbance, nausea, agranulocytosis
Mycophenolate mofetil	1000 mg once or twice daily	Inhibits inosine monophosphate dehydrogenase (blocks guanosine nucleotide, purine and DNA synthesis) and thereby blocks T and B cell proliferation and leukocyte recruitment. May take several months to have real effect. More gastrointestinal, haematological effects (red cell aplasia) and infections than with azathioprine. No liver or kidney damage. Contraindicated in pregnancy
Pentoxifylline	400 mg twice daily	A xanthine derivative, a cyclic nucleotide phosphodiesterase inhibitor that improves blood flow through blood vessels, and inhibits proinflammatory cytokine (TNF) production, leukocyte–endothelial cell adhesion, chemokines and leukocyte–keratinocyte adhesion. Common adverse reactions are nausea, dysphagia, and flushing. Contraindicated in cerebrovascular haemorrhage, myocardial infarction

Table 5.7 Systemic immunomodulatory agents*—Cont'd

Agent	Dosage	Comments (see Tables 5.18 and 5.19)
Prednisolone (give as enteric coated prednisolone with meals)	Initially 30–80 mg orally each day in divided doses, reducing as soon as possible to 10 mg/day	Limit dosage in hypertension and diabetes mellitus. May produce adrenal suppression. May cause weight gain, osteoporosis
Tacrolimus	100 mg/kg daily	Used in transplants mainly. Contraindicated in pregnancy. May cause cardiomyopathy
Thalidomide	50–200 mg/day at night initially, then alternate-day therapy	Originally used as a sedative, thalidomide was withdrawn in 1961 because of birth defects when given to pregnant women. It suppresses TNF-α synthesis and modulates interferon-gamma, producing CD3$^+$ cells. Patients given thalidomide may need a pregnancy test to check this is negative before starting thalidomide treatment, must take effective contraceptive measures while taking thalidomide and for 3 months after finishing the tablets, and must not get pregnant. Peripheral neuropathy (which may be permanent) can occur during thalidomide treatment. Nerve conduction tests are needed before the start of treatment, and these should be repeated every 6 months. Nerve damage will recover on stopping the treatment in approximately 50% of cases. Thalidomide makes most people feel drowsy. It should be taken at night. Drowsiness persisting during the day makes it unsafe for patients to drive or operate machinery, and may impair alertness and ability to think clearly. Alcohol must be avoided. Thalidomide may predispose to venous or arterial thromboembolism, including myocardial infarction and CVEs. Antithrombotic prophylaxis for at least 5 months is indicated. Thalidomide may also predispose to other identified serious, or potentially serious, adverse effects, including: neutropenia; thrombocytopenia; syncope and bradycardia; and serious skin reactions, including Stevens–Johnson syndrome. May take 2–3 months to have real effect. Other effects include constipation, rash, oedema and reversible lymphopenia

*Many can increase liability to infection and, long term, possibly also neoplasia.

- Hypertension: the blood pressure must always be monitored.
- Precipitation of diabetes: the blood glucose must always be monitored.
- Cataract: ophthalmological monitoring is indicated.
- Osteoporosis: patients on protracted courses should have bone densitometry monitoring and be given bisphosphonates and calcium.
- Avascular necrosis of the femoral head.
- Psychoses.

Alternate-day administration after breakfast reduces the adverse effects of corticosteroids (**Table 5.8**). Patients should always be given a steroid card, warned of possible adverse reactions, and warned of the need for an increase in the dose if ill or traumatized, or having an operation.

CORTICOSTEROID-SPARING IMMUNOSUPPRESSANTS

Because of possible adverse reactions of corticosteroids, drugs with alternative modes of action are used as alternatives or in combination with corticosteroids and are termed 'steroid-sparing' immunosuppressants. However, most of these drugs may have serious, adverse effects in addition to those noted above, and so they are used by specialists.

Of these steroid-sparing drugs (**Tables 5.7**, **5.9** and **5.10**), dapsone most require monitoring for potential adverse effects.

BIOLOGICS

Generated by recombinant biotechnology, biologic agents target specific steps in pro-inflammatory pathways and are thus increasingly used in the treatment of a variety of inflammatory immune-mediated conditions. Three broad classes exist (**Table 5.10**):

- Lymphocyte modulators (e.g. rituximab (anti-CD20)).
- Tumour necrosis factor-alpha (TNF-α) cytokine inhibitors include the monoclonals infliximab (Remicade), etanercept (Enbrel), or adalimumab (Humira).
- Interleukin inhibitors such as ustekinumab (which inhibits IL-12/IL-23).

Table 5.8 Reducing course of systemic corticosteroid
Short-course treatment schedule: 105 prednisolone (enteric-coated) 5 mg tablets to cover an almost 4-week period

Day	1	3	5	7	9	11	13	15	17	19	21	23
No. of tablets to take after breakfast	12	12	12	9	9	9	9	6	6	6	6	3
Steroid dose over 2 days (mg)	60	60	60	45	45	45	45	30	30	30	30	15

Table 5.9 Immune suppressant and antiinflammatory agents

	Latency (wks)	Pregnancy (FDA)*	Adverse effects			
			Blood	Liver	Cancer	Main others
Azathioprine	4-8	D	+	+	+	Blood
Ciclosporin	1-2	C	-	+	+	Hypertension Nephrotoxic
Colchicine	2-4	C	+	-	-	Blood Neuromyopathy
Corticosteroids	1-2	C	-	-	+/-	Osteoporosis Hypertension Weight
Cyclophosphamide	2-4	D	+	+	+ Bladder	Cystitis Leukaemia
Dapsone	50-100	C	+	+	-	Idiosyncrasy
Mycophenolate	8-12	D	+	+	+/-	Gastrointestinal

*FDA guidance against use in pregnancy

Table 5.10 Emerging biologic agents

Main action upon	Examples
B cells	Rituximab
T cells	Abatecept
TNF	Adalimumab Certolizumab Etanercept Golimumab Infliximab
IL-1	Anakinra
IL-6	Tocilizumab
IL-12 and IL-23	Ustekinumab

These agents have been used in a wide variety of diseases, including some oral conditions. Safety concerns are such that their use requires precautionary considerations, including screening for co-existing medical conditions and an appreciation of potential adverse effects.

Potential adverse effects of biologics may include:

- Infections: screening for mycobacterial infections with consideration of prophylactic anti-TB therapy if there is evidence of latent disease, and definitive treatment in active disease, and for risk factors for HBV, HCV and HIV infection should be performed prior to anti-TNF therapy. Other opportunistic bacterial and fungal infections are also more prevalent in patients receiving TNF-α inhibitors, most frequently histoplasmosis and invasive candidosis.
- Cardiac failure: potentiated with TNF-α blockade, so the agents should be used with caution and it would seem prudent to monitor cardiac function in patients receiving therapy, and discontinue treatment if cardiac function declines.
- Increased risk of malignancy: for non-melanoma skin cancer and possibly for melanoma and lymphoma.

- Pregnancy and paediatric considerations: there is a potential increased occurrence of congenital abnormalities with TNF-α inhibitors used in pregnancy, in particular those of the VACTERL spectrum, and a possible increased risk of spontaneous abortion.
- Adverse drug reactions: range from minor reactions at injection sites to hypersensitivity reactions and anaphylaxis, including some oral adverse effects (Ch. 54).

Lymphocyte modulators carry similar adverse reactions which are well illustrated in the case of efalizumab, initially approved for the treatment of psoriasis, where safety concerns, primarily related to the risk of progressive multifocal leukoencephalopathy (PML), led to licence withdrawal by the FDA and EMA. Of this group, only rituximab is licenced. Rituximab concerns include:

- Infections
- Immune toxicity
- Severe infusion reactions
- Tumour lysis syndrome with hyperkalaemia and acute renal failure and arrhythmias
- Cardiac arrest
- Lung toxicity.

RETINOIDS

Tretinoin as a 0.1% cream or 0.01% gel, or acitretin (pro-drug of etretinate) 10–50 mg/day orally, may be of value in controlling lichen planus. Systemic retinoids however, are teratogenic and may disturb liver function and blood lipids.

ANTIMICROBIALS

ANTIBACTERIAL THERAPY

- The bacteria which cause most odontogenic infections are sensitive to penicillins.
- Anaerobes have now been implicated in many odontogenic infections, and these often respond to penicillins or metronidazole.

Table 5.11   Main antifungal agents

Agent	Dosage and duration (continue for at least 48h after lesions have cleared)*	Comments (see Tables 5.18 and 5.19)†
Topical		
Chlorhexidine	0.12–0.2% mouth rinse twice daily	Tooth staining, especially if the patient drinks tea, coffee or red wine
Nystatin	100 000 IU/mL of suspension**. 100 000 IU 6-hourly for at least 14–21 days	Topical use – often no problems, but may cause unpleasant taste, nausea or gastrointestinal disturbance. Suspension contains sucrose
Clotrimazole	10 mg 6-hourly for at least 14 days	Difficult to dissolve if mouth dry. Contains sucrose. Not available in the UK
Miconazole	20 mg mucoadhesive buccal tablet, 25 mg/mL gel. 50 mg daily for at least 14–21 days** 50 mg/g denture lacquer; apply weekly for at least 2 weeks. Not available in the USA	Available topically but may be absorbed systemically. May interact with many drugs, including anticoagulants, antidiabetic drugs, ciclosporin, cisapride, midazolam, phenytoin, statins and terfenadine. May impair oral contraceptive. Avoid in pregnancy and porphyria
Oral		
Fluconazole	50–200 mg/day capsules or suspension** 50 mg/5 mL for at least 14 days	Less toxic than ketoconazole. May interact with many drugs, including anticoagulants, antidiabetic drugs, ciclosporin, cisapride, midazolam, phenytoin repaglinide, rifabutin, statins, sulphonylureas, tacrolimus, terfenadine, theophylline and zidovudine. Avoid in pregnancy and porphyria. May impair oral contraceptive. May sometimes be hepatotoxic and myelosuppressive. Expensive. Avoid in pregnancy, infants and andrenal disease
Itraconazole	100–200 mg/day for at least 14 days capsule or 10 mg/mL liquid** 10 mL twice daily for at least 14 days	Expensive. May impair oral contraceptive. May cause cardiac failure. May interact with many drugs, including anticoagulants, antidiabetic drugs, ciclosporin, cisapride, midazolam, phenytoin repaglinide, rifabutin, statins, sulphonylureas, tacrolimus, terfenadine, theophylline, zidovudine, digoxin and sertindole. Not absorbed in achlorhydria. Avoid in cardiac disease, pregnancy and porphyria
Ketoconazole	200–400 mg/day for at least 14 days	Hepatotoxic. Expensive. May interact with many drugs, including anticoagulants, antidiabetics, ciclosporin, cimetidine, cisapride, isoniazid, midazolam, phenytoin, ranitidine, rifampicin, sertindole, statins and terfenadine. Enhances nephrotoxicity of ciclosporin. May impair oral contraceptive. Avoid in pregnancy and porphyria. Not absorbed in achlorhydria
Posaconazole	400 mg twice daily for at least 14 days available as suspension** 200 mg/5 mL	Posaconazole is the newest azole antifungal approved by the US FDA. Broad spectrum of activity against numerous yeasts and filamentous fungi. Available as an oral suspension and is generally well tolerated. It is used routinely and effectively for the prophylaxis of invasive fungal infections in immunosuppressed hosts and is an effective treatment of oral candidosis, including azole-resistant disease. May interact with many drugs, including anticoagulants, antidiabetic drugs, ciclosporin, cisapride, midazolam, phenytoin repaglinide, rifabutin, statins, sulphonylureas, tacrolimus, terfenadine, theophylline and zidovudine. Contraindicated in cardiac disease, liver disease, porphyria and pregnancy. Avoid in breastfeeding
Voriconazole	100–200 mg/every 12 hrs for at least 14 days available as suspension** 200 mg/5 ml	For fluconazole resistant *C. albicans* or *C. krusei* infections. May interact with many drugs, including anticoagulants, antidiabetic drugs, ciclosporin, cisapride, midazolam, phenytoin repaglinide, rifabutin, statins, sulphonylureas, tacrolimus, terfenadine, theophylline and zidovudine. Contraindicated in cardiac disease, liver disease and pregnancy. May prolong QT interval. Avoid in breastfeeding. Wide range of possible adverse effects. May cause nausea, neuropathy and rash

Table 5.11 Main antifungal drugs—Cont'd

Agent	Dosage and duration (continue for at least 48h after lesions have cleared)*	Comments (see Tables 5.18 and 5.19)†
Intravenous		
Amphotericin	0.5mg/kg for at least 10–14 days	Expensive. May cause nephrotoxicity, arrhythmias, neuropathies and anaphylactoid reactions. Avoid in pregnancy. Liposomal amphotericin may be safer
Caspofungin	Infusion 50 mg i.v. daily	For fluconazole resistant *C. albicans*. Contraindicated in cardiac disease, liver disease and pregnancy. Avoid in breastfeeding. Wide range of possible adverse effects including anaphylaxis
Micafungin	Infusion 100 mg i.v. daily	Prophylaxis of candidosis in haematopoietic stem cell transplantation when fluconazole, itraconazole of posaconazole cannot be used. Significantly hepatotoxic. Contraindicated in liver disease, renal disease and pregnancy. Avoid in breastfeeding

*The higher doses are used in HIV infection.
**Do not take with food; swish around mouth and swallow; for additional topical effect do not rinse mouth or eat or drink for 30 min.
†Check pharmacopoeia for other contraindications, cautions and interactions.

- Amoxicillin 500 mg three times daily is effective, and produces high blood antimicrobial levels, with good patient compliance.
- Flucloxacillin 500 mg four times daily is also effective against many oral bacterial infections.
- If the patient is allergic, has had penicillin within the previous month (resistant bacteria) or has meticillin-resistant *Staphylococcus aureus* (MRSA) a different antimicrobial should be used.
- Drainage must be established if there is pus; antimicrobials will not remove pus.
- A sample of pus (as much as possible) should be sent for culture and sensitivities, but, if antimicrobials are indicated, they should be started immediately and in adequate doses.
- If a lesion fails to respond to an antimicrobial reconsider possible:
  - inadequacy of drainage
  - inappropriateness of the antimicrobial
  - inadequate antimicrobial dose
  - antimicrobial insensitivity of causal micro-organism, e.g. staphylococci are now frequently resistant to penicillin and some show multiple resistances (e.g. MRSA) when vancomycin is usually effective
  - patient non-compliance
  - local factors (e.g. foreign body)
  - unusual type of infection
  - impaired host defences (unusual and opportunistic infections are increasingly identified, particularly in the immunocompromised patient)
  - non-infective cause for the condition.

In serious, unusual or unresponsive cases of infection, consult the clinical microbiologist.

Indications for the use of antibacterials

Infections (together with appropriate surgical or other measures), such as:

- cervical fascial space infections
- osteomyelitis

- odontogenic infections in ill or toxic patients (e.g. if the patient is immunocompromised)
- acute ulcerative gingivitis
- specific infections, such as tuberculosis and syphilis.

Antimicrobials should be used in some instances of surgical conditions if they do not respond to local measures:

- pericoronitis
- dental abscess
- dry socket.

Antimicrobials should be used for prophylaxis:

- of infective endocarditis in at-risk patients having invasive oral procedures
- in cerebrospinal rhinorrhoea
- in most facial or compound skull fractures
- in major oral, maxillofacial and craniofacial surgery (e.g. osteotomies or tumour resection)
- in surgery involving bone in immunocompromised or debilitated patients
- in surgery involving bone in patients who have been taking bisphosphonates
- in surgery involving bone following radiotherapy to the jaws
- possibly in patients with hydrocephalus shunts having invasive oral procedures
- possibly in some patients with prosthetic joint replacements having invasive oral procedures, especially following rheumatoid arthritis.

Using antibacterials

- The practitioner should attempt to obtain relevant specimens before commencing therapy.
- For most infections, a 5-day course of antibiotics is adequate.
- Antibiotic prescriptions should be reviewed at 48h and 5 days, and in the light of microbiology results.

- Most infections should be treated with a single antibiotic only. Exceptions include endocarditis prophylaxis, tuberculosis treatment and some infections in immunocompromised persons.
- Always enquire first about allergies and other contraindications.

ANTIFUNGAL THERAPY

Antifungals (**Table 5.11**) are used:

- to treat oral or oropharyngeal fungal infections, but underlying predisposing factors should be corrected first
- until there is no evidence of residual clinical lesions or symptoms, and should be continued for at least 2 weeks more, to reduce the risk of recurrence
- topically often effectively and, importantly, they are without serious adverse effects apart from occasional drug interactions (e.g. topical miconazole can enhance the effect of warfarin)
- systemically and though sometimes more effective against *Candida*, systemic use can be associated with adverse effects or drug interactions.

Polyene antifungal agents

These include the following:

- **Nystatin** is antifungal by interfering with fungal cell membranes. It binds to ergosterol, an essential component of fungal cell membranes, disrupting the cell membrane and leading to potassium leakage and fungal inhibition. Nystatin, topically, used at least four times daily, 500 000 units for adults and 100 000 units for children. Higher doses may be required in immunocompromised patients. Compliance can be a problem because of the taste, but suspensions often overcome this disadvantage. Nystatin, if swallowed, may lead occasionally to gastrointestinal side-effects, such as nausea, vomiting and diarrhoea.
- **Amphotericin** has a similar mode of action to nystatin. It can be given intravenously for systemic candidosis, but there is then a considerable risk of toxicity, which may manifest as fever, vomiting, and renal, bone marrow, cardiovascular and neurological toxicity.

Azole antifungal agents

Azoles are synthetic antifungals with broad-spectrum activity and are fungistatic, but are expensive and usually used mainly systemically, though miconazole in particular is often used topically. Liquid or suspension forms can also be used for topical effect (**Table 5.11**). Azoles inhibit the fungal cytochrome P450 dependent enzymes, which are essential catalysts for the 14-demethylation of lanosterol in sterol biosynthesis, and, therefore, block the synthesis of ergosterol, the principal sterol in fungal cell membranes. One adverse effect of azoles, therefore, is the accumulation of precursors of ergosterol. Azoles include:

- imidazoles (clotrimazole, econazole, ketoconazole and miconazole)
- triazoles (fluconazole, itraconazole, voriconazole and posaconazole). Fluconazole, voriconazole and posaconazole are available as suspensions, and itraconazole as a liquid; preparations which may find favour for use in patients with dry mouths and for use as topical therapy.

The absorption of ketoconazole and itraconazole is dependent on gastric acid and so any drugs that increase gastric pH (e.g. H_2 antagonists, proton pump inhibitors), and antacids, metal ion containing drugs (e.g. sulcralfate), and vitamin supplements can decrease antifungal absorption. P-glycoprotein (P-gp) – a versatile drug transporter – functions as a 'detoxification' pump that expels drugs back into the intestinal lumen. P-gp also works in concert with the cytochrome P450 (CYP) 3A4 enzymes in intestine and liver where drug metabolites are produced for renal elimination. Ketoconazole and itraconazole not only affect P-gp but are highly dependent upon metabolism through several CYP 450 pathways including CYP 3A4. Fluconazole, on the other hand, is more readily cleared from the body. Co-administration of azoles with drugs that induce or accelerate strongly CYP-450 metabolism can result in low or undetectable levels of the azole antifungal. Higher antifungal dosages (particularly of ketoconazole, itraconazole, voriconazole) cannot overcome this interaction. All azoles are also reversible inhibitors of CYP enzymes. Thus important drug interactions with azole antifungals arise from inhibition of CYP 3A4, which plays a critical role in the metabolism of a range of drugs used for cardiovascular disease, endocrine disorders including hyperglycaemia, anaesthesia, psychiatric disorders, epilepsy, cancer chemotherapy, and treatment of infectious diseases. There can be interactions with bortezomib, bosutinib, carbamazepine, closporin, H_2 receptor antagonists, isoniazid, phenobarbitone, phenytoin, rifampicin, statins, sucralfate, terfenadine, tricyclic antidepressants and warfarin. Rifampicin, rifabutin and phenytoin can decrease antifungal levels.

The imidazoles (ketoconazole and miconazole) have more effect on cytochromes than do the triazoles, and the latter thus tend to have less severe adverse effects. However, none of the azoles are entirely benign; hepatotoxicity may be common to all, and the potential for endocrine toxicities exists, particularly at high doses.

Finally, azole resistance is increasingly reported. The development of cross-resistance of *C. albicans* to different azoles during treatment with a single derivative has been described. Azoles may thus:

- be hepatotoxic
- displace protein-bound drugs and, thus, enhance the activity of, for example, anticoagulants, producing a bleeding tendency
- interact with a number of drugs. An important interaction is to produce arrhythmias with terfenadine (and in the past with astemizole and cisapride). They may also interfere with the oral contraceptive
- cause antifungal resistance (to ketoconazole, fluconazole, miconazole and itraconazole) and this is now becoming a significant problem in immunocompromised persons, especially those with a severe immune defect, who may show *Candida* species resistant to fluconazole and, sometimes, to other azoles. Voriconazole may then be effective.

CLOTRIMAZOLE

Clotrimazole is used only topically as a 10 mg troche three times daily, because it has gastrointestinal and neurological toxicity. It is less effective than other azoles in patients with HIV infection.

KETOCONAZOLE

Ketoconazole is usually used systemically, 200–400 mg/day taken orally with food, since gastric acid is essential for its dissolution. Absorption can be enhanced by taking orange juice, carbonated beverages or glutamic acid. Ketoconazole is poorly absorbed from an empty stomach in HIV/AIDS because of gastric atrophy and reduced acid production, or if there is concurrent use of medications, such as cimetidine, ranitidine and other antacids. It is also poorly absorbed if rifampicin or phenytoin are given. Adverse effects may include nausea, rashes, abdominal pain and pruritus, but especially liver damage. Transient disturbance of liver function (e.g. increased serum aminotransferase concentrations) is so common that regular monitoring with liver function tests is essential in all patients on systemic ketoconazole for more than a few days. Severe liver damage may sometimes occur. Ketoconazole also blocks hormone steroid synthesis and reduces testosterone levels. Adrenocortical suppression may also develop. Drug interactions with ketoconazole are shown in **Tables 5.18** and **5.19**. These adverse effects have restricted its use.

MICONAZOLE

Miconazole is used mainly for topical treatment of various forms of candidosis, such as angular stomatitis. Miconazole buccal tablets exhibit few drug interactions because of low systemic absorption and are generally well tolerated with a safety profile similar to comparators. The once-daily dosing schedule may improve patient adherence compared with topical alternatives. Miconazole is effective for the treatment of chronic atrophic candidosis; chewing gum may be effective against intraoral candidosis.

Miconazole is also available for parenteral use against systemic mycoses, but the injection contains polyethoxylate castor oil, which may provoke allergic reactions. Intravenous miconazole may also cause liver damage and pruritus, nausea, blood dyscrasias, hyponatraemia, hyperlipidaemia and arrhythmias.

FLUCONAZOLE

Fluconazole, unlike some other azoles, has little affinity for cytochromes, which is thought to explain its lower toxicity. Fluconazole is active against most *C. albicans*, though resistance may appear (see below) and it is less active against some *non-albicans Candida* species. It tends to be active against *C. parapsilosis* and *C. tropicalis*, but less active against *C. glabrata*, and is inactive against *C. krusei*. Fluconazole is well absorbed from the gut, even in the absence of gastric acidity, and absorption is rapid and nearly complete within 2 h. Fluconazole appears to undergo relatively little metabolism in the body, elimination being predominantly renal with a half-life of approximately 30 h, meaning that fluconazole can be given once daily, in a dose of 50–100 mg. It also enters saliva. Fluconazole has generally been well tolerated, toxicity is mild and infrequent and, with usual doses, fluconazole does not appear to suppress the synthesis of corticosteroid hormones. Drug interactions present less difficulties than those associated with ketoconazole (see **Table 5.18** and Ch. 5). An oral suspension of fluconazole is also available. Chronic use of fluconazole in high doses (400–800 mg/day) during the first trimester of pregnancy may be associated with certain birth defects in infants. The risk does not appear to be associated with a single, low dose of fluconazole (150 mg). According to the FDA, 'a few published case reports describe a rare pattern of distinct congenital anomalies in infants exposed in utero to high-dose maternal fluconazole (400–800 mg/day) during most or all of the first trimester'. The features seen in these infants include brachycephaly, abnormal facies, abnormal calvarial development, cleft palate, femoral bowing, thin ribs and long bones, arthrogryposis, and congenital heart disease.

Table 5.12 Antivirals against herpesviruses

Virus	Disease	Otherwise healthy patient[a]	Immunocompromised patient[b]
Herpes simplex 1 and 2	Primary herpetic gingivostomatitis	Consider oral 100–200 mg aciclovir tablets 5 times daily, or oral suspension (200 mg/5 mL) 5 times daily for 7 days	Consider aciclovir 250 mg/m² i.v. every 8 h. Famciclovir 250 mg three times daily. Caution in renal disease, older patients and pregnancy. Occasionally causes nausea and headache. Valaciclovir 1000 mg can be given orally 2 times daily
	Recurrent herpes labialis	1% penciclovir cream every 2 h while awake, or 5% aciclovir cream every 4 h	Aciclovir tablets 5 times daily, or oral suspension (200 mg/5 mL) 5 times daily. Consider aciclovir 250 mg/m² i.v. every 8 h
	Recurrent herpetic ulcers	Aciclovir tablets 5 times daily, or oral suspension (200 mg/5 mL) 5 times daily	Consider aciclovir 250 mg/m² i.v. every 8 h
Herpes varicella zoster	Chickenpox	Consider oral 100–200 mg aciclovir tablets 5 times daily, or oral suspension (200 mg/5 mL) 5 times daily for 7 days	Aciclovir 500 mg/m² (5 mg/kg) i.v. every 8 h
	Zoster (shingles)	Consider oral 400–800 mg aciclovir tablets 5 times daily, or oral suspension (800 mg/5 mL) 5 times daily for 7 days. 3% aciclovir ophthalmic ointment for shingles of trigeminal ophthalmic division	Famciclovir 500 mg three times daily. Caution in renal disease, older patients and pregnancy. Occasionally causes nausea and headache. Valaciclovir 2000 mg can be given orally three times daily

[a]In neonate, treat as if immunocompromised,
[b]Aciclovir (systemic preparations): caution in renal disease and pregnancy. Occasional increase in liver enzymes and urea, rashes and CNS effects.

ITRACONAZOLE

Itraconazole is an orally active triazole available in 50 mg and 100 mg capsules and as a 10 mg/mL oral solution. Itraconazole has a long half-life and fewer side-effects than ketoconazole, but is expensive, is eliminated hepatically and its use is contraindicated in liver disease. Itraconazole is well absorbed, but absorption is impaired when gastric acid is reduced or when antacids, rifampicin or phenytoin are given. Adverse effects of itraconazole have included altered liver function (but hepatotoxicity is less than that of ketoconazole) and hypokalaemia with hypertension due to accumulation of corticosteroids with an aldosterone-like activity, mild leukopenia, nausea, epigastric pain, headache and oedema. Itraconazole can aggravate or cause cardiac failure, especially in the older patient or one on calcium channel blockers. Drug interactions are shown in **Table 5.12**.

VORICONAZOLE

Voriconazole is a relatively new triazole antifungal agent, effective against candida species but mainly indicated for the primary treatment of acute invasive aspergillosis. Elevated liver function tests, cardiac QT interval, rash and visual disturbances are the main treatment-related adverse events. Drug interactions are shown in **Table 5.11**.

POSACONAZOLE

Posaconazole is a relatively new triazole antifungal agent, probably more effective than the others against invasive fungal infections but with more severe adverse effects. Posaconazole acts by disrupting phospholipids, impairing certain enzyme systems such as ATPase and the electron transport system and thus inhibiting synthesis of ergosterol by inhibiting lanosterol 14α-demethylase and accumulation of methylated sterol precursors. Posaconazole can cause QT prolongation, liver dysfunction, rashes and allergies. Drug interactions are shown in **Table 5.12**.

ANTIVIRAL THERAPY

- Most antivirals (**Table 5.12**) achieve maximum benefit if given early in the disease.
- Most acute viral infections resolve naturally, though in immunocompromised persons they may be severe, widespread or persistent.
- Immunocompromised patients with viral infections may thus benefit from active antiviral therapy.
- Antiviral resistance is now becoming a significant problem to immunocompromised persons, especially those with a severe immune defect.
- Some antivirals active against herpesviruses and some active against retroviruses, such as HIV, are available, but there are few other antiviral agents of proven efficacy.

ANTIVIRALS ACTIVE AGAINST HERPESVIRUSES

Antivirals are usually nucleoside analogues, which compete with natural nucleosides to block virus DNA synthesis, or pro-drugs which generally produce greater bioavailability of the active agent. Antivirals include the following:

- Aciclovir, a guanosine analogue selectively phosphorylated to active form by herpesvirus thymidine kinases has proven efficacy in herpes simplex virus (HSV) infections, including herpes labialis and is fairly safe, though neurotoxic if given intravenously. It is given 5 times daily. Aciclovir is not effective against cytomegalovirus (which has no such thymidine kinase).
- Valaciclovir is a pro-drug of aciclovir; it has the advantage of a 2 or 3 times daily dosing only.
- Penciclovir is a synthetic acyclic guanine derivative which possesses the same antiviral spectrum as, and a similar mechanism of action to that of aciclovir, in that it undergoes phosphorylation in response to HSV viral thymidine kinase and is then further phosphorylated by host cell enzymes into a triphosphate, which selectively inhibits HSV viral DNA replication. It has considerably more bioavailability and a longer intracellular effect than aciclovir, and is generally more effective topically than topical aciclovir, is cheaper than aciclovir but only available as a cream.
- Famciclovir, a pro-drug of penciclovir, is a guanosine analogue, that is particularly useful against HSV and varicella-zoster virus (VZV), but produces DNA mutations that may predispose to cancer of the breast or testis.
- Ganciclovir, a guanosine analogue, is active against cytomegalovirus (CMV), but is more toxic than aciclovir, can produce neutropenia, may have carcinogenic activity and, if given with zidovudine, can produce profound myelosuppresssion.
- Cidofovir is a DNA polymerase chain inhibitor, active against CMV and human papillomaviruses (HPV), but is nephrotoxic and may produce eye damage.

Other antiherpes agents

- Docosanol is an aliphatic alcohol that inhibits fusion between the plasma membrane and the HSV envelope, thereby preventing viral entry into cells and viral replication. A 10% docosanol cream is available for treating herpes labialis.
- Inosine pranobex (isoprinosine, methisoprinolol) is a stimulator of immunity via actions like thymic hormones, active against HSV and HPV. It should be used with caution in gout or renal disease.
- Foscarnet is an organic analogue of inorganic pyrophosphate that selectively inhibits the pyrophosphate-binding site on viral DNA polymerases and can be used for HSV or CMV infections. It is potentially nephrotoxic.

ANTIRETROVIRAL AGENTS

Antiretroviral therapy (ART) includes agents (**Tables 5.13–5.16**) developed in the past decades, and though effective all are liable to fairly severe adverse reactions and resistance and many can cause drug interactions: The current philosophy is to start ART early in HIV infection.

Nucleoside reverse transcriptase inhibitors

Nucleoside reverse transcriptase inhibitors (NRTIs) block HIV reverse transcriptase activity by competing with natural substrates and being incorporated into viral DNA where they act as chain terminators in the synthesis of pro-viral

Table 5.13 Antiretroviral drugs: nucleoside reverse transcriptase inhibitors (NRTIs)*

Proper name (abbreviation)	Trade name	Possible orofacial adverse effects	Other main adverse effects
Abacavir (ABC)	Ziagen	Erythema multiforme	Lactic acidosis, nausea, diarrhoea
Didanosine (DDI)	Videx	Erythema multiforme, dry mouth	Nausea, diarrhoea, lactic acidosis, mitochondrial dysfunction leading to pancreatitis, abnormal liver function, peripheral neuropathy, retinal damage
Emtricitabine (FTC)	Emtriva	–	Similar to lamivudine. Pruritus, hyperpigmentation
Lamivudine (3TC)	Epivir	dry mouth	Nausea, diarrhoea, mitochondrial dysfunction leading to pancreatitis, abnormal liver function
Stavudine (D4T)	Zerit	Lipodystrophy	Neuropsychiatric reactions, mitochondrial dysfunction leading to pancreatitis, abnormal liver function
Tenofovir disoproxil (TDF)	Viread	–	Renal tubular damage, hypophosphataemia
Zidovudine (azidothymidine; AZT, ZDV)	Retrovir	Erythema multiforme, hyperpigmentation	Nausea, diarrhoea, myelotoxic, lactic acidosis, myopathy

*Also available in combinations.

Table 5.14 Antiretroviral drugs: non-nucleoside reverse transcriptase inhibitors (NNRTIs)

Proper name (abbreviation)	Trade name	Possible orofacial adverse effects	Other main adverse effects
Efavirenz (EFV)	Sustiva	Erythema multiforme	Interferes with liver drug-metabolizing enzymes, neuropsychiatric reactions
Etravirine (ETV)	Intelence	Erythema multiforme, ulcers	Hypersensitivity
Nevirapine (NVP)	Viramune	Erythema multiforme, ulcers	Induces liver drug-metabolizing enzymes, abnormal liver function

nucleic acids. The NRTIs often produce adverse effects and, perhaps more significantly, HIV-resistance may arise. Among the common effects of many are haematological toxicity, neurological toxicity (including effects on memory, cognition, motor and peripheral nerve function) and enhanced risk of dry mouth ulcers and erythema multiforme (**Table 5.13**).

Non-nucleoside reverse transcriptase inhibitors

Non-nucleoside reverse transcriptase inhibitors (NNRTIs) directly bind to HIV reverse transcriptase to inhibit it. NNRTIs suffer from similar disadvantages to NRTIs, especially rashes (**Table 5.14**).

Protease inhibitors

Protease inhibitors (PIs) can be anti-HIV (there are also PIs that are anti-HCV (Boceprevir)). Anti-HIV PIs competitively inhibit an HIV aspartyl protease without affecting the human enzyme, and they induce a profound and sustained fall in HIV viral load and restore T-cell counts. Drug-induced lipodystrophy may cause dyslipidaemia and facial lipoatrophy. Taste abnormalities are common and oral and perioral paraesthesia can be disturbing adverse effects. Indinavir, which has activity related to vitamin A analogues, can also produce cheilitis (**Table 5.15**).

Entry inhibitors

Entry inhibitors prevent HIV attachment by attaching themselves to CD4 cell surface proteins or proteins on the surface of HIV. Some entry inhibitors target the gp120 or gp41 proteins on HIV.

CCR5 receptor antagonists

These cells target CD4 protein or the CCR5 or CXCR4 receptors on CD4 (**Table 5.16**).

Table 5.15 Antiretroviral drugs: protease inhibitors*

Proper name (abbreviation)	Trade name	Possible orofacial adverse effects	Other main adverse effects
Atazanavir (ATV)	Reyataz	Ulcers	Prolongs QR interval, jaundice, neurological effects
Darunavir (DRV)	Prezista	Dry mouth	ECG changes, neuropathy, weight changes
Fosamprenavir (FPV)	Telzir	Perioral paraesthesia, parotid lipomatosis	Interferes with liver drug-metabolizing enzymes, dyslipidaemia
Indinavir (IDV)	Crixivan	Cheilitis, parotid lipomatosis, dry mouth, taste disturbance	Nephrolithiasis in 40%, interferes with liver drug-metabolizing enzymes, oesophagitis, haemolysis
Nelfinavir (NFV)	Viracept	Parotid lipomatosis, dry mouth	Nausea, diarrhoea, interferes with liver drug-metabolizing enzymes, dyslipidaemia
Ritonavir (RTV)	Norvir	Perioral paraesthesia, parotid lipomatosis, dry mouth, taste disturbance, facial oedema	Nausea, diarrhoea, interferes with liver drug-metabolizing enzymes, flushing, dyslipidaemia
Saquinavir (SQV)	Fortovase, Invirase	Erythema multiforme, ulcers, parotid lipomatosis, dry mouth	Nausea, diarrhoea, interferes with liver drug-metabolizing enzymes, dyslipidaemia
Tipranavir (TPV)	Aptivus	-	Hepatotoxicity and bleeding tendency

*Also available in combinations.

Table 5.16 Antiretroviral drugs: fusion entry inhibitors

Proper name (abbreviation)	Trade name	Possible orofacial adverse effects	Other main adverse effects
Enfuvirtide (ENF)	Fuzeon	?	Hypersensitivity, pancreatitis, hypertriglyceridaemia
Maraviroc (MVC)	Selzentry Celsentri	Taste disturbance	Cough, liver dysfunction

Integrase inhibitors

These inhibit integration of viral nucleic acids into the host cells. Raltegravir (isentress) can cause abdominal pain, diarrhea, erythema multiforme and dry mouth. Dolutegravis is a newer integrase inhibitor.

Maturation inhibitors

These block production of HIV capsid protein p24. Alpha interferon has this effect as do bevirimat and Vivecon.

Combination therapies

Highly active antiretroviral therapies (HAART) are combinations (CART), involving a protease inhibitor and other antiretroviral drugs, and these have reduced the incidence of opportunistic infections, extended life substantially and decreased the infective load of HIV and other viruses. Such has been the effect of ART and HAART, that orofacial disease caused by HIV/AIDS has now been significantly reduced.

Conversely, oral and perioral adverse effects can arise and may sometimes result in patient non-adherence to anti-HIV therapy.

Immune reconstitution syndrome (IRIS) is the term given when ART provokes an inflammatory reaction against residual micro-organisms. Long-term use of ART has been associated with oral warts, erythema multiforme, hyposalivation, toxic epidermal necrolysis, lichenoid reactions, exfoliative cheilitis, oral ulceration and paraesthesia.

TREATMENTS APPROPRIATE FOR PRIMARY OR SECONDARY CARE

Treatments appropriate for primary care are shown in **Table 5.17**. A specialist opinion may also be called for in the case of other disorders (Ch. 4).

Contraindications and the most important interactions for drugs used by dental clinicians in primary care are shown in **Table 5.18** and for medical clinicians and secondary care management in **Table 5.19**.

FOLLOW-UP OF PATIENTS

Though it is desirable to offer active treatment for oral lesions, this is not always possible or indicated, and, sometimes, watchful waiting is required, by following up the patient. Sometimes, for example in suspected traumatic ulceration, the diagnosis can only be decided by removing predisposing factors, and then checking progress in 2 weeks to see if the lesion is healing. Patients with chronic conditions can often be followed up in a primary care setting but frequently the care is best shared between the specialist and the primary dental and/ or medical practitioner. Follow-up in secondary care may be indicated when there is:

- a complicated or serious diagnosis (notably Behçet syndrome, cancer, erythroplakia or other potentially malignant disorder with severe dysplasia, HIV infection, pemphigus, etc.)
- a situation where investigations are required, but not possible or appropriate to carry out in a primary care setting
- a situation where therapy may not be straightforward and may require potent agents not available or appropriate to be prescribed in a primary care setting.

PATIENT INFORMATION SHEET

Corticosteroid treatment (this sheet is for systemic corticosteroids only)

Please read this information sheet. If you have any questions, particularly about the treatment of potential side-effects, please ask your doctor.

- Corticosteroids are very helpful, but must be used with caution.
- Always tell an attending doctor or dentist you are on corticosteroids.
- Always carry your steroid card.
- The steroid dose must usually be increased if you:
  - are ill
  - have an accident
  - have an operation.

Adverse effects seen on treatment for over 4 weeks can include:

- weight gain and fat re-distribution
- hypertension (high blood pressure)
- precipitation of diabetes
- osteoporosis
- mood changes
- liability to fungal and viral infection.

Alternate-day dosing reduces the adverse effects of corticosteroids.

Table 5.17 Primary care diagnosis and management of main oral medicine conditions (see Tables 5.18 and 5.19)

Condition	Typical main clinical features	Investigations that may be indicated for diagnosis in addition to history and examination	Therapeutic protocols	High levels of available evidence
Acute necrotizing ulcerative gingivitis	Pain, ulcerations, bleeding, halitosis	Full blood count Consider HIV	Debridement Metronidazole or amoxicillin	Yes
Aphthous stomatitis	Recurrent oral ulcers only	Full blood count Exclude underlying systemic disease (e.g. transglutaminase for coeliac disease; haematinic assys)	Vitamin B12, aqueous chlorhexidine, corticosteroids topically (e.g. hydrocortisone, betamethasone), amlexanox or, only in adults, topical tetracycline (doxycycline)	Yes (for all)
Allergic reactions	Swelling, erythema or erosions	Allergy testing	Avoid precipitant Consider antihistamines (e.g. loratidine)	Yes
Atypical (idiopathic) facial pain	Persistent dull ache typically in one maxilla in an older female	Clinical and imaging to exclude organic disease	Reassurance, CBT GMPs or specialists may use SSRIs or tricyclic antidepressants	Yes (for CBT and tricyclics)
Burning mouth syndrome	Glossodynia	Full blood picture, thyroid function, electrolytes	Reassurance, CBT Topical capsaicin GMPs or specialists may use tricyclic antidepressants or SSRIs	Yes
Candidosis (including angular stomatitis and denture-related stomatitis)	White or red persistent lesions	Consider smear, or biopsy Consider immune defect	Antifungals Leave out dental appliances, allowing the mouth to heal Disinfect the appliance Use intraorally antifungal creams, gels or tablets (e.g. miconazole) or suspensions (e.g. nystatin or fluconazole) regularly for up to 4 weeks Miconazole or fucidin cream (with or without hydrocortisone) applied to commissures	Yes
Chapped lips	Dry, flaking lips	–	Topical petrolatum gel or bland creams	No
Dental infections and pain	Pain usually aggravated by pressure or heat	Oral examination ± radiology	Restorative dentistry; possibly amoxicillin or metronidazole for 5 days	Yes
Erythema migrans	Desquamating patches on tongue	–	Reassurance ± benzydamine	No
Halitosis	Oral malodour	Oral/ENT examination and radiography	Treat underlying cause	No
Herpes simplex infection	Oral ulcers, gingivitis, fever	Sometimes PCR or immunostain	Symptomatic ± aciclovir suspension or tablets	Yes
Herpes labialis	Lip blisters	–	Antiviral cream (penciclovir or aciclovir)	Yes

Table 5.17   Primary care diagnosis and management of main oral medicine conditions (see Tables 5.18 and 5.19)—Cont'd

Condition	Typical main clinical features	Investigations that may be indicated for diagnosis in addition to history and examination	Therapeutic protocols	High levels of available evidence
Hyposalivation	Dry mouth May be dry eyes, or a connective tissue disease	Assess salivary flow rate Exclude drugs, diabetes, Sjögren syndrome (serology – SS-A (Ro) and SS-B (La) antibodies), HCV, HIV Ultrasound Consider labial gland biopsy, sialography or scintiscan	Preventive dentistry; mouth wetting agents (artificial salivas, of which there are several available) and artificial tears; salivary stimulants (sialogogues) – such as sugar-free chewing gum, or systemic pilocarpine or cevimeline	Yes
Keratosis	Flat, raised or warty white lesion	Biopsy	Stop tobacco, betel or alcohol use Excise if dysplastic	No
Leukoplakia	Flat, raised or warty white or white and red lesion (erythroleukoplakia)	Biopsy	Stop tobacco, betel or alcohol use Excise if dysplastic	No
Lichen planus	Mucosal white or other lesions Polygonal purple pruritic papules on skin May be genital, skin or adnexal involvement	Biopsy ± immunofluorescence	Corticosteroids (e.g. betamethasone or clobetasol propionate) topically. Aloe vera gel may be tried Stop tobacco or any causal drug use	Yes (for corticosteroid and aloe vera)
Pemphigoid	Blisters, mainly in mouth occasionally on conjunctivae, genitals or skin Scarring	Biopsy ± immunostaining	Topical corticosteroids (e.g. betamethasone or clobetasol propionate) Specialists may use tetracycline, dapsone, systemic corticosteroids or other immunosuppressives	Yes
Sinusitis	Pain, nasal discharge	Imaging	Nasal decongestants (e.g. ephedrine) Amoxicillin, doxycycline or clarithromycin for 7 days	Yes
TMJ pain-dysfunction	TMJ pain, click, limitation of movement	Rarely imaging or arthroscopy	Reassurance, occlusal splint (overlay appliance), anxiolytics or muscle relaxants (e.g. benzodiazepines such as diazepam or temazepam). Topical NSAIDs	No

CBT, cognitive behavioural therapy; ENT, ear, nose and throat; GMP, general medical practice; PCR, polymerase chain reaction; SSRI, selective serotonin reuptake inhibitor.
Adapted from Scully, Bagan, Carrozzo, Flaitz and Gandolfo, *Pocket Guide to Oral Diseases*, 2013, Elsevier.

Table 5.18   Primary care management: main drug contraindications and interactions*

Drug	Contraindications in addition to allergies to the agent, and possibly pregnancy and breastfeeding	Cautions	Most important potential interactions
Aciclovir (topical)	–	–	–
Aloe vera	–	Anorexia Inflammatory bowel disease	Digoxin Diuretics Glyburide Hydrocortisone
Amoxicillin	–	Chronic lymphocytic leukaemia Gout Infectious mononucleosis	Anticoagulants Methotrexate
Antihistamines (e.g. promethazine, loratidine)	–	Asthma Cardiac disease Diabetes Driving or operating machinery Epilepsy Glaucoma Liver disease Prostatic hypertrophy Renal disease	Alcohol Azithromycin Bepridil Clarithromycin CNS depressants Dicyclomine Disopyramide Erythromycin Itraconazole Ketoconazole Maprotiline MAOI Phenothiazines Pimozide procainamide Quinidine Tricyclic antidepressants
Aspirin	Asthma Children	Bleeding tendency Peptic ulcer	Alcohol Antacids Anticoagulants Cilostazol Clopidogrel Corticosteroids Iloprost Lithium Methotrexate Metoclopramide Mifepristone NSAIDs Oral hypoglycaemics Paracetamol Phenylbutazone Phenytoin Probenecid Sodium valproate SSRIs Subitramine Sulphinpyrazone Venlafaxine Zafirlukast
Benzydamine	–	–	–
Capsaicin	–	–	–
Carbamazepine	Patients with HLA-B1502	Porphyria Blood dyscrasias Cardiac disease Driving or operating machinery Glaucoma Liver disease Renal disease	Alcohol Anticonvulsants Antidepressants Antimalarials Calcium channel blockers Ciclosporin Cimetidine Clarithromycin CNS depressants

Table 5.18 Primary care management: main drug contraindications and interactions*—Cont'd

Drug	Contraindications in addition to allergies to the agent, and possibly pregnancy and breastfeeding	Cautions	Most important potential interactions
			Contraceptive pill Danazol Dextropropoxyphene Diltiazem Diuretics Doxycycline Erythromycin Fluconazole Fluoxetine Gefitinib Irinotecan Isoniazid Lithium MAOI Miconazole Paracetamol Phenytoin Protease inhibitors Sodium valproate Tricyclic antidepressants Verapamil
Chlorhexidine	–	–	–
Corticosteroids topically	–	Candidosis	–
Diazepam	Children Glaucoma Porphyria	Cerebrovascular disease Depression Driving or operating machinery Epilepsy Hypothyroidism Liver disease Myasthenia gravis Obesity Old people Parkinsonism Renal disease Respiratory disease	Alcohol Aspirin Clozapine CNS depressants Droperidol Fluvoxamine Grapefruit juice Olanzapine Propoxyphene
Dihydrocodeine		Asthma, Children Hypothyroidism Pancreatitis Renal disease	Alcohol
Ephedrine	Hypertension	Cardiac disease Diabetes Glaucoma Prostatic hypertrophy Adrenal disorders Seizures Stroke Hyperthyroid Severe asthma	Beta blockers Bromocriptine Catechol-O-methyltransferase (COMT) inhibitors (e.g. entacapone) Digoxin Droxidopa Cocaine Furazolidone Guanadrel Guanethidine Indometacin Mecamylamine Methyldopa MAOI Oxytocic medicines (e.g. oxytocin) Rauwolfia derivatives (e.g. reserpine) Tricyclic antidepressants

Table 5.18 Primary care management: main drug contraindications and interactions*—Cont'd

Drug	Contraindications in addition to allergies to the agent, and possibly pregnancy and breastfeeding	Cautions	Most important potential interactions
Fluconazole	Porphyria	Cardiac 'long QT syndrome' or arrhythmia Liver disease Renal disease	Antacids, Anticoagulants Anticonvulsants Antidiabetics Bortezomib Bosutinib Calcium channel blockers Carbamazepine Celecoxib Ciclosporin Cisapride Digoxin H$_2$ receptor antagonists Isoniazid Midazolam Mizolastine Oral contraceptive Parecoxib Phenobarbitone Phenytoin Pimozide Protease inhibitors Quinidine Rifabutin Rifampicin Sirolimus Statins Sucralfate Terfenadine Tricyclic antidepressants Vincristine Zidovudine
Fucidin (topical)	–	–	–
Ibuprofen	Arrhythmias Cardiac infarction	Aspirin hypersensitivity Asthma Bleeding problems Cardiac disease Liver disease Older patients Peptic ulcer Renal	Angiotensin II antagonists Anticoagulants Baclofen Cardiac glycosides Ciclosporin Clopidogrel Corticosteroids Diuretics Erlotinib Haloperidol Lithium Methotrexate Nitrates Pentoxifylline Prasugrel SSRIs Sulfonylureas Tacrolimus Venlafaxine Zidovudine
Metronidazole	Alcoholism Porphyria	CNS disease Epilepsy Liver disease Renal disease	Alcohol Anticoagulants Anticonvulsants Cimetidine Fluorouracil Lithium

Table 5.18 Primary care management: main drug contraindications and interactions*—Cont'd

Drug	Contraindications in addition to allergies to the agent, and possibly pregnancy and breastfeeding	Cautions	Most important potential interactions
Miconazole	Porphyria	Liver disease Neuromuscular diseases	Antacids Anticoagulants Antidiabetic drugs Bortezomib Bosutinib Carbamazepine Ciclosporin Cisapride H_2 receptor antagonists Isoniazid Midazolam Oral contraceptive Phenobarbitone Phenytoin Rifabutin Rifampicin Statins Sucralfate Terfenadine Tricyclic antidepressants
Mouth wetting agents	–	Certain cultures	–
Nystatin	–	Gastrointestinal disturbance	–
Paracetamol	–	Alcoholism Anorexia Liver disease Renal disease	Alcohol Anticoagulants Anticonvulsants Busulphan Carbamazepine Cholestyramine Domperidone Isonicotinic hydrazide Metoclopramide Zidovudine
Penciclovir (topical)	–	–	–
Temazepam	–	Depression Driving or operating machinery Glaucoma Liver disease Myasthenia gravis Renal disease Respiratory problems	Alcohol CNS depressants Fluvoxamine Itraconazole Ketoconazole Nefazodone
Tetracyclines (e.g. doxycycline)	Children Myasthenia gravis	Lupus erythematosus Neuromuscular diseases Photosensitivity Renal disease	ACE inhibitors Antacids Anticoagulants Barbiturates Ciclosporin Cimetidine Iron Lithium Methotrexate Methoxyflurane Milk Oral contraceptive Retinoids Sulfonylureas
Vitamin B_{12}	–	–	–

*This list is not complete and there may be other drugs that can interact, including over-the-counter medications, vitamins, minerals, or herbal products. Always check BNF or other sources before use. See also http://www.drugs.com/drug-interactions.
MAOI, monoamine oxidase inhibitors; NSAIDs, nonsteroidal antiinflammatory drugs; SNRI, selective noradrenaline reuptake inhibitor; SSRI, selective serotonin reuptake inhibitor.

Table 5.19 Primary medical care or secondary care management (in addition to Table 5.18)*

Drug	Contraindications in addition to allergies to the agent, and possibly pregnancy and breastfeeding	Cautions	Most important potential interactions
Antimicrobials			
Clarithromycin	Children Myasthenia gravis Porphyria	Cardiac 'long QT syndrome' (personal or family history) Kidney disease Liver disease	Anticoagulants Antihistamines Antimuscarinics Artemeter Carbamazepine Ciclosporin Cisapride Clozapine Colchicine Corticosteroids Digoxin Dronedarone Droperidol Eletriptan Eplerenone Ergot Ivabradine Midazolam Moxifloxacin Nilotinib Omeprazole Pazopanib Phenytoin Pimozide Ranolazine Reboxetine Repaglinide Rifabutin Sulpride Sildenafil Sirolimus Statins Tacrolimus Tadalafil Vinorelbine
Analgesics			
Codeine phosphate	Liver disease	Cardiac arrhythmias	Alcohol MAOIs
Mefenamic acid	Epilepsy Inflammatory bowel disease Porphyria	Asthma Bleeding tendency Cardiac disease Liver disease Older patients Peptic ulcer Renal disease	Alcohol Anticoagulants Oral hypoglycaemics
Nefopam	Convulsive disorders Myocardial infarction	Liver disease Older patients Renal disease Urinary retention	Alcohol
Pentazocine	Children Hypertension Respiratory depression Head injuries or raised intracranial pressure		Alcohol Diazepam
Analgesics (opioids)			
Buprenorphine	Patients with head injury (interferes with pupillary responses and respiration) Liver disease Renal disease	Older patients May affect driving and skilled tasks	Alcohol Anaesthetics (general) Diazepam Grapefruit juice MAOIs

Table 5.19   Primary medical care or secondary care management (in addition to Table 5.18)*—Cont'd

Drug	Contraindications in addition to allergies to the agent, and possibly pregnancy and breastfeeding	Cautions	Most important potential interactions
Fentanyl	Patients with head injury (interferes with pupillary responses and suppresses respiration) Liver disease Renal disease	Cerebral tumour Diabetes Older patients May affect driving and skilled tasks	Alcohol Anaesthetics (general) Diazepam MAOIs
Methadone	Cardiac conduction issues especially long QT Phaeochromocytoma	Older patients May affect driving and skilled tasks	Alcohol Anaesthetics (general) Diazepam Grapefruit juice
Oxycodone	Patients with head injury (interferes with pupillary responses and suppresses respiration) Liver disease Porphyria Renal disease	Pancreatitis Psychoses Older patients May affect driving and skilled tasks	Alcohol Anaesthetics (general) Diazepam MAOIs
Pethidine	Patients with head injury (interferes with pupillary responses and suppresses respiration) Liver disease Renal disease	May cause arrhythmias, cor pulmonale, neurotoxicity Older patients May affect driving and skilled tasks	Alcohol Anaesthetics (general) Diazepam MAOIs Phenothiazines
Anxiolytics			
Buspirone	Epilepsy Liver disease	Non-benzodiazepine May affect driving and skilled tasks	Alcohol Grapefruit juice
Zopiclone	Liver disease Renal disease Respiratory or neuromuscular disease	Non-benzodiazepine Older patients May affect driving and skilled tasks	Alcohol
Antidepressants			
Amitriptyline	Arrhythmias Liver disease Porphyria Recent myocardial infarction	Diabetes Epilepsy Glaucoma Older patients Urinary retention May affect driving and skilled tasks Avoid sudden withdrawal	Alcohol Anaesthetics (general) Antiarrhythmics Anticoagulants Antidepressants Anticonvulsants Antihistamines Antipsychotics Anxiolytics Baclofen Cimetidine Lithium Sibutramine
Clomipramine	Arrhythmias Liver disease Porphyria Recent myocardial infarction	Diabetes Epilepsy Glaucoma Older patients Urinary retention May affect driving and skilled tasks Avoid sudden withdrawal	Alcohol Anaesthetics (general) Antiarrhythmics Anticoagulants Antidepressants Anticonvulsants Antihistamines Antipsychotics Anxiolytics Baclofen Cimetidine Lithium Sibutramine

Continued

Table 5.19 Primary medical care or secondary care management (in addition to Table 5.18)*—Cont'd

Drug	Contraindications in addition to allergies to the agent, and possibly pregnancy and breastfeeding	Cautions	Most important potential interactions
Dosulepin (dothiepin)	Arrhythmias Liver disease Porphyria Recent myocardial infarction	Diabetes Epilepsy Glaucoma Older patients Urinary retention May affect driving and skilled tasks Avoid sudden withdrawal	Alcohol Anaesthetics (general) Antiarrhythmics Anticoagulants Antidepressants Anticonvulsants Antihistamines Antipsychotics Anxiolytics Baclofen Cimetidine Lithium Sibutramine
Doxepin	Arrhythmias Liver disease Porphyria Recent myocardial infarction	Diabetes Epilepsy Glaucoma Older patients Urinary retention May affect driving and skilled tasks Avoid sudden withdrawal	Alcohol Anaesthetics (general) Antiarrhythmics Anticoagulants Antidepressants Anticonvulsants Antihistamines Antipsychotics Anxiolytics Baclofen Cimetidine Lithium Sibutramine
Fluoxetine	Mania Arrhythmias Liver disease Porphyria Recent myocardial infarction	Epilepsy Cardiac disease Glaucoma Liver disease Renal disease May affect driving and skilled tasks Avoid sudden withdrawal	Alcohol Anaesthetics (general) Antiarrhythmics Anticoagulants Antidepressants Anticonvulsants Antihistamines Antipsychotics Anxiolytics Carbamazepine Cimetidine Dopaminergics Lithium MAOIs Sibutramine Sumatriptan
Nortryptiline	Arrhythmias Liver disease Porphyria Recent myocardial infarction	Diabetes Epilepsy Glaucoma Older patients Urinary retention May affect driving and skilled tasks Avoid sudden withdrawal	Alcohol Anaesthetics (general) Antiarrhythmics Anticoagulants Antidepressants Anticonvulsants Antihistamines Antipsychotics Anxiolytics Baclofen Cimetidine Lithium Sibutramine

Table 5.19 Primary medical care or secondary care management (in addition to Table 5.18)*—Cont'd

Drug	Contraindications in addition to allergies to the agent, and possibly pregnancy and breastfeeding	Cautions	Most important potential interactions
Venlafaxine	Arrhythmias Hypertension	Bleeding tendency Epilepsy Cardiac disease Glaucoma Liver disease Mania Renal disease May affect driving and skilled tasks Avoid sudden withdrawal	Alcohol Anticoagulants Antidepressants Antipsychotics Dopaminergics Lithium NSAIDs Sibutramine
Antineuralgics			
Baclofen	Peptic ulceration	Common adverse effect of sedation Avoid abrupt withdrawal	ACE inhibitors Alcohol NSAIDs
Gabapentin	Diabetes Psychiatric disease Renal disease	Similar adverse effects to carbamazepine Headache common Avoid sudden withdrawal	Alcohol
Phenytoin	Han Chinese or other patients with HLA-B1502 Liver disease Porphyria	Similar adverse effects to carbamazepine Produces gingival swelling Avoid sudden withdrawal	Alcohol Aspirin Azoles Baclofen Carbamazepine Cimetidine Clarithromycin Disulphiram INAH Midazolam NSAIDs
Topiramate	Glaucoma Porphyria	Avoid abrupt withdrawal May cause glaucoma Caution in renal or hepatic disease	Alcohol
Immuno-modulators			Other immunosuppressants (increase the risk of infection)
Azathioprine	Low TPMT	Myelotoxic May also cause liver dysfunction, arrhythmias, hypotension, nephritis Increased liability to infection and, long term, possibly also neoplasia	ACE inhibitors Allopurinol (increases the effect of azathioprine) Aspirin (bleeding) Clozapine Co-trimoxazole Rifampicin Trimethoprim Warfarin
Ciclosporin (cyclosporin)	Hypertension Infections Malignant disease Porphyria Renal disease	Nephrotoxic Hepatotoxic May cause hypertension, blood dyscrasias, gingival swelling Increased liability to infection and, long term, possibly also neoplasia	ACE inhibitors Aciclovir Allopurinol, analgesics and antifungals (increase ciclosporin toxicity) Aminoglycosides Antibacterials (clarithromycin, erythromycin, doxycycline) Anticonvulsants (reduced efficiency) Azoles Carbamazepine Clarithromycin Colchicine Corticosteroids Diclofenac Erythromycin NSAIDs

Continued

Table 5.19 Primary medical care or secondary care management (in addition to Table 5.18)*—Cont'd

Drug	Contraindications in addition to allergies to the agent, and possibly pregnancy and breastfeeding	Cautions	Most important potential interactions
Colchicine	Cardiac disease Liver disease Older patients Renal disease	Myelotoxicity	Ciclosporin Clarithromycin Erythromycin Statins
Corticosteroids systemically	–	Adrenal suppression Diabetes Glaucoma Hypertension Mental health problems Osteoporosis Peptic ulcers Tuberculosis Malignant neoplasms	ACE inhibitors Aminoglycosides Anticoagulants Antidiabetics Aspirin/NSAIDS
Cyclophosphamide	Haemorrhagic cystitis	Leukopenia always (but reversible) Liver disease Renal disease Increase liability to infection and, long term, possibly also neoplasia	Clozapine Digoxin Itraconazole Phenytoin

Dapsone	Allergies to:
	  Naphthalene
	  Niridazole
	  Nitrofurantoin
	  Phenylhydrazine
	  Sulfa drugs
	  Primaquine
	Anaemia
	Glucose-6-phosphate dehydrogenase (G6PD) deficiency
	Liver disease
	Methaemoglobin reductase deficiency
	Porphyria
		Complications:
		Haematological (Agranulocytosis, Haemolysis, Methaemoglobinaemia)
		Liver dysfunction
		Renal dysfunction
		Hypersensitivity
		Photosensitivity
		Headaches
			Trimethoprim and methotrexate (increase risk of haematological complications)
			Rifamycin

Hydroxychloroquine	Liver disease Renal disease	May cause retinal damage May be myelotoxic Increased liability to infection and, long term, possibly also neoplasia	Amiodarone Anticonvulsants Ciclosporin Droperidol
Leflunomide		Hepatotoxic Myelotoxic	Never use with methotrexate Anticoagulants Phenytoin
Levamisole		May cause agranulocytosis	Alcohol Anticoagulants Phenytoin
Mycophenolate mofetil		May cause red cell aplasia and other blood dyscrasias Increased liability to infection and, long term, possibly also neoplasia	Aciclovir Antacids Metronidazole
Pentoxifylline	Cerebrovascular haemorrhage Myocardial infarction Porphyria Retinal haemorrhage	Caution in renal and hepatic disease Increased liability to infection and, long term, possibly also neoplasia	NSAIDs

Table 5.19 Primary medical care or secondary care management (in addition to Table 5.18)*—Cont'd

Drug	Contraindications in addition to allergies to the agent, and possibly pregnancy and breastfeeding	Cautions	Most important potential interactions
Tacrolimus		Cardiomyopathy Drowsiness may interfere with driving Increased liability to infection and, long term, possibly also neoplasia	Aciclovir Antifungals Ciclosporin Clarithromycin Erythromycin Grapefruit juice NSAIDS Omeprazole phenytoin
Thalidomide	Pregnancy	Caution in renal or liver disease Must take effective contraceptive measures while taking thalidomide and for 3 months after finishing tablets, and must not get pregnant Nerve damage Thromboses Thalidomide makes people feel drowsy. It should be taken at night. Drowsiness during the day makes it unsafe for patients to drive or operate machinery, and may impair alertness and ability to think clearly	Alcohol must be avoided

Antifungals

Drug	Contraindications in addition to allergies to the agent, and possibly pregnancy and breastfeeding	Cautions	Most important potential interactions
Fluconazole	Porphyria Renal disease	May be hepatotoxic and myelosuppressive	Anticoagulants Anticonvulsants Antidiabetic drugs Calcium channel blockers Carbamazepine Ciclosporin Cisapride Digoxin Midazolam Mizolastine Oral antidiabetics Oral contraceptive Parecoxib Phenytoin Pimozide Protease inhibitors Quinidine Rifampicin Sirolimus Statins Tacrolimus Terfenadine Vincristine Zidovudine
Ketoconazole	Liver disease Porphyria	Hepatotoxic Not absorbed in achlorhydria	Anticoagulants Antidiabetics drugs Carbamazepine Ciclosporin Cimetidine Cisapride Isoniazid Midazolam Phenytoin Ranitidine Rifampicin Sertindole Statins

Continued

Table 5.19 Primary medical care or secondary care management (in addition to Table 5.18)*—Cont'd

Drug	Contraindications in addition to allergies to the agent, and possibly pregnancy and breastfeeding	Cautions	Most important potential interactions
			Terfenadine Enhances nephrotoxicity of ciclosporin May impair oral contraceptive
Itraconazole	Cardiac failure Porphyria	Not absorbed in achlorhydria.	Anticoagulants Carbamazepine Ciclosporin Cisapride Digoxin Sertindole Midazolam Oral contraceptive Phenytoin Simvastatin Statins Terfenadine
Posaconazole	Cardiac disease Liver disease Porphyria		Anticoagulants Carbamazepine Ciclosporin Cisapride Digoxin Midazolam Oral contraceptive Phenytoin Sertindole Simvastatin Statins Terfenadine
Voriconazole	Cardiac disease – may prolong QT interval Liver disease Porphyria	Renal disease	Astemizole Carbamazepine Cisapride Terfenadine
Antiherpes agents (systemic)			
Aciclovir		Older patients Renal disease	Ciclosporin Mycophenolate NSAIDs Tacrolimus Zidovudine
Famciclovir		Renal disease	Probenecid
Valaciclovir		Renal disease	Ciclosporin Mycophenolate Tacrolimus
Sialogogues			
Pilocarpine	Asthma COPD Glaucoma	Driving or operating machinery	Alcohol Atropinics Beta blockers Biperiden Chlorphenamine Clozapine Dicyclomine Diuretics Procainamide Quinidine

*This list is not complete and there may be other drugs that can interact, including over-the-counter medications, vitamins, minerals, or herbal products. Always check BNF or other sources before use. See also http://www.drugs.com/drug-interactions.

COPD, chronic obstructive pulmonary disease; MAOI, monoamine oxidase inhibitors; NSAIDs, nonsteroidal antiinflammatory drugs; SNRI, selective noradrenaline reuptake inhibitor; SSRI, selective serotonin reuptake inhibitor.

USEFUL WEBSITES

Healthline, Drug Interaction Checker. http://www.
healthline.com/druginteractions/

Medscape, Multi-Drug Interaction Checker. http://
reference.medscape.com/drug-interactionchecker/

RxList, The Internet Drug Index. http://www.
rxlist.com/

Treatment Action Group, http://www.
treatmentactiongroup.org/publications

FURTHER READING

Meggitt, S.J., Anstey, A.V., Mohd Mustapa, M.F., et al.,
2011. British Association of Dermatologists' guidelines
for the safe and effective prescribing of azathioprine
2011. Br. J. Dermatol 165, 711–734.

O'Neill, I.D., 2008. Off-label use of biologicals in the
management of inflammatory oral mucosal disease.
J. Oral Pathol. Med 37 (10), 575–581.

O'Neill, I., Scully, C., 2012. Biologies in oral medicine:
principles of use and practical considerations. Oral
Dis. Mar 15 Epub.

O'Neill, I., Scully, C., 2012. Biologies in oral medicine:
ulcerative disorders. Oral Dis. Mar 13 Epub.

O'Neill, I., Scully, C., 2012. Biologies in oral medicine:
oral Crohn's disease and orofacial granulomatosis.
Oral Dis. Mar 13 Epub.

O'Neill, I., Scully, C., 2012. Biologies in oral medicine;
Sjognen syndrome. Oral Dis. Mar 13 Epub.

COMMON COMPLAINTS

When you treat a disease, first treat the mind.
Chen Jen

Cervical lymphadenopathy

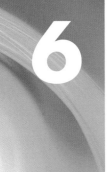

INTRODUCTION

Discrete swellings in the neck are often due to lymph node enlargement (cervical lymphadenopathy) but may occasionally be caused by disorders in:

- the salivary glands
- the thyroid gland
- other structures.

More diffuse swelling of the neck may be caused by obesity or:

- oedema (inflammatory or allergic)
- haematoma
- malignant infiltration
- surgical emphysema.

The location of a lump or swelling in the neck will often give a good indication of the tissue of origin, and the age of the patient may also help suggest the most likely diagnoses (**Box 6.1**). The duration of the lesion is also relevant: one that has been present since an early age is likely to be of congenital origin, while a lump appearing in later life and persisting may be malignant.

Although a wide range of diseases may present with lesions in the neck (**Fig. 6.1**), the most common complaint is of swelling and/or pain in the cervical lymph nodes (**Box 6.2**, **Algorithm 6.1**). This chapter concentrates on these. Over a quarter of the lymph nodes in the body are connected with lymph nodes situated in the head and the neck. The tonsil

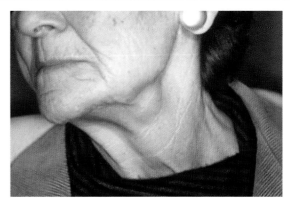

Fig. 6.1 Visible swelling in the submandibular triangle of the neck

---

BOX 6.1 Most common causes of swellings in the neck at different ages

Child (first decade)
- Lymphadenitis due to viral respiratory tract infection
- Kawasaki disease

Adolescent and teenager (second decade)
- Lymphadenitis due to viral respiratory tract infection
- Bacterial infection
- Glandular fever syndromes, including HIV infection
- Toxoplasmosis

Adult (third and fourth decades)
- Lymphadenitis
- Glandular fever syndromes, including HIV infection
- Malignancy

After fourth decade
- Lymphadenitis
- Malignancy

BOX 6.2 Main causes of cervical lymph node enlargement

Infections
- Viral upper respiratory tract: an enlarged jugulodigastric (tonsillar) lymph node, is common
- Oral or local bacterial in the drainage area (dental, scalp, ear, nose or throat): including cat-scratch fever and staphylococcal and mycobacterial lymphadenitis
- Systemic:
  - viral (e.g. infectious mononucleosis, cytomegalovirus, HIV infection)
  - bacterial, including syphilis, tuberculosis, brucellosis
  - fungal, including histoplasmosis
  - parasitic; toxoplasmosis, leishmaniasis, tularaemia

Malignant disease
- In the drainage area (usually oral, scalp, ear, nose or throat; rarely thyroid or gastric)
- Lymphoreticular (leukaemia, lymphoma)
- Langerhans histiocytosis

Inflammatory disorders
- Connective tissue disorders
- Orofacial granulomatosis
- Crohn disease
- Sarcoidosis

Others
- Drug-induced hypersensitivity syndrome (e.g. phenytoin) (see Table 24.26)
- Mucocutaneous lymph node syndrome (Kawasaki disease)

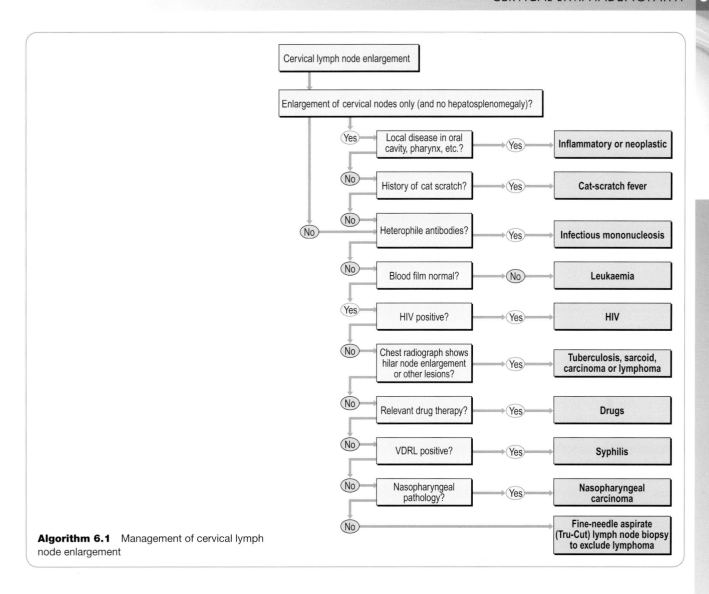

Algorithm 6.1 Management of cervical lymph node enlargement

is lymphoid tissue located between the pillars of the fauces, and there is similar material in the posterior third of the tongue (lingual tonsil) and the posterior wall of the pharynx (adenoids). These three areas form a ring of lymphoid tissue around the oropharynx (Waldeyer ring). It is not surprising then, that many diseases of the lymphoid tissue present primarily in the head and neck.

The dental surgeon can often detect serious disease through neck node examination. Tenderness, consistency and mobility should be documented. Both anterior and posterior cervical nodes should be examined as well as other nodes, liver and spleen if systemic disease is a possibility. Generalized lymphadenopathy with or without enlargement of other lymphoid tissue such as liver and spleen (hepatosplenomegaly) suggests a systemic cause.

their presence. The history should include: date of onset of symptoms; details of any swelling, such as duration and character; and any details of pain experienced, such as duration, character, radiation, aggravating and relieving factors, and associated phenomena.

Lymph nodes that are tender and mobile may be inflammatory (lymphadenitis). Lymph nodes swollen from acute infections are usually tender, soft and discrete, while chronic infections give firm lymph nodes. In the systemic infective disorders the nodes are usually firm, discrete, tender and mobile.

Nodes that are increasing in size and are hard, or fixed to adjacent tissues may be malignant. Nodes that are enlarged and firm and matted or rubbery may be due to leukaemia. In the lymphomas particularly, the nodes may be rubbery, matted together and fixed to deeper structures.

CLINICAL FEATURES

The patient may be aware that they have lymphadenopathy, usually termed 'glands in the neck'. The main complaint with respect to cervical lymph nodes is usually of swelling. Tenderness may have drawn the patient's attention to

AETIOLOGY AND PATHOGENESIS

Lymph nodes can enlarge in a number of disorders (see **Box 6.2**), often because of disease in the local area of drainage, sometimes because of disease affecting the wider lymphoreticular system (lymph nodes, liver and spleen).

83

Enlargement of the cervical lymph nodes alone usually arises because they are involved in an immune response to an infectious agent in the area of drainage which is anywhere on the face, scalp and nasal cavity, sinuses, ears, pharynx and oral cavity. Such lymphadenitis only rarely leads to suppuration. The local cause may not always be found however, despite a careful search; for example, young children (especially those of African heritage) occasionally develop a *Staphylococcus aureus* lymphadenitis (see below) or a similar problem due to atypical *Mycobacteria* (non-tuberculous mycobacteria; NTM) (usually in a submandibular node) in the absence of any obvious portal of infection or any clear explanation for their susceptibility. *Mycobacterium avium-intracellulare* complex (MAC) is the main organism involved but sometimes *M. kansasii* or *M. scrofulaceum* are implicated. These bacteria are common in soil and infection may be via the oral cavity; chemotherapy with antituberculous agents may be used but most lesions clear spontaneously over several months.

Enlargement of cervical lymph nodes alone may also occur when there is reactive hyperplasia to a malignant tumour in the drainage area, or metastatic infiltration. The latter may cause the node to feel distinctly hard, and it may become bound down to adjacent tissues ('fixed'), it may not be discrete, and may even, in advanced cases, ulcerate through the skin. Most disease is detected in nodes in the anterior triangle of the neck, which is bounded superiorly by the mandibular lower border, posteriorly and inferiorly by the sternomastoid muscle, and anteriorly by the midline of the neck. Nodes in this site drain most of the head and neck except the occiput and back of the neck. Lymphadenopathy in the anterior triangle of the neck alone is often due to local disease, especially if the nodes are enlarged on only one side.

Generalized lymph node enlargement, including cervical nodes, sometimes with liver and/or spleen involvement, may occur in:

- Systemic infections, such as the glandular fever syndromes. Lymphadenitis in tuberculosis may also lead to neck swelling (scrofula) and suppuration (cold abscess).
- Inflammatory lesions, such as connective tissue diseases and granulomatous conditions (Crohn disease, orofacial granulomatosis and sarcoidosis); and mucocutaneous lymph node syndrome (Kawasaki disease).
- Drug reactions (see Page 83).
- Neoplasms of the lymphoreticular system, such as lymphomas, leukaemias and histiocytoses (see **Box 6.2**). In some there is clinical involvement of the whole reticuloendothelial system, with generalized lymph node enlargement (detectable clinically in the neck, groin and axilla) and enlargement of both liver and spleen (hepatosplenomegaly). Rosai–Dorfman disease is a rare, non-neoplastic histiocytosis most commonly characterized by painless, massive cervical lymphadenopathy.

INFECTIVE INFLAMMATORY CONDITIONS
Viral infections with predominantly upper respiratory and oral manifestations

- Usually cause fever and malaise.
- Usually several anterior triangle nodes – especially the jugulodigastric nodes – are enlarged, often bilaterally.

Posterior triangle nodes are not enlarged and there is, of course, no generalized lymph node enlargement nor hepatosplenomegaly unless there are systemic complications or lesions elsewhere.

- Any viral upper respiratory infection from the common cold to viral tonsillitis can be responsible for enlarged cervical nodes (see **Box 6.2**).
- Oral viral infections that may cause cervical lymph node swelling are mainly those that also produce mouth ulcers such as:
  - herpes simplex stomatitis
  - herpangina
  - occasionally, herpes zoster of the trigeminal nerve (see Ch. 43).

Viral infections with multiple systemic manifestations

In these disorders there are typically fever and malaise and perhaps a rash, and there are usually several anterior and often posterior triangle nodes enlarged, with generalized enlargement and, in some instances, hepatosplenomegaly. Infections implicated are mainly:

- hand, foot and mouth disease (see Ch. 57)
- viral exanthemata (chickenpox, measles, rubella)
- glandular fever syndromes (Epstein–Barr virus, human herpesvirus 6, cytomegalovirus infections and HIV/AIDS).

Acute non-specific bacterial infections

Any bacterial infection in the area of drainage, such as an odontogenic infection (e.g. dental abscess, pericoronitis), sinusitis, or a boil in the nose, can cause enlargement of anterior cervical lymph nodes. Usually only one or two nodes are enlarged, often unilaterally and only in the anterior triangle in most instances. However, lesions on the back of the scalp or neck may cause enlargement of posterior cervical nodes.

Acute specific bacterial infections

Occasionally, specific acute bacterial infections involve lymph nodes, particularly in young children who can develop acute lymphadenitis caused by *Staphylococcus aureus* in the absence of any detectable entry point for the organism. These infections, usually of a submandibular lymph node, should be treated with antibiotics – usually flucloxacillin because the *S. aureus* is often penicillinase-producing. If the lesion is fluctuant and pointing, surgical drainage is needed.

Chronic specific bacterial infections

- Tuberculosis and atypical mycobacterial (non-tuberculous) infections (see Ch. 57).
- Secondary syphilis (see Ch. 57).
- Brucellosis.
- Cat-scratch disease (see Ch. 57).

Chronic granulomatous disease (CGD)

A rare genetic immune defect of leukocyte function in which neutrophils and macrophages fail to kill catalase-positive bacteria, such as staphylococci. Patients suffer from recurrent pyogenic infections and may develop suppurating cervical lymph nodes showing granulomas on biopsy.

Parasitic: toxoplasmosis, Leishmaniasis

For these conditions see Ch. 57.

NON-INFECTIVE INFLAMMATORY CONDITIONS

- Connective tissue diseases: cervical lymph nodes may be enlarged in rheumatoid arthritis or lupus erythematosus.
- Mucocutaneous lymph node syndrome (MLNS): Kawasaki disease (see Ch. 56).
- Granulomatous diseases: sarcoidosis (see Ch. 57), Crohn disease (see Ch. 57), orofacial granulomatosis (see Ch. 46).
- Drug-induced hypersensitivity syndrome (DIHS): also therefore called drug rash with eosinophilia and systemic symptoms (DRESS), is a severe immune-mediated reaction involving macrophage and T-lymphocyte activation and cytokine release, usually characterized by fever, rash, and multiorgan failure, occurring 1–8 weeks after exposure to various drugs (see Table 54.26). Diagnosis is supported by a finding of eosinophilia and abnormal liver function tests. There may be reactivation of herpesviruses including HHV-6, HHV-7, CMV and/or EBV. The mortality from drug hypersensitivity syndrome is estimated at around 8%. Specialist medical care is indicated with immediate withdrawal of all suspect medicines, followed by supportive care, typically with systemic corticosteroids.
- Others (e.g. Kikuchi disease: a self-limiting illness characterized by pyrexia, neutropenia and cervical lymphadenopathy in young women of Asian descent).

NEOPLASTIC CONDITIONS
Metastases

The neoplasms that usually metastasize to cervical lymph nodes are mainly head and neck cancers including:
- Oral squamous carcinoma (**Fig. 6.2**; see Ch. 31): usually one or more anterior cervical nodes are involved, often unilaterally in oral neoplasms anteriorly in the mouth, but otherwise not infrequently bilaterally.
- Tonsillar: clinically unsuspected tonsillar cancer is the commonest cause of metastasis in a cervical node of unidentified origin. Blind biopsy of the tonsil may reveal a hitherto unsuspected malignancy.
- Nasopharyngeal: clinically unsuspected nasopharyngeal cancer is a common cause of metastasis in a cervical node of unidentified origin. Blind biopsy of the nasopharynx, particularly the fossa of Rosenmuller or tonsil, may reveal a hitherto unsuspected malignancy.
- Laryngeal.
- Thyroid.
- Skin.

Other metastatic neoplasms (other than lymphoid)

Rarely, cervical metastases from the stomach or even testicular tumours to the lower cervical nodes, especially the

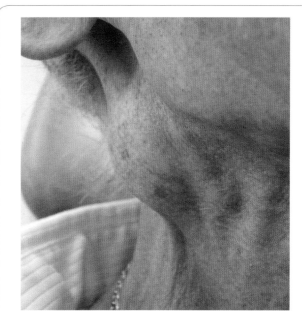

Fig. 6.2 Enlarged jugulodigastric lymph node from metastatic oral squamous cell carcinoma

supraclavicular nodes. In occasional patients with a malignant cervical lymph node, the primary tumour is never located.

Lymphoid malignancies

In lymphoid malignancies there is usually swelling both of anterior and posterior cervical lymph nodes together with generalized lymph node enlargement and often hepatosplenomegaly.

Histiocytoses

Management should be of the underlying Langerhans histiocytosis or Rosai–Dorfman disease (see Ch. 56).

MANAGEMENT OF A PATIENT WITH CERVICAL LYMPHADENOPATHY

Most enlarged lymph nodes have an infectious aetiology. A full blood count, ESR, serology and SACE levels may help the diagnosis (**Table 6.1**). If aspects of the clinical picture suggest chronic infection or malignancy, such as persistent fevers or weight loss, chest imaging, MRI scan and lesional biopsy should be pursued sooner (**Table 6.2**). Fine-needle aspiration (FNA) of the cervical lymph nodes is the most reliable diagnostic method for many disorders, including tuberculosis (see Ch. 57). If TB is suspected, though few patients have positive chest radiographs, and there is a variable response to the tuberculin skin test, and often a negative culture for mycobacterial organisms, these investigations are indicated, as are DNA studies.

Table 6.1 Aids that might be helpful in diagnosis/prognosis/management in some patients with cervical lymphadenopathy thought related to infection/inflammation*

In most cases	In some cases
Full blood picture	ESR
	ANA
	RF
	SACE
	Serology and DNA studies for viral or bacterial diseases, or toxoplasmosis
	Tuberculin test
	US-FNA
	Chest imaging
	MRI neck
	Biopsy

*See text for details and glossary for abbreviations.

Table 6.2 Aids that might be helpful in diagnosis/prognosis/management in some patients with cervical lymphadenopathy thought related to malignant disease*

In most cases	In some cases
Full blood picture	ESR
Ultrasound	Thyroid scan
FNA	Examination under anaesthetic
MRI	Blind biopsy of nasopharynx/tonsil
Biopsy	

*See text for details and glossary for abbreviations.

FURTHER READING

Alawi, F., Robinson, B.T., Carrasco, L., 2006. Rosai–Dorfman disease of the mandible. Oral Surg. Oral Med. Oral Pathol. Oral Radiol. Endod. 102 (4), 506–512.

Chang, J.T., Huang, Y.F., Lin, Y.T., et al., 2006. *Mycobacterium abscessus* cervical lymphadenitis: an immunocompetent child. Kaohsiung J. Med. Sci. 22 (8), 415–419.

Chuang, C.H., Hsiao, M.H., Chiu, C.H., et al., 2006. Kawasaki disease in infants three months of age or younger. J. Microbiol. Immunol. Infect. 39 (5), 387–391.

Connor, S.E., Olliff, J.F., 2000. Imaging of malignant cervical lymphadenopathy. Dentomaxillofac. Radiol. 29, 133–143.

Freeman, A.F., Shulman, S.T., 2006. Kawasaki disease: summary of the American Heart Association guidelines. Am. Fam. Phys. 74 (7), 1141–1148.

Helvaci, S., Gedikoglu, S., Akalin, H., et al., 2000. Tularemia in Bursa, Turkey: 205 cases in ten years. Eur. J. Epidemiol. 16, 271–276.

Kanlikama, M., Mumbuc, S., Bayazit, Y., et al., 2000. Management strategy of mycobacterial cervical lymphadenitis. J. Laryngol. Otol. 114, 274–278.

Kundu, S.S., Das, B.K., Talukdar, A., et al., 2006. Pyrexia of unknown origin with neutropenia, cervical lymphadenopathy, pneumonia and marrow hypoplasia. J. Assoc. Physicians India 54, 661.

Morais, A., Figueiredo, S., Moreira, E., et al., 2005. Clinical aspects and characteristics at presentation in sarcoidosis patients. Rev. Port. Pneumo 11 (6 Suppl. 1), 31–32.

Thavagnanam, S., McLoughlin, L.M., Hill, C., Jackson, P.T., 2006. Atypical Mycobacterial infections in children: the case for early diagnosis. Ulster. Med. J. 75 (3), 192–194.

Vasallo Morillas, J.R., Perera Penate, J., Osorio Acosta, A., et al., 2000. Inflammatory pseudotumor of the lymph nodes. A case report. Acta Otorrinolaringol. Esp 51, 88–91.

Weiler, Z., Nelly, P., Baruchin, A.M., et al., 2000. Diagnosis and treatment of cervical tuberculous lymphadenitis. J. Oral Maxillofac. Surg. 58, 477–481.

Drooling and sialorrhoea

INTRODUCTION

Drooling is defined as saliva beyond the margins of the lips. Increased salivary flow is termed sialorrhoea or ptyalism.

INCIDENCE

People at the extremes of age, the chronically debilitated, or those in chronic care facilities, especially when associated with cerebrovascular events and oesophageal cancer, are especially affected by drooling. True sialorrhoea is rare.

AGE

Drooling is perfectly normal in healthy infants, but usually stops by about 18 months of age and is considered abnormal if it persists beyond the age of 4 years.

GENDER

Drooling can occur in either gender.

GEOGRAPHIC

Drooling has no known geographic incidence.

PREDISPOSING FACTORS

Drooling is a problem for many children with cerebral palsy, intellectual disability and other neurological conditions, and in adults who have Parkinson disease or have cerebral palsy, intellectual disability, or have had a stroke (cerebrovascular event; CVE), pseudobulbar palsy, or bulbar palsy.

AETIOLOGY AND PATHOGENESIS

Drooling is caused either by increased saliva flow (sialorrhoea) that cannot be compensated for by swallowing, or by poor oral and facial muscle control in patients with swallowing dysfunction (secondary sialorrhoea), or by anatomic or neuromuscular anomalies (**Table 7.1**).

CLINICAL FEATURES

Drooling (**Fig. 7.1**) impacts on patients, families, and/or caregivers:

- Functionally: saliva soils clothing (of patient, peers, siblings, parents and caregivers), furniture, carpets, teaching materials, communicative devices and toys.
- Socially: embarrassment may make it difficult for patients to interact with their peers and can lead to isolation.
- Psychologically: stigmatism is common.
- Clinically: drooling persons are at increased risk of skin maceration, infection periorally and on the neck, chest, and hands and aspiration-related respiratory infections. Pulmonary complications are greatest in those with a diminished sensation of salivary flow and hypopharyngeal retention.

DIAGNOSIS

History helps assess the severity and frequency of drooling, and the effect on the quality of life of patient and family. Quantitative measurements can be helpful for guiding treatment decisions (**Table 7.2**): counting the number of bibs or items of clothing soiled each day provides a subjective estimate. Examination should include:

- head position and control
- perioral skin condition
- dentition and occlusion: malocclusion, particularly an open bite deformity, is common in patients with cerebral palsy and can make proper oral hygiene difficult to maintain
- tongue size and control and the presence of thrusting behaviours
- tonsil and adenoid size
- gag reflex and intraoral tactile sensitivity
- mouth breathing, nasal obstruction and appearance of tissues upon anterior rhinoscopy
- swallowing efficiency: determined by observation, barium swallow, or fibreoptic endoscopic evaluation of swallowing
- neurologic examination: cranial nerve examination.

Investigations (**Table 7.3**) may include:

- Flexible nasopharyngoscopy, lateral neck radiography or MRI to detect adenoid hypertrophy.
- Modified barium swallow to help rule out the contraindications to surgical therapy, including oesophageal motility disorders, oesophageal spasm or aspiration.

Table 7.1 Causes of drooling

Excessive saliva production (sialorrhoea)	Decreased swallowing	Anatomic abnormalities	Neuromuscular diseases
Oral lesions or foreign bodies Neurologic disorders (especially Riley–Day syndrome, Ch. 56) Otolaryngologic diseases Pregnancy Gastrointestinal causes Liver disease Drugs and poisons parathion, strychnine, (Table 54.6)	Oropharyngeal infections and obstruction	Macroglossia or tongue thrusting Surgical defects following major head and neck surgery	Parkinson disease, cerebral palsy, intellectual impairment, stroke, pseudobulbar palsy, bulbar palsy, anterior opercular syndrome (Foix–Chavany–Marie syndrome, Ch. 56) Rabies

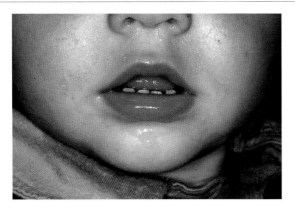

Fig. 7.1 Drooling

Table 7.3 Aids that might be helpful in diagnosis/prognosis/management in some patients with drooling and sialorrhoea*

In most cases	In some cases
Sialometry	Psychological assessment Flexible nasopharyngoscopy Lateral neck radiography MRI Modified barium swallow Radiosialography Audiography

*See text for details and glossary for abbreviations.

Table 7.2 Quantitation of drooling

Condition	Description
Dry	Never drools
Mild	Only lips wet Occasional drooling – not every day
Moderate frequent drooling	Lips and chin wet – every day
Constant drooling	Severe – clothing soiled Profuse – hands moist and wet

- Radiosialography, a dynamic study of the salivary glands by 99m Tc-pertechnetate for evaluating salivary secretory function.
- Audiography to detect unilateral hearing impairment in patients considered for tympanic neurectomy or chorda tympani nerve section (because of the risk of hearing loss associated with these procedures).

TREATMENT (see also Chs 4 and 5)

- Treatment is best by a team approach, including at least an otolaryngologist, neurologist, surgeon, dentist, orthodontist, and speech, occupational and physical therapists.
- The impact of drooling on the quality of life is the most important factor in determining the treatment needs.

- The goal is to reduce drooling whilst maintaining a moist, healthy oral cavity.
- Treatment options include medical therapy, radiotherapy and surgery.

MEDICAL THERAPY

- Oral motor training: exercises to improve muscle tone, increase lip closure, and promote swallowing.
- Behaviour therapy: biofeedback and automatic cueing techniques.
- Medication to reduce saliva to amounts that can be swallowed (to prevent 'pool and drool') without producing hyposalivation (**Table 7.4**), by:
  - reducing cholinergic activity, either systemically (e.g. atropine-related anticholinergics orally), hyoscine transdermal patch, or more locally (e.g. sublingual ipratropium spray). These drugs are contraindicated in patients with asthma, or ocular problems such as glaucoma, or synechia (adhesions) between the iris and lens.
  - increasing adrenergic activity (e.g. clonidine patch)
  - botulinum toxin type A injected under ultrasound guidance into the parotid and submandibular glands.

RADIOTHERAPY

Irradiation of the major salivary glands has been used to reduce salivation, but has variable success, and potential risks of late malignancy.

Table 7.4 Medications used to reduce drooling/sialorrhoea

Agent	Adult dosage	Potential adverse effects apart from hyposalivation
Botulinum toxin A	Single injections of 10–40 units, under US guidance, into major glands	Pain at injection site
Clonidine	0.25 mg twice daily	May cause drowsiness and interfere with driving
Glycopyrrolate*	Start 0.5 mg orally, one to three times daily; titrate to effectiveness and tolerability	Constipation, urinary retention, blurred vision, hyperactivity, irritability
Ipratropium*	Spray 250 µg/mL sublingually as needed	Nausea, urinary retention, blurred vision, glaucoma
Scopolamine (hyoscine)*	One 1.5 mg patch every day	Pruritus at patch site, urinary retention, irritability, blurred vision, dizziness, glaucoma
Trihexyphenidyl (benzhexol)*	1 mg daily	Drowsiness, vertigo, headache, glaucoma, urinary retention

*Atropinics – care in patients with cardiovascular disease, older patients, glaucoma or urinary obstruction; caution with driving; avoid in gastrointestinal obstruction and myasthenia gravis.

SURGERY

Surgery (**Table 7.5**) is indicated where drooling:

- persists after at least 6 months of conservative therapy; or
- is moderate to profuse and in a patient whose cognitive function precludes use of conservative therapy.

Surgical procedures to control drooling are aimed at decreasing salivary flow, or redirecting it to a location more advantageous to promote swallowing. Procedures include salivary:

- gland excision
- duct re-routing
- duct ligation or
- nerve sectioning (neurectomy), or combinations of the above.

Table 7.5 Surgical treatment of drooling/sialorrhoea

Surgical therapy	Advantages	Disadvantages
Submandibular gland excision	Good reduction in salivation	General anaesthesia usually needed External scar Potential for dental caries
Submandibular duct re-routing	Redirects saliva flow No external scar	General anaesthesia usually needed Potential for anterior dental caries Potential for aspiration Without sublingual gland excision, patient may develop ranula
Parotid duct re-routing	Redirects saliva flow	General anaesthesia usually needed Risk of sialocele Potential for aspiration
Parotid duct ligation	Does not require general anaesthesia Simple procedure	Risk of sialocele
Transtympanic neurectomy	Does not require general anaesthesia Technically simple, fast procedure Useful in older patients	Predictable return of salivary function Requires repeating

Adapted from Hockstein et al 2004.

FURTHER READING

Arbouw, M.E., Movig, K.L., Koopmann, M., et al., 2010. Glycopyrrolate for sialorrhea in Parkinson disease: a randomized, doubleblind, crossover trial. Neurology 74 (15), 1203–1207.

Arvedson, J., Clark, H., Lazarus, C., 2010. The effects of oral-motor exercises on swallowing in children: an evidence-based systematic review. Dev. Med. Child Neurol. 52 (11), 1000–1013.

Carranza del Rio, J., Clegg, N.J., Moore, A., et al., 2011. Use of trihexyphenidyl in children with cerebral palsy. Pediatr. Neurol. 44 (3), 202–206.

Crysdale, W.S., Raveh, E., McCann, C., et al., 2001. Management of drooling in individuals with neurodisability: a surgical experience. Dev. Med. Child Neurol. 43, 379–383.

Fairhurst, C.B.R., Cockerill, H., 2011. Management of drooling in children. Arch. Dis. Child Educ. Pract. Ed. 96, 25–30.

Freudenreich, O., 2005. Drug-induced sialorrhea. Drugs Today (Barc) 41 (6), 411–418.

Hockstein, N.G., Samadi, D.S., Gendron, K., Handler, S.D., 2004. Sialorrhea: a management challenge. Am. Fam. Phys. 69, 2628–2634.

Inga, C.J., Reddy, A.K., Richardson, S.A., Sanders, B., 2001. Appliance for chronic drooling in cerebral palsy patients. Pediatr. Dent. 23, 241–242.

Lamey, P.J., Clifford, T.J., El-Karim, I.A., Cooper, C., 2006. Personality analysis of patients complaining of sialorrhoea. J. Oral Pathol. Med. 35 (5), 307–310.

Mato, A., Limeres, J., Tomás, I., et al., 2010. Management of drooling in disabled patients with scopolamine patches. Br. J. Clin. Pharmacol. 69 (6), 684–688.

Meningaud, J.P., Pitak-Arnnop, P., Chikhani, L., Bertrand, J.C., 2006. Drooling of saliva: a review of the etiology and management options. Oral Surg. Oral Med. Oral Pathol. Oral Radiol. Endod. 101 (1), 48–57.

Mier, R.J., Bachrach, S.J., Lakin, R.C., et al., 2000. Treatment of sialorrhea with glycopyrrolate: a double-blind, dose-ranging study. Arch. Pediatr. Adolesc. Med. 154, 1214–1218.

Panarese, A., Ghosh, S., Hodgson, D., et al., 2001. Outcomes of submandibular duct re-implantation for sialorrhoea. Clin. Otolaryngol. 26, 143–146.

Porta, M., Gamba, M., Bertacchi, G., Vaj, P., 2001. Treatment of sialorrhoea with ultrasound guided botulinum toxin type A injection in patients with neurological disorders. J. Neurol. Neurosurg. Psychiat. 70, 538–540.

Praharaj, S.K., Verma, P., Roy, D., Singh, A., 2005. Is clonidine useful for treatment of clozapine-induced sialorrhea? J. Psychopharmacol 19 (4), 426–428.

Reddihough, D., Erasmus, C.E., Johnson, H., et al., 2010. Botulinum toxin assessment, intervention and aftercare for paediatric and adult drooling: international consensus statement. Eur. J. Neurol. 17, 109–121.

Reed, J., Mans, C.K., Brietzke, S.E., 2009. Surgical management of drooling: a meta-analysis. Arch. Otolaryngol. Head Neck Surg. 135 (9), 924–931.

Scully, C., Limeres, J., Gleeson, M., et al., 2009. Drooling. J. Oral Pathol. Med. 38 (4), 321–327.

Serrano-Duenas, M., 2003. Treatment of sialorrhea in Parkinson's disease patients with clonidine. Double-blind, comparative study with placebo. Neurologia 18 (1), 2–6.

Thomsen, T.R., Galpern, W.R., Asante, A., et al., 2007. Ipratropium bromide spray as treatment for sialorrhea in Parkinson's disease. Mov. Disord. 22 (15), 2268–2273.

Wong, V., Sun, J.G., Wong, W., 2001. Traditional Chinese medicine (tongue acupuncture) in children with drooling problems. Pediatr. Neurol. 25, 47–54.

Dry mouth (xerostomia and hyposalivation)

INTRODUCTION

Saliva is essential to oral health, and patients who have decreased salivary flow (hyposalivation) suffer from lack of oral lubrication, affecting many functions, and may develop infections as a consequence of the reduced defences.

Dry mouth (xerostomia) is a complaint that is the most common salivary problem and is the subjective sense of dryness which may be due to:

- reduced salivary flow (hyposalivation)
- changed salivary composition.

Advancing age is increasingly associated with dry mouth, but this is usually due to medication or disease, rather than age *per se*. Age does, however, result in an increase in adipose tissue and in a reduction of salivary acini, in salivary secretory reserve and in proteins such as MG1 and MG2 mucins.

AETIOLOGY AND PATHOGENESIS

Dry mouth is common in mouth-breathers and during periods of anxiety. Salivation is significantly reduced during sleep. Other than these, the causes can be remembered from the mnemonic 'men can see dangerous practices' (**Box 8.1**).

The main causes of dry mouth are iatrogenic (Ch. 54) and salivary gland diseases:

- Drugs with anticholinergic or sympathomimetic or diuretic activity are the most common cause (**Box 8.2** and **Fig. 8.1**). There is usually a fairly close temporal relationship between starting the drug treatment or increasing the dose, and experiencing the dry mouth. However, the cause for which the drug is being taken may also be important; for example, patients with anxiety or depressive conditions may complain of dry mouth even in the absence of drug therapy (or evidence of reduced salivary flow).

BOX 8.1   Main causes of dry mouth

- Medications
- Cancer treatments
- Salivary disease
- Dehydration
- Psychogenic

- Irradiation involving the salivary glands can produce profound hyposalivation, such as in treatment for neoplastic conditions in the head and neck, or in mantle irradiation in lymphomas, or total body irradiation (TBI) before haematopoietic stem cell transplant (bone marrow transplant). Chemotherapy and graft-versus-host disease (GVHD) can also produce hyposalivation (Ch. 54).
- Dehydration, as in diabetes mellitus, diabetes insipidus, hyperparathyroidism or any fever, is an occasional cause of hyposalivation.
- Disorders affecting salivary glands such as Sjögren syndrome, sarcoidosis and some viral infections (e.g. EBV, CMV, HIV, HCV) may cause hyposalivation.
- Psychogenic causes may underlie the complaint of dry mouth; objective evidence for hyposalivation may be lacking.
- Rarely there is salivary gland aplasia, or cholinergic dysfunction (congenital or autoimmune).

CLINICAL FEATURES

The patient with hyposalivation may complain of dry mouth alone, or combined with other features, such as dryness of the eyes and other mucosae (nasal, laryngeal, genital), with other eye complaints (inability to cry, blurring, light intolerance, burning, itching or grittiness), and sometimes voice or other changes (see Sjögren syndrome, Ch. 50).

In hyposalivation there may be:

- difficulty in swallowing- especially in eating dry foods, such as biscuits (the cracker sign)
- difficulty in controlling dentures
- difficulty in speaking, as the tongue tends to stick to the palate; this can lead to 'clicking' speech
- mouth soreness
- unpleasant taste or change in or loss of sense of taste
- a dry mucosa (**Fig. 8.2**) – the lips adhere one to another and an examining dental mirror may stick to the mucosa
- lipstick or food debris sticking to the teeth (**Fig. 8.3**)
- lack of the usual pooling of saliva in the floor of the mouth
- thin lines of frothy saliva may form along lines of contact of the oral soft tissues or in the vestibule
- saliva not expressible from the salivary ducts
- a characteristic lobulated tongue, usually red, with partial or complete depapillation
- complications of hyposalivation.

BOX 8.2   More advanced list of causes of dry mouth

Iatrogenic causes: drugs (Table 54.4)
- Atropine, atropinics and hyoscine
- Antidepressants: tricyclic (e.g. amitriptyline, nortriptyline, clomipramine and dosulepin), selective serotonin re-uptake inhibitors (e.g. fluoxetine), lithium and some other antidepressants
- Antihypertensives: may also cause a compositional change in saliva. α_1-Antagonists (e.g. terazosin and prazosin) and α_2-agonists (e.g. clonidine) may reduce salivary flow. Beta blockers (e.g. atenolol and propranolol) reduce protein levels
- Opioids
- Cytotoxic drugs
- Many others

Other iatrogenic causes
- Irradiation
- External beam
- Radioiodine
- Graft-versus-host disease

Dehydration (e.g. diabetes, hypercalcaemia, renal disease, diarrhoea and vomiting)

Salivary gland disease
- Aplasia (agenesis)
- Cystic fibrosis
- Deposits (haemochromatosis, hyperlipidaemia, amyloidosis)
- Ectodermal dysplasia
- IgG4 syndrome
- Infections (HIV, hepatitis C, EBV, CMV, human T lymphotropic virus 1 (HTLV-1))
- Parotidectomy
- Primary biliary cirrhosis
- Sarcoidosis
- Sjögren syndrome

Neural
- Alzheimer disease
- Anxiety states
- Autonomic cholinergic dysfunction
- Bulimia
- Dysautonomia (Allgrove syndrome (Ch. 56), diabetes, dysautonomia, hypothyroidism)
- Psychogenic

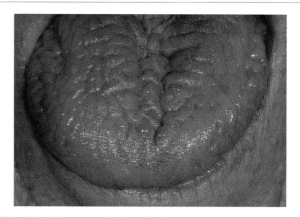

Fig. 8.2   Dryness evident on the tongue

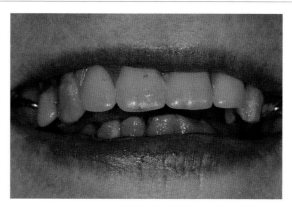

Fig. 8.3   Dryness causing lipstick and food retention

ORAL COMPLICATIONS

Oral complications of hyposalivation may also include:

- halitosis (oral malodour) (Ch. 9)
- dental caries, which tends to involve smooth surfaces and areas otherwise not very prone to caries – such as the lower incisor region. Caries can also involve roots and be severe and difficult to control
- candidosis (Ch. 39), which may cause:
  - burning sensation
  - taste changes
  - intolerance of acids and spices
  - mucosal erythema
  - lingual filiform papillae atrophy
  - angular stomatitis (angular cheilitis)
- ascending (suppurative) sialadenitis (Ch. 15), which presents with pain and swelling of a major salivary gland, and sometimes purulent discharge from the duct.

DIAGNOSIS

Hyposalivation is a clinical diagnosis, made predominantly on the basis of the history and examination and measurement of salivary flow (sialometry). The aims are to document the degree of salivary dysfunction and to determine the cause (**Algorithm 8.1**).

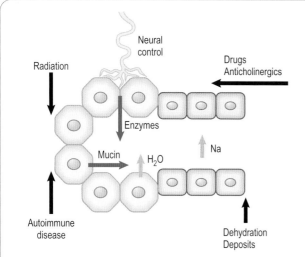

Fig. 8.1   Dry mouth; causes

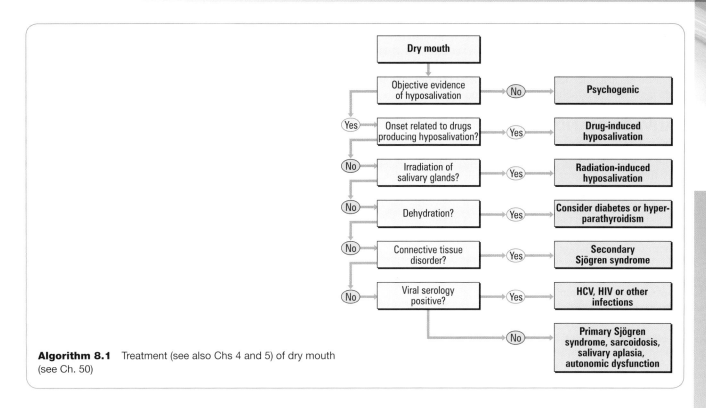

Algorithm 8.1 Treatment (see also Chs 4 and 5) of dry mouth (see Ch. 50)

SALIVARY STUDIES

It can be helpful to document salivary function by salivary function studies, especially studies of the salivary flow rates (sialometry). Ultrasonography is also useful. Other studies such as sialography, salivary scintiscanning and salivary biopsy, are less commonly used. Sialoendoscopy has no role in assessment of hyposalivation.

SALIVARY FLOW RATES (SIALOMETRY)

Salivary flow rate estimation (**Fig. 8.4**) is simple, non-invasive, inexpensive but not especially sensitive and a non-specific indicator of salivary gland dysfunction usually carried out by one of two possible methods:

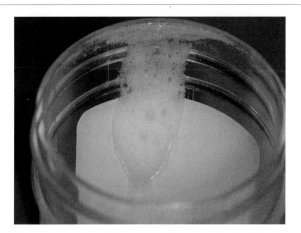

Fig. 8.4 Dryness evident on unstimulated whole sialometry

- Unstimulated whole saliva flow rate (this more closely correlates with symptoms of hyposalivation than do stimulated flow rates). The test should be standardized by being carried out first thing in morning after overnight fasting; no food or drink for at least 1 h before the test; no smoking for at least 1 h before the test. Allow the patient to dribble into a measuring container over 15 min. A resting secretion rate of <1.5 mL in 15 min indicates hyposalivation: in a normal person the unstimulated whole saliva flow rate exceeds 1.5 mL/15 min (0.1 mL/min).
- Stimulated saliva flow rate. Use various means of stimulation, such as 10% citric acid dropped onto the tongue, and collect parotid saliva using a Carlsson–Crittenden cup placed over Stensen papilla. A flow of <0.5 mL per gland in 5 min or <1 mL per gland in 10 min is decreased. In normal persons the flow should well exceed 1 mL/min.

ULTRASONOGRAPHY

Ultrasonography provides information about the changes to major salivary glands during inflammation. It reveals for example, decreased echogenicity and volume of submandibular glands in patients with Sjögren syndrome, with a high specificity and moderate sensitivity.

SIALOGRAPHY

Sialography, in which radio-opaque dye, often iodine-based, is introduced into the salivary duct, is non-specific. It may be of value if there is dilatation or duct obstruction (e.g. by a calculus, though this rarely causes dryness), but carries risks of discomfort and infection.

SALIVARY SCINTISCANNING

Salivary scintiscanning non-invasively examines all major salivary glands simultaneously, but is associated with a small radiation hazard since technetium-99 m, a γ-emitting radionuclide is used. It is not always available and is expensive.

SALIVARY GLAND BIOPSY

Although it is perfectly possible to biopsy the parotid or other major gland, there is a small risk of nerve damage or salivary fistula, and an extraoral approach will leave a small scar. Therefore, biopsy of minor salivary glands is usually done. Minor glands in the palate and lower lip are accessible, but the latter site is preferred both from the aspects of patient comfort and access for the operator, and also because the extent and pattern of histopathological changes on labial salivary gland (LSG) biopsy correlate with those in major glands. Glands in the lower labial mucosa are selected, since they are readily biopsied through a simple incision in the labial mucosa under local analgesia. The incision is paramedian, placed in the lower labial mucosa (avoiding any clinically obvious mucosal lesions, which could confuse the diagnosis) and is thus not visible externally. Four to six lobules of salivary glands should be removed. The wound is closed with one or two sutures and, apart from mild discomfort in many and anaesthesia or hypoaesthesia in some cases, complications are rare.

DETERMINATION OF THE CAUSE OF XEROSTOMIA

The history and examination may help to determine the cause of a complaint of xerostomia, and determine whether or not there is objective evidence of hyposalivation. It is important to recognize that some patients complaining of dry mouth have no evidence of reduced salivary flow or a salivary disorder; there may then be a psychogenic reason for the complaint.

If there is hyposalivation, investigations may be indicated to exclude systemic causes noted above. Commonly indicated investigations may thus include the following (**Table 8.1**):

- Eye tests, using Schirmer test of lacrimal flow (**Fig. 8.5**), and slit-lamp examination, mainly to exclude Sjögren syndrome (see Ch. 50).
- Urinalysis, mainly to exclude diabetes.
- Blood tests:
  - ESR, CRP or PV – non-specific tests mainly to exclude Sjögren syndrome or sarcoidosis
  - antinuclear antibodies (ANA) – including SS-A and SS-B antibodies, mainly to exclude Sjögren syndrome and lupus erythematosus (see Ch. 50)
  - rheumatoid factor (RF), mainly to exclude Sjögren syndrome
  - serum liver function tests, and antimitochondrial autoantibodies to exclude primary biliary cirrhosis
  - serum immunoglobulin levels, a non-specific test mainly to exclude connective tissue diseases
  - serum immunoglobulin IgG4 levels, to exclude IgG4 syndrome (see Ch. 50)
  - serum angiotensin-converting enzyme (SACE), mainly to exclude sarcoidosis
  - serum calcium and phosphate, mainly to exclude hyperparathyroidism

Table 8.1 Aids that might be helpful in diagnosis/prognosis/management in some patients with dry mouth (xerostomia and hyposalivation)*

In most cases	In some cases
Sialometry	Sialography
Antinuclear antibodies (ANA) SS-A and SS-B antibodies	Salivary scintiscanning
	Salivary gland biopsy
	Eye tests, e.g. Schirmer
Blood glucose	Urinalysis
ESR	Serum ferritin, vitamin B$_{12}$ and corrected whole blood folate levels
Full blood picture	
Rheumatoid factor (RF)	
	Blood CD4 cell counts
	Complement levels
	Serum immunoglobulin levels
	Serum immunoglobulin IgG4 levels
	Serum liver function tests, and antimitochondrial autoantibodies
	Serum angiotensin-converting enzyme (SACE)
	Serum calcium and phosphate
	Serology-viral (HCV, HIV)
	Thyroid function tests
	Chest radiography
	Ultrasonography
	MRI
	Psychological assessment

*See text for details and glossary for abbreviations.

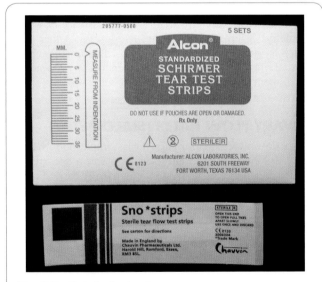

Fig. 8.5 Tests for lacrimation

  - serology, to exclude viral causes
  - blood glucose, to exclude diabetes.
- Imaging:
  - chest radiography, mainly to exclude sarcoidosis
  - ultrasonography, mainly to exclude Sjögren syndrome or neoplasia
  - MRI, mainly to exclude Sjögren syndrome.
- Salivary biopsy may be indicated if there is suspicion of organic disease of the salivary glands.

TREATMENT (see also Chs 4 and 5)

- If there is objective evidence of hyposalivation, any underlying cause should, if possible, be rectified; for example, hyposalivation-producing drugs may be changed for an alternative, and causes such as diabetes should be treated.
- Efforts should be made to avoid factors that may increase dryness, such as:
  - dry hot environments
  - dry foods such as biscuits
  - drugs (e.g. tricyclic antidepressants or diuretics)
  - alcohol (including alcohol-based mouthwashes)
  - smoking
  - beverages that produce diuresis (coffee and tea).
- The mouth should be hydrated as regularly as possible. The lips may become dry, atrophic and susceptible to cracking and thus should be kept moist using a water-based lubricant or a lanolin-based product rather than one containing petroleum-derived lubricants (e.g. Vaseline). Olive oil, vitamin E or lip balm may help.
- Mouth wetting agents (salivary substitutes) may help symptomatically. Various are available, including:
  - water or ice chips: frequent sips of water are generally more effective than synthetic salivary substitutes
  - synthetic salivary substitutes, which vary in properties and patient acceptability, fluoride content and pH (**Table 8.2**). Synthetic salivary substitutes usually contain: carboxymethylcellulose (UK: Glandosane, Luborant (contains fluoride), Salivace, Saliveze. USA: Moi-Stir, Orex, Salivart, Xero-Lube, Mouth-Kote), mucin (Saliva Orthana; also contains xylitol and fluoride) or glycerate polymer (Oral Balance; also contains xylitol, glucose

oxidase and lactoperoxidase). A home preparation can be made using ¼ teaspoon of glycerine in 8 ounces of water (approximately 250 mL).
- Salivation may be promoted by using a stimulant: (sialogogue) such as;
  - chewing gums (containing sorbitol or xylitol, not sucrose)
  - diabetic sweets
  - cholinergic drugs such as pilocarpine, bethanecol, cevimeline or anetholetrithione.
- Oral complications, such as dental caries, should be prevented and treated with:
  - dietary control of sucrose intake
  - regular dental checks and monitoring of *Streptococcus mutans* counts
  - topical fluorides (reduce caries risk by reducing demineralization and by increasing remineralization)
  - full-strength fluoride toothpastes containing 1000–1500 ppm fluoride should be used at least twice daily. Higher content pastes may be indicated
  - fluoride rinses of 0.05% sodium fluoride (used before retiring to bed at night)
  - fluoride gel products provided in tightly adapted vacuform mouth guard carriers are also useful. Fluorides may be usefully applied in the dental office, and daily at home (sodium fluoride gels or 0.4% stannous fluoride gels)
  - amorphous calcium phosphate (ACP)
  - glass ionomer restorations can be useful since they release fluoride
  - it is best to wait until a year of no new caries has elapsed before constructing new crowns.
- Oral complications such as candidosis should be treated:

Table 8.2 Some salivary stimulants (sialogogues) and salivary replacements (mouth wetting agents or artificial salivas)

Agent	Use	Comments
Sialogogues		
Pilocarpine (Salagen), or cevimeline	5 mg up to 3 times daily with food	Patient may be unable to see well enough to drive or operate machinery Contraindicated in asthma, chronic obstructive airways disease, glaucoma and pregnancy Care with cardiac disease
Chewing gum	Regularly	Inexpensive, no adverse effects
Salivix	Malic acid	Pastille
Salivary replacements		
Glandosane	Sodium carboxymethylcellulose base	Spray
Luborant	Sodium carboxymethylcellulose base	Spray
Oralbalance	Lactoperoxidase, glucose oxidase and xylitol	Gel
Saliva orthana	Mucin	Spray containing fluoride, or lozenge May be unsuitable if there are religious objections to porcine mucin
Salivace	Sodium carboxymethylcellulose base	Spray
Saliveze	Sodium carboxymethylcellulose base	Spray

- a rinse or swab from the oral mucosa should be taken to confirm candidosis if there is soreness and signs of inflammation. A commercial kit such as Ori-cult may be helpful
- dentures should be left out of the mouth at night and stored in sodium hypochlorite solution, benzalkonium chloride or chlorhexidine
- chlorhexidine, used in aqueous solution as a mouth rinse, has both antibacterial and antifungal effects, and there may be advantages to its use in dentate patients, due to some effect of chlorhexidine against cariogenic bacteria as well as *Candida*
- antifungals should be used, until there is no evidence of mucosal erythema and symptoms, and should be continued for at least 2 weeks more, to reduce the risk of recurrence. Topical antifungals tend to be most effective, since salivation is low and thus salivary antifungal delivery is not good. Topical antifungals are available as gels or tablets which can be allowed to dissolve intraorally, resulting in contact with mucosa while dissolving in the mouth. However, if the mouth is extremely dry, tablets may not dissolve, and in these cases liquid products such as suspensions or gels are best. The polyene, nystatin, is effective topically and available as a suspension. Azoles can be given as a suspension or liquid, used as a mouthwash and then swallowed (Ch. 5). Fluconazole, itraconazole and posaconazole are available as suspensions effective against oropharyngeal candidosis, and voriconazole as a liquid – preparations which may find favour for use in patients with dry mouths. An antifungal, such as miconazole gel, should be spread on dentures or appliances before re-insertion.
- Oral complications such as bacterial sialadenitis should be treated:
  - a swab should be collected of any pus expressed from the salivary duct, for bacterial culture and antibiotic sensitivities
  - acute sialadenitis needs treating, usually with a penicillinase-resistant antibiotic, such as flucloxacillin.

PATIENT INFORMATION SHEET

Dry mouth

▼ Please read this information sheet. If you have any questions, particularly about the treatment or potential side-effects, please ask your doctor.
- Saliva usually helps swallowing, talking and taste, and protects the mouth and teeth.
- Where saliva is reduced there is a risk of dental decay (caries), halitosis, altered taste sensation, mouth soreness and infections.
- Saliva may be reduced after radiotherapy or chemotherapy or the use of various drugs, after bone marrow transplants, in diabetes, in some viral infections, in anxiety/stress/depression, or in some salivary gland disorders.

Diagnosis

This is a clinical diagnosis mainly, but investigations may be indicated, including:

- blood tests
- eye tests
- urine analysis
- salivary flow rate tests
- salivary gland biopsy.
  A simple biopsy, under local anaesthesia, of small glands inside the lower lip is quick and has few adverse effects except occasional minor anaesthesia.
- X-rays or scans.
- Chest X-ray.
- Sialography – your saliva is dyed and the amount measured.
- Scintiscanning – your saliva is radioactively marked and the amount measured.
- Ultrasound, like an X-ray but for the soft tissues.

10 steps to manage dry mouth

- Sip on juices and other fluids throughout the day. Dryness can be combated by rinsing with water. Take small sips of fluids with each bite of food at meal times. Keep water at your bedside.
- Replace missing saliva with salivary substitutes (Artificial Saliva, Glandosane, Luborant, Oralbalance, Saliva Orthana, Salivace, Saliveze).
- Stimulate saliva with:
  - sugar-free chewing gums (EnDeKay or Orbit)
  - diabetic sweets
  - Salivix, if advised
  - drugs that stimulate salivation (Salagen) if advised by the specialist.
- Avoid spicy or dry foods or hard crunchy foods such as biscuits even when dunked in liquids. Take small bites and eat slowly. Eat soft, creamy foods (casseroles, soups), or cool foods with a high liquid content (melon, grapes, ice cream). Moisten foods with gravies, sauces, extra oil, margarine, salad dressings, sour cream, mayonnaise or yogurt. Pineapple has an enzyme that helps clean the mouth.
- Always take water or non-alcoholic drinks with meals.
- Avoid anything that may worsen dryness, such as:
  - drugs (e.g. antidepressants, unless they are necessary)
  - alcohol (including in mouthwashes)
  - smoking
  - caffeine (coffee, some soft drinks)
  - mouth-breathing.
- Protect against dental caries by avoiding sugary foods/drinks and by:
  - reducing sugar intake (avoid snacking and eating last thing at night)
  - avoiding sticky foods such as toffee
  - keeping your mouth very clean (twice daily toothbrushing and flossing)
  - using a fluoride toothpaste
  - using fluoride gels or mouthwashes daily before going to bed
  - having regular dental checks.
- Protect against thrush and halitosis by:
  - keeping your mouth very clean
  - keeping your mouth as moist as possible
  - rinsing twice daily with chlorhexidine (Chlorohex, Corsodyl, Eludril)
  - leaving dentures out at night
  - disinfecting dentures in hypochlorite (e.g. Milton, Dentural)
  - using antifungals if recommended by a specialist.
- Protect the lips with a lip salve.
- Consider a humidifier for the bedroom.

FURTHER READING

Baker, S.R., Pankhurst, C.L., Robinson, P.G., 2007. Testing relationships between clinical and non-clinical variables in xerostomia: a structural equation model of oral health-related quality of life. Qual. Life Res. 16, 297–308.

Braam, P.M., Terhaard, C.H., Roesink, J.M., Raaijmakers, C.P., 2006. Intensity-modulated radiotherapy significantly reduces xerostomia compared with conventional radiotherapy. Int. J. Radiat. Oncol. Biol. Phys. 66, 975–980.

Dirix, P., Nuyts, S., Van den Bogaert, W., 2006. Radiation-induced xerostomia in patients with head and neck cancer: a literature review. Cancer 107, 2525–2534.

Eveson, J.W., 2008. Xerostomia. Periodontol 48, 85–91.

Heath, N., Macleod, I., Pearce, R., 2006. Major salivary gland agenesis in a young child: consequences for oral health. Int. J. Paediatr. Dent. 16 (6), 431–434.

Ishii, M., Kurachi, Y., 2006. Muscarinic acetylcholine receptors. Curr. Pharm. Des. 12 (28), 3573–3581.

Leung, W.K., Dassanayake, R.S., Yau, J.Y., et al., 2000. Oral colonization, phenotypic, and genotypic profiles of Candida species in irradiated, dentate, xerostomic nasopharyngeal carcinoma survivors. J. Clin. Microbiol. 38, 2219–2226.

Lopez-Jornet, P., Camacho-Alonso, F., Bermejo-Fenoll, A., 2006. A simple test for salivary gland hypofunction using Oral Schirmer's test. J. Oral Pathol. Med. 35 (4), 244–248.

Mandel, S.J., Mandel, L., 2007. False-positive xerostomia following radioactive iodine treatment: case report. Oral Surg. Oral Med. Oral Pathol. Oral Radiol. Endod. 103, e43–e47.

Papas, A.S., Sherrer, Y.S., Charney, M., et al., 2004. Successful treatment of dry mouth and dry eye symptoms in Sjögren's syndrome patients with oral pilocarpine: a randomized, placebo-controlled, dose-adjustment study. J. Clin. Rheumatol. 10 (4), 169–177.

Porter, S.R., Scully, C., Hegarty, A., 2004. An update of the etiology and management of xerostomia. Oral Surg. Oral Med. Oral Pathol. Oral Radiol. Endod. 97, 28–46.

Prager, T.M., Finke, C., Miethke, R.R., 2006. Dental findings in patients with ectodermal dysplasia. J. Orofac. Orthop. 67 (5), 347–355.

Scully, C., 2001. The role of saliva in oral health problems. Practitioner 245, 841–856.

Scully, C., 2003. Drug effects on salivary glands; dry mouth. Oral Dis. 9, 165–1176.

Scully, C., 2003. Oral medicine for the general practitioner: part five: dry mouth. Independent Dent 8, 45–50.

Scully, C., Felix, D.H., 2005. Oral medicine – update for the dental practitioner. 3. Dry mouth and disorders of salivation. Br. Dent. J. 199, 423–4437.

Sully, C., Luker, J., 2011. Dry mouth. In Bradley, P.J., Guntinas-Lichius, O. Disorders and Diseases of the Salivary Glands. Thieme, Stuttgart, 123–128.

Shimizu, M., Okamura, K., Yoshiura, K., et al., 2006. Sonographic diagnostic criteria for screening Sjögren's syndrome. Oral Surg. Oral Med. Oral Pathol. Oral Radiol. Endod. 102 (1), 85–93.

Thomson, W.M., Lawrence, H.P., Broadbent, J.M., Poulton, R., 2006. The impact of xerostomia on oral-health-related quality of life among younger adults. Health Qual. Life Outcomes 4 (1), 86.

von Bültzingslöwen, I., Sollecito, T.P., Fox, P.C., Daniels, T., 2007. Salivary dysfunction associated with systemic diseases: systematic review and clinical management recommendations. Oral Surg. Oral Med. Oral Pathol. Oral Radiol. Endod. 103 (S57), e1–e15.

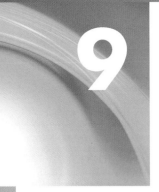

9 Halitosis (oral malodour)

INTRODUCTION

Halitosis, from the Latin for breath *halitus*, is oral malodour. Halitosis is a problem analogous to body odour and is the cause for serious concern by many sufferers since it has negative connotations, affecting not only the patient's self image, but also others' attitudes towards the patient. It is a fairly common complaint, found mainly in adults. Up to 30% of adults over 60 years old report either being conscious of their oral malodour, or having been told by others they have it.

Oral malodour is common on awakening (morning breath) and is then usually a consequence of low salivary flow and oral cleansing during sleep. This is termed 'physiological halitosis', rarely has any special significance, and can be readily rectified by eating, oral cleansing and rinsing the mouth with fresh water. Malodour at other times is often the consequence of habits such as smoking or drinking alcohol, or of eating various foods such as especially durian, garlic, onion or spices, and to some extent cabbage, cauliflower or radish. The avoidance of these habits and foods is the best prevention.

Halitosis is also more common:

- in starvation, probably partly due to oral stagnation
- in the ovulation phase of the menstrual cycle
- in use of certain drugs:
  - amphetamines
  - chloral hydrate
  - cytotoxic agents
  - dimethyl sulphoxide (DMSO)
  - disulfiram
  - nitrates and nitrites
  - phenothiazines
  - solvent abuse.

AETIOLOGY AND PATHOGENESIS

Halitosis that is not due to the above causes is termed 'pathological halitosis' and is most often a consequence of oral bacterial activity (**Fig. 9.1**). More than 85% of cases are due to oral causes (oral malodour) . In most cases the aetiology is from anaerobes in the tongue coating or periodontal pockets, or arising from:

- poor oral hygiene (**Figs 9.2** and **9.3**)
- gingivitis (especially necrotizing gingivitis)
- periodontitis

- pericoronitis and other types of oral sepsis
- infected extraction sockets
- residual blood postoperatively
- debris under bridges or appliances
- ulcers
- dry mouth.

There is no single micro-organism incriminated. Bacteria (especially anaerobes) appear to be the main culprits, the main organisms implicated including:

- *Porphyromonas gingivalis*
- *Prevotella intermedia*
- *Fusobacterium nucleatum*
- *Bacteroides forsythus*
- *Treponema denticola.*

Others such as *Solobacterium moorei, Peptostreptococcus, Eubacterium, Selenomonas, Centipeda,* have also been incriminated in halitosis. The predominant bacteria found in the control samples in one study were *Lysobacter*-type species, *Streptococcus salivarius, Veillonella dispar*, an unidentified oral bacterium, *Actinomyces odontolyticus, Atopobium parvulum* and *Veillonella atypical* while in the samples from people with halitosis, *Lysobacter*-type species, *S. salivarius, Prevotella melaninogenica*, an unidentified oral bacterium, *Prevotella veroralis* and *Prevotella pallens* were the most common species. The story is not yet complete, but in any event, the responsible anaerobes produce chemicals that cause the malodour in many instances, and these include:

- volatile sulphur compounds (VSCs) (mainly methyl mercaptan, hydrogen sulphide and dimethyl sulphide)
- volatile aromatic compounds (indole, skatole)
- polyamines (putrescine and cadaverine)
- short-chain fatty acids (butyric, valeric, acetic and propionic acids).

Halitosis in a very few cases originates distal to the tonsils (**Box 9.1**). Such causes that may be responsible for malodour include the following:

- Respiratory disease: nasal sepsis or foreign bodies, or infection of the paranasal sinuses or respiratory tract may be a cause. In children, the insertion of foreign bodies, such as small toys into the nose, and subsequent sepsis, is a common cause of halitosis. At any age infections in the respiratory tract, such as tonsillitis, bronchitis, bronchiectasis or other lung infections, or tumours in the respiratory tract, may be responsible.

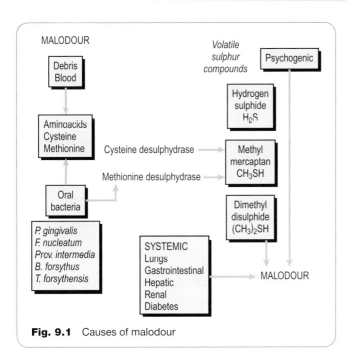

Fig. 9.1 Causes of malodour

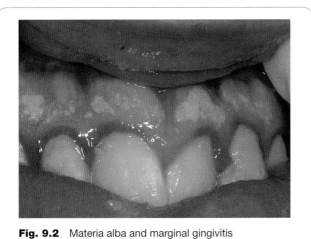

Fig. 9.2 Materia alba and marginal gingivitis

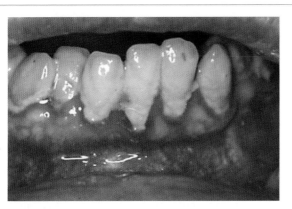

Fig. 9.3 Plaque accumulation and gingivitis.

BOX 9.1 Causes of halitosis

- Dry mouth
- Starvation
- Smoking
- Some foods
- Drugs (see Ch. 54 and Algorithm 9.1)
- Oral sepsis
- Systemic disease:
  - respiratory and nasal disease
  - gastrointestinal disease
  - diabetic ketosis
  - hepatic failure
  - renal failure
  - trimethylaminuria
- Psychogenic factors

- Gastrointestinal disease: gastro-oesophageal reflux may be responsible. Although *Helicobacter pylori* has been suspected as a cause, it is an uncommon aetiology.
- Metabolic disorders:
  - diabetic ketosis: the breath may smell of ketones, especially acetone
  - hepatic failure: caused by dimethyl sulfide and to a lower extent by ketones in alveolar air
  - renal failure: dialysis helps reduce halitosis.
- Trimethylaminuria: fish and eggs may produce malodour in this rare metabolic syndrome.
- Psychogenic or psychosomatic factors: not all persons who believe they have halitosis actually have any objectively confirmed malodour, and the halitosis may then be attributed to a form of delusion, obsessive compulsive disorder or monosymptomatic hypochondriasis (*halitophobia*). Such patients rarely wish to visit a psychological specialist because they fail to recognize their own psychological condition and never doubt they have oral malodour. Attempting to persuade them otherwise is usually futile. Other people's behaviour, or perceived behaviour, such as apparently covering the nose or averting the face, is typically misinterpreted by these patients as an indication that their breath is indeed offensive. Such patients may have latent psychosomatic illness tendencies and may be mentally immature. Anxiety may also increase malodour.

DIAGNOSIS

Diagnosis (**Algorithm 9.1**; **Table 9.1**) is mainly clinical, made from:

- Full history: many patients will adopt behaviour to minimize their problem, such as covering the mouth when talking, avoiding or keeping a distance from other people, using chewing gum, mints, mouthwashes or sprays designed to reduce malodour, or excessively cleaning their tongue or mouth.
- Examination: the Winkel tongue coating index (WTCI) or a digital tongue imaging system (DTIS) can be used to calculate tongue coating area.
- Assessment of halitosis: usually by simply smelling the exhaled air (organoleptic method) first from the mouth (with nose closed by pinching nostrils) then from the nose (with patient's mouth

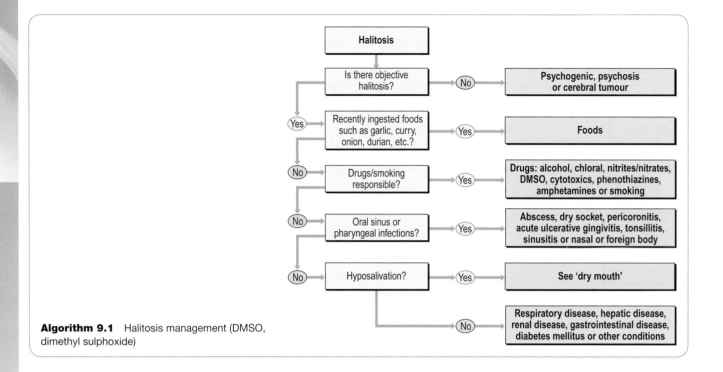

Algorithm 9.1 Halitosis management (DMSO, dimethyl sulphoxide)

Table 9.1 Aids that might be helpful in diagnosis/prognosis/management in some patients with halitosis (oral malodour)*

In most cases	In some cases
Halimetry or organoleptic assessment	Full blood picture
	Blood glucose
	Serum ferritin, vitamin B_{12} and corrected whole blood folate levels
	ESR
	BANA (benzoyl-arginine-naphthyl-amide) test
	Dark field microscopy
	Oral imaging
	Sinus imaging
	Nasendoscopy
	Chest radiography
	Helicobacter pylori serum antibody or endoscopy and rapid urease test or biopsy
	Liver function tests
	Renal function tests
	Urinalysis for the ratio of trimethylamine to trimethylamine oxide
	Psychological assessment

*See text for details and glossary for abbreviations.

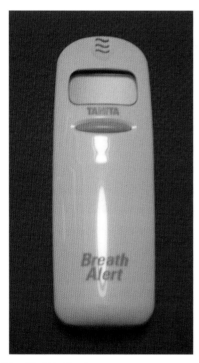

Fig. 9.4 Hand held halimeter

closed). Some centres are able to also undertake objective measurements of the agents responsible, such as:

- volatile sulphur compounds, using a halimeter (Interscan Corp., Chatsworth, CA, USA) (**Figs 9.4** and **9.5**) or using OralChroma™ a portable gas chromatograph (**Fig. 9.6**). Compounds other than VSCs, however, are not detectable
- oral flora, such as by the BANA (benzoyl-arginine-naphthyl-amide) test or dark field microscopy, which can be helpful, at least for patient education.

Systemic causes if suspected need the opinion of the relevant specialist and possibly, investigations such as nasendoscopy, chest imaging, *Helicobacter pylori* serum antibody or endoscopy and rapid urease test or biopsy, liver and renal function tests, and urinalysis for the ratio of trimethylamine to trimethylamine oxide.

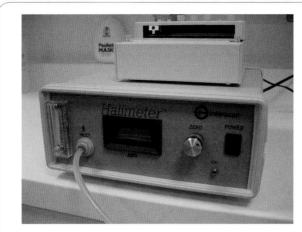

Fig. 9.5 Halimeter

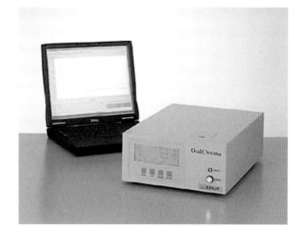

Fig. 9.6 OraChroma machine

TREATMENT (see also Chs 4 and 5)

The management of halitosis currently includes the following:

- Patient education.
- Treating the cause: medical help may be required to manage patients with a systemic background to their complaint.
- Avoiding smoking, and foods such as onions, garlic, durian, cabbage, cauliflower and radish.
- Eating regular meals and finishing meals with fibrous fruits/vegetables (e.g. carrots, pineapple).
- Ensuring good oral hygiene: dental prophylaxis, toothbrushing, flossing and tongue cleaning (with a brush or scraper; this is best done before going to bed since scraping early during the day may induce retching).
- Using oral healthcare products: there is evidence of benefit mainly from the use of toothpastes and mouthwashes containing:
  - chlorhexidine digluconate, or
  - triclosan, or
  - amine fluoride/stannous fluoride, or
  - metal ions.
- Oral antiseptics such as chlorhexidine (which is effective but may cause tooth-staining and occasional other adverse effects), triclosan, cetylpyridinium, essential oils or products with zinc or stannous ions can be helpful. All are reportedly effective at reducing malodour for at least 3 h. Generally, it is recommended that mouthwashes should be used two or three times daily for at least 30 s.

Some products appear effective for longer, such as a toothpaste containing triclosan and a copolymer; and a two phase mouthwash consisting of natural essential oils, triclosan and cetylpyridinium chloride, plus sodium fluoride.

Using oral deodorants (oral malodour counteractives (OMC)). Chewing gum, parsley, mint, cloves or fennel seeds and the use of proprietary 'fresh breath' preparations may help mask malodour.

- In recalcitrant cases, the specialist empirically may use a 1-week course of metronidazole 200 mg three times daily in an effort to eliminate unidentified anaerobic infections.
- Emergent therapies include the use of chemicals, natural products, or probiotics to inhibit the bacterial enzymes responsible for production of odiferous substances, and even vaccines prepared against the responsible bacteria.
- A multitude of anti-malodour products is also available over the counter, testimony to the extent of the perceived or, indeed real, problem of halitosis and also to the fact that few of the preparations are reliably effective.
- Patients with halitophobia may benefit from specialist mental healthcare, possibly including medication with, for example, paroxetine.

PATIENT INFORMATION SHEET
Oral malodour (halitosis)

▼ Please read this information sheet. If you have any questions, particularly about the treatment or potential side-effects, please ask your doctor.

Halitosis

- Is common on awakening.
- Is often far more obvious to the sufferer than others.
- If real is usually caused by diet, habits, dental plaque or oral disease.
- Can be measured with a halimeter.
- Often improves with oral hygiene.
- Can sometimes be caused by conditions of the sinuses, nose or throat.
- Is rarely caused by more serious disease.

10 steps to control breath odour

- Treat any identifiable cause (this may need antimicrobials).
- Avoid odiferous foods such as onions, garlic and spices.
- Avoid habits that may worsen breath odour, such as:
  - alcohol
  - smoking.
- Take regular meals.
- Eat fresh fruit regularly: pineapple has an enzyme that helps clean the mouth.
- Brush your teeth after eating.
- Keep oral hygiene regular and good by:
  - prophylaxis
  - toothbrushing
  - flossing
  - rinsing twice daily with chlorhexidine (Chlorohex, Corsodyl, Eludril) cetylpyridinium, Listerine or other mouthwashes.
- Brush your tongue before going to bed: use a tongue scraper if that helps.
- Keep your mouth as moist as possible by using:
  - sugar-free chewing gums
  - diabetic sweets.
- Use proprietary 'fresh breath' preparations.
- If you have dentures, leave them out at night and in hypochlorite or chlorhexidine.

FURTHER READING

Calil, C.M., Marcondes, F.K., 2006. Influence of anxiety on the production of oral volatile sulfur compounds. Life Sci. 79 (7), 660–664.

Di Fede, O., Di Liberto, C., Occhipinti, G., et al., 2008. Oral manifestations in patients with gastro-oesophageal reflux disease: a single-center case-control study. J. Oral Pathol. Med. 37 (6), 336–340.

Eldarrat, A.H., 2011. Influence of oral health and lifestyle on oral malodour. Int. Dent. J. 61 (1), 47–51.

Farrell, S., Baker, R.A., Somogyi-Mann, M., et al., 2006. Oral malodor reduction by a combination of chemotherapeutical and mechanical treatments. Clin. Oral Invest. 10 (2), 157–163.

Faveri, M., Hayacibara, M.F., Pupio, G.C., et al., 2006. A cross-over study on the effect of various therapeutic approaches to morning breath odour. J. Clin. Periodontol. 33 (8), 555–560.

Hartley, M.G., McKenzie, C., Greenman, J., et al., 2000. Tongue microbiota and malodour; effects of metronidazole mouth rinse on tongue microbiota and breath odour levels. Microb. Ecol. Health Dis. 11, 226–233.

Hughes, F.J., McNab, R., 2008. Oral malodour–a review. Arch. Oral Biol. 53 (Suppl. 1), S1–S7.

Kawamoto, A., Sugano, N., Motohashi, M., Matsumoto, S., Ito, K., 2010. Relationship between oral malodor and the menstrual cycle. J. Periodontal. Res. 45 (5), 681.

Keles, M., Tozoglu, U., Uyanik, A., et al., 2011. Does peritoneal dialysis affect halitosis in patients with end-stage renal disease? Perit. Dial. Int. 31 (2), 168.

Kim, J., Jung, Y., Park, K., Park, J.-W., 2009. A digital tongue imaging system for tongue coating evaluation in patients with oral malodour. Oral Dis. 15, 565–569.

Kinberg, S., Stein, M., Zion, N., Shaoul, R., 2010. The gastrointestinal aspects of halitosis. Can. J. Gastroenterol. 24 (9), 552.

Krespi, Y.P., Shrime, M.G., Kacker, A., 2006. The relationship between oral malodor and volatile sulfur compound-producing bacteria. Otolaryngol. Head Neck Surg. 135 (5), 671–676.

Lee, H., Kho, H.S., Chung, J.W., et al., 2006. Volatile sulfur compounds produced by *Helicobacter pylori*. J. Clin. Gastroenterol. 40 (5), 421–426.

Mackay, R.J., McEntyre, C.J., Henderson, C., et al., 2011. Trimethylaminuria: causes and diagnosis of a socially distressing condition. Clin. Biochem. Rev. 32 (1), 33–43.

Moshkowitz, M., Horowitz, N., Leshno, M., Halpern, Z., 2007. Halitosis and gastroesophageal reflux disease: a possible association. Oral Dis. 13 (6), 581.

Nachnani, S., 2011. Oral malodor: causes, assessment, and treatment. Compend. Contin. Educ. Dent. 32 (1), 22–24, 26–28, 30–31.

Outhouse, T.L., Al-Alawi, R., Fedorowicz, Z., Keenan, J.V., 2006. Tongue scraping for treating halitosis. Cochrane Database Syst. Rev. 19 (2), CD005519.

Porter, S.R., Scully, C., 2006. Oral malodour (halitosis). BMJ 333 (7569), 632–635.

Riggio, M., Lennon, A., Rolph, H., et al., 2008. Molecular identification of bacteria on the tongue dorsum of subjects with and without halitosis. Oral. Dis. 14, 251–258.

Scully, C., Felix, D.H., 2005. Oral medicine – update for the dental practitioner. 4. Oral malodour. Br. Dent. J. 199, 498–500.

Scully, C., Greenman, J., 2012. Halitology (breath odour aetiopathogenisis and management). Oral Dis. 18, 333–345.

Scully, C., Porter, S.R., 2006. Halitosis. Clin. Evid. 15, 472–473.

Scully, C., Rosenberg, M., 2003. Halitosis. Dent. Update 30, 205–210.

Seemann, R., 2006. Tongue scrapers may reduce halitosis in adults. Evid. Based Dent. 7 (3), 78.

Seemann, R., Bizhang, M., Djamchidi, C., et al., 2006. The proportion of pseudo-halitosis patients in a multidisciplinary breath malodour consultation. Int. Dent. J. 56 (2), 77–81.

Souza, C.M., Braosi, A.P., Luczyszyn, S.M., et al., 2008. Oral health in Brazilian patients with chronic renal disease. Rev. Med. Chil. 136 (6), 741.

Suzuki, N., Yoneda, M., Naito, T., et al., 2011. Association between oral malodour and psychological characteristics in subjects with neurotic tendencies complaining of halitosis. Int. Dent. J. 61 (2), 57–62.

Tanaka, M., Toe, M., Nagata, H., et al., 2010. Effect of eucalyptus-extract chewing gum on oral malodor: a double-masked, randomized trial. J. Periodontol. 81 (11), 1564.

Tangerman, A., Winkel, E.G., 2010. Extra-oral halitosis: an overview. J. Breath Res. 4 (1), 017003.

Van Den Broek, A., Feenstra, L., De Baat, C., 2008. A review of the current literature on management of halitosis. Oral Dis. 14, 30–39.

Van der Sleen, M.I., Slot, D.E., Van Trijffel, E., et al., 2010. Effectiveness of mechanical tongue cleaning on breath odour and tongue coating: a systematic review. Int. J. Dent. Hyg. 8 (4), 258.

Van Steenberghe, D., 2004. Breath malodor: a step-by-step approach. Quintessence Books, Coppenhagen.

Xu, X., Zhou, X.D., Wu, C.D., 2010. Tea catechin EGCg suppresses the mgl gene associated with halitosis. J. Dent. Res. 89 (11), 1304.

Yaegaki, K., Coil, J.M., 2000. Examination, classification, and treatment of halitosis; clinical perspectives. J. Can. Dent. Assoc. 66, 257–261.

Lumps and swellings

INTRODUCTION

Swelling and lumps in the mouth are common, and the tongue often detects even very small swellings or patients may notice a lump because it is sore. Some individuals discover and worry about normal anatomical features, such as the parotid papilla, foliate papillae on the tongue, or the pterygoid hamulus. Some examine their mouths out of idle curiosity, and some through fear (perhaps after hearing of someone with 'mouth cancer'). In contrast, many oral cancers are diagnosed far too late, often after being present several months, because the patient ignores the swelling. Some 'lumps' become ulcers, as in various bullous lesions, infections and in malignant neoplasms.

Many different conditions may present as oral lumps or swellings, causes including the following:

- The mouth's normal anatomy, such as tongue foliate or circumvallate papillae (**Figs 10.1** and **10.2**).
- Developmental lumps: unerupted teeth, and tori are common causes of hard swellings related to the jaws. Cysts and hamartomas may present as a swelling. Hamartomas include lymphangiomas and haemangiomas (angiomas). Lymphangiomas are hamartomas or benign neoplasms of lymphatic channels that present as a colourless, sometimes finely nodular soft mass. Bleeding into lymphatic spaces causes sudden purplish discolouration. If in the tongue and extensive, it is a rare cause of macroglossia. If in the lip, it is a rare cause of macrocheilia. Diagnosis can be confirmed, if necessary, by excision biopsy.

Haemangiomas are vascular malformations that are red, purple or blue, painless, soft and sometimes fluctuant and usually blanch on pressure. Most appear in infancy, but about 15% develop later. Haemangiomas are common on the tongue, lip vermilion, or buccal mucosa. Diagnosis may be assisted by aspiration, ultrasonography, radiography, angiography, MRI, and MRI-angiography. Differentiation is from lymphangioma, telangiectasia, purpura, Kaposi sarcoma and epithelioid angiomatosis. Management may be active, with removal of the haemangioma, or simple observation (since some 50% regress spontaneously in childhood). Cryosurgery or laser (Nd-YAG, carbon dioxide, pulsed tuneable dye or copper vapour) are the main treatments. Alternatively, sclerosant injection (boiling water, absolute alcohol, sodium tetradecyl sulphate, sodium morrhuate, or ethanolamine oleate (or propranolol)), compression sutures (Popescu) or (rarely) arterial embolization are used.

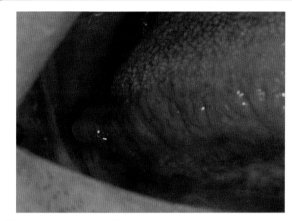

Fig. 10.1 Foliate papillae

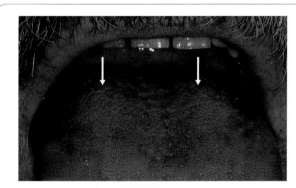

Fig. 10.2 Circumvallate papillae

- Inflammatory lumps: dental abscess is one of the most common causes of oral swelling. Parasites are rare. Non-infective inflammatory causes include fibrous lumps, Crohn disease, orofacial granulomatosis and sarcoidosis. Salivary gland inflammation can cause swelling in sialadenitis.
- Fibrous lump or nodule ('fibroepithelial polyp'): this is a pedunculated or broadly sessile, sometimes ulcerated, firm or soft, lump seen mainly on the buccal mucosa usually with a normal overlying mucosa. It is termed 'epulis' if on the gingival margin. It is common and is probably caused by chronic irritation causing fibrous hyperplasia. Excision biopsy helps

differentiate it from any other soft tissue tumour. The flange of a denture impinging on the vestibular mucosa may stimulate a similar reactive hyperplasia – the so-called denture granuloma or denture-induced hyperplasia (denture granuloma; epulis fissuratum). This is a painless, firm swelling with a smooth pink surface usually in the buccal sulcus related to an ill-fitting lower complete denture, especially anteriorly lying parallel with the alveolar ridge and sometimes grooved or ulcerated by the denture flange. Several leaflets with a fairly firm consistency may develop. Common, mainly in middle-aged or older patients, the diagnosis is clear-cut if the lesion is in relation to a denture flange. If ulcerated, it may mimic carcinoma (rarely). Diagnosis is clinical, but excision biopsy may be indicated. The denture flange should be relieved, to prevent recurrence.

- Allergic: angioedema can produce diffuse swelling, typically of rapid onset. Oedema of slower onset may be orofacial granulomatosis.
- Traumatic: haematoma may cause a swelling at the site.
- Hormonal: pregnancy may result in generalized gingival swelling (pregnancy gingivitis) or a discrete lump (pregnancy epulis – really a pyogenic granuloma). Diabetes predisposes to periodontal abscesses and occasionally giant cell lesions are seen in hyperparathyroidism. Sialosis is a painless swelling of major salivary glands that often has a hormonal basis, for example in diabetes.
- Drug induced: a range of drugs can produce gingival swelling – most commonly implicated are phenytoin, ciclosporin and calcium channel blockers. Drugs, such as chlorhexidine occasionally cause salivary gland swelling.
- Benign neoplasms, such as fibromas or salivary gland tumours may be seen. Malignant neoplasms may include carcinoma (**Fig. 10.3**), lymphoma, Kaposi sarcoma, malignant salivary gland tumours and others (**Fig. 10.4**). Occasionally metastatic malignant disease or leukaemia may present as a lump.
- Viral lesions: mumps virus can cause acute sialadenitis. Papillomas (**Fig. 10.5**), common warts (verruca vulgaris), genital warts (condyloma acuminatum) and focal epithelial hyperplasia (Heck disease) are all caused by human papilloma viruses (HPV). A higher prevalence is seen in patients with sexually shared infections or in people who

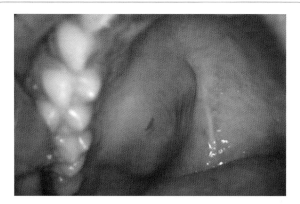

Fig. 10.4 Salivary neoplasm causing palatal swelling

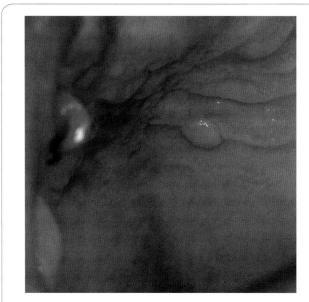

Fig. 10.5 Papilloma causing palatal swelling

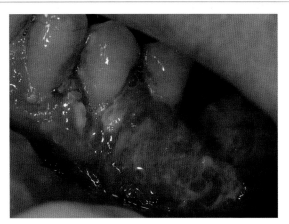

Fig. 10.3 Carcinoma causing gingival swelling

are immunocompromised, as in HIV/AIDS. Papillomas are uncommon in the mouth, but typically seen on the fauces, soft palate or tongue, usually <5 mm diameter and with whitish filiform projections. Warts are rare in the mouth: verrucae vulgaris are usually transmitted from skin lesions, and found predominantly on the lips whereas condyloma acuminata, transmitted from genital or anal lesions, are found mainly on the tongue or palate. Diagnose by biopsy to differentiate from other tumours and manage with podophyllum or imiquimod, excision, laser, or electro- or cryosurgery.

- Pyogenic granuloma (**Fig. 10.6**).
- Fibro-osseous lesions: fibrous dysplasia and Paget disease can result in hard jaw swellings.
- Deposits: amyloid disease and other deposits can cause swellings.
- Obstruction to salivary glands can cause swellings (mucoceles or obstructive sialadenitis).

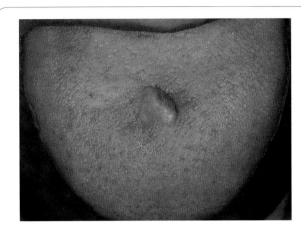

Fig. 10.6 Pyogenic granuloma on the tongue

DIAGNOSIS

- Position: the anatomical position of the lump should be defined as accurately as possible. The proximity of the lump to other structures (e.g. teeth, dentures) should be noted. Does the swelling have an orifice, or sinus? If fluid is draining from the opening, is it clear, cloudy or purulent? Other similar or relevant changes elsewhere in the oral cavity should be noted (**Box 10.1**).
- Midline lesions tend to be developmental in origin (e.g. torus palatinus; see Ch. 13).
- Determine whether the lump is bilateral, since most neoplastic lumps are unilateral.
- Number of swellings, particularly with regard to whether the lesion is bilaterally symmetrical and thus possibly anatomical. Multiple or extraoral lesions suggest an infective or occasionally developmental origin.
- Size: the size should always be measured and recorded. A diagram may be helpful. Thus, significant changes that may occur later can be recognized. In contrast, vague comments describing the swelling as 'medium' or 'large' are unhelpful.
- Shape: many swellings have characteristic shapes that point towards the diagnosis. Thus swelling of the parotid gland often fills in the space between the posterior border of the mandible and the mastoid process.
- Colour and temperature: brown or black pigmentation may be due to a variety of causes, such as melanoma. Purple

or red may be due to an angioma (**Fig. 10.6**) or Kaposi sarcoma. Is the lump pale in colour (suggesting underlying fibrosis, or soft tissues stretched over bony enlargement); red (suggesting inflammation); or deep red (suggesting haemangioma or giant-cell epulis)? Any variations in colour within the lump (e.g. a 'pointing' abscess) should be observed. The skin and mucosa overlying acute inflammatory lesions, such as an abscess, is frequently red and warm.

- Tenderness: inflammatory swellings, such as an abscess, are characteristically tender, although clearly palpation must be gentle to avoid excessive discomfort to the patient.
- Discharge: note any discharge from the lesion (e.g. clear fluid, pus, blood).
- Movement: the mobility of any swelling should be tested to determine if it is fixed to adjacent structures or the overlying skin/mucosa, such as often happens with a malignant neoplasm.
- Consistency: lumps may vary from soft and fluctuant to hard. Fluctuation refers to the presence of fluid within a swelling, such as a cyst, and is a sign elicited by detecting movement of fluid when the swelling is compressed. Palpation may then help assessment of its contents and these can be put into such categories as fluid (fluctuant because of cyst fluid, mucus, pus or blood), soft, firm, or hard like a carcinoma (indurated). Palpation may cause the release of fluid (e.g. pus from an abscess) or cause the lesion to blanch (vascular) or occasionally cause a blister to appear or expand (Nikolsky sign). Sometimes palpation causes the patient pain (suggesting an inflammatory lesion). The swelling overlying a bony cyst may crackle (like an egg-shell) when palpated. Palpation may disclose an underlying structure (e.g. the crown of a tooth under an eruption cyst) or show that the actual swelling is in deeper structures (e.g. submandibular calculus). Bimanual palpation should be used when investigating lesions in the floor of the mouth, cheek, and occasionally the tongue.
- Surface texture: the surface of a swelling may vary from the uniform smooth texture of many fibrous lumps to the grossly irregular. The surface characteristics should be noted: papillomas have an obvious anemone-like appearance; carcinomas and other malignant lesions tend to have a pebbly surface and may ulcerate. Abnormal blood vessels suggest a neoplasm.
- Ulceration: some swellings may develop superficial ulceration, such as squamous cell carcinoma. The character of the edge of the ulcer and the appearance of the ulcer base should also be recorded. Ulcers should be examined for induration, which is indicative of malignancy.
- Margin: the margins of the swelling may be well or poorly defined. This may give some indication of the underlying pathology. Thus, ill-defined margins are frequently associated with malignancy, whereas clearly defined margins are more suggestive of a benign growth.
- Associated swelling: some conditions are associated with multiple swellings of a similar nature inside or outside the mouth (e.g. neurofibromatosis).
- The nature of many lumps cannot be established without further investigation:
- Any teeth adjacent to a lump involving the jaw should be tested for vitality, and any caries or suspect restorations investigated.
- The periodontal status of any involved teeth should also be determined.

BOX 10.1 Causes of oral lumps and swellings

- Normal anatomy
- Lesions:
  - developmental
  - inflammatory
  - allergic
  - traumatic
  - hormonal
  - drug-induced
  - neoplasms
  - fibro-osseous lesions
  - others

BOX 10.2 More advanced list of conditions that may present as oral lumps or swellings

Normal
- Pterygoid hamulus
- Parotid papillae
- Foliate papillae
- Unerupted teeth

Developmental
- Haemangioma
- Lymphangioma
- Maxillary and mandibular tori
- Hereditary gingival fibromatosis
- von Recklinghausen neurofibromatosis

Cystic
- Eruption cysts
- Developmental cysts
- Cysts of infective origin

Inflammatory
- Abscess
- Pyogenic granuloma
- Crohn disease
- Orofacial granulomatosis
- Sarcoidosis
- Wegener granulomatosis
- Infections
- Insect bites
- Others

Traumatic
- Haematoma
- Epulis
- Epithelial polyp
- Denture granulomas

Hormonal
- Pregnancy epulis/gingivitis
- Oral contraceptive (pill gingivitis)
- Brown tumour of hyperparathyroidism

Drugs
- Phenytoin
- Ciclosporin
- Calcium channel blockers

Neoplasms
- Benign (and warts)
- Malignant

Fibro-osseous lesions
- Fibrous dysplasia
- Paget disease

Deposits
- Amyloidosis
- Hypoplasminogenaemia (fibrin deposits)
- Other deposits

Others
- Angioedema

- Imaging is required whenever lumps involve the jaws, or may so do, and should show the full extent of the lesion and possibly other areas. Special radiographs (e.g. of the skull, sinuses and salivary gland function), CT scans, MRI or ultrasonography may, on occasions, be indicated. Photographs may be useful for future comparison.

- The medical history should be fully reviewed, as systemic disorders may be associated with intra-oral or facial swellings (**Box 10.2**). Blood tests may be needed, particularly if there is suspicion that a blood dyscrasia or endocrinopathy may underlie the development of the lump.

FURTHER READING

Leão, J.C., Hodgson, T., Scully, C., Porter, S.R., 2004. Review article: orofacial granulomatosis. Aliment. Pharmacol. Ther. 20, 1019–1027.

Scully, C., 2002. Oral medicine for the general practitioner: part three: lumps and swellings. Independent Dent. 7 (10), 25–32.

Scully, C., Felix, D.H., 2005. Oral medicine – update for the dental practitioner. 8. Lumps and swellings. Br. Dent. J. 199, 763–770.

Scully, C., Porter, S.R., 2000. Orofacial disease: update for the dental clinical team. 11. Cervical lymphadenopathy. Dent. Update 27, 44–47.

Scully, C., Porter, S., 2000. ABC of Oral Health. 6. Swellings, and red: white, and pigmented lesions. BMJ 321, 225–228.

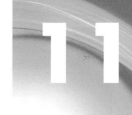

Lumps and swellings in the lip

INTRODUCTION

Lip or facial swelling may be diffuse or localized (**Boxes 11.1** and **11.2**).

- Lip or facial swelling that appears rapidly over a few minutes or hours may be caused by an insect bite or sting, or angioedema.
- Lip or facial swelling that appears over a few hours or days is most commonly inflammatory in origin, often caused by trauma or infection (cutaneous, dental (odontogenic) or rarely systemic).
- Lip or facial swelling that appears over days or weeks may occasionally be caused by granulomatous disorders (e.g. Crohn disease, orofacial granulomatosis or sarcoidosis) (**Fig. 11.1**).
- Facial swelling that appears over weeks or months is occasionally due to systemic infections (such as tuberculosis, Leishmaniasis or a deep mycosis), a neoplasm (such as lymphoma or salivary gland tumour), deposits such as amyloidosis, or endocrine conditions (e.g. corticosteroid therapy, Cushing disease, hypothyroidism, acromegaly, diabetes mellitus).
- Facial swelling is commonly of very slow onset in masseteric hypertrophy and in obesity.
- Facial swelling that is persistent is rarely caused by
  - fluid as in vascular lesions or lymphangiomas
  - solids such as primary neoplasms or metastases, deposits (e.g. amyloidosis) or foreign material (as in lip augmentation with silicone or other fillers).

BOX 11.1 Main causes of swelling of lips/face

- Haemangioma
- Mucocele
- Allergy
- Inflammation
- Trauma
- Granulomatous condition (e.g. Crohn disease, orofacial granulomatosis, sarcoid) including foreign bodies
- Neoplasm (e.g. carcinoma, salivary gland neoplasm, lymphoma)

BOX 11.2 More advanced list of causes of swelling of lips/face

Lip swelling is most commonly inflammatory in origin – caused by cutaneous or dental (odontogenic) infections or trauma.

Congenital (e.g. haemangioma, lymphangioma, Ascher syndrome (see Ch. 56))
- Cysts in soft tissues or bone (especially mucocele or cystic neoplasm)

Infective
- Oral or cutaneous infections, cellulitis, fascial space infections
- Systemic infections
- Insect bites/stings
- Papillomas and warts

Traumatic
- Traumatic or post-operative oedema or haematoma
- Surgical emphysema

Immunological
- Allergic angioedema (see also Drugs: Table 54.20)
- C1 esterase inhibitor deficiency (hereditary angioedema)
- Crohn disease, orofacial granulomatosis or sarcoidosis
- Cheilitis glandularis

Endocrine and metabolic
- Cushing syndrome and disease
- Myxoedema
- Nephrotic syndrome
- Obesity
- Systemic corticosteroid therapy
- Neoplasms
- Carcinomas
- Lymphoma
- Oral, salivary and antral tumours

Foreign bodies (including cosmetic fillers)
- Deposits
- Amyloidosis

Others
- Masseteric hypertrophy (facial rather than lip swelling)
- Bone disease
- Fibrous dysplasia
- Paget disease

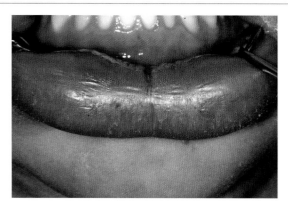

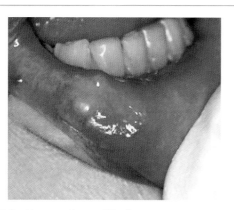

Fig. 11.1 Lip and gingival swelling in orofacial granulomatosis

Fig. 11.2 Haemangioma of the lip

- Localized swellings in the lip or face may be congenital as in haemangioma (**Fig. 11.2**) or lymphangioma but more usually are seen after trauma, or in infections, inflammatory conditions such as granulomatous disorders, or pyogenic granuloma, foreign bodies (including fillers) or caused by neoplasms or deposits.

- Pyogenic granuloma is a possibly reactive vascular lesion, sometimes associated with pregnancy. Typically, a pyogenic granuloma is a small (< 3 cm) red painless mass that bleeds easily, ulcerates and grows rapidly, and is frequently seen on the lip, gingival margin or tongue. Treatment is excision to exclude angiomatous proliferations, chancre, carcinoma or Kaposi sarcoma.

FURTHER READING

Alves, L.A., Di Nicoló, R., Ramos, C.J., et al., 2010. Retention mucocele on the lower lip associated with inadequate use of pacifier. Dermatol. Online J. 16 (7), 9.

Azevedo, L.R., Dos Santos, J.N., De Lima, A.A., et al., 2008. Canalicular adenoma presenting as an asymptomatic swelling of the upper lip: a case report. J. Contemp. Dent. Pract. 9 (1), 91–97.

Bajwa, S.S., Panda, A., Bajwa, S.K., et al., 2011. Anesthetic and airway management of a child with a large upper-lip hemangioma. Saudi J. Anaesth. 5 (1), 82–84.

Cotter, A., Treacy, A., O'Keane, C., et al., 2008. Cutaneous T-cell lymphoma presenting as a ten month history of unilateral facial swelling. Ir. Med. J. 101 (5), 151–152.

Crincoli, V., Scivetti, M., Di Bisceglie, M.B., et al., 2008. Unusual case of adverse reaction in the use of sodium hypochlorite during endodontic treatment: a case report. Quintessence Int. 39 (2), e70–e73.

Dougherty, A.L., Rashid, R.M., Bangert, C.A., 2011. Angioedema-type swelling and herpes simplex virus reactivation following hyaluronic acid injection for lip augmentation. J. Am. Acad. Dermatol. 65 (1), e21–e22.

Ekşi, E., Oztop, I., 2010. Nerve sheath myxoma of the upper lip: a case report. Kulak Burun Bogaz Ihtis. Derg. 20 (6), 318–320.

Jham, B.C., Meiller, T.F., King, M., Scheper, M.A., 2008. A diffuse but subtle swelling of the upper lip. Oral. Surg. Oral. Med. Oral. Pathol. Oral. Radiol. Endod. 106 (6), 773–777.

Kapferer, I., Berger, K., Stuerz, K., Beier, U.S., 2010. Self-reported complications with lip and tongue piercing. Quintessence Int. 41 (9), 731–737.

Leão, J.C., Hodgson, T., Scully, C., Porter, S.R., 2004. Review article: orofacial granulomatosis. Aliment. Pharmacol. Ther. 20, 1019–1027.

McCartan, B., Healy, C., McCreary, C., et al., 2011. Characteristics of patients with orofacial granulomatosis. Oral. Dis. 17 (7), 696–704.

Michailidou, E., Arvanitidou, S., Lombardi, T., et al., 2009. Oral lesions leading to the diagnosis of Crohn disease: report on 5 patients. Quintessence Int. 40 (7), 581–588.

Patel, H., Bhatia, L., McQueen, G., Moorman, J., 2008. Persistent upper lip swelling caused by foreign body infection: a case report. South Med. J. 101 (6), 651–653.

Praessler, J., Elsner, P., Ziemer, M., 2007. Persistent non-tender swelling of the upper lip. Diagnosis: cheilitis granulomatosa. Am. J. Clin. Dermatol. 8 (4), 251–253.

Ramesh, B.A., 2011. Ascher syndrome: Review of literature and case report. Indian J. Plast. Surg. 44 (1), 147–149.

Scully, C., 2002. Oral medicine for the general practitioner: part three: lumps and swellings. Independent Dent. 7 (10), 25–32.

Scully, C., Felix, D.H., 2005. Oral medicine – update for the dental practitioner. 8. Lumps and swellings. Br. Dent. J. 199, 763–770.

Scully, C., Porter, S.R., 2000. ABC of Oral Health. 6. Swellings, and red, white, and pigmented lesions. BMJ 321, 225–228.

Scully, C., Porter, S.R., 2000. Orofacial disease: update for the dental clinical team. 11. Cervical lymphadenopathy. Dent. Update 27, 44–47.

Srivastava, N., Mishra, N., Singh, S., 2008. Erythematous indurated swelling on nose and upper lip. Cutaneous T cell lymphoma. Dermatol. Online J. 14 (8), 16.

Stanton, D.C., Chou, J.C., Sollecito, T.P., et al., 2008. Recurrent lower lip swelling in a 62-year-old African American female. Cheilitis glandularis. J. Oral. Maxillofac. Surg. 66 (12), 2585–2591.

Sumer, A.P., Celenk, P., Sumer, M., et al., 2010. Nasolabial cyst: case report with CT and MRI findings. Oral. Surg. Oral. Med. Oral. Pathol. Oral. Radiol. Endod. 109 (2), e92–e94.

Tackett, A.E., Smith, K.M., 2008. Bupropion-induced angioedema. Am. J. Health Syst. Pharm. 65 (17), 1627–1630.

Tiago, R.S., Maia, M.S., Nascimento, G.M., et al., 2008. Nasolabial cyst:diagnostic and therapeutical aspects. Braz. J. Otorhinolaryngol. 74 (1), 39–43.

Vasudevan, B., Bahal, A., 2011. Leishmaniasis of the lip diagnosed by lymph node aspiration and treated with a combination of oral ketaconazole and intralesional sodium stibogluconate. Indian J. Dermatol. 56 (2), 214–216.

Veraldi, S., Bottini, S., Persico, M.C., Lunardon, L., 2007. Case report: Leishmaniasis of the upper lip. Oral. Surg. Oral. Med. Oral. Pathol. Oral. Radiol. Endod. 104 (5), 659–661.

Weinberg, M.J., Solish, N., 2009. Complications of hyaluronic acid fillers. Facial Plast. Surg. 25 (5), 324–328.

Lumps and swellings in the gingiva

INTRODUCTION

Gingival swelling is often very localized (then sometimes termed an 'epulis' from the Greek, meaning 'upon the gum'; plural 'epulides'), but may be more generalized, or can involve most of the gingivae. Imaging and biopsy may be required for diagnosis.

Epulides are common, but rarely are they true neoplasms (**Box 12.1**).

Most gingival lumps originate in the gingival tissues but some arise from the underlying tissues such as from the bone (**Box 12.2**).

More generalized gingival swelling is fairly common, often localized to the maxillary anterior gingivae in hyperplastic gingivitis arising as a consequence of mouth-breathing. Generalized gingival swelling is commonly drug-induced, usually aggravated by poor oral hygiene and starting interdentally, especially labially. Affected papillae are firm, pale and enlarge to form false vertical clefts. Granulomatous disorders such as orofacial granulomatosis (Ch. 46) Wegener granulomatosis (Ch. 56), and plasma cell gingivitis may present with localized or more generalized swelling.

Generalized gingival swelling may occasionally be congenital (hereditary gingival fibromatosis) which usually presents with firm pink slow-growing swellings; due to deposits such as fibrin in the rare condition hypoplasminogenaemia; or due for example, to leukaemia – when there may be other features such as purpura and/or ulceration.

EPULIDES (LOCALIZED GINGIVAL SWELLINGS)

The main types of epulis include:

- *Fibrous epulides* (irritation fibromas; fibroepithelial polyp) are most common; they typically form narrow, firm, pale swellings of an anterior interdental papilla and may ulcerate (**Fig. 12.1**). Fibrous epulides may result from local gingival irritation, leading to fibrous hyperplasia. They are usually pink and firm but cannot be distinguished clinically with certainty from neoplastic epulides or the usually softer and redder pyogenic granulomas, or giant cell granulomas.
- *Pyogenic granulomas* (see Ch. 10) are common lesions, especially in children and teens, where there are local factors, including inadequate oral hygiene, malocclusion and orthodontic appliances, and in pregnancy (pregnancy epulis; epulis gravidarum) (lesions themselves not histologically distinguishable). Pyogenic granuloma commonly affects the gingiva, the lip or the tongue. It may be caused by chronic irritation and appears predisposed in patients who have had organ transplantation.
- *Giant cell epulides* (giant cell granulomas) are reactive lesions seen mainly in children, caused by local irritation or resulting from proliferation of giant cells persisting after resorption of deciduous teeth. Classically, a giant cell epulis is a swelling with a deep-red colour (although older lesions tend to be paler) and it often arises interdentally, but only anterior to the permanent molar teeth.
- *Neoplastic epulides* may be carcinomas, lymphomas, sarcomas or represent metastatic disease.

DIAGNOSIS

Radiography and excision biopsy.

MANAGEMENT

Excision and removal of local irritants (e.g. calculus).

DRUG-INDUCED GINGIVAL OVERGROWTH (DIGO)

INTRODUCTION

DIGO can be caused by a number of disparate drugs (Table 54.19), mainly phenytoin, ciclosporin and calcium channel blockers, as an adverse reaction. Swelling typically arises from the interdental papillae and is aggravated by poor oral hygiene.

AETIOLOGY AND PATHOGENESIS

The multidrug resistance 1 (MDR1) gene may modify the inflammatory response to drugs and thereby play a role in the pathogenesis. Causal drugs may include the following:

- Phenytoin: which is used mainly for the control of grand mal epilepsy. Histology shows marked thickening of epithelium

---

BOX 12.1 Main causes of gingival lumps or swelling

- Inflammation
- Granulomatous conditions (e.g. Crohn disease, sarcoidosis or orofacial granulomatosis)
- Neoplasms
- Drugs

BOX 12.2 More advanced causes of lumps on the gingiva

Gingival origin
- Inflammation
- Irritation fibroma (fibrous hyperplasia)
- Hyperplastic gingivitis
- Fibrous epulis (fibroepithelial polyp)
- Pyogenic granuloma
- Pregnancy tumour
- Peripheral giant cell granuloma
- Peripheral ossifying fibroma
- Abscesses
- Chronic gingivitis
- Granulomatous conditions
    - Crohn disease
    - Orofacial granulomatosis
    - Sarcoidosis
    - Wegener granulomatosis (Ch. 56)
    - Tuberculosis
    - Deep mycoses
- Neoplasms
    - Carcinoma
    - Leukaemia
    - Lymphoma
    - Kaposi sarcoma
    - Melanoma
    - Metastasis
    - Papilloma
    - Traumatic neuroma
    - True fibroma
    - Verruciform xanthoma
- Drugs
    - Phenytoin
    - Ciclosporin
    - Calcium channel blockers
- Deposits
    - Amyloidosis
    - Hypoplasminogenaemia
    - Oral focal mucinosis
- Cysts
    - Gingival cysts
    - Lateral periodontal cyst
    - Inflammatory cysts
    - Peripheral odontogenic keratocyst
- Exostoses
- Fibrous epulis
- Giant cell tumour
- Hereditary
    - Hereditary gingival fibromatosis
    - Torus
    - Exostosis
    - Naevus

Central lesions perforating the jaw bone
- Odontogenic tumours
- Adenomatoid odontogenic tumour
- Ameloblastoma
- Ameloblastic fibroma
- Calcifying epithelial odontogenic tumour
- Odontogenic fibroma
- Squamous odontogenic tumour
- Calcifying odontogenic cyst
- Odontoma
- Malignant neoplasms

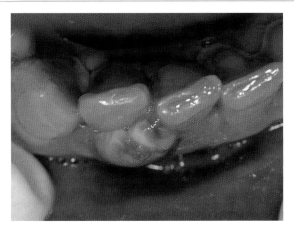

Fig. 12.1 Fibrous epulis

with long overgrowths into the connective tissue. Fibroblasts show increased mitotic activity, but are not increased in number, and the collagen fibre component is not increased.
- Ciclosporin (cyclosporin): an immunosuppressive drug particularly used to suppress the cell-mediated response after organ transplants, but only one-third of patients may be affected, more commonly children.
- Calcium-channel blockers (especially nifedipine): which are mainly used as anti-hypertensive agents. Increased numbers of fibroblasts containing strongly sulphated muco-polysaccharides may be demonstrated histochemically; their cytoplasm contains numerous secretory granules, suggesting an increased production of acid mucopolysaccharides.
- Amphetamines.

CLINICAL FEATURES

Drug-induced gingival swelling usually starts interdentally, the palatal and lingual gingiva being usually involved less than buccal and labial gingiva. Papillae are firm, pale and enlarge to form false vertical clefts (**Fig. 12.2**), which may later involve the marginal and even attached gingiva. The enlargement rarely affects edentulous sites.

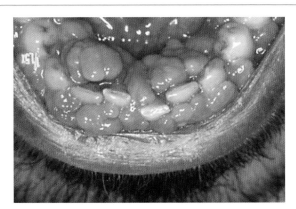

Fig. 12.2 Ciclosporin-induced gingival swelling (extreme example)

The earlier lesions may be softer and redder, sometimes giving the impression of 'bubbling up' behind the existing papillae. The enlargement is characteristically firm, pale, and tough with coarse stippling, but these features may take several years to develop. Older lesions may become red if inflamed.

There is no correlation between the extent of overgrowth and the drug dose, its serum level, or the age and gender of the patient. The swelling is aggravated if oral hygiene is poor; there is a positive correlation between the severity of overgrowth and gingival inflammation, plaque score, calculus accumulation and pocket depths.

Excessive body hair growth (hypertrichosis) is commonly associated.

DIAGNOSIS

This is usually a clinical diagnosis.

TREATMENT (see also Chs 4 and 5)

Treatment of drug-induced gingival overgrowth often poses problems as the patient often really needs to be on the responsible medication. The patient's level of plaque control often needs improvement and a chlorhexidine mouthwash may be helpful. Excision of enlarged tissue may be indicated, but difficult if the tissue is very firm and fibrous. Healing may be slow, possibly hampered by infection of the large wound. Unfortunately, the gingival enlargement readily recurs, although this is less likely with meticulous oral hygiene, particularly if the drug has been stopped. The physician may be willing to substitute another drug. Therefore:

- treat predisposing factors
- improve oral hygiene
- undertake gingivoplasty where indicated.

Follow-up of patients

Long-term follow-up as shared care is usually appropriate.

HEREDITARY GINGIVAL FIBROMATOSIS

Hereditary gingival fibromatosis (HGF) presents with gingival enlargement which begins in puberty, is painless, slowly progressive and dependent to a great extent on oral hygiene. The hyperplastic tissues are usually firm to palpation. It is not unusual for the fibromatosis to completely cover the teeth.

Symmetrical fibromatosis of the tuberosities presents as a generalized, soft, smooth-surfaced, painless enlargement of the tissues – usually over the posterior maxillary alveolus and typically bilaterally.

The most common form of HGF (HGF-1) maps to chromosome 2p21 and is caused by mutation in the SOS1 (Son of sevenless-1) gene (a guanine nucleotide-exchange factor that mediates the coupling of receptor tyrosine kinases to Ras gene activation) or to chromosome 5q13-q22. An autosomal dominant form of HGF may be associated with hypertrichosis.

Syndromic forms of HGF (e.g. Rutherford, Cross, Laband and Ramon syndromes) have other types of inheritance and associations (Ch. 56).

FURTHER READING

Ajura, A.J., Lau, S.H., 2007. Gingival myofibroma in children: report of 4 cases with immunohistochemical findings. Malays. J. Pathol. 29 (1), 53–56.

Angiero, F., Stefani, M., 2008. Metastatic embryonal carcinoma in the maxillary gingiva. Anticancer Res. 28 (2B), 1181–1186.

Buddula, A., Assad, D., 2011. Peripheral T-Cell lymphoma manifested as gingival enlargement in a patient with chronic lymphocytic leukemia. J. Indian Soc. Periodontol. 15 (1), 67–69.

Bulut, S., Uslu, H., Ozdemir, B.H., Bulut, O.E., 2006. Analysis of proliferative activity in oral gingival epithelium in immunosuppressive medication induced gingival overgrowth. Head Face Med. 19 (2), 13.

Dos Santos, J.N., Gurgel, C.A., Ramos, E.A., et al., 2009. Gingival cyst of the adult: a case report and immunohistochemical investigation. Gen. Dent. 57 (5), e41–e45.

Doufexi, A., Mina, M., Ioannidou, E., 2005. Gingival overgrowth in children: epidemiology, pathogenesis, and complications. A literature review. J. Periodontol. 76 (1), 3–10.

Groselj, D., Grabec, I., Seme, K., et al., 2008. Prediction of clinical response to anti-TNF treatment by oral parameters in Crohn's disease. Hepatogastroenterology 55 (81), 112–119.

Hasan, A.A., Ciancio, S., 2004. Relationship between amphetamine ingestion and gingival enlargement. Paediat. Dent. 26, 396–400.

Hirshberg, A., Shnaiderman-Shapiro, A., Kaplan, I., Berger, R., 2008. Metastatic tumours to the oral cavity – pathogenesis and analysis of 673 cases. Oral. Oncol. 44 (8), 743–752.

Hubácek, M., Dostálová, T., Bartonová, M., et al., 2008. Giant cell reparative granuloma in the mandible–case report and review of the literature. Acta. Chir. Plast. 50 (2), 59–63.

Jainkittivong, A., Swasdison, S., Thangpisityotin, M., Langlais, R.P., 2009. Oral squamous cell carcinoma: a clinicopathological study of 342 Thai cases. J. Contemp. Dent. Pract. 10 (5), e33–e40.

Johnson, T.M., Demsar, W.J., Herold, R.W., et al., 2011. Pyogenic granuloma occurring in a postmenopausal woman on hormone replacement therapy. US Army Med. Dep. J. Jan–Mar, 86–90.

Kataoka, M., Kido, J., Shinohara, Y., Nagata, T., 2005. Drug-induced gingival overgrowth – a review. Biol. Pharm. Bull. 28 (10), 1817–1821.

Küpers, A.M., Andriessen, P., van Kempen, M.J., et al., 2009. Congenital epulis of the jaw: a series of five cases and review of literature. Pediatr. Surg. Int. 25 (2), 207–210.

Lourenço, S.V., Lobo, A.Z., Boggio, P., et al., 2008. Gingival manifestations of orofacial granulomatosis. Arch. Dermatol. 144 (12), 1627–1630.

Madrid, C., Aziza, J., Hlali, A., et al., 2010. Melanotic neuroectodermal tumour of infancy: a case report and review of the aetiopathogenic hypotheses. Med. Oral. Patol. Oral. Cir. Bucal. 15 (5), e739–e742.

Matsumoto, N., Ohki, H., Mukae, S., et al., 2008. Anaplastic large cell lymphoma in gingiva: case report and literature review. Oral. Surg. Oral. Med. Oral. Pathol. Oral. Radiol. Endod. 106 (4), e29–e34.

Meisel, P., Giebel, J., Kunert-Keil, C., et al., 2006. MDR1 gene polymorphisms and risk of gingival hyperplasia induced by calcium antagonists. Clin. Pharmacol. Ther. 79 (1), 62–71.

Morisaki, I., Dol, S., Ueda, K., et al., 2001. Amlodipine-induced gingival overgrowth: periodontal responses to stopping and restarting the drug. Spec. Care Dentist. 21, 60–62.

Sharma, S., Dasroy, S.K., 2000. Images in clinical medicine. Gingival hyperplasia induced by phenytoin. N. Engl. J. Med. 342, 325.

Sumanth, S., Bhat, K.M., Bhat, G.S., 2007. Clinical management of an unusual case of gingival enlargement. J. Contemp. Dent. Pract. 8 (4), 88–94.

Thompson, A.L., Herman, W.W., Konzelman, J., Collins, M.A., 2004. Treating patients with drug-induced gingival overgrowth. J. Dent. Hyg. 78 (4), 12.

13 Lumps and swellings in the palate

INTRODUCTION

Lumps in the palate are usually due to unerupted teeth, or bone conditions (especially torus palatinus) (**Fig. 13.1**). Other lumps, which warrant imaging and often biopsy, can be due to fibrous lumps, papillomas, odontogenic infections (**Fig. 13.2**), odontogenic cysts, nasopalatine cyst, granulomatous disorders (e.g. sarcoidosis), lymphoid hyperplasia, and neoplasms (e.g. carcinoma, melanoma, salivary neoplasms, antral neoplasms, disseminated neoplasms, lymphomas, Kaposi sarcoma) (**Box 13.1**).

Many of these conditions are described elsewhere in the text.

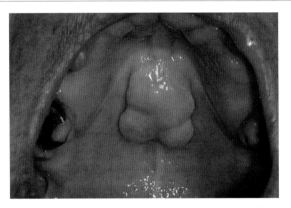

Fig. 13.1   Torus palatinus; a central lobulated bony lesion

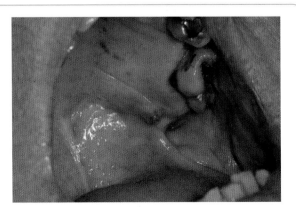

Fig. 13.2   Dental abscess arising from the non-vital third molar

---

BOX 13.1   Main causes of a lump in the palate

- Unerupted tooth
- Torus palatinus
- Dental abscess
- Fibrous lump (fibroepithelial polyp)
- Papilloma
- Neoplasm (e.g. carcinoma, lymphoma, salivary gland neoplasm, Kaposi sarcoma, antral neoplasm)
- Others (e.g. allergies, syphilis, sarcoidosis and other granulomas, follicular lymphoid hyperplasia, necrotizing sialometaplasia)

FIBROUS LUMP OR NODULE ('FIBROEPITHELIAL POLYP')

Fibrous lump or nodule ('fibroepithelial polyp') is usually a pedunculated or broadly sessile, sometimes ulcerated, hard or soft, lump in the palate. It may resemble a papilloma. Excision biopsy is warranted.

PAPILLOMA

Papilloma is a benign epithelial neoplasm with an anemone-like appearance, caused by human papillomavirus: HPV 6 or 11. Common in HIV-infected people and increased after therapy with HAART (Ch. 53), papilloma is often a small, white or pink, cauliflower-like, sessile or pedunculated lesion, <1 cm in diameter. Most common at the junction of the hard and soft palate, the lip, gingiva or tongue may occasionally be affected. Papillomas in the mouth appear to be and remain, benign, unlike papillomas of the larynx or bowel, which may undergo malignant transformation but they are best removed and examined histologically to establish the diagnosis. Excision must be total, deep and wide enough to include any abnormal cells beyond the zone of the pedicle. Cryosurgery or pulse dye laser or carbon dioxide (CO_2) laser may be used. Some use salicylic acid, imiquimod or topical podophyllum resin paint but the latter is potentially teratogenic and toxic to brain, kidney and myocardium.

FOLLICULAR LYMPHOID HYPERPLASIA

Follicular lymphoid hyperplasia of the palate is a rare benign lymphoproliferative lesion that closely resembles lymphomas, clinically and/or histopathologically. It presents as a firm, painless, nonulcerated, nonfluctuant and slowly growing swelling of the palate. The typical histologic features include multiple germinal centres with a rim of well-differentiated B lymphocytes together with a mixed, mainly mononuclear infiltrate with plasmacytoid lymphocytes.

LYMPHOMAS

(See also Burkitt lymphoma, Hodgkin disease and non-Hodgkin lymphoma (Chs 56 and 57).)

Lymphomas are malignant tumours that originate in lymph nodes and lymphoid tissue, and can originate from any type of lymphocyte, but mostly from B cells. HIV/AIDS and immunosuppression predispose. Painless enlarged cervical lymph nodes are the initial complaint in 50% of cases, but a lymphoma may occasionally produce primary or secondary oral tumours appearing as swellings, often of the pharynx, palate, tongue, gingivae or lips. Involvement of Waldeyer ring is common in non-Hodgkin lymphomas.

Patients with lymphoma develop a secondary immunodeficiency, when herpes zoster, herpetic stomatitis and oral candidosis may be seen. Diagnosis is from clinical findings (generalized lymph node enlargement and hepatosplenomegaly), imaging (hilar and abdominal lymph node enlargement), lymphangiography and biopsy (lymph node or lesional). Treatment is usually with chemotherapy.

KAPOSI SARCOMA (KS)

Kaposi sarcoma is a malignant neoplasm of endothelial cells caused by KSHV (Kaposi sarcoma herpes virus – also known as HHV-8 or human herpesvirus 8). KS is seen especially in HIV/AIDS when this is contracted sexually or via blood-borne routes, and also in other immunosuppressed patients. Usually oral lesions are part of more widespread disease. KS early oral lesions are red, purple or brown macules (**Fig. 13.3**), later becoming nodular, extending, ulcerating and disseminating. KS typically involves the palate or gingivae. Diagnosis is confirmed by biopsy: epithelioid angiomatosis, haemangiomas, lymphomas and purpura may need to be differentiated.

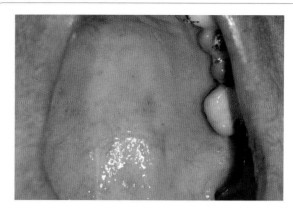

Fig. 13.3 Kaposi sarcoma – early lesions present as bluish macules over the greater palatine vessels. Later, swelling appears.

Management is treatment of the underlying predisposing condition if possible, and then radiotherapy or vinca alkaloids systemically or intralesionally.

ANTRAL CARCINOMA

Antral carcinoma is rare, usually squamous carcinoma, seen mainly in older males – the only identified predisposing factor being occupational exposure to wood dust. Initially asymptomatic, it may cause swelling or pain in the face or palate when the carcinoma invades. Symptoms depend on the main direction of spread:

- Oral invasion: causes pain and swelling of palate, alveolus or sulcus; teeth may loosen.
- Ocular invasion: causes pain and swelling, ipsilateral epiphora, diplopia or proptosis.
- Nasal invasion: causes nasal pain and swelling, obstruction or a blood-stained discharge.

Diagnose from radiographs, MRI (opaque antrum and later destruction of antral wall or floor), and biopsy. Manage by surgery (sometimes with radiotherapy). Prognosis is 10–30% 5-year survival.

FURTHER READING

Accurso, B., Allen, C., Chacon, G., 2008. A woman with a palatal swelling. J. Am. Dent. Assoc. 139 (11), 1493–1495.

Alcoceba, E., Gonzalez, M., Gaig, P., et al., 2010. Edema of the uvula: etiology, risk factors, diagnosis, and treatment. J. Investig. Allergol. Clin. Immunol. 20 (1), 80–83.

Amaral, M.B., Buchholz, I., Freire-Maia, B., et al., 2008. Treatment of an enlarged uvula. Br. J. Oral. Maxillofac. Surg. 46 (6), 490–491.

Bakshi, J., Virk, R.S., Verma, M., 2009. Pyogenic granuloma of the hard palate: a case report and review of the literature. Ear Nose Throat J. 88 (9), e4–e5.

Bascones-Martínez, A., Muñoz-Corcuera, M., Cerero-Lapiedra, R., et al., 2011. Case report of necrotizing sialometaplasia. Med. Oral. Patol. Oral. Cir. Bucal. 16 (6), e700–e703.

Farina, D., Gavazzi, E., Avigo, C., et al., 2008. Case report. MRI findings of necrotizing sialometaplasia. Br. J. Radiol. 81 (966), e173–e175.

Femiano, F., Lanza, A., Buonaiuto, C., et al., 2008. Oral malignant melanoma: a review of the literature. J. Oral. Pathol. Med. 37 (7), 383–388.

Frei, M., Dubach, P., Reichart, P.A., et al., 2010. Diffuse swelling of the buccal mucosa and palate as first and only manifestation of an extranodal non-Hodgkin 'double-hit' lymphoma: report of a case. Oral. Maxillofac. Surg. Oct 28 [Epub ahead of print].

Jham, B.C., Binmadi, N.O., Scheper, M.A., et al., 2009. Follicular lymphoid hyperplasia of the palate: case report and literature review. J. Craniomaxillofac. Surg. 37 (2), 79–82.

Kharkar, V., Gutte, R.M., Khopkar, U., et al., 2009. Kaposi's sarcoma: a presenting manifestation of HIV infection in an Indian. Indian J. Dermatol. Venereol. Leprol. 75 (4), 391–393.

Kolokotronis, A., Dimitrakopoulos, I., Asimaki, A., 2003. Follicular lymphoid hyperplasia of the palate: report of a case and review of the literature. Oral. Surg. Oral. Med. Oral. Pathol. Oral. Radiol. Endod. 96 (2), 172–175.

Kyo, C., Kawaoka, Y., Kinoshita, K., Ohno, H., 2010. Mantle cell lymphoma presenting with a tumor of the hard palate. Intern. Med. 49 (15), 1663–1666.

Martins, C.R., Horta, M.C., 2008. Advanced osteosarcoma of the maxilla: a case report. Med. Oral. Pathol. Oral. Cir. Bucal. 13 (8), e492–e495.

Pahwa, R., Khurana, N., Chaturvedi, K.U., 2004. Angiomyoma of the palate – a case report. Indian J. Pathol. Microbiol. 47 (2), 229–230.

Phipps, W., Ssewankambo, F., Nguyen, H., et al., 2010. Gender differences in clinical presentation and outcomes of epidemic Kaposi sarcoma in Uganda. PLoS One 5 (11), e13936.

Rabbels, J., Scheer, M., Heibel, H., et al., 2005. Neurinoma of the hard palate in an 11-year-old girl. Case report. Mund Kiefer Gesichtschir. 9 (6), 400–403.

Rapidis, A.D., 2009. Orbitomaxillary mucormycosis (zygomycosis) and the surgical approach to treatment: perspectives from a maxillofacial surgeon. Clin. Microbiol. Infect. 15 (Suppl. 5), 98–102.

Scolozzi, P., Martinez, A., Richter, M., Lombardi, T., 2008. A nasopalatine duct cyst in a 7-year-old child. Pediatr. Dent. 30 (6), 530–534.

Scully, C., 2002. Oral medicine for the general practitioner: part three: lumps and swellings. Independent Dent. 7 (10), 25–32.

Scully, C., Felix, D.H., 2005. Oral medicine – update for the dental practitioner. 8. Lumps and swellings. Br. Dent. J. 199, 763–770.

Scully, C., Porter, S., 2000. ABC of Oral Health. 6. Swellings, and red: white, and pigmented lesions. BMJ 321, 225–228.

Shakib, K., McCarthy, E., Walker, D.M., Newman, L., 2009. Post operative maxillary cyst: report of an unusual presentation. Br. J. Oral. Maxillofac. Surg. 47 (5), 419–421.

Urs, A.B., Shetty, D., Praveen Reddy, B., Sikka, S., 2011. Diverse clinical nature of cavernous lymphangioma: report of two cases. Minerva Stomatol. 60 (3), 149–153.

Werder, P., Altermatt, H.J., Zbären, P., et al., 2010. Palatal swelling as the first and only manifestation of extranodal follicular non-Hodgkin lymphoma: a case presentation. Quintessence Int. 41 (2), 93–97.

Lumps and swellings in the tongue

INTRODUCTION

Tongue swelling is usually because of an isolated lump typically acquired and caused by trauma, infection or a neoplasm (**Box 14.1, Figs 14.1–14.3**). Biopsy and other investigations are usually indicated. Ectopic thyroid tissue in the tongue is rare, and usually presents as a persistent single symptomless nodule in the posterior midline dorsum of tongue lingual thyroid. It is important not to remove this without establishing there is adequate thyroid tissue present in the neck.

Diffuse swelling is usually acquired and caused by trauma, infection or allergy (angioedema). Sudden swelling of the

---

BOX 14.1 Main causes of enlarged tongue

- Allergy
- Trauma
- Infection
- Angioma
- Neoplasm

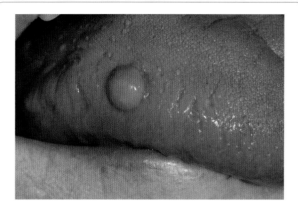

Fig. 14.2 Fibrous lump on the tongue

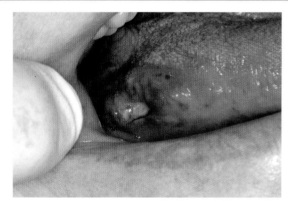

Fig. 14.3 Tongue cancer, presenting as a persistent lump that has ulcerated

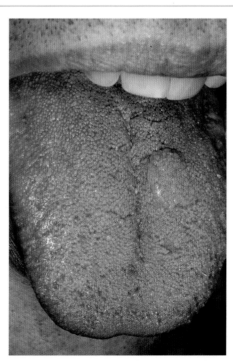

Fig. 14.1 Lingual lump caused by abnormal healing after trauma

tongue can arise due to an allergic reaction or an adverse drug effect. Rare acquired causes are of slow onset over weeks or months and include amyloidosis (then often with purpura; Ch. 57) and other deposits (**Box 14.2**), or parasites such as cysticercosis.

Diffuse swelling of the tongue (macroglossia) may occasionally have congenital causes including: lymphangioma (see Ch. 57); haemangioma (see Ch. 57); neurofibromatosis (see Ch. 57); Down syndrome; cretinism; Hurler syndrome (a mucopolysaccharidosis) and multiple endocrine adenomatosis (Ch. 57).

BOX 14.2   **More advanced list of causes of tongue swelling/lumps**

- Acromegaly
- Allergic reaction (see also Drugs: Ch. 54)
- Amyloidosis
- Angioedema
- Beckwith syndrome
- Congenital micrognathia
- Deep mycosis
- Down syndrome
- Fibrous lump
- Foreign body
- Granular cell tumour
- Granulomatous conditions (Crohn disease, OFG, Sarcoidosis)
- Median rhomboid glossitis
- Haemangioma
- Hypothyroidism
- Infection
- Leishmaniasis
- Leukaemia

- Lymphangioma
- Lingual thyroid
- Mucopolysaccharidosis
- Multiple endocrine neoplasia syndrome
- Neoplasms (carcinoma, lymphoma, Kaposi sarcoma, salivary gland neoplasms, metastases others)
- Oedema
- Papilloma
- Pellagra
- Pernicious anaemia
- Pyogenic granuloma
- Simpson–Golabi–Behmel syndrome (Ch. 56)
- Syphilis
- Trauma
- Tuberculosis
- TUGSE (traumatic ulcerative granuloma with stromal eosinophilia)

The tongue may get somewhat wider in edentulous persons who do not wear dentures (false macroglossia):

- In true macroglossia, the tongue is indented by teeth, or too large to be contained in the mouth.

- Severe macroglossia can cause cosmetic and functional difficulties including in speaking, eating, swallowing and sleeping. Surgery may be indicated.

FURTHER READING

Abdel-Aziz, M., Ibrahim, N., Ahmed, A., et al., 2011. Lingual tonsils hypertrophy; a cause of obstructive sleep apnea in children after adenotonsillectomy: Operative problems and management. Int. J. Pediatr. Otorhinolaryngol. 75 (9), 1127–1131.

Bezerra, M.F., Costa, F.W., Pereira, K.M., et al., 2010. Chondrolipoma of the posterior tongue. J. Craniofac. Surg. 21 (6), 1982–1984.

Breik, O., Hay, K.D., 2008. Migrating foreign body in the tongue. N. Z. Dent. J. 104 (2), 62–64.

Cohen, M., Wang, M.B., 2009. Schwannoma of the tongue: two case reports and review of the literature. Eur. Arch. Otorhinolaryngol. 266 (11), 1823–1829.

Eley, K.A., Afzal, T., Shah, K.A., Watt-Smith, S.R., 2010. Alveolar soft-part sarcoma of the tongue: report of a case and review of the literature. Int. J. Oral. Maxillofac. Surg. 39 (8), 824–826.

Furugen, M., Nakamura, H., Tamaki, Y., et al., 2009. Tuberculosis of the tongue initially suspected of tongue cancer: a case report – including the search for recent 16 cases in Japan. Kekkaku 84 (8), 605–610.

Groh, O.R., Southwold, A., Verbeek, P.C., 2010. A foreign body in the tongue. Ned. Tijdschr. Tandheelkd. 117 (9), 433–434.

Gupta, R., Gupta, K., Gupta, R., 2009. Polymorphous low-grade adenocarcinoma of the tongue: a case report. J. Med. Case Reports 3, 9313.

Kapferer, I., Berger, K., Stuerz, K., Beier, U.S., 2010. Self-reported complications with lip and tongue piercing. Quintessence Int. 41 (9), 731–737.

Karaca, C.T., Habesoglu, T.E., Naiboglu, B., et al., 2010. Schwannoma of the tongue in a child. Am. J. Otolaryngol. 31 (1), 46–48.

Kumar Choudhury, B., Kaimal Saikia, U., Sarma, D., et al., 2011. Dual ectopic thyroid with normally located thyroid: a case report. J. Thyroid Res. 2011, 159–703.

Leszczyńska, M., Borucki, L., Popko, M., 2008. Head and neck amyloidosis. Otolaryngol. Pol. 62 (5), 643–648.

Merz, H., Marnitz, S., Erbersdobler, A., Goektas, O., 2010. Schmincke's Tumor, Carcinoma of the Base of the Tongue c T1-2, cN2c M0 - A Case Report. Case Rep. Oncol. 3 (1), 77–82.

Mukozawa, M., Kono, T., Fujiwara, S., Takakura, K., 2011. Late onset tongue edema after palatoplasty. Acta Anaesthesiol. Taiwan 49 (1), 29–31.

Ottomeyer, C., Sick, C., Hennerici, M.G., Szabo, K., 2009. Orolingual angioedema under systemic thrombolysis with rt-PA: an underestimated side effect. Nervenarzt 80 (4), 459–463.

Prlesi, L., Plakogiannis, R., 2010. Angioedema after nonsteroidal antiinflammatory drug initiation in a patient stable on an angiotensin-converting-enzyme inhibitor. Am. J. Health Syst. Pharm. 67 (16), 1351–1353.

Sánchez Barrueco, A., Melchor Díaz, M.A., Jiménez Huerta, I., et al., 2012. Recurrent lingual abscess. Acta Otorrinolaringol. Esp. 63 (4), 318–320.

Sarwar, A.F., Ahmad, S.A., Khan, M.H., et al., 2010. Swelling of vallate papillae of the tongue following arsenic exposure. Bangladesh Med. Res. Counc. Bull. 36 (1), 1–3.

Scully, C., 2002. Oral medicine for the general practitioner: part three: lumps and swellings. Independent Dent. 7 (10), 25–32.

Scully, C., Felix, D.H., 2005. Oral medicine – update for the dental practitioner. 8. Lumps and swellings. Br. Dent. J. 199, 763–770.

Scully, C., Porter, S., 2000. ABC of Oral Health. 6. Swellings, and red: white, and pigmented lesions. BMJ 321, 225–228.

Scully, C., Porter, S.R., 2000. Orofacial disease: update for the dental clinical team. 11. Cervical lymphadenopathy. Dent. Update. 27, 44–47.

Sood, A., Kumar, R., 2008. The ectopic thyroid gland and the role of nuclear medicine techniques in its diagnosis and management. Hell. J. Nucl. Med. 11 (3), 168–171.

Urs, A.B., Shetty, D., Praveen Reddy, B., Sikka, S., 2011. Diverse clinical nature of cavernous lymphangioma: report of two cases. Minerva Stomatol. 60 (3), 149–153.

Watanabe, T., Fujiwara, T., Toyama, M., et al., 2011. Case of sublingual hematoma following difficult laryngoscopy in a patient on anticoagulant therapy. Masui 60 (1), 100–103.

Lumps and swellings in the salivary glands

INTRODUCTION

Swelling in the region of the salivary glands may arise from the gland or in an intra-salivary lymph node, or in other tissue (**Box 15.1**). Ultrasonography, other imaging and biopsy are often indicated.

The most common salivary lesion causing a swelling is the mucocele, usually caused by extravasation of saliva from a damaged minor salivary gland duct and seen in the lower labial mucosa, sometimes caused by retention within a gland (**Fig. 15.1**). In the floor of mouth a large mucocele may be termed a 'ranula' from its likeness to the belly of a frog (Latin rana = frog).

Sialadenitis (inflammation of the salivary gland) is another common cause of salivary gland swelling (**Box 15.2**). Sialadenitis may be caused by infection, or may be non-infective (e.g. in Sjögren syndrome or sarcoidosis).

In children and young people, the most common cause of swelling of one or more the major glands, is viral sialadenitis (mumps).

In older children, recurrent sialadenitis (juvenile recurrent parotitis), is of uncertain cause but is probably a group of conditions

BOX 15.1   Main causes of salivary gland swelling

- Obstruction
- Sialadenitis
- Sjögren syndrome
- Sialosis
- Neoplasm

BOX 15.2   More advanced list of lumps in the salivary glands

Salivary gland swellings may be caused mainly by lymph nodes or other lesions, or salivary:
- Cyst (mucocele or cystic neoplasm)
- Calculus or other obstruction to salivary flow
- Deposits (e.g. amyloidosis, haemochromatosis)
- Hamartoma (branchial cyst, angioma, lymphangioma)
- Hypersensitivity (allergic sialadenitis)
- IgG4 syndrome (Kuttner tumour – chronic sialadenitis)
- Infection (usually bacterial or viral sialadenitis)
- Necrotizing sialometaplasia
- Neoplasm (epithelial or mesenchymal)
- Sarcoidosis
- Sialosis
- Sjögren syndrome

variously caused by genetic factors, ductal obstruction, ductal ectasia (dilatations), or diseases such as Sjögren syndrome or sarcoidosis.

In adults, salivary swelling is most commonly obstructive (e.g. a salivary stone or calculus (sialolith)) or inflammatory in origin (e.g. infective sialadenitis, sclerosing sialadenitis (IgG4 syndrome), Sjögren syndrome and sarcoidosis) (**Fig. 15.2**).

- Salivary swelling may be caused rarely by systemic infections such as tuberculosis.
- Salivary swelling may be caused by neoplastic disease: when it is typically a unilateral lump (**Fig. 15.3**), or other disorders (e.g. sialosis) when it is typically diffuse and often bilateral.

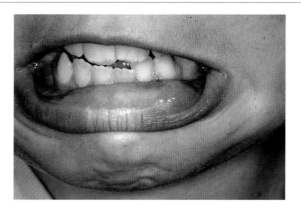

Fig. 15.1   Mucocele in a typical site – the lower labial mucosa

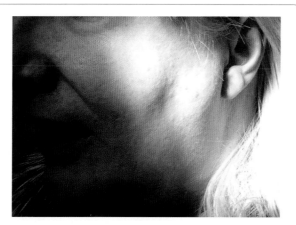

Fig. 15.2   Parotid salivary gland enlargement

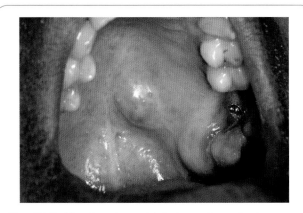

Fig. 15.3 Neoplasm in a palatal minor salivary gland

- Salivary swelling may be painful or painless and this may help differential diagnosis (**Table 15.1**). Salivary swelling can also be caused by:
  - fluid: as in trauma (oedema or haematoma), mucocele or vascular lesions
  - solids: such as deposits (e.g. amyloidosis, heamochromatosis) or foreign material
  - swelling of intra-salivary lymph nodes.

The main conditions apart from salivary gland neoplasms (Ch. 49) causing swellings are summarized alphabetically below.

MUCOCELES

Cystic lesions of minor salivary glands, that mostly appear in the lower labial mucosa, buccal mucosa or ventrum of tongue; mucoceles are fluctuant bluish lesions mostly caused by trauma to the duct, leading to mucous extravasation (extravasation mucoceles). This type of mucocele is not, however, lined by epithelium, and, therefore, is not a true cyst. Occasional mucoceles are caused by saliva retention (retention mucoceles), especially in the floor of mouth when they may resemble a frog belly and are termed 'ranula'. Mucoceles are diagnosed clinically but it is important to differentiate from a cystic neoplasm, this being most likely in the upper lip (usually a canalicular adenoma).

Most mucoceles either resolve spontaneously or can be excised, ligated or removed with cryosurgery. Ranula may respond to the sclerosant picibanil.

Minor salivary gland outlet obstruction is most commonly encountered when a mucocele is present, although smoking and its accompanying nicotinic stomatitis produces transient palatal minor gland outlet obstruction also.

Superficial mucoceles may be seen in lichen planus.

MUMPS (ACUTE VIRAL SIALADENITIS; EPIDEMIC PAROTITIS)

A common acute viral disease, which principally affects the parotid salivary glands, mumps is:

- caused by an RNA paramyxovirus (the mumps virus)
- transmitted by direct contact or by droplet spread from saliva
- characterized by a longish incubation period of 2–3 weeks
- followed by immunity to further attacks.

Typically the patient with mumps suffers an acute onset of:

- painful salivary swelling (parotitis), usually bilaterally, although in the early stages only one parotid gland may appear to be involved. There is no significant hyposalivation. In approximately 10% of cases, the submandibular glands are also affected; rarely, these may be the only glands involved. Generally, the salivary swelling persists for about 7 days and then gradually subsides
- trismus
- fever
- malaise.

Mumps less commonly (and mainly in adults) has extrasalivary manifestations involving organs other than the salivary glands, including:

- orchitis; rarely, oophoritis and thyroiditis; ensuing infertility is rare
- pancreatitis
- meningoencephalitis

Table 15.1 Differentiation of salivary lumps

Type of swelling	Diffuse		Discrete	
Symptoms	**Painful**	**Painless**	**Painful**	**Painless**
Main causes	Sialadenitis Lymphadenitis Neoplasm	Sialadenitis Sialosis Neoplasm Sarcoidosis Sjögren syndrome Hamartoma (e.g. angioma) Deposits (e.g. amyloidosis, haemochromatosis)	Abscess Neoplasm Sialometaplasia	Cyst Neoplasm Hamartoma (e.g. angioma)
Investigations	US FNAC MRI or CT Biopsy Sialoendoscopy if obstructive	US FNAC Biopsy Chest radiography Serology SACE Adenosine deaminase	US FNAC MRI or CT	US FNAC

The diagnosis is on clinical grounds, but confirmation, if needed, is by demonstrating a fourfold rise in serum antibody titres to mumps S and V antigens between acute serum and convalescent serum collected 3 weeks later. Other viruses can rarely produce parotitis. No specific antiviral agents are available, so treatment is symptomatic involving:

- analgesics
- adequate hydration
- reducing the fever.

Patient isolation for 6–10 days may be advisable since virus is in saliva during this time.

OBSTRUCTION (OBSTRUCTIVE SIALADENITIS; 'MEALTIME SYNDROME')

Obstruction of a minor salivary gland duct or a ductal tear may produce a mucocele (see above). Obstruction is fairly common in the submandibular duct or gland (calculus is the usual cause) and rare in parotid (more likely to be a mucus plug, fibrous stricture or neoplasm) (see also Ch. 49). Uncommon causes of duct obstruction include:

- oedema from irritation of the duct by, for example, a denture clasp
- 'physiological' duct obstruction due either to duct spasm or an abnormal passage of the parotid duct through the buccinator or in relation to the masseter muscles
- neoplasm
- stricture.

Obstruction may be asymptomatic but typically there is pain and swelling of gland at meals ('mealtime syndrome') and there can be a consequent bacterial sialadenitis. Prolonged duct obstruction produces atrophy, particularly of serous acini, such as in the parotid gland:

It is important to differentiate from other causes of salivary swelling:

- inflammatory: mumps, bacterial sialadenitis,
- Sjögren syndrome, sarcoidosis: duct obstruction; neoplasms (see Ch. 49); others including sialosis, drugs
- Mikulicz disease (sclerosing sialadenitis, IgG4 syndrome).

It is occasionally possible clinically to determine the cause of major duct obstruction if a calculus is palpable or visible. Ultrasound may help but sialoendoscopy, radiography (but 40% of stones are radiolucent) can be diagnostic, and MRI/ CT or sialography if necessary. Management is the surgical removal of the obstruction (lithotripsy, interventional sialoendoscopy, Storz balloon or Dormia basket removal, or incisional removal).

SARCOIDOSIS

An uncommon chronic granulomatous reaction of unknown aetiology, prevalent particularly in black females, sarcoidosis may present with cervical lymphadenopathy, enlarged salivary glands and hyposalivation. Other oral lesions may occasionally precede systemic involvement but Heerfordt syndrome (salivary and lacrimal swelling, facial palsy and uveitis), mucosal nodules, gingival hyperplasia or labial swelling are rare.

Diagnosis is by lesional biopsy, chest radiography, gallium scan, raised serum angiotensin converting enzyme and adenosine deaminase, to differentiate from Crohn disease, tuberculosis and foreign body reactions. Biopsy of minor salivary glands reveals granulomas in up to 20% of patients with sarcoidosis, particularly in those with hilar lymphadenopathy. Management is with intralesional corticosteroids; systemic corticosteroids if the lung or eye are involved.

SIALADENITIS (BACTERIAL)

Sialadenitis most commonly manifests in the parotid gland (parotitis). The organisms most commonly isolated from bacterial ascending sialadenitis are α-haemolytic streptococci, such as *Streptococcus viridans* and *Staphylococcus aureus*, the latter frequently being penicillin-resistant. Reduced salivary flow allows retrograde access of bacteria from the oral cavity, associated with:

- dehydration: such as following gastrointestinal surgery
- radiotherapy for oral or salivary tumours
- salivary gland or duct abnormalities or obstruction
- Sjögren syndrome.

Acute parotitis presents with:

- painful, swollen salivary gland
- the overlying skin may be reddened
- pus may exude from the parotid duct (if the infection localizes as a parotid abscess it may point externally through the overlying skin or, rarely, into the external acoustic meatus)
- trismus
- pyrexia
- cervical lymphadenopathy
- leukocytosis.

Diagnosis is on clinical grounds but US may help. Investigations may be needed to exclude hyposalivation. Management is as follows:

- Collect pus for a stained smear, culture and antibiotic sensitivity testing.
- Body temperature should be noted.
- Cervical lymphadenopathy should be excluded.
- Antibiotic therapy should be commenced orally. The antibiotic of choice is flucloxacillin, with erythromycin as an alternative if the patient is penicillin-allergic.
- Any fluctuant swelling should be surgically drained.
- Supportive therapy, such as ensuring an adequate fluid intake, analgesics and attention to good oral hygiene, is important.

Once the acute condition has resolved, correctable factors, such as mucus plugs, strictures or calculi should be treated. If treatment is inadequate, or predisposing factors are not eliminated chronic bacterial sialadenitis may develop. Unfortunately, serous acini may atrophy when salivary outflow is chronically obstructed and this further reduces salivary function.

SIALADENOSIS (SIALOSIS)

Sialadenosis is an uncommon, benign, non-inflammatory, non-neoplastic bilaterally symmetrical and painless enlargement of salivary glands. A variety of causes are recognized, most associated with autonomic neuropathy, including:

- drugs (sympathomimetic agents such as isoprenaline, phenylbutazone, isoprenaline, antithyroid drugs and phenothiazines)
- alcohol abuse with or without accompanying liver cirrhosis
- endocrine conditions:
  - diabetes mellitus
  - pregnancy
  - acromegaly
  - following oophorectomy
- nutritional disorders:
  - malnutrition
  - anorexia nervosa
  - bulimia
  - cystic fibrosis and pancreatitis.

Sialadenosis usually affects both parotids with soft, painless general enlargement of the glands. A useful guide to whether the patient is simply obese or has parotid enlargement is to observe the outward deflection of the ear lobe, which is seen in true parotid swelling. The diagnosis of sialadenosis is one of exclusion, based mainly on history and clinical examination. Investigations indicated may include:

- Blood tests: for raised glucose levels or abnormal liver function.
- Ultrasound: rarely, a bilateral space-occupying lesion such as a salivary neoplasm, cyst or lymphoid neoplasm may present difficulties in differentiation from sialadenosis, and then ultrasound may help.
- Sialography: reveals enlarged but otherwise normal glands, although salivary secretion is not impaired. However, if a bilateral space-occupying lesion, such as a salivary neoplasm, cyst or lymphoid neoplasm presents difficulties in differentiation, sialography or MRI may help.
- Biopsy is rarely needed. The affected glands show acinar hypertrophy, which appears related to an autonomic neuropathy.
- Sialochemistry shows raised potassium and calcium levels, which are not found in other causes of parotid enlargement.

No treatment is available. If investigations have revealed a likely cause such as alcoholism or diabetes, then sialadenosis may resolve when alcohol intake is reduced or glucose control is instituted.

FURTHER READING

Berardi, D., Scoccia, A., Perfetti, G., Berardi, S., 2009. Recurrence of pleomorphic adenoma of the palate after sixteen years: case report and an analysis of the literature. J. Biol. Regul. Homeost. Agents 23 (4), 225–229.

Bradley, P., Huntinas-Lichius, O., 2011. Salivary Gland Disorders and Diseases: Diagnosis and Management. Thieme, Stuttgart.

Cherian, S., Kulkarni, R., Bhat, N., 2010. Epithelial-myoepithelial carcinoma in the hard palate: a case report. Acta Cytol. 54 (Suppl. 5), 835–839.

Dhanuthai, K., Sappayatosok, K., Kongin, K., 2009. Pleomorphic adenoma of the palate in a child: a case report. Med. Oral. Patol. Oral. Cir. Bucal. 14 (2), e73–e75.

Jaber, M.A., 2006. Intraoral minor salivary gland tumors: a review of 75 cases in a Libyan population. Int. J. Oral. Maxillofac. Surg. 35 (2), 150–154.

Jaguar, G.C., da Cruz Perez, D.E., de Lima, V.C., et al., Palatal ulcerations and midfacial swelling. Oral. Surg. Oral. Med. Oral. Pathol. Oral. Radiol. Endod. 108 (4), 483–487.

Magliocca, K.R., Leung, E.M., Desmond, J.S., 2009. Parotid swelling and facial nerve palsy: an uncommon presentation of sarcoidosis. Gen. Dent. 57 (2), 180–182.

Rocha, L.A., Brasil Moreira, A.E., Pereira Neto, J.S., et al., 2010. Mucoepidermoid carcinoma diagnosed in orthodontic patients. Am. J. Orthod. Dentofacial. Orthop. 138 (3), 349–351.

Scully, C., 2002. Oral medicine for the general practitioner: part three: lumps and swellings. Independent Dent. 7 (10), 25–32.

Scully, C., Bagán, J.V., Eveson, J.W., et al., 2008. Sialosis: 35 cases of persistent parotid swelling from two countries. Br. J. Oral. Maxillofac. Surg. 46 (6), 468–472.

Scully, C., Felix, D.H., 2005. Oral medicine – update for the dental practitioner. 8. Lumps and swellings. Br. Dent. J. 199, 763–770.

Scully, C., Porter, S., 2000. ABC of Oral Health. 6. Swellings, and red: white, and pigmented lesions. BMJ 321, 225–228.

Werder, P., Altermatt, H.J., Zbären, P., et al., 2010. Palatal swelling as the first and only manifestation of extranodal follicular non-Hodgkin lymphoma: a case presentation. Quintessence Int. 41 (2), 93–97.

Lumps and swellings in the jaws

INTRODUCTION

Jaw swelling is most often caused by developmental enlargements (e.g. tori or exostoses), which are benign, painless, broad-based and self-limiting, usually with normal overlying mucosa and typically require no intervention.

Jaw swelling is less commonly due to odontogenic causes (unerupted teeth, infections, cysts or neoplasms) (**Box 16.1**).

Jaw swelling may occasionally be caused by non-odontogenic inflammatory or neoplastic disorders, or metabolic or fibro-osseous diseases (**Box 16.2**).

Metastasis to the mouth is rare but is typically to the jaws, especially the posterior mandible.

Imaging and other investigations (often biopsy) are almost invariably required to assist the diagnosis of a jaw swelling.

Many of these conditions are discussed elsewhere in the text. Here we discuss alphabetically other relevant but uncommon or rare, conditions.

BOX 16.1 **Main causes of jaw swelling**

- Congenital (torus palatinus, torus mandibularis, exostosis)
- Odontogenic (teeth, infections, cysts or neoplasms)

BOX 16.2 **More advanced list of causes of jaw swellings**

- Congenital (e.g. torus, exostosis)
  - Odontogenic
  - Cysts
  - Infections
  - Neoplasms
  - Post-operative or post-traumatic oedema or haematoma
  - Unerupted teeth
- Non-odontogenic
  - Infections
  - Cysts
  - Neoplasms (e.g. myeloma, histiocytoses)
  - Pseudotumours (e.g. haemophilic pseudotumour)
  - Foreign bodies
  - Bone disease
    - Fibrous dysplasia
    - Cherubism
    - Neoplasms (e.g. sarcomas)
    - Osteomas (and Gardner syndrome)
    - Paget disease

ANEURYSMAL BONE CYST

Aneurysmal bone cyst is a rare lesion, which is actually not a cyst. The aetiology remains obscure: approximately one-third appear to be associated with other bone disorders, such as a giant cell lesion, fibrous dysplasia and ossifying fibromas. This rare lesion presents as an asymptomatic hard swelling of the jaw, sometimes following a history of trauma. It may occur in any part of the skeleton. Radiographs show a unilocular, or multilocular translucency with a honeycomb or soap-bubble appearance. Preoperative aspiration shows bloody fluid with a low haematocrit, differentiating it from undiluted blood in a vascular anomaly, such as haemangioma. Diagnosis is confirmed by histology, which shows numerous capillaries and blood-filled spaces, areas of haemorrhage associated with multinucleated giant cells and irregular areas of osteoid. Treat by thorough curettage or excision.

CHERUBISM

Cherubism is a rare genetically determined jaw disease, which closely resembles fibrous dysplasia except for the autosomal dominant inheritance (but variable expression) and association with chromosome 4p and mutated gene SH3BP2 which codes for a c-abl-binding protein. Painless symmetrical enlargement at the angles of the mandible and in the maxilla leads to the typical 'cherubic' facial appearance. Cherubism presents at 2–4 years of age, lesions growing progressively until puberty when they arrest or regress. Expansion of the alveolar bone results in irregular spacing and premature loss of teeth and possibly disturbances to a developing dentition. Imaging shows well-defined multilocular radiolucencies in the mandible, but maxillary lesions are less clearly defined. Blood chemistry is normal, although there may a raised alkaline phosphatase during active growth periods. Histologically, the lesions consist of loose vascular connective tissue with numerous multinucleated giant cells and, as in fibrous dysplasia, there is fibrous replacement of bone (**Fig. 16.1**). Other fibro-osseous lesions and giant cell lesions of bone (giant cell granuloma, hyperparathyroidism, giant cell tumours) should be excluded. Treatment of cherubism is as for fibrous dysplasia (see also Noonan syndrome, Ch. 56).

EXOSTOSES

Bone prominences are not uncommon in the jaws and are given different names which are site-specific. Torus palatinus is found only in the midline of the hard palate (see below).

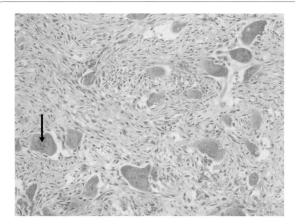

Fig. 16.1 Cherubism showing multinucleated giant cells (arrowed) in fibrous stroma

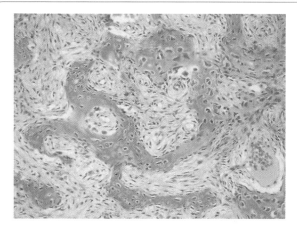

Fig. 16.2 Fibrous dysplasia: Chinese characters formed by bone

Torus mandibularis is found only on the lingual surface of the mandible, near the premolar teeth. Buccal exostosis is found only on the facial surface of the alveolar bone, usually in the maxilla. Exostoses typically appear in early adulthood, are painless and may slowly enlarge over time. Bone prominences usually require no treatment, and have no malignant potential.

Bony proliferations in other sites are considered to be usually either trauma-induced inflammatory periosteal reactions (exostoses), or true neoplasms (osteomas). Unless such a bony prominence is specifically located, is pedunculated or is associated with an osteoma-producing syndrome such as Gardner syndrome (Ch. 56), there is no way to differentiate exostosis from osteoma, even histopathologically.

FIBROUS DYSPLASIA

Fibrous dysplasia is an uncommon disorder characterized by the replacement of an area of bone with fibrous tissue. Mutations in signalling protein gene GNAS 1 may be involved. Fibrous dysplasia usually presents as a painless bony hard swelling, most often in a child and in the maxilla or adjacent bones. The maxillary sinus is often involved, when there may be encroachment on the orbit (causing proptosis) and nasal cavity (causing obstruction). Expansion of the alveolar bone leads to disruption of occlusion, displacement of teeth and possibly failure of eruption of teeth. Lesions appear to stabilize with skeletal maturation.

Three types of fibrous dysplasia (FD) are recognized:

- Monostotic (MFD), in which there is a single lesion in only one bone.
- Polyostotic (PFD), in which several lesions are present in one or more bones.
- McCune–Albright syndrome, PFD plus cutaneous pigmentation (cafe-au-lait type) on the same side as the bony lesion, and precocious puberty (see Section 6).

Radiographically, there is either a translucent cystic appearance in the affected bone, or mottled opaque areas likened to ground glass. The lesions are often ill-defined and may extend to, but not cross, suture lines. Serum calcium and phosphate levels are normal but, in many, the serum alkaline phosphatase level is high and urinary hydroxyproline is increased (findings similar to those in Paget disease). Microscopically, the lesion consists of fibrous tissue that replaces the normal bone and gives rise to osseous trabeculae by metaplasia (**Fig. 16.2**). The osseous tissue is composed of irregular ('Chinese characters') trabeculae of woven bone lined by osteoblasts. Focal degeneration of fibrous tissue accounts for the cystic spaces seen macroscopically. The treatment of choice to correct any cosmetic defect is conservative surgery, preferably after the cessation of normal skeletal growth. The lesion is not radio-sensitive; irradiation may cause sarcomatous change.

GIANT CELL GRANULOMA

The central giant cell granuloma is an uncommon lesion only seen in the tooth-bearing regions of the jaws, most commonly in the mandible and typically in the second and third decades. The true nature of these lesions is unknown but, as they are invariably destructive, the term 'reparative' giant cell granuloma would appear to be inappropriate. Lesions may be symptomless or simulate a malignant neoplasm clinically and radiographically. Occasionally, the lesion erodes through the cortical bone where it presents as a domed, purplish submucosal swelling. Radiography shows an ill-defined area of radiolucency and there may be resorption of the roots of related teeth. Microscopy shows multinucleated giant cells irregularly distributed in a cellular stroma of plump, spindle-shaped cells which is often highly vascular. There may be areas of new and old haemorrhage with haemosiderin pigment deposition. These microscopic features are indistinguishable from the focal lesions of hyperparathyroidism, which can only be excluded by the appropriate serological tests (calcium and phosphate levels and alkaline phosphatase). Although central giant cell granulomas may recur following curettage, they virtually never metastasize.

METASTATIC TUMOURS IN THE JAWS

The jaws are not a common site for clinically obvious metastases ('secondaries') but it is probable that sub-clinical secondary deposits are not rare. The mandible is involved four times as frequently as the maxilla, especially in the premolar and molar region. In up to one-third of patients, the jaw lesions are the first manifestation of a tumour. Most metastases originate from primary cancers of the breast, lung, kidney, thyroid, stomach, liver, colon, bone or prostate via lymphatic or haematogenous spread, and present as a lumps, ulceration, pain, swelling, tooth loosening, sensory change or pathological fracture. Metastases from the bronchus, breast, kidney or thyroid gland are usually destructive and osteolytic. Prostatic metastases tend to be osteoblastic and may be confused radiographically with chronic osteomyelitis, Paget disease or cemental lesions.

OSTEOID OSTEOMA AND OSTEOBLASTOMA

These are benign bone tumours that are uncommon in the skeleton generally and rare in the jaws, and their microscopic features are similar, with a vascular stroma in which there are trabeculae of osteoid surrounded by numerous, and darkly staining, osteoblasts, but they have distinctive clinical and radiological features.

Osteoid osteoma is usually seen in adolescents and young adults, most frequently in the femur and fibia, is often painful (particularly at night) and has a characteristic central radiolucent area or nidus surrounded by a rim of densely sclerotic bone of variable thickness.

Osteoblastoma, on the other hand, shows progressive growth without the osteosclerotic rim and is rarely painful.

OSTEOMA

Osteoma is a benign bone neoplasm which grows by the continuous formation of lamellar bone. Osteomas are usually unilateral, painless, hard smooth swellings covered by normal oral mucosa. Multiple osteomas, cutaneous cysts or fibromas and polyposis coli are features of Gardner syndrome; an autosomal dominant syndrome in which the polyps in the large bowel may become malignant. Should a patient have multiple bony growths or lesions not in the classic torus or buccal exostosis locations, Gardner syndrome should be excluded.

PAGET DISEASE OF BONE

Paget disease of bone affects mainly older males. The aetiology is unclear and incidence appears to be decreasing. Viruses, particularly paramyxoviruses such as canine distemper or measles virus, have been implicated – but with little evidence. There is a strong genetic component; 15–20% have a first-degree relative with Paget disease. Mutations in sequestosome 1/p62 gene (SQSTM1/p62) are seen in about one-third, and in 5–15% of patients with no family history. SQSTM1/p62 protein is a selective activator of the transcription factor NFB, which plays an important role in osteoclast differentiation and activation in response to the cytokines RANK-ligand and interleukin-1.

Paget disease is characterized by the total disorganization of the normally orderly remodelling of bone and an anarchic alternation of bone resorption and apposition ('reversal lines')

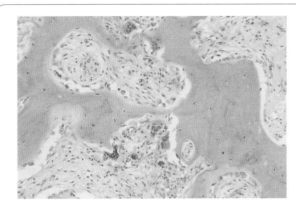

Fig. 16.3 Paget disease showing bone reversal lines from resorption/deposition with a 'mosaic pattern' (arrowed)

(**Fig. 16.3**) often with severe bone pain. In early lesions, bone destruction predominates (osteolytic stage) and there is bowing of long bones, especially the tibia, pathological fractures, broadening/flattening of chest and spinal deformity. If Paget disease is widespread, the increased bone vascularity can lead to high output cardiac failure. As disease activity declines, bone apposition increases (osteosclerotic stage) and bones enlarge. If the skull is affected, the patient may notice hat becomes tight. Constriction of skull foraminae may cause cranial neuropathies. The maxilla often enlarges, particularly in the molar region, with widening of the alveolar ridge and any dentures may appear to become too tight. The dense bone, hypercementosis and loss of lamina dura make extractions difficult, and there is a liability to haemorrhage and infection. Diagnosis is supported by imaging, biochemistry and histopathology. In early lesions, large irregular areas of relative radiolucency (osteoporosis circumscripta) are seen, but later there is increased radio-opacity, with appearance of an irregular 'cotton wool' pattern. There is progressive thickening of the diploe and base of the skull as well as the sphenoid, orbital and frontal bones. Isotope bone scanning shows localized areas of very high uptake. Increase in plasma alkaline phosphatase and urine hydroxyproline levels, but little or no changes in serum calcium or phosphate levels. Differential diagnosis includes other fibro-osseous lesions, such as fibrous dysplasia, and conditions with a raised alkaline phosphatase, such as osteomalacia, hyperparathyroidism and osteoblastic metastatic deposits (e.g. prostate carcinoma). Bisphosphonates are the treatment.

TORUS PALATINUS AND MANDIBULARIS

Torus palatinus and mandibularis are common developmental benign exostoses more common in Asians, especially Koreans. They appear in late teens or adulthood and may become more apparent with increasing age. They have a smooth or nodular surface, and are of no consequence apart from occasionally interfering with denture construction. The two types are not necessarily associated one with another:

- Torus palatinus occurs in the centre of the hard palate, is of variable size and configuration (**Fig. 16.4**).
- Torus mandibularis is lingual to the lower premolars and usually bilateral (**Fig. 16.5**).

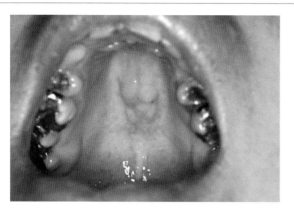

Fig. 16.4 Torus palatinus: central palatal symptomless bony mass

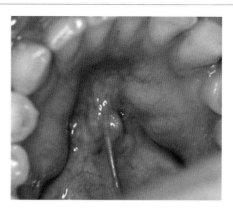

Fig. 16.5 Torus mandibularis: symptomless, bilateral bony masses

FURTHER READING

Ajura, A.J., Lau, S.H., 2010. A retrospective clinicopathological study of 59 osteogenic sarcoma of jaw bone archived in a stomatology unit. Malays. J. Pathol. 32 (1), 27–34.

Akinbami, B.O., 2009. Metastatic carcinoma of the jaws: a review of literature. Niger J. Med. 18 (2), 139–142.

Angadi, P.V., Rekha, K., Shetty, S.R., 2010. 'An exophytic mandibular brown tumor': an unusual presentation of primary hyperparathyroidism. Oral. Maxillofac. Surg. 14 (1), 67–69.

Chang, C.C., Hung, H.Y., Chang, J.Y., et al., 2008. Central ossifying fibroma: a clinicopathologic study of 28 cases. J. Formos. Med. Assoc. 107 (4), 288–294.

Cox, D.P., Solar, A., Huang, J., Chigurupati, R., 2011. Pseudotumor of the Mandible as First Presentation of Hemophilia in a 2-Year-Old Male: A Case Report and Review of Jaw Pseudotumors of Hemophilia. Head Neck Pathol. 5 (3), 226–232.

De, S., Ghosh, S., Mondal, D., Sur, P.K., 2010. Osteosarcoma of the mandible–second cancer in a case of Hodgkin's lymphoma post-chemotherapy. J. Cancer Res. Ther. 6 (3), 336–338.

Duggan, D., MacLeod, I., 2010. An osteosarcoma, presenting as a loose maxillary bridge, with pain and swelling. Dent. Update 37 (6), 400–402.

El Fares, N., El Bouihi, M., Zouhair, K., et al., 2011. Maxillary bone sarcoidosis. Rev. Stomatol. Chir. Maxillofac. 112 (2), 121–124.

Jiang, J.Y., Zhu, Z.Y., Geng, N., et al., 2009. Central mucoepidermoid carcinoma of the jaws: a clinical and pathological analysis of eight cases. Zhonghua Kou Qiang Yi Xue Za Zhi 44 (10), 614–618.

Kruse, A., Pieles, U., Riener, M.O., et al., 2009. Craniomaxillofacial fibrous dysplasia: a 10-year database 1996-2006. Br. J. Oral. Maxillofac. Surg. 47 (4), 302–305.

Kumar Dutta, H., 2009. Jaw and gum tumours in children. Pediatr. Surg. Int. 25 (9), 781–784.

Küpers, A.M., Andriessen, P., van Kempen, M.J., et al., 2009. Congenital epulis of the jaw: a series of five cases and review of literature. Pediatr. Surg. Int. 25 (2), 207–210.

Kyo, C., Kawaoka, Y., Kinoshita, K., Ohno, H., 2010. Mantle cell lymphoma presenting with a tumor of the hard palate. Intern. Med. 49 (15), 1663–1666.

Li, Y., Li, L.J., Huang, J., Han, B., Pan, J., 2008. Central malignant salivary gland tumors of the jaw: retrospective clinical analysis of 22 cases. J. Oral. Maxillofac. Surg. 66 (11), 2247–2253.

Lloyd, T.E., Drage, N., Cronin, A.J., 2009. Chondrosarcoma of the jaws. Dent. Update 36 (10), 632–634.

MacDonald-Jankowski, D.S., 2009. Ossifying fibroma: a systematic review. Dentomaxillofac. Radiol. 38 (8), 495–513.

Macdonald-Jankowski, D.S., Li, T.K., 2009. Fibrous dysplasia in a Hong Kong community: the clinical and radiological features and outcomes of treatment. Dentomaxillofac. Radiol. 38 (2), 63–72.

MacDonald-Jankowski, D.S., Li, T.K., 2010. Orthokeratinized odontogenic cyst in a Hong Kong community: the clinical and radiological features. Dentomaxillofac. Radiol. 39 (4), 240–245.

Mizbah, K., Barkhuysen, R., Weijs, W.L., et al., 2010. Painless swelling proved to be a central giant cell granuloma. Ned. Tijdschr Tandheelkd. 117 (11), 557–559.

Motamedi, M.H., Navi, F., Eshkevari, P.S., et al., 2008. Variable presentations of aneurysmal bone cysts of the jaws: 51 cases treated during a 30-year period. J. Oral. Maxillofac. Surg. 66 (10), 2098–2103.

Muramatsu, T., Hall, G.L., Hashimoto, S., et al., 2010. Clinico-pathologic conference: case 4. Langerhans cell histiocytosis (LCH). Head Neck Pathol 4 (4), 343–346.

Park, J.W., Chung, J.W., 2010. Long-term treatment of Langerhans cell histiocytosis of the mandibular condyle with indomethacin. Oral. Surg. Oral. Med. Oral. Pathol. Oral. Radiol. Endod. 109 (4), e13–e21.

Pechalova, P.F., Bakardjiev, A.G., Beltcheva, A.B., 2011. Jaw cysts at children and adolescence: A single-center retrospective study of 152 cases in southern Bulgaria. Med. Oral. Patol. Oral. Cir. Bucal. 16 (6), e767–e771.

Scully, C., 2002. Oral medicine for the general practitioner: part three: lumps and swellings. Independent Dent. 7 (10), 25–32.

Scully, C., Felix, D.H., 2005. Oral medicine – update for the dental practitioner. 8. Lumps and swellings. Br. Dent. J. 199, 763–770.

Scully, C., Porter, S., 2000. ABC of Oral Health. 6. Swellings, and red: white, and pigmented lesions. BMJ 321, 225–228.

Seehra, J., Horner, K., Sloan, P., 2009. The unusual cyst: solitary bone cyst of the jaws. Dent. Update 36 (8), 502–504, 507–508.

Sheth, M.B., Sujan, S.G., Poonacha, K.S., 2010. Maxillary aneurysmal bone cyst: report of a rare case. J. Indian Soc. Pedod. Prev. Dent. 28 (4), 307–310.

Sopta, J., Dražić, R., Tulić, G., et al., 2011. Cemento-ossifying fibroma of jaws–correlation of clinical and pathological findings. Clin. Oral. Investig. 15 (2), 201–207.

Sun, K.T., Chen, M.Y., Chiang, H.H., Tsai, H.H., 2009. Treatment of large jaw bone cysts in children. J. Dent. Child. (Chic) 76 (3), 217–222.

Sun, Z.J., Zhao, Y.F., Yang, R.L., Zwahlen, R.A., 2010. Aneurysmal bone cysts of the jaws: analysis of 17 cases. J. Oral. Maxillofac. Surg. 68 (9), 2122–2128.

Yamada, T., Mishima, K., Ota, A., et al., 2010. A case of ATLL (adult T-cell leukemia/lymphoma) mimicking odontogenic infection. Oral. Surg. Oral. Med. Oral. Pathol. Oral. Radiol. Endod. 109 (6), e51–e55.

Yoon, H.J., Hong, S.P., Lee, J.I., et al., 2009. Ameloblastic carcinoma: an analysis of 6 cases with review of the literature. Oral. Surg. Oral. Med. Oral. Pathol. Oral. Radiol. Endod. 108 (6), 904–913.

Yoshitake, Y., Nakayama, H., Takamune, Y., et al., 2011. Haemophilic pseudotumour of the mandible in a 5-year-old patient. Int. J. Oral. Maxillofac. Surg. 40 (1), 120–123.

INTRODUCTION

Pain in the head, face, mouth, or teeth is the main reason why many patients consult their dental professional.

Pain is an unpleasant sensory and emotional experience associated with actual or potential tissue damage, or described in terms of such damage. Pain relation with tissue damage may not be constant and it is often associated with affective and cognitive responses.

The pain pathway starts at nociceptors and is transmitted via sensory nerves, the spinal cord dorsal horn, midbrain, thalamus and hypothalamus eventually to be perceived in the brain in the cerebral cortex (somatosensory and limbic) (**Fig. 17.1**).

Modulation, either enhancing or inhibiting nociception, is also crucial to pain perception.

The initial steps relate to the neurochemical signals of actual or impending tissue damage (nociceptive stimuli); nociception is the physiological process of activation of specialized neural pathways, specifically by tissue damaging or potentially damaging stimuli. These include injury, which releases algogenic substances or tissue autocoids, such as bradykinin and prostaglandins from damaged cells, platelets or mast cells. Prostaglandins stimulate nerves at the site of injury and can cause inflammation and fever. Cytokines can trigger pain by promoting inflammation. Injury also releases peptides (tachykinins) (such as substance P (SP) and neurokinin A) which play a role in pain responses by activating pain receptors (nociceptors). SP acts on mast cells to release histamine and on vessels to release bradykinin. Other relevant small peptides found in nervous tissue, function as synaptic neurotransmitters, and include:

- inhibitory neuropeptides: somatostatin, enkephalins
- somatostatin, calcitonin gene-related peptide (CGRP), vasoactive intestinal polypeptide (VIP), cholecystokinin, neuropeptide Y.

Other small peptides act in a paracrine fashion as diffusible hormones that affect many neurones over great distance (neurohormones like endorphins and enkephalins – natural painkillers).

OROFACIAL PAIN

Most orofacial pain (probably over 95%) arises from diseases of the teeth and is thus termed 'odontogenic' (**Fig. 17.2**). There

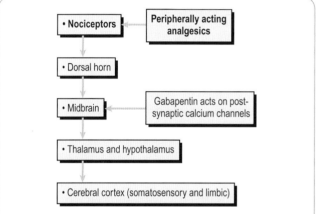

Fig. 17.1 Pain pathway modulation by peripherally acting analgesics and gabapentin

are also non-odontogenic causes that can be of organic origin (neurological, vascular or referred) or non-organic (psychogenic or 'functional'). Most orofacial pain and most recurrent headaches (tension-type, migraine and cluster headaches) are not life threatening, but these conditions can interfere with the quality of life.

The causes of orofacial pain can be remembered from the mnemonic; 'let veterans read news papers' (local, vascular, referred, neurological, psychogenic). (**Box 17.1** and **Box 17.2**).

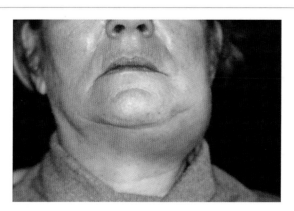

Fig. 17.2 Dental abscess; odontogenic causes are the main reasons for orofacial pain

DIAGNOSIS OF PAIN

The most important means of diagnosis of orofacial pain is the history. Indeed, there are no investigations available to prove that the patient is suffering pain, or the severity of it.

In order to differentiate the widely disparate causes, it is essential to determine key points about the pain (**Box 17.3**): which can be remembered by the acronym 'SOCRATES'.

- Site: valuable information can be obtained by watching the patient when asked if the pain is localized or diffuse. For example, patients frequently point with one finger when describing trigeminal neuralgia, but atypical (idiopathic) facial pain is much more diffuse and may radiate.
- Onset: the average duration of each episode may help diagnosis. For example, pain from exposed dentine is fairly transient, lasting only for seconds, while the pain from pulpitis lasts for a longer period. Trigeminal neuralgia is a brief lancinating pain lasting up to about 5 s, migrainous neuralgia lasts 30–45 min, migraine lasts hours or days, while atypical (idiopathic) facial pain is persistent.
- Character: patients should be asked about the severity and whether the pain is 'sharp', 'dull', 'aching', 'throbbing' or 'shooting'. Trigeminal neuralgia is sharp and shooting (lancinating); odontogenic pain often throbbing; giant cell arteritis is 'burning' while atypical (idiopathic) facial pain is typically dull.
- Radiation: is the pain referred elsewhere?
- Associated features: some types of pain may be associated with other features that are helpful diagnostically. These include a swollen face in dental abscess, nausea and vomiting in migraine, a history of nasal stuffiness or lacrimation in migrainous neuralgia, or a number of other complaints such as dry mouth, bad taste, irritable bowel syndrome, back pain, etc., in some patients with atypical (idiopathic) facial pain.
- Time course: determine whether the pain occurs at specific times. A pain diary can help. For example, the pain of sinusitis is often aggravated by lying down, while periodic migrainous neuralgia frequently disturbs the patient's sleep at a specific time each night, around 2.00 a.m. The pain of temporomandibular joint pain–dysfunction syndrome may be more severe on waking whereas atypical (idiopathic) facila pain tends to worsen through the day.
- Exacerbating and relieving factors: ask if any factors influence the pain. For example, temperature often aggravates dental pain, touching a trigger zone may precipitate trigeminal neuralgia attacks, stress may worsen atypical (idiopathic) facial pain, and alcohol may induce migrainous neuralgia episodes. Exercise may induce cardiac anginal pain referred to the mouth. It may be necessary to resort to leading questions, asking about the effects of temperature, biting, posture, analgesics, alcohol, etc.

BOX 17.1   Main causes of orofacial pain

- Local
- Vascular
- Referred
- Neurological
- Psychogenic

BOX 17.2   More advanced list of causes of orofacial pain

Local disorders
- Teeth and supporting tissues
- Jaws
- Maxillary antrum
- Salivary glands
- Nose and pharynx
- Eyes

Vascular disorders
- Migraine
- Giant cell arteritis
- Neuralgia-inducing cavitational osteonecrosis (NICO)

Neurological disorders
- Idiopathic trigeminal neuralgia
- Malignant neoplasms affecting the trigeminal nerve
- Glossopharyngeal neuralgia
- Herpes zoster (including post-herpetic neuralgia)
- Multiple (disseminated) sclerosis
- Post-stroke pain
- Migrainous neuralgia
- Paroxysmal hemicrania
- SUNCT (severe unilateral neuralgia and conjunctival tearing) syndrome
- Trigeminal autonomic cephalgias

Possible psychogenic causes
- Atypical (idiopathic) facial pain
- Burning mouth syndrome
- Temporomandibular pain-dysfunction

Referred pain
- Sinuses
- Eyes
- Ears
- Neck
- Nasopharynx
  - Chest
  - cardiac (including angina)
  - respiratory (including lung cancer)

BOX 17.3   Pain assessment

Site
Onset
Character
Radiation
Associations
Time course
Exacerbating/ relieving factor
Severity

- Severity: Ask the patient to rate the pain severity on a scale of zero (no pain) to 10 (most severe pain that the patient has experienced), or ask them to mark this on a line divided into 10 equal sections (visual analogue scale) or use an assessment instrument such as the McGill pain questionnaire. These help assess the severity, accepting always that it is subjective, and may also be useful in monitoring the response to treatment. Disturbance of the normal sleep pattern by pain is also useful in assessing the severity.

Thus, the answers to a series of features may be needed, including:

- Previous history
- Character:
  - continuous
  - very severe
  - dull
  - throbbing
  - lancinating
  - burning sensation
  - interferes with sleep
- Provoking or relieving factors:
  - worse with hot/cold
  - worse on biting
  - worse with exercise
  - worse on moving head
  - trigger point
  - other provoking factors known
  - stress related
  - alcohol changes pain
- Other features:
  - ocular or nasal symptoms
  - neurological signs or symptoms
  - nausea/vomiting
  - relieved by analgesics/drugs
  - weight loss
  - temporomandibular click
  - trismus.

Various instruments, such as IMPATH and the TMJ scale, are available to assess behavioural and psychological factors.

LOCAL CAUSES OF OROFACIAL PAIN

Most orofacial pain is related to dental disease – odontogenic causes.

DENTINAL PAIN

Pain originating in dentine:

- is sharp and deep
- is usually evoked by an external stimulus (normally food and drinks which are hot, cold, sweet, sour or, sometimes, salty). Although extreme changes in temperature (e.g. hot soup followed by ice-cream) may cause pain in intact, non-diseased teeth, pain evoked by natural stimuli usually indicates a hyperalgesic state of the tooth
- usually subsides within a few seconds of withdrawal of stimulus
- may be poorly localized, often only to an approximate area within two to three teeth adjacent to the affected tooth. Sometimes, the patient is unable to distinguish whether the pain originates from the lower or the upper jaw. Pain from affected posterior teeth is more difficult to localize than that from anterior teeth. However, patients rarely make localization errors across the midline.

PULPAL PAIN

Vitalometry using a pulp vitality tester may be indicated. Pain associated with pulp disease:

- is spontaneous: pain may be described by patients in different ways, and a continuous dull ache can periodically be exacerbated (by stimulation or spontaneously) for short (minutes) or long (hours) periods. The pain of pulpitis is frequently discontinuous and abates spontaneously; the precise explanation for such abatement is not clear
- is strong, and can be excruciating for many minutes
- is often throbbing
- is typically exacerbated by temperature change and pressure on a carious lesion
- may increase and throb when the patient lies down, and in many instances wakes the patient from sleep
- outlasts the stimulus (unlike stimulus-induced dentinal pain)
- is poorly localized, particularly when pain becomes more intense
- tends to radiate or refer to the ipsilateral ear, temple and cheek, but does not cross the midline.

PERIODONTAL PAIN

Pain originating in the periodontium:

- is more readily localized than is pulpal pain. The improved ability to localize the source of pain may be attributed to the proprioceptive and mechanoreceptive sensibility of the periodontium that is lacking in the pulp. However, although localization of the affected tooth is often precise, in up to half of cases the pain is diffuse and radiates into the jaw on the affected side
- may be less severe than pulpal pain
- is often associated with tenderness to pressure on the affected teeth
- is usually not aggravated by heat or cold.

ACUTE PERIAPICAL PERIODONTITIS

Pain associated with acute periapical inflammation:

- is spontaneous in onset
- is moderate to severe in intensity
- persists for long periods of time (hours)
- is exacerbated by biting on the tooth and, in more advanced cases, even by closing the mouth and bringing the affected tooth gently into contact with the opposing teeth. In these cases, the tooth feels 'high' (extruded) and is very sensitive to touch
- has often been preceded by pulpal pain
- is usually better tolerated than the paroxysmal and excruciating pain of pulpitis
- is usually precisely localized and the patient is able to indicate the affected tooth. During examination the affected tooth is located readily by means of tooth percussion
- is usually associated with a non-vital tooth
- is usually associated with tenderness to palpation in the periapical buccal vestibular area
- may be associated with swelling of the face, caused by oedema and cellulitis or sometimes connected with fever and malaise. Usually, when the face swells, pain diminishes in intensity due to rupture of the pus through the periosteum of the bone around the affected tooth and the consequent decrease in pressure of the tooth apex.

LATERAL PERIODONTAL ABSCESS

- The pain is similar to that of acute periapical periodontitis, though often less severe, and is well localized and with swelling and redness of the gingiva.
- However, the swelling is usually located more gingivally than in the case of an acute periapical lesion.
- The affected tooth is sensitive to percussion and is often mobile and slightly extruded, and there is a deep periodontal pocket. Probing the pocket may cause pus exudation and subsequent relief from pain.
- The tooth pulp is usually vital.

FOOD IMPACTION

The cause of food impaction is usually a faulty contact between the teeth because of caries or poor restorations. Examination shows a faulty contact between two teeth and often food trapped between these teeth; the gingival papilla is tender to touch and bleeds easily.

Food impaction interdentally can cause:

- localized pain that develops between or in two adjacent teeth after meals, especially when food is fibrous (e.g. meat)
- pain associated with a feeling of pressure and discomfort, which may gradually disappear until being evoked again at the next meal, or may be relieved immediately by removing the impacted food
- the adjacent teeth to be sensitive to percussion
- oral malodour.

CRACKED TOOTH

Examination may fail to elicit the cause of pain. Cracks may be revealed by biting on rubber or a Tooth Slooth or Fracfinder, by fibre-optic or blue light illumination or by staining with, for example, disclosing solution. Teeth can crack under trauma and can give rise to pain, which is:

- severe
- worse on biting
- often precipitated by hot or cold.

PERICORONITIS

Acute pericoronal infections are common, and are related to incompletely erupted teeth partially covered by flaps of gingival tissue (operculum), particularly lower third molars. Pain is spontaneous and is often exacerbated by closing the mouth. In more severe cases, pain may be aggravated by swallowing, and there may be trismus and, occasionally, fever, lymphadenopathy and malaise. Examination shows an operculum that is acutely inflamed, red and oedematous. Frequently, an opposing upper tooth indents or ulcerates the oedematous operculum.

ACUTE NECROTIZING GINGIVITIS

Examination shows necrosis and ulceration of the gingival papilla with different degrees of marginal gingival destruction. Similar features but with more intense pain may be seen in necrotizing periodontitis in HIV/AIDS. Acute necrotizing gingivitis may cause:

- soreness and pain. In the early stages some patients may complain of a feeling of tightness around the teeth. Pain is fairly well localized to the affected areas
- profuse gingival bleeding
- halitosis, usually
- metallic taste, sometimes
- fever and malaise, sometimes.

MUCOSAL PAIN

Pain from oral mucosal lesions can be either localized or diffuse. Localized pain is usually associated with an erosion or ulcer. Diffuse pain may be associated with a widespread infection, mucosal atrophy or erosion, a systemic underlying deficiency disease or other factors, and is usually described as 'soreness' or sometimes 'burning'. Mucosal pain may be aggravated mechanically by touch, or by sour, spicy, salty or hot foods.

OTHER LOCAL CAUSES OF OROFACIAL PAIN

Jaws

Pain from the jaws can be caused by acute infection, malignancies, Paget disease and direct trauma. Lesions such as cysts, retained roots and impacted teeth are usually painless unless associated with infection or fracture of the jaw. Odontogenic and other benign tumours of the bone do not normally produce pain, but malignant tumours usually produce deep, boring pain, sometimes associated with paraesthesia, hypoaesthesia or anaesthesia. Radiation therapy or bisphosphonate may result in severe pain due to infection associated with osteonecrosis.

Temporomandibular joint

Pain from the temporomandibular joint may result from dysfunction, trauma, acute or chronic inflammation, or primary or secondary malignant tumours. Examination may reveal the masticatory muscles tender to palpation or occasionally the joint swollen and warm to touch or tender to palpation via the external auditory meatus. Pain from the temporomandibular joint:

- is usually dull
- is usually caused by muscle spasm. Nociceptors may be triggered by release of substances such as cytokines (interleukin-1 and IL-6, and tumor necrosis factor), lactic acid, potassium ions, prostaglandin E2, bradykinin, leukotriene B4, serotonin, neuropeptides such as substance P (SP), neuropeptide Y, calcitonin gene-related peptide (CGRP) or somatostatin
- is usually poorly localized
- may radiate widely
- is usually intensified by movement of the mandible
- may be associated with trismus because of the spasm in the masticatory muscles.

Salivary glands

Examination usually reveals the salivary gland swollen and sensitive to palpation. In acute parotitis, mouth-opening causes severe pain, and thus there is a degree of trismus. Salivary flow from the affected gland is usually reduced. Pain may be associated with fever and malaise. In children, the most common cause is mumps. In adults, pain from salivary glands results usually from blockage of a salivary duct by calculus or a mucus plug, or sialadenitis, when pus may exude from the duct orifice. Pain from salivary gland disorders:

- is localized to the affected gland
- may be quite severe
- may be intensified by increased salivation, such as before and with meals – the pain may wane in the minutes/hours following such salivary stimulation.

Sinuses and pharynx

Disease of the paranasal sinuses and nasopharynx can cause oral and/or facial pain. In acute sinusitis there has usually been a preceding 'cold' followed by local pain and tenderness (but not swelling) and radio-opacity of the affected sinuses, sometimes with an obvious fluid level. Transillumination from a light in the oral cavity may show a fluid level. With maxillary sinusitis, pain may be felt in related upper molars and premolars, any of which may be tender to percussion. The pain of ethmoidal or sphenoidal sinusitis is deep in the nose. Pain in any type of acute sinusitis may be aggravated by a change of position of the head.

Tumours of the sinuses or nasopharynx can also cause facial pain. These tumours are often carcinomas that infiltrate various branches of the trigeminal nerve and can remain undetected until too late. Nasopharyngeal carcinoma often presents late, with facial pain, paraesthesia, ipsilateral deafness and/or cervical lymph node enlargement (Trotter syndrome).

Pressure on the mental nerve

Rarely, pain is caused by pressure from a denture on the nerve, which comes to lie on the crest of the ridge as the alveolar bone is resorbed in the edentulous mandible. Either the denture should be relieved from the area or, occasionally, it is necessary to re-site the nerve surgically.

VASCULAR CAUSES OF OROFACIAL PAIN

Disorders in which the most obvious organic feature is vascular dilatation or constriction cause orofacial pain. The pain is usually obviously in the face or head rather than in the mouth, but occasionally can involve both, and can be difficult to differentiate from other causes of orofacial pain (**Table 17.1**). These include the following disorders.

MIGRAINE

Migraine is a common problem mainly for women, especially past middle age, and typically causes recurrent headache rather than facial pain. The headache is often incapacitating not least as it can be associated with nausea and photophobia, to the extent that the sufferer may need to retire to rest in a darkened environment. It appears related to 5-HT (serotonin) release, cerebral arterial dilatation and increased midbrain periaqueductal grey matter metabolic activity (the endogenous pain control pathway). Attacks may be precipitated by stress, alcohol, various foods such as ripe bananas or chocolate, or the contraceptive pill. Preceding warning symptoms (an aura) of visual, sensory,

Table 17.1 Differential diagnosis of oral pain

Source of pain	Character	Exacerbating factors	Localization	Associated with	Pain provoked by	Radiography
Dental						
Dentinal	Evoked, does not outlast	Hot/cold, sweet/sour	Poor	Caries, defective restorations, exposed dentine	Hot/cold, probing dentine	May show interproximal caries, defective restorations
Pulpal	Severe, intermittent, throbbing	Hot/cold, sometimes biting	Poor	Deep caries, extensive restoration	Hot/cold, probing, sometimes percussion	May show deep caries or deep restoration
Periodontal						
Periapical	For hours at same intensity; deep, boring	Biting	Good	Periapical swelling and redness, tooth mobility	Percussion, palpation of periapical area	Periapical views may show periapical changes
Lateral	For hours at same level, boring	Biting	Good	Periodontal, boring, deep pockets with pus exuding, tooth mobility	Percussion, palpation of periodontal area	Useful when X-rayed with probe inserted into pocket
Gingival	Pressing, annoying	Food impaction, toothbrushing	Good	Acute gingival inflammation	Touch, percussion	Not applicable
Mucosal						
Mucosal	Burning, sharp	Sour, sharp and hot food	Good	Erosive or ulcerative lesions, redness	Palpation	Not applicable

motor or speech disturbances. Visual phenomena often of zig-zag coloured lights (fortification spectra) or transient visual defects. Headache is severe, usually unilateral (hemicranial) and lasts for hours or days. Photophobia, nausea or vomiting may occur. The number, frequency and intensity of attacks decrease with increasing age and spontaneous remissions are not uncommon. Diagnosis is clinical. Management is aspirin or paracetamol, or lysine acetylsalicylate with metoclopramide in acute attacks. Patients usually prefer to lie in a quiet, dark room. Other treatments are directed at 5-HT receptors or uptake by blood platelets. Dihydroergotamine (interacts with 5-HT receptors) or sumatriptan (or other triptan-5-HT agonists which stimulate 5-HT receptors; see migrainous neuralgia, below), tricyclic antidepressants or phenelzine may also help intractable migraine. Prophylaxis is with cyproheptadine, pizotifen, propranolol, tricyclics or calcium channel blockers.

GIANT CELL ARTERITIS

Giant cell arteritis is an immunological disorder in which there is inflammation of medium sized arteries especially in the head and neck ('cranial arteritis'), such as the superficial temporal artery (an alternative term is 'temporal arteritis'). Giant cell arteritis affects old people, more women than men, and is characterized by a severe burning pain in the distribution of the vessels affected, which may be in the temple, tongue or masticatory muscle regions. The headache is intense, deep and aching, throbbing in nature and persistent, frequently made worse when the patient lies flat in bed and may be exacerbated or reduced by digital pressure on the artery involved. Occasionally the affected artery may be enlarged and tender. There may be jaw claudication (pain on chewing) or even pain and necrosis in the tongue or lip. The condition can affect the retinal artery in the eye and lead to blindness; and therefore is an emergency. There may also be malaise, weakness, weight loss, anorexia, fever, and sweating; and polymyalgia rheumatica is often associated.

Diagnosis is clinical, supported by a raised ESR, and arterial biopsy, which shows the arterial elastic tissues to be fragmented, with giant cells numerous in the region of the deranged internal elastic lamina. Because of the hazard to vision, management is urgent treatment with systemic corticosteroids (enteric-coated prednisolone) starting at 60 mg daily until the pain subsides.

Neuralgia-inducing cavitational osteonecrosis (NICO) is controversial and, if it does exist, this rare condition is said to be related to disorders in blood coagulation, and it may also cause jaw pain.

REFERRED CAUSES OF OROFACIAL PAIN

Pain may occasionally be referred to the mouth, face or jaws from any pathology affecting the trigeminal nerve and from the following:

- Sinuses
- Eyes: pain from the eyes can arise from disorders of refraction, retrobulbar neuritis (e.g. in disseminated sclerosis), or glaucoma (raised intraocular pressure), and can radiate to the orbit or frontal region.
- Ears: middle-ear disease may cause headaches. Conversely, oral disease not infrequently causes pain referred to the ear,

particularly from lesions of the posterior tongue. The classic picture is an older man with an undiagnosed tongue cancer who complains of earache.

- Neck: cervical vertebral disease, especially cervical spondylosis, very occasionally causes pain referred to the face.
- Pharynx: carcinoma of the pharynx may cause facial pain.
- Oesophagus: pain plus sialorrhoea may result from oesophageal lesions.
- Styloid process (stylalgia): eagle syndrome, a rare disorder due to an elongated styloid process, may cause pain on chewing, swallowing or turning the head.
- Heart, in patients with angina: the latter pain usually affects the mandible, is initiated by exercise (especially in the cold) and abates quickly on rest.
- Lungs: orofacial pain emanating from lung cancer is a well-recognized entity and has been misdiagnosed as temporomandibular joint pain or idiopathic facial pain.

NEUROLOGICAL (NEUROPATHIC) CAUSES OF OROFACIAL PAIN

Sensory innervation of the mouth, face and scalp depends on the trigeminal nerve, so that disease affecting this nerve can cause orofacial pain or, indeed, sensory loss – sometimes with serious implications.

FACIAL NEURALGIA CAUSED BY TUMOURS OR OTHER LESIONS

Any lesion affecting the trigeminal nerve, whether it be traumatic, cerebrovascular disease, disseminated sclerosis, infections such as HIV/AIDS or Lyme disease, inflammatory or neoplastic (e.g. a nasopharyngeal or antral carcinoma), may cause pain, often with physical signs, such as facial sensory or motor impairment.

TRIGEMINAL NEURALGIAS

Severe lancinating unilateral orofacial pain may be of idiopathic origin and, in the absence of identifiable organic cause is termed 'idiopathic trigeminal neuralgia' (see Ch. 52).

TRIGEMINAL AUTONOMIC CEPHALGIAS (TACs)

Similar pain as that reported in trigeminal neuralgia is experienced in paroxysmal hemicranias; the rare idiopathic short-lasting, unilateral, neuralgiform headache attacks with conjunctival injection and tearing (abbreviated to SUNCT syndrome); and in cluster headaches (commonly termed migrainous neuralgia). The International Headache Society classification defines these trigeminal autonomic cephalgias (TACs) as strictly unilateral headaches. TACs are characterized by episodic, stereotypic attacks and, often prominent, cranial autonomic symptoms, such as lacrimation, conjunctival injection and/or rhinorrhea. TACs involve afferent activation of the trigeminal innervation of intracranial pain-producing structures, or the perception of that activation, and reflex activation of the facial, seventh cranial, nerve outflow pathway. This excess reflex trigeminal-autonomic activation seems to be permitted by dysfunction in the brain, specifically in the posterior hypothalamic grey matter.

Paroxysmal hemicranias

Characterized by frequent short-lasting attacks of unilateral pain usually in the orbital, supraorbital or temporal region paroxysmal hemicranias typically last minutes only. The attack frequency usually ranges from 5–40 attacks per day. The pain is severe and associated with autonomic symptoms such as conjunctival injection, lacrimation, nasal congestion, rhinorrhoea, ptosis or eyelid oedema. Almost all reported cases respond to treatment with indometacin, but respond poorly to other treatments including other NSAIDs.

SUNCT syndrome

SUNCT is a distinctive rare condition characterized by pain less severe than hemicrania but often triggered by cutaneous stimuli, with marked autonomic activation and often intractable to therapy.

Migrainous neuralgia

Cluster headaches; histamine cephalgia; Sluder's headaches. Affecting men mainly, often precipitated by alcohol, and typically producing pain in the maxilla or behind the eye, notably in the very early morning hours, migrainous neuralgia attacks may occur repeatedly over several days ('cluster headaches'). The pain is defined by the International Headache Society as unilateral excruciatingly severe attacks of pain in the ocular, frontal and temporal areas, recurring in separate bouts with daily or almost daily attacks for weeks or months usually with ipsilateral lacrimation, conjunctival injection, photophobia and nasal stuffiness and/or rhinorrhoea. Less common than migraine, attacks often begin at about middle age. Generally, attacks last <1 h (usually 30–45 min), commence and often terminate suddenly, and often awaken the patient at night or in the early morning hours (2.00 a.m. to 3.00 a.m.). The fact that pain is always located periorbitally-frontally, implicates trigeminal nociceptive mechanisms with autonomic manifestations ipsilateral to the pain which seem to involve both parasympathetic (lacrimation and rhinorrhoea) and sympathetic (ptosis and miosis) systems, and the periodicity of the attacks and seasonal recurrence of the cluster periods suggest involvement of the hypothalamus. There is vasodilatation in the extracranial carotid arteries and increased hypothalamic metabolic activity. Attacks are sometimes precipitated by hypoxaemia in REM sleep or at high altitudes, or where there is vasodilatation induced by alcohol, histamine or nitroglycerin. Diagnosis is clinical but, as similar symptoms may be related to tumours around the cavernous sinus and craniospinal junction, CT and/or MRI are indicated. Similar pain has also been reported in patients with lung cancer, and thus chest imaging is indicated. Management is with oxygen inhalations, and a triptan (e.g. sumatriptan). Prophylaxis includes lithium, verapamil, nifedipine, diltiazem or ergotamine.

Glossopharyngeal and postherpetic neuralgias may also cause orofacial pain.

Table 17.2 Medically unexplained symptoms – pain at various sites

System	Examples
Chest	Tietze syndrome
Gastrointestinal	Irritable bowel syndrome
Musculoskeletal	Low back pain
Ear, nose and throat	Dysphagia (globus hystericus)
Orofacial	Idiopathic facial pain/oral dysaesthesia

POSSIBLE PSYCHOGENIC CAUSES OF OROFACIAL PAIN

The mouth and perioral soft tissues have among the richest sensory innervation in the body. Furthermore, a large part of the sensory homunculus on the cerebral cortex receives information from orofacial structures. Right from infancy, the mouth is concerned intimately with the psychological development of the individual, and disorders of structures, such as the lips, teeth and oral mucosa can hold enormous emotional significance. It is hardly surprising, therefore, that there is a range of psychogenic types of orofacial pain, sometimes termed 'medically unexplained symptoms' (MUS), features of which include the following (**Table 17.2**):

- Many patients are female
- Constant chronic discomfort or pain
- Pain often of a dull boring or burning type
- Pain that is poorly localized (it may cross the midline to involve the other side or may move elsewhere)
- Pain that rarely wakens the patient from sleep; however, sleep disturbances are common
- Total lack of objective signs of organic disease
- All investigations are also negative
- There are often recent adverse 'life events', such as bereavement or family illness
- There are often multiple oral and/or other MUS, such as headaches, chronic back or neck pain, irritable bowel syndrome, insomnia, numbness or dysmenorrhoea (**Table 17.2**)
- Cure is uncommon in most, yet few of those suffering seem to try or persist in using medication.

MUS are commonplace in from 50% in primary care, to 15% in hospital outpatients, especially manifesting as chest pain, dyspnoea, dizziness, or headache. The reasons for MUS may include the following:

- Possible links between neurohumoral mechanisms and altered CNS function
- The heightening of bodily sensations (lowered pain threshold) as a consequence of physiological processes, such as autonomic arousal, muscle tension, hyperventilation or inactivity
- Misattribution of normal sensations to serious physical disorders.

Psychogenic (tension) headaches are well-recognized and common, especially in young adults. The headache, which is caused by anxiety or stress-induced muscle tension, affects the frontal, occipital and/or temporal muscles, and is felt as a constant ache or band-like pressure. The pain is often worse by the evening, but does not waken the patient. Reassurance may be effective, but the pain may be helped by massage, warmth, NSAIDs, or benzodiazepines, such as diazepam, as this is both anxiolytic and a mild muscle relaxant.

Psychogenic types of orofacial pain include:

- atypical (idiopathic) facial pain and atypical odontalgia
- oral dysaesthesia (burning mouth syndrome)
- temporomandibular pain-dysfunction
- the syndrome of oral complaints.

Multiple pains and other complaints may occur simultaneously or sequentially and relief is rarely found (or admitted). Patients may bring diaries of their symptoms to emphasize their problem. Some have termed this the 'malady of small bits of paper' (la maladie du petit papier) and, though there is not always a psychogenic basis, such notes characterize patients with non-organic complaints. An anecdotal example is a 35-year-old woman who sequentially 'developed' right submandibular gland pain, right glossopharyngeal neuralgia (her words!), left glossopharyngeal neuralgia and left

submandibular pain over a period of 15 years, during which time she appeared not to develop signs of neurological disease or to deteriorate physically. On the other hand, written notes kept by the patient can be of considerable help to the clinician. Occasional patients quite deliberately induce painful oral lesions and some have Munchausen syndrome, where they behave in such a fashion as to appear to want operative intervention.

DIAGNOSIS OF OROFACIAL PAIN

The cause of orofacial pain is established mainly from the history and examination findings, but it is important to consider the usefulness of additional investigations, particularly imaging of the head and neck, using MRI or CT, and chest imaging (**Algorithms 17.1–17.3**). It is important not to miss detecting serious organic disease and thus mislabelling the patient as having psychogenic pain (**Tables 17.1–17.4**). Even patients with psychogenic disorders can suffer organic pain.

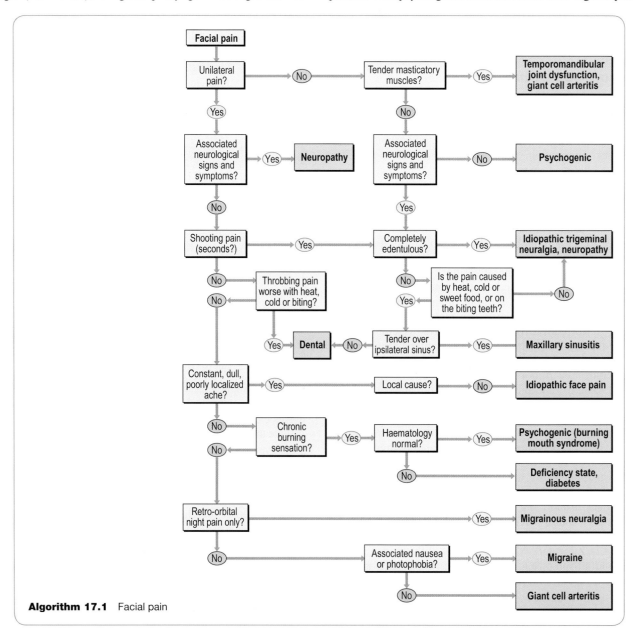

Algorithm 17.1 Facial pain

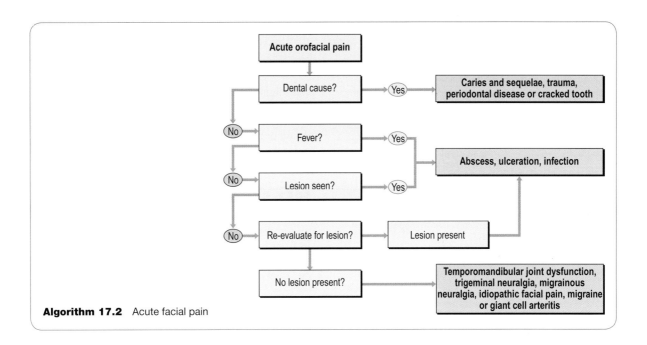

Algorithm 17.2   Acute facial pain

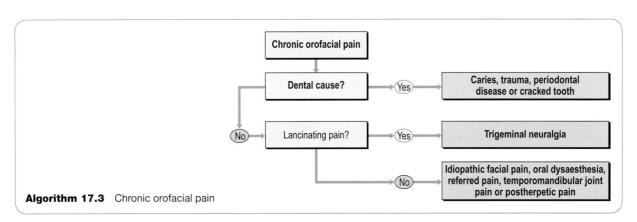

Algorithm 17.3   Chronic orofacial pain

Table 17.3   Differentiation of important types of facial pain

	TMJ pain-dysfunction	Migraine	Idiopathic (atypical) facial pain	Migrainous neuralgia	Idiopathic trigeminal neuralgia	Giant cell arteritis
Age (years)	15–30	Any	30–50	30–50	50	60–80
Gender	F>M	F>M	F>M	M>F	F>M	F>M
Site	Unilateral Temporal Jaw Ear	Any, especially supraorbital	± Bilateral, maxilla	Retro-orbital	Unilateral, mandible or maxilla	Temple
Associated features	Click Limited movements	± Photophobia ± nausea ± vomiting	± Depression	Conjunctival injection ± lacrimation ± nasal congestion	–	Polymyalgia
Character	Dull	Throbbing	Dull	Boring	Lancinating	Burning
Duration	Weeks to months	Hours (usually daytime)	Continual	Few hours (usually night)	Brief (seconds)	Hours
Precipitating factors	Trauma	± Foods	None	± Alcohol	Trigger areas	None
Relieving factors	Rest	Sumatriptan, clonidine; ergot derivatives	Antidepressants	Oxygen, sumatriptan, clonidine, ergot derivatives, verapamil	Carbamazepine	Corticosteroids

Table 17.4 Aids that might be helpful in diagnosis/prognosis/management in some patients with orofacial pain*

In most cases	In some cases
Tooth vitality testing	Neurological opinion
Oral radiography	Nasendoscopy
	MRI of head
	Blood pressure
	ESR
	Temporal artery biopsy
	Chest imaging
	Serology (Lyme disease)
	ANA
	Psychological assessment

*See text for details and glossary for abbreviations.

TREATMENT (see also Chs 4 and 5) OF OROFACIAL PAIN

Pain is the most important symptom suggestive of orofacial disease, but absence of pain does not exclude organic disease and presence of pain does not necessarily mean organic disease. There is also considerable individual variation in response to pain, and the threshold is lowered by tiredness, and psychogenic and other factors:

- Simple analgesics, such as NSAIDs, should be used initially, before embarking on more potent preparations. Chronic pain requires regular analgesia (not just as required). Details are given in Ch. 5.
- Anticonvulsants may help in neuropathic pain (neuralgias).
- Opioids may help in cancer and in mucositis pain.
- Antidepressants may help in orofacial pain of psychogenic origin.

It is important also:

- where possible, to identify and treat the cause of pain
- to relieve factors that lower the pain threshold (fatigue, anxiety and depression)
- to avoid polypharmacy.

CHRONIC POST-TRAUMATIC HEADACHE

Most persons who have had head injuries have local pain or tenderness at the site of impact for a few hours or even for a few days, after which many become symptom-free. However, up to one-half of all persons who injure their heads sufficiently to warrant hospitalization develop chronic post-traumatic headaches. A small number of patients with headaches that persist after head injury have pain due to bleeding in the epidural, subdural or subarachnoid spaces, which is potentially lethal and needs urgent neurological attention. The headache of subdural haematoma begins at the time of trauma or the regaining of consciousness and persists, often for weeks or months, until the haematoma is removed. Blood in the subarachnoid space may induce headache, as may adhesions after head injury involving pain-sensitive structures in the arachnoid. However, most patients with post-traumatic headaches that persist or recur for long periods after head injury have no identifiable intracranial abnormalities to explain their pain and some of these have a 'compensation neurosis' – a psychogenic type of pain.

CAUSALGIA

Causalgia is a persistent burning pain, often in the mandible, that follows surgery or trauma. The cause is unclear and there is no good evidence that it is related to a peripheral nerve lesion or to psychogenic causes.

If a local anaesthetic injection relieves causalgia then cryoanalgesia may effect relief, but neurosurgery may be required.

FREY SYNDROME

Frey syndrome (auriculotemporal syndrome, see Ch. 56) is a paroxysmal burning pain, usually in the temporal area or in front of the ear, associated with flushing and sweating on eating, which often follows parotid surgery and appears to be due to abnormal reinnervation.

OTHER CAUSES OF HEADACHE OR OROFACIAL PAIN

Headaches often have an obvious, but unimportant cause (e.g. hangovers). Most acute head pain has a simple cause and there are no serious sequelae but some, such as an acute ('thunderclap') headache or progressive subacute headache may have sinister implications and can be life threatening, such as an intracranial haemorrhage or meningitis, and warrants urgent investigation. Any patient older than 50 years who develops headaches for the first time or who has a change in a chronic headache pattern should be investigated for an underlying cause. One of these, giant cell arteritis, needs to be recognized and treated promptly with corticosteroids to avoid loss of vision. Other causes of headache that are more common in older people include subdural haematomas, herpes zoster infection, malignancies and trigeminal neuralgia (Ch. 52).

Headache or orofacial pain is occasionally the presenting feature of:

- raised intracranial pressure: this is one of the most serious, but also the least common causes of headache. The headache is severe, worse on waking and decreases during the day. It is aggravated by straining, coughing, sneezing or lying down. Nausea and vomiting are common. Neurological attention and examination for papilloedema is essential, since this may be caused by malignant hypertension, a tumour, abscess or haematoma. When no specific cause can be found it is termed 'idiopathic ('benign') intracranial hypertension', which may be precipitated by tetracyclines, vitamin A, nitrofurantoin and nalidixic acid and is associated with partial thrombosis of the superior sagittal sinus
- meningeal irritation: severe headache with nausea, vomiting, neck pain or stiffness (with inability to kiss the knees) or pain on raising the straightened legs (Kernig sign) implies meningeal irritation. Urgent neurological attention is needed, since the pain may indicate meningitis, metastases or subarachnoid haemorrhage
- fever
- hypertension
- exertion (including postcoital headache)
- coughing as in chronic obstructive airways disease
- stress
- a range of other causes including some cerebrovascular events, endocrinopathies, such as diabetes; HIV infection; drug use (e.g. nitrites, phenothiazines vinca alkaloids, see Table 54.23) or Paget disease.

USEFUL WEBSITES

International Association for the Study of Pain: http://www.iasp-pain.org/

FURTHER READING

Bussone, G., Usai, S., 2004. Trigeminal autonomic cephalalgias: from pathophysiology to clinical aspects. Neurol. Sci. 25 (Suppl. 3), S74–S76.

Christoforidou, A., Bridger, M.W., 2006. Angina masquerading as sinusitis. J. Laryngol. Otol. 120 (11), 961–962.

Clark, G.T., 2006. Persistent orodental pain, atypical odontalgia, and phantom tooth pain: when are they neuropathic disorders? J. Calif. Dent. Assoc. 34 (8), 599–609.

Cohen, A.S., Matharu, M.S., Goadsby, P.J., 2006. Short-lasting unilateral neuralgiform headache attacks with conjunctival injection and tearing (SUNCT) or cranial autonomic features (SUNA) – a prospective clinical study of SUNCT and SUNA. Brain 129 (Pt 10), 2746–2760.

Evans, R.W., Agostoni, E., 2006. Persistent idiopathic facial pain. Headache 46 (8), 1298–1300.

Goadsby, P.J., 2005. Trigeminal autonomic cephalalgias. Pathophysiology and classification. Rev. Neurol. (Paris) 161 (6–7), 692–695.

Graff-Radford, S.B., 2000. Facial pain. Curr. Opin. Neurol. 13, 291–296.

Israel, H.A., Scrivani, S.J., 2000. The interdisciplinary approach to oral, facial and head pain. J. Am. Dent. Assoc. 131, 919–926.

Lance, J.W., 2000. Headache and face pain. Med. J. Aust. 172, 450–455.

Obermann, M., 2010. Treatment options in trigeminal neuralgia. Ther. Adv. Neurol. Disord. 3 (2), 107–115.

Padilla, M., Clark, G.T., Merrill, R.L., 2000. Topical medications for orofacial neuropathic pain: a review. J. Am. Dent. Assoc. 131, 184–195.

Ram, S., Kumar, S.K., Clark, G.T., 2006. Using oral medications, infusions and injections for differential diagnosis of orofacial pain. J. Calif. Dent. Assoc. 34 (8), 645–654.

Sciubba, J., 2009. Neuralgia-inducing cavitational osteonecrosis: a status report. Oral. Dis. 15, 309–312.

Scully, C., 2002. Oral medicine for the general practitioner: part one: pain. Independent Dent. 7 (8), 47–54.

Scully, C., Felix, D.H., 2006. Oral medicine – update for the dental practitioner. 10. Oral pain. Br. Dent. J. 200, 75–80.

Sessle, B.J., 2000. Acute and chronic craniofacial pain: brainstem mechanisms of nociceptive transmission and neuroplasticity, and their clinical correlates. Crit. Rev. Oral. Biol. Med. 11, 57–91.

Shintaku, W., Enciso, R., Broussard, J., Clark, G.T., 2006. Diagnostic imaging for chronic orofacial pain, maxillofacial osseous and soft tissue pathology and temporomandibular disorders. J. Calif. Dent. Assoc. 34 (8), 633–644.

Smith, L., Osborne, R.F., 2006. Facial sarcoidosis presenting as atypical facial pain. Ear Nose Throat J. 85 (9), 574–578.

Tarabichi, M., 2000. Characteristics of sinus-related pain. Otolaryngol. Head Neck Surg. 122, 842–847.

Yi, H.J., Kim, C.H., Bak, K.H., et al., 2000. Metastatic tumors in the sellar and parasellar regions: clinical review of four cases. J. Korean Med. Sci. 15, 363–367.

18 Pigmented brown or black lesions

INTRODUCTION

Oral mucosal discolouration, which ranges from brown to black may be due to superficial (extrinsic) or deep (intrinsic in or beneath mucosa) causes, the latter usually being more important.

AETIOLOGY AND PATHOGENESIS

Causes are shown in **Boxes 18.1** and **18.2**.

EXTRINSIC DISCOLOURATION

Extrinsic discolouration is rarely of serious consequence, usually being caused by coloured foods, drinks or drugs, when both mucosae and teeth may be discoloured. Causes include:

- Foods and beverages, such as beetroot, red wine, fruit juices, coffee and tea.
- Confectionery, such as liquorice and coloured candies.
- Drugs, such as chlorhexidine, iron salts, griseofulvin, crack cocaine, minocycline, bismuth subsalicylate, lansoprazole and HRT, and stains such as gentian violet and toluidine blue.
- Tobacco: may cause extrinsic brown staining and may also cause intrinsic pigmentary incontinence, with pigment cells increasing and appearing in the lamina propria– especially in persons who smoke with the lighted end of the cigarette within the mouth (reverse smoking), as practised mainly in some Asian communities. Tobacco is a risk factor for potentially malignant disorders and cancer.

> **BOX 18.1 Main causes of brown pigmented mucosal lesions:**
>
> **Increased melanin:**
> - Drugs
> - Ephelis (freckle)
> - Hypoadrenalism (Addison disease)
> - Malignant melanoma
> - Melanotic macule
> - Naevus
> - Pigmentary incontinence
> - Racial
>
> **Exogenous pigments:**
> - Amalgam tattoo
> - Drugs and heavy metals
> - Smoking

> **BOX 18.2 More advanced list of causes of hyperpigmentation**
>
> **Localized**
> - Amalgam, graphite, carbon, dyes, inks or other tattoos
> - Ephelis (freckle)
> - Epithelioid angiomatosis
> - Kaposi sarcoma
> - Malignant melanoma
> - Melanoacanthoma
> - Melanotic macule
> - Naevus
> - Pigmented neuroectodermal tumour
> - Verruciform xanthoma
>
> **Multiple or generalized**
> - Genetic:
>   - Carney syndrome (Ch. 56)
>   - isolated mucocutaneous melanotic pigmentation (IMMP) (Ch. 57)
>   - Laugier–Hunziker syndrome (Ch. 56)
>   - Lentiginosis profusa
>   - Leopard syndrome (Ch. 56)
>   - Peutz–Jeghers syndrome
>   - racial
> - Drugs: (Table 54.17)
> - Metals (bismuth, mercury, silver, gold, arsenic, copper, chromium, cobalt, manganese)
> - Smoking
> - Endocrine:
>   - Addison disease
>   - Albright syndrome
>   - Nelson syndrome
>   - pregnancy
>   - postinflammatory
> - Others:
>   - Gaucher disease
>   - generalized neurofibromatosis
>   - haemochromatosis
>   - HIV
>   - incontinentia pigmenti
>   - thalassaemia
>   - Whipple disease
>   - Wilson disease

- Betel: this may cause a brownish-red extrinsic discolouration, mainly on the teeth and in the buccal mucosa, with an irregular epithelial surface that has a tendency to desquamate. Betel chewing is seen mainly in women from South and Southeast Asia; the mucosa epithelium is often hyperplastic, and histologically brownish amorphous material from the betel quid may be seen on the epithelial surface and intra- and intercellularly, with ballooning of epithelial cells. This betel chewer's mucosa is not known to be precancerous, but betel use predisposes to submucous fibrosis and potentially malignant disorders and to cancer.

- Black or brown hairy tongue (**Fig. 18.1**). Black hairy tongue affects mainly the posterior tongue; the filiform papillae are excessively long. The discolouration may vary from yellow to brown to black and usually involves the anterior and middle thirds of the dorsal tongue. It appears to be caused by the accumulation of epithelial squames and proliferation of chromogenic micro-organisms. It is more common:
  - in smokers
  - in people with hyposalivation
  - where the diet is soft
  - where various agents are used antimicrobials (penicillin, cephalosporin, chloramphenicol, streptomycin, and tetracycline), corticosteroids, oxygenating mouth rinses, NSAIDs and psychotropics
  - where oral hygiene is wanting and also seen with much greater frequency in drug addicts, alcoholics, and patients infected with HIV.

The discontinuation of smoking, oxygenating mouth rinses, and antibiotics may help the condition resolve. Patients with black hairy tongue may also find the condition improved by:
- increasing their oral hygiene
- using a tongue scraper
- brushing the tongue before retiring at night, with a hard toothbrush and cold water
- using sodium bicarbonate mouthwashes
- eating pineapple or sucking a peach stone
- chewing gum.

Superficial transient brown discolouration of the dorsum of the tongue and sometimes other soft tissues may be caused by cigarette smoking, tobacco or betel chewing, some drugs (such as iron salts), some foods and beverages (such as coffee and tea), liquorice and chlorhexidine. Such discolouration is easily brushed off. Topical podophyllin and tretinoin have been advocated by some.

INTRINSIC DISCOLOURATION

Intrinsic discolouration may have more significance than the extrinsic type. Normal intrinsic pigmentation is due to melanin, produced by melanocytes – dendritic cells prominent in the basal epithelium. This originates from the amino acid tyrosine, which is converted to dihydroxyphenylalanine (DOPA) and thence to melanin. The colour can vary from brown to blue or black, depending on the amount and location of the melanin. Increased melanin or number of melanocytes, or other materials can cause intrinsic (endogenous) hyperpigmentation.

GENERALIZED HYPERPIGMENTATION

Generalized pigmentation, often affecting the gingivae mainly, is common in persons of colour, and is racial (**Figs 18.2** and **18.3**).

- Racial pigmentation: this is the most usual cause of patchy or generalized brown oral mucosal pigmentation, caused by melanin. Seen mainly in people of African or Asian heritage it can also be noted in patients of Mediterranean descent,

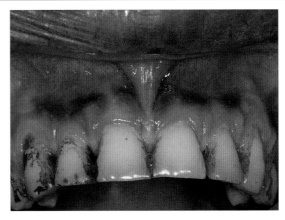

Fig. 18.2 Racial pigmentation (the teeth are stained from betel chewing and poor oral hygiene)

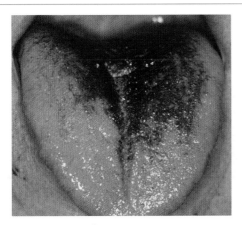

Fig. 18.1 Black hairy tongue

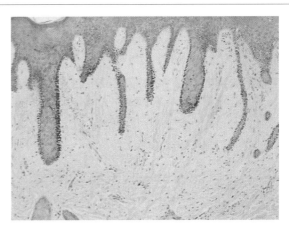

Fig. 18.3 Racial pigmentation showing melanin-containing cells in the basal epithelium

sometimes even in some fairly light-skinned people. It is most obvious in the anterior labial gingivae and palatal mucosa, and the pigmentation is usually symmetrically distributed. Patches may be seen elsewhere. Pigmentation may be first noted by the patient in adult life and then incorrectly assumed to be acquired rather than congenital in origin.

- Chronic inflammation, such as in lichen planus, can result in melanin drop-out, especially in persons with pigmented skin. This oral pigmentation (pigmentary incontinence) is often gingival or buccal.
- Drugs: generalized hyperpigmentation or pigmentation may be induced sometimes with pigmentation of skin or other areas:
  - smoking tobacco is a fairly common cause (smoker's melanosis)
  - antimalarials produce a variety of colours in the mucosa, ranging from yellow with mepacrine to blue-black with amodiaquine
  - zidovudine and ACTH therapy may both produce brown pigmentation
  - busulphan, some other cytotoxic drugs, oral contraceptives, phenothiazines and anticonvulsants may also occasionally produce, or increase, brown pigmentation
  - minocycline may cause blackish discolouration of the teeth, gingivae and bone, skin, sclera and even breast milk
  - gold may produce purplish gingival discolouration
  - many of the other heavy metals formerly implicated in producing oral pigmentation (such as mercury, lead and bismuth) are not used therapeutically now, although industrial or accidental exposures still occur, fortunately rarely. Metallic sulphides deposited in the tissues are seen especially where oral hygiene is poor, and bacteria produce sulphides, resulting in pigmentation at the gingival margin (e.g. lead line).
- Hypoadrenalism (Addison disease): uncommon, but may cause generalized or patchy hyperpigmentation due to excessive production of ACTH, which has activities similar to MSH. Addison disease is usually autoimmune (idiopathic), but hypoadrenalism may be seen in HIV disease. Hyperpigmentation is generalized, but is most obvious in areas normally pigmented (e.g. the areolae of nipples, genitalia), skin flexures and sites of trauma. The oral mucosa may show patchy hyperpigmentation. Patients with Addison disease also typically have weakness and weight loss, and hypotension.
- Nelson syndrome: this is a rare condition caused by ACTH overproduction in response to adrenalectomy, usually for breast cancer.
- Melanin pigmentation increases under hormonal stimulation, either by MSH, or in pregnancy, or rarely due to the action of adrenocorticotrophic hormone (ACTH), the molecule of which is similar to MSH, or under the influence of other factors (e.g. smoking).
- Peutz–Jeghers syndrome: a rare autosomal-dominant condition, in which oral and circumoral patchy brown pigmentation is seen with small-intestinal polyps (circumoral melanosis with intestinal polyposis). A similar condition without intestinal polyps has been termed isolated mucocutaneous melanotic pigmentation (IMMP); both conditions may be associated with various malignant neoplasms (see Chs 56 and 57).

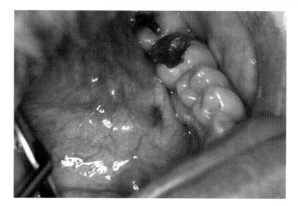

Fig. 18.4 Amalgam tattoo

LOCALIZED AREAS OF PIGMENTATION

Localized areas of pigmentation may be caused by the above but are usually caused by:

- Embedded amalgam (**Fig. 18.4**). Amalgam tattoo is the most common cause of a single patch of macular blue-black pigmentation, does not change significantly in size or colour, is painless and is usually seen in the mandibular gingiva or at least close to the teeth or an apicectomy where there has been a retrograde amalgam root end filling. The diagnosis is clinical but the lesion may be radio-opaque. Tattoos are best excised to confirm the diagnosis and exclude naevi or melanoma.
- Embedded graphite (graphite tattoo) may be seen, for example, where a pencil lead has broken off in the mucosa. Tattoos are best excised to exclude naevi or melanoma.
- Other foreign bodies.

LOCAL IRRITATION/INFLAMMATION

- Melanotic macules (**Fig. 18.5**): these are usually single, brown, collections of melanin-containing cells. Melanotic macules are flat and mostly smaller than 1 cm and contain increased melanin, do not change rapidly in size or colour, are painless and are seen particularly on the vermilion border of the lip and on the palate. They are seen mainly in white people and are innocuous. Most arise slowly, but occasionally they rapidly appear. They are best removed to exclude melanoma.
- Naevi: these are blue-black lesions formed from increased melanin-containing cells (naevus cells) usually smaller than

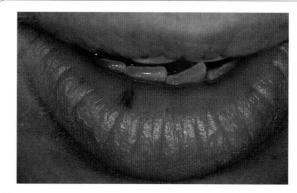

Fig. 18.5 Labial melanotic macule

1 cm. Some 60% are papular, they do not change rapidly in size or colour, are painless and are seen particularly on the palate. Approximately half of naevi are histologically of the intradermal (intramucosal) type when the melanin is in the lamina propria, one-third are blue naevi, others are compound naevi, and some are junctional. There is no evidence that naevi, except rare junctional naevi, progress to melanoma. However, naevi may clinically resemble melanomas and are therefore usually best removed to exclude melanoma. The melanocyte-specific gene (MSG-1) is expressed in some cases of malignant melanoma, but is absent in all benign naevi.

- Malignant melanoma: this is rare but may arise in apparently normal mucosa or in a pre-existent pigmented naevus, usually in the palate or maxillary gingivae. About one-third of melanomas arise in areas of hyperpigmentation. Features suggestive of malignancy include a rapid increase in size, change in colour, ulceration, pain, the occurrence of satellite pigmented spots or regional lymph node enlargement. However, up to 15% of melanomas are amelanotic. Superficial melanomas have a better prognosis than nodular ones. Radical excision is indicated.
- Other neoplasms, such as Kaposi sarcoma, pigmented neuroectodermal tumour, or palatal pigmentation from ACTH-producing bronchogenic carcinoma.
- Melanoacanthoma: in some adults of African descent, larger lesions, from 5–20 mm in diameter, termed 'melanoacanthomas', may be seen. These are seen mainly in the buccal mucosa or palate in females, may appear rapidly, and are probably reactive rather than neoplastic lesions. They are best removed.

DIAGNOSIS

The nature of hyperpigmentation can sometimes only be established after further investigation (**Table 18.1**).

PATIENTS WITH GENERALIZED OR MULTIPLE HYPERPIGMENTATION

Systemic causes should be excluded, and therefore, the following may be indicated:

- Blood pressure: to exclude Addison disease (hypotension is characteristic).
- Plasma cortisol levels: to exclude Addison disease (low levels found).
- An adrenocorticotrophic hormone stimulation (ACTH: Synacthen) test: to exclude Addison disease (an impaired response is typical).
- Endocrinological or gastroenterological opinions.
- HIV serology or opinion.
- Bone imaging to exclude Albright syndrome (Ch. 56).

Table 18.1 Aids that might be helpful in diagnosis/prognosis/management in some patients with pigmented lesions*

In many cases	In some cases
Biopsy	Blood pressure
	Full blood picture
	Serum ferritin, vitamin B_{12} and corrected whole blood folate levels
	HIV test
	Plasma cortisol
	ACTH stimulation test
	Oral radiography
	Chest radiography
	Urinary catecholamines
	Endocrine opinion
	Gastroenterological opinion

*See text for details and glossary for abbreviations.

PATIENTS WITH LOCALIZED HYPERPIGMENTATION

- Radiographs may be helpful, as they can sometimes show amalgam, graphite or a foreign body, or (in pigmented neuroectodermal tumour of infancy) bone rarefaction. In the latter, the urinary catecholamines are raised.
- Biopsy. If early detection of oral melanomas is to be achieved, all pigmented oral cavity lesions should be viewed with suspicion. The consensus of opinion is that a lesion with the following clinical features is seriously suggestive of being a malignant melanoma; and is best biopsied at the time of definitive operation:
  - a solitary raised lesion
  - a rapid increase in size
  - change in colour
  - ulceration
  - pain
  - evidence of satellite pigmented spots
  - regional lymph node enlargement.
- Photographs may be useful for future comparison of size and colour.

MANAGEMENT

Management is of the underlying condition. Excision biopsy of isolated hyperpigmented lesions is often recommended to exclude malignancy, and because of the malignant potential of some others (particularly the junctional naevus) and for cosmetic reasons. This is particularly important if the lesions are raised or nodular or have clinical features as above seriously suggestive of being malignant melanoma.

FURTHER READING

Boardman, L.A., Pittelkow, M.R., Couch, F.J., et al., 2000. Association of Peutz-Jeghers-like mucocutaneous pigmentation with breast and gynecologic carcinomas in women. Medicine (Baltimore) 79 (5), 293–298.

Ciçek, Y., Ertaş, U., 2003. The normal and pathological pigmentation of oral mucous membrane: a review. J. Contemp. Dent. Pract. 4 (3), 76–86.

Femiano, F., Lanza, A., Buonaiuto, C., et al., 2008. Oral malignant melanoma: a review of the literature. J. Oral. Pathol. Med. 37 (7), 383–388.

Fernandez, G.T., 2000. Pigmented lesion of the oral cavity with eight years follow-up. P. R. Health Sci. J. 19, 165–168.

Flaitz, C.M., Baker, K.A., 2000. Treatment approaches to common symptomatic oral lesions in children. Dent. Clin. North Am. 44, 671–696.

Kumar, S.K., Shuler, C.F., Sedghizadeh, P.P., Kalmar, J.R., 2008. Oral mucosal melanoma with unusual clinicopathologic features. J. Cutan. Pathol. 35 (4), 392–397.

Meleti, M., Vescovi, P., Mooi, W.J., van der Waal, I., 2008. Pigmented lesions of the oral mucosa and perioral tissues: a flow-chart for the diagnosis and some recommendations for the management. Oral. Surg. Oral. Med. Oral. Pathol. Oral. Radiol. Endod. 105 (5), 606–616.

Müller, S., 2010. Melanin-associated pigmented lesions of the oral mucosa: presentation, differential diagnosis, and treatment. Dermatol. Ther. 23 (3), 220–229.

Noonan, V.L., Kabani, S., 2005. Diagnosis and management of suspicious lesions of the oral cavity. Otolaryngol. Clin. North Am. 38 (1), 21–35.

Reichart, P.A., 2000. Oral mucosal lesions in a representative cross-sectional study of aging Germans. Community Dent. Oral. Epidemiol. 28 (5), 390–398.

Sarswathi, T.R., Kumar, S.N., Kavitha, K.M., 2003. Oral melanin pigmentation in smoked and smokeless tobacco users in India. Clinico-pathological study. Indian J. Dent. Res. 14 (2), 101–106.

Scully, C., 2003. Oral medicine for the general practitioner: part four: red, white and coloured lesions. Independent Dent. 8, 87–94.

Scully, C., Felix, D.H., 2005. Oral medicine – update for the dental practitioner. 6. Red and pigmented lesions. Br. Dent. J 199 (10), 639–645.

Sedghizadeh, P.P., Williams, J.D., Allen, C.M., Prasad, M.L., 2005. MSG-1 expression in benign and malignant melanocytic lesions of cutaneous and mucosal epithelium. Med. Sci. Monit. 11 (7), BR189–BR194.

Tran, H.T., Anandasabapathy, N., Soldano, A.C., 2008. Amalgam tattoo. Dermatol. Online J. 14 (5), 19.

INTRODUCTION

Red oral lesions are commonplace in the mouth and usually caused by inflammation in, for example, mucosal infections, such as candidosis (**Fig. 19.1**). However, they can also be sinister and signify severe epithelial dysplasia or malignant neoplasms. Red lesions, especially if persistent, can be:

- Focal: the lesion of most concern is erythroplasia, since it is usually dysplastic. Carcinoma or telangiectasia can also cause red lesions.
- Multifocal: these lesions are often caused by candidosis or lichen planus.
- Discoid: these are prominent on the dorsum of the tongue in erythema migrans (geographic tongue).
- Diffuse: candidosis is the most common cause, but these lesions may be caused by mucositis, haematinic deficiency states and infections.
- Linear: these may be seen on the tongue in deficiency states.

The causes of red lesions can be remembered from the acronym BLING (Blood disorders, Lichen planus, Infection or inflammation, Neoplastic and pre-neoplastic and Geographic tongue).

AETIOLOGY AND PATHOGENESIS

MUCOSAL INFLAMMATION

Most red lesions are inflammatory (**Box 19.1**), the most common being caused by:

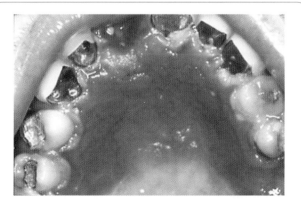

Fig. 19.1 Denture-related stomatitis; red lesions are usually inflammatory in origin

---

> ### BOX 19.1   Main causes of oral red lesions
>
> - Blood disorders
> - Lichen planus
> - Infection or inflammation
> - Neoplastic and pre-neoplastic
> - Geographic tongue

- Viral stomatitis (e.g. herpes simplex stomatitis) (Ch. 43).
- Candidosis (Ch. 39):
  - denture-related stomatitis is a form of mild chronic atrophic candidosis consisting of inflammation of the mucosa beneath a dental appliance (usually a complete upper denture), such that the hard palate is red (**Fig. 19.1**)
  - acute oral candidosis may complicate corticosteroid or antibiotic therapy, particularly with long-term, broad-spectrum antimicrobials, and causes widespread erythema and soreness of the oral mucosa, sometimes with thrush
  - erythematous oral candidosis may complicate HIV disease, and causes focal or widespread erythema and soreness of the oral mucosa, often in the palate, and sometimes with thrush.
  - Median rhomboid glossitis is usually detected by the patient or dental professional as a persistent red, rhomboidal depapillated area in the midline of the dorsum of the tongue, just anterior to the circumvallate papillae.
- Deep mycoses, which are rare in the developed world, except in HIV disease and other immunocompromised persons:
  - histoplasmosis
  - cryptococcosis
  - blastomycosis
  - paracoccidioidomycosis
  - iatrogenic
  - radiation-induced mucositis (mucosal barrier injury or MBI) is common after irradiation of tumours of the head and neck, if the radiation field involves the oral mucosa. Arising within 3 weeks of the irradiation, there is generalized erythema, and sometimes ulceration
  - chemotherapy-induced mucositis is common after chemotherapy. Fluorouracil and cisplatin almost always cause mucositis. Etoposide, melphalan, doxorubicin, vinblastine, taxanes and methotrexate are also particularly stomatotoxic. Arising within 1–2 weeks of the therapy, there is generalized erythema, and sometimes ulceration
- Immunological reactions, such as lichen planus, plasma cell gingivostomatitis, granulomatous disorders (sarcoidosis, Crohn disease, orofacial granulomatosis), amyloidosis and graft-versus-host disease.

REACTIVE LESIONS

These include for example pyogenic granulomas and peripheral giant cell granulomas.

EROSIONS

These are caused by burns, and vesiculobullous disorders, such as lichen planus, erythema multiforme, pemphigoid and pemphigus.

ATROPHY

These are caused by:

- erythroplasia: one of the more important causes of a localized red lesion, since it is pre-neoplastic
- erythema migrans (geographic tongue): manifests with irregular depapillated red areas, which change in size and shape, usually in the dorsum of the tongue
- lichen planus and lupus erythematosus: may present with atrophic red areas in some forms
- desquamative gingivitis: A fairly common problem in which the gingivae show chronic desquamation and is a term that denotes a particular clinical picture and not a diagnosis in itself. Many of the patients are middle-aged women. Desquamative gingivitis is mainly a manifestation of:

    - mucocutaneous disorders, usually. Most gingival involvement in the vesiculobullous or skin diseases (dermatoses) is related to lichen planus or pemphigoid, but pemphigus, dermatitis herpetiformis, linear IgA disease, chronic ulcerative stomatitis and other conditions may need to be excluded. Most of these conditions are acquired, but a few are congenital with a strong hereditary predisposition, such as epidermolysis bullosa
    - chemical damage, such as reactions to sodium lauryl sulphate in toothpastes
    - allergic responses
    - drugs
    - psoriasis
    - pyostomatitis vegetans.

Some patients make no complaint, but others complain of persistent gingival soreness, worse when eating spices, or acidic foods, such as tomatoes or citrus fruits. Most patients are seen only when vesicles and bullae have broken down to leave desquamation, and the clinical appearance is thus of erythematous gingivae, mainly labially, the erythema and loss of stippling extending apically from the gingival margins to the alveolar mucosae. The desquamation may vary from mild almost insignificant small patches to widespread erythema with a glazed appearance. In addition to a full history and examination, biopsy examination and histopathological and immunological investigations are frequently indicated. Conditions which should be excluded include:

- reactions to mouthwashes, chewing gum, medications and dental materials
- candidosis
- lupus erythematosus
- plasma cell gingivitis
- Crohn disease, sarcoidosis and orofacial granulomatosis
- leukaemias
- factitial (self-induced) lesions.

The treatment of desquamative gingivitis consists of:

- improving the oral hygiene
- minimizing irritation of the lesions
- specific therapies for the underlying disease where available
- local or systemic immunosuppressive or dapsone therapy, notably corticosteroids.

Corticosteroid creams used overnight in a soft polythene splint may help.

- iron or vitamin deficiency states: may cause glossitis or other red lesions.

PURPURA

Bleeding into the skin and mucosa is usually caused by trauma (**Box 19.2**), occasional small traumatic petechiae at the occlusal line (or elsewhere) are seen in otherwise healthy patients (**Fig. 19.2**). Less common causes include (**Box 19.3**):

- suction (e.g. fellatio may produce bruising in the soft palate)
- localized oral purpura or angina bullosa haemorrhagica: an idiopathic, fairly common, cause of purpura or blood blisters, seen only in the mouth, pharynx or oesophagus, mainly in the soft palate, in older persons

---

BOX 19.2 More advanced list of causes of red lesions

Localized

- Inflammatory
- Herpes or other viral infections
- Candidosis
- Other mycoses
- Granulomatous conditions (Crohn disease, orofacial granulomatosis, sarcoidosis)
- Plasma cell gingivitis
- Reiter syndrome (reactive arthritis) (Ch. 56)
- Graft-versus-host disease
- Drugs (e.g. causing candidosis, mucositis or lichenoid lesions)
- Epithelioid angiomatosis
- Reactive lesions:
    - pyogenic granulomas
    - peripheral giant cell granulomas
- Atrophic lesions
    - Geographic tongue
    - Lichen planus
    - Lupus erythematosus
    - Erythroplasia
    - Avitaminosis B_{12}
- Burns
- Vascular anomalies (e.g. angiomas)
- Purpura
- Telangiectases (hereditary haemorrhagic telangiectasia or scleroderma)
- Angiokeratomas (Fabry disease) (Ch. 56)
- Neoplasms
    - Giant cell tumour
    - Squamous carcinoma
    - Kaposi sarcoma
    - Wegener granulomatosis

Generalized

- Candidosis
- Avitaminosis B complex
- Mucositis irradiation or chemotherapy-induced
- Polycythaemia

BOX 19.3 Causes of oral purpura

- Trauma
- Suction or trauma from:
  - appliances
  - habits
  - coughing
  - fellatio
  - cunnilingus
  - vomiting
- Localized oral purpura (angina bullosa haemorrhagica)
- Platelet disorders
- Autoimmune thrombocytopenia (idiopathic thrombocytopenic purpura)

- Drugs
- Aplastic anaemia
- Leukaemia
- Amyloidosis
- Infections:
  - infectious mononucleosis
  - rubella
  - HIV infection
- Gammopathies
- Vascular disorders
- Scurvy
- Ehlers–Danlos syndrome

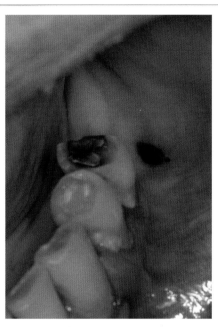

Fig. 19.2 Petechiae from trauma

- a blood platelet disorder such as thrombocytopenia: red or brown pinpoint lesions (petechiae) or diffuse bruising (ecchymoses) are seen, mainly at sites of trauma, such as at the junction of the hard and soft palate (and often extraorally).

VASCULAR ANOMALIES (ANGIOMAS AND TELANGIECTASIA)

These can be caused by:

- dilated lingual veins (varices): these may be conspicuous in the older in the ventrum of the tongue and may cause unnecessary alarm. Similar lesions may be seen in the lip
- haemangiomas: these are usually small isolated developmental anomalies, or hamartomas. Rarely, orofacial angiomas may be more extensive and part of the Sturge–Weber syndrome (haemangioma with epilepsy and hemiplegia; see Ch. 56)
- telangiectasias (dilated capillaries): these may be seen after irradiation of the mouth and in various systemic disorders,

such as hereditary haemorrhagic telangiectasia, systemic sclerosis and primary biliary cirrhosis.

NEOPLASMS

Red neoplasms include the following:

- Peripheral giant cell tumour
- Angiosarcomas, such as Kaposi sarcoma: a common neoplasm in HIV/AIDS, appears in the mouth as red or purplish areas or nodules, especially seen on the palate
- Squamous cell carcinoma
- Wegener granulomatosis
- Lymphoma.

DIAGNOSIS

Diagnosis of red lesions is mainly clinical; lesions should also be sought on the skin or other mucosae. It may be necessary to take a blood picture (including blood and platelet count) and assess haemostatic function or exclude vitamin deficiencies, and/or aspiration, biopsy or imaging may be indicated (**Algorithm 19.1** and **Table 19.1**).

TREATMENT (see also Chs 4 and 5)

Treatment is of the underlying cause.

Table 19.1 Aids that might be helpful in diagnosis/ prognosis/management in some patients with persistent red lesions*

In most cases	In some cases
Biopsy	Aspiration
	Diascopy (blanching on pressure)
	Full blood picture
	Serum ferritin, vitamin B_{12} and corrected whole blood folate levels
	ESR
	Microbiological swabs

*See text for details and glossary for abbreviations.

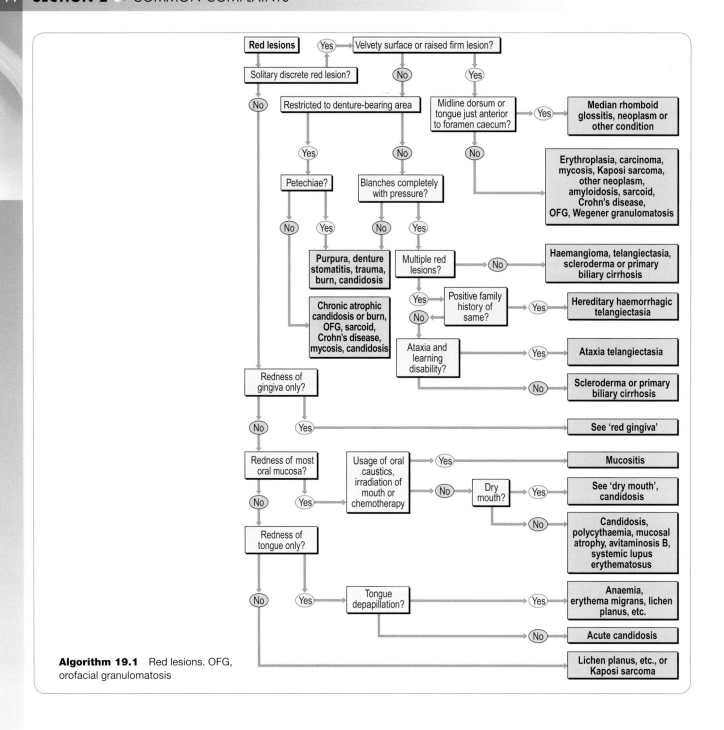

Algorithm 19.1 Red lesions. OFG, orofacial granulomatosis

FURTHER READING

Flaitz, C.M., Baker, K.A., 2000. Treatment approaches to common symptomatic oral lesions in children. Dent. Clin. North Am. 44, 671–696.

Gillenwater, A.M., Chambers, M.S., 2006. Diagnosis of premalignant lesions and early cancers of the oral cavity. Tex. Dent. J. 123 (6), 512–520.

Noonan, V.L., Kabani, S., 2005. Diagnosis and management of suspicious lesions of the oral cavity. Otolaryngol. Clin. North Am. 38 (1), 21–35.

Reichart, P.A., 2000. Oral mucosal lesions in a representative cross-sectional study of aging Germans. Community Dent. Oral. Epidemiol. 28 (5), 390–398.

Reichart, P.A., Philipsen, H.P., 2005. Oral erythroplakia – a review. Oral. Oncol. 41 (6), 551–561.

Scully, C., Felix, D.H., 2005. Oral medicine – update for the dental practitioner. 6. Red and pigmented lesions. Br. Dent. J. 199 (10), 639–645.

Scully, C., Newman, L., Bagan, J.V., 2005. The role of the dental team in preventing and diagnosing cancer: 3. Oral cancer diagnosis and screening. Dent. Update 32 (6), 326–328, 331–332, 335–337.

Warnakulasuriya, K.A., Ralhan, R., 2007. Clinical, pathological, cellular and molecular lesions caused by oral smokeless tobacco – a review. J. Oral. Pathol. Med. 36 (2), 63–77.

Sensory and motor changes

20

INTRODUCTION

Sensory, motor or autonomic neuropathies may affect the orofacial region. The main orofacial sensory and motor lesions are shown in **Table 20.1**.

Sensory changes most frequently follow nerve damage from trauma. Weakness of the facial muscles is most commonly seen in neurological disorders and presents with paralysis (palsy) but is also seen in primary muscle disease and neuromuscular junction disorders, is then usually symmetrical, and the uncommon causes include:

- myasthenia gravis
- dystrophia myotonica
- facioscapulohumeral dystrophy.

SENSORY CHANGES

Normal facial sensation, mediated by the trigeminal nerve, is important to protect the skin, mucosae and especially the cornea of the eye from damage. Facial sensory changes, which can be caused by lesions of a sensory branch of the trigeminal nerve or the central connections (**Fig. 20.1**), may lead to sensory awareness that is:

- completely lost (anaesthesia)
- partially lost (hypoaesthesia)
- altered (paraesthesia) – often 'pins and needles' or similar discomfort – which may arise during recovery from nerve damage
- increased (hyperaesthesia).

Sensory defects may lead to unrecognized damage from trauma or burns ('trophic lesions'), and are occasionally associated with hyperaesthesia (i.e. the patient has a decreased sensory perception, but when sensation is perceived, it may cause discomfort).

Table 20.1 Main orofacial neuropathies

Features	V	VII
Major	Sensory loss in face	Weak muscles of facial expression
Minor	Jaw movements impaired	Reduced sense of taste in anterior ⅔ of tongue

AETIOLOGY AND PATHOGENESIS

Causes of lesions affecting the trigeminal nerve are shown in **Boxes 20.1** and **20.2**.

EXTRACRANIAL CAUSES

Extracranial causes of facial sensory loss are most common and include damage to the trigeminal nerve from the following causes.

Trauma

This is the usual cause of sensory loss – especially after orthognathic or cancer surgery. Ipsilateral hypoaesthesia or anaesthesia usually result. If the nerves are stretched or compressed (neuropraxia), there is often only hypoaesthesia, and recovery of sensation is speedy, typically within days. However, if the nerves are severed (neurotmesis), anaesthesia is profound and recovery is delayed for months accompanied by paraesthesia or hyperaesthesia. Recovery is sometimes not complete: repair may be indicated:

- Trauma to the mandibular division can have a variety of causes:
  - inferior alveolar local analgesic injections
  - fractures of the mandibular body or angle
  - surgery (particularly surgical extraction of lower third molars, osteotomies or jaw resections) or even endodontics or implants.
- Trauma to the mental nerve can have a variety of causes:
  - operations in the region
  - pressure from a denture – the mental foramen is close beneath a lower denture and there is anaesthesia of the lower lip on the affected side.
- Trauma to the lingual nerve can arise especially during resections or removal of lower third molars, particularly when the lingual split technique is used.
- Trauma to branches of the maxillary division of the trigeminal nerve may be caused by direct trauma or fractures (usually Le Fort II or III middle-third facial fractures) or surgery.

Bone disease

- Osteomyelitis in the mandible may affect the inferior alveolar nerve to cause labial anaesthesia.
- Osteochemonecrosis.
- Paget disease.
- Osteopetrosis.

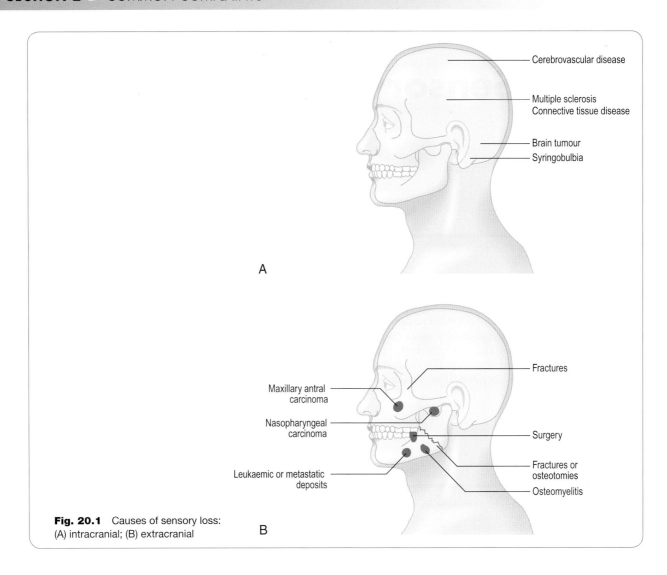

Fig. 20.1 Causes of sensory loss: (A) intracranial; (B) extracranial

---

BOX 20.1 Main causes of sensory loss

BOX 20.1 **Main causes of sensory loss**

- Trauma (e.g. surgical, fractures)
- Infections or inflammatory
- Disseminated sclerosis
- Neoplastic
- Cerebrovascular disease
- Psychogenic

Neuropathies

- Drugs occasionally produce hypoaesthesia (**Box 20.1**).
- Disseminated (multiple) sclerosis may cause sensory loss.
- Diabetes may produce a neuropathy.
- Infections such as syphilis, leprosy, Lyme disease or herpesviruses are rare causes.

Neoplastic disease

- Oral carcinomas may invade the jaws to cause anaesthesia.
- Skull base or central malignancies such as osteosarcoma may produce a similar pattern.
- Nasopharyngeal carcinomas may invade the pharyngeal wall to infiltrate the mandibular division of the trigeminal

nerve, causing pain and sensory loss in the region of the inferior alveolar, lingual and auriculotemporal nerve distributions; invade the levator palati to cause soft palate immobility; and, by occluding the Eustachian tube, cause deafness (Trotter syndrome).
- Leukaemia, myeloma or metastases (usually from breast, lung, stomach or colon cancer) may cause deposits in the mandible and labial hypoaesthesia.
- Carcinoma of the maxillary antrum may produce ipsilateral upper labial hypoaesthesia or anaesthesia.

Intracranial lesions

Intracranial lesions affecting the trigeminal nerve or connections are uncommon but often serious.
Causes include:

- Trauma including surgical treatment of trigeminal neuralgia.
- Inflammatory disorders:
  - disseminated sclerosis
  - sarcoidosis
  - infections (e.g. HIV, syphilis)
  - connective tissue disorders.
- Neoplasms, such as brain tumours (often metastases).

BOX 20.2   More advanced list of causes of facial sensory loss

Extracranial

- Trauma (e.g. surgical, fractures) to inferior dental, lingual, mental or infraorbital nerves
- Inflammatory:
  - osteomyelitis
  - infections – neurosyphilis, HIV infection, herpesviruses, tuberculosis, leprosy, diphtheria, Lyme disease
- Neoplastic:
  - carcinoma of antrum or nasopharynx
  - metastatic tumours
  - leukaemic deposits
  - paraneoplastic syndrome

Intracranial

- Trauma (e.g. surgical treatment of trigeminal neuralgia)
- Inflammatory:
  - disseminated sclerosis
  - sarcoidosis
  - connective tissue disorders
  - infections
- Neoplastic:
  - cerebral tumours (metastases, glioma, meningioma, acoustic neuroma)
- Vascular:
  - cerebrovascular disease
  - aneurysms
- Syringobulbia
- Drugs: (see Table 54.21)
- Others:
  - Bone disease
  - Paget disease
  - osteopetrosis
  - benign trigeminal neuropathy
  - idiopathic (connective tissue diseases)
- Psychogenic:
  - hysteria
  - hyperventilation syndrome
- Metabolic and endocrine disease:
  - diabetes
  - chronic kidney disease

- Cerebrovascular disease:
  - since other cranial nerves are anatomically close, there may be associated neurological deficits in intracranial causes of facial sensory loss. Thalamic strokes in particular can cause facial sensory loss
  - in posterior cranial fossa lesions, for example, there may be cerebellar features, such as ataxia
  - in middle cranial fossa lesions there may be associated neurological deficits affecting cranial nerve VI and thus mediolateral eye movements.
- Brainstem lesions that may involve the fifth nuclei and central connections include brainstem:
  - glioma
  - disseminated sclerosis
  - infarction
  - syringobulbia: this leads to sensory loss spreading from the periphery of the face inwards towards the nose, plus a lower motor nerve lesion of the vagus, hypoglossal and accessory nerves, leading to disturbances of speech and swallowing, and bilateral upper motor neurone lesions affecting all limbs. A 'syringomyelia-like' syndrome has been infrequently reported in neurological disorders such as Tangiers disease, lepromatous leprosy and a novel syndrome termed 'facial onset sensory and motor neuronopathy syndrome' (FOSMN).
- Cerebellopontine angle lesions that can compress the trigeminal nerve and as they enlarge, affect the neighbouring seventh and eighth nerves, producing facial weakness and deafness include:
  - acoustic neuroma
  - meningioma
  - metastases.
- Petrous temporal bone lesions may cause pain and also affect the sixth nerve (Gradenigo's syndrome) and include the following.

INFECTION SPREADING FROM THE MIDDLE EAR
Metastases

- Cavernous sinus lesions can compress the trigeminal (Gasserian) ganglion and these include:
  - internal carotid artery aneurysm
  - cavernous sinus thrombosis
  - invasion from a pituitary neoplasm
  - metastasis.
- Benign trigeminal neuropathy is a transient sensory loss in one or more divisions of the trigeminal nerve. It seldom occurs until the second decade or affects the corneal reflex. The aetiology is unknown, though some patients prove to have connective tissue disorder.
- Hysteria, and particularly hyperventilation syndrome, may underlie some causes of facial anaesthesia/hypoaesthesia. Typically the 'anaesthesia' is bilateral and associated with bizarre neurological complaints.

CLINICAL FEATURES

Central (brainstem) lesions of the lower trigeminal nuclei (e.g. in syringobulbia), produce a characteristic circumoral sensory loss. When the spinal tract (or spinal nucleus) alone is involved, the sensory loss is restricted to loss of pain and temperature sensation, but normal touch sensation, i.e. it is dissociated. A complete fifth nerve lesion causes unilateral sensory loss on the face, tongue and buccal mucosa. Diminution of the corneal reflex is an early, and sometimes isolated sign of a fifth nerve lesion.

DIAGNOSIS

Trigeminal functions that should be tested include the following (**Table 20.2**):

- Skin sensation testing is subjective but done simply by having the patient close their eyes and respond affirmatively to touch with a light wisp of cotton over the three divisions of the trigeminal nerve, the patient being asked to compare the perception on the two sides. It is important to define the pattern and distribution of sensory alteration, using various stimuli:
  - light touch (cotton wool)
  - pin point (sterile needle)

Table 20.2 Aids that might be helpful in diagnosis/prognosis/management in some patients with sensory changes*

In most cases	In some cases
Neurological testing	Psychological assessment Blood pressure Full blood picture Serum ferritin, vitamin B$_{12}$ and corrected whole blood folate levels ESR Blood glucose SACE Serology (HIV, HTLV-1, HSV, VZV, HCV, Lyme disease, syphilis) ANA RF Nasendoscopy Audiometry Radiography (panoral, occipitomental, lateral and postero-anterior skull) MRI Lumbar puncture

*See text for details and glossary for abbreviations.

- temperature
- vibration
- two-point discrimination.
- Corneal reflex testing is much more objective (this tests fifth and seventh cranial nerves); touching the cornea gently with sterile cotton wool should produce a blink. Asymmetries of this reflex are a good sign of sensory impairment in the distribution of the trigeminal ophthalmic division.

If there is objective facial sensory and corneal reflex loss, a full neurological assessment must be undertaken, unless the loss is unequivocally related to local trauma (**Algorithm 20.1**). Spreading numbness is of particular significance. On the other hand, occasional patients feign sensory loss and this then often has a bizarre distribution such as a hairline or perfect midline demarcation.

Trigeminal motor function is to the muscles of mastication:

- masseters
- temporalis
- pterygoids.

Function is tested by palpating the muscles during function, and performing the jaw jerk. The latter may be impaired if there is a trigeminal nerve lesion, or increased if there is a lesion above the pons nucleus, and weak in lesions of brain stem or cortex. Unilateral cerebral lesions do not affect jaw movements. In trigeminal lesions there may be atrophy of the masseter and/or temporalis muscles.

Possible investigations in patients with facial sensory loss include:

- imaging (panoral, occipitomental, lateral and postero-anterior skull, and MRI/CT). Diffusion-weighted MRI can be especially helpful.
- a full blood count, ESR; random blood sugar level; syphilis and Lyme disease serology and possibly viral serology (e.g. herpesviruses or HIV); autoantibodies to exclude connective tissue diseases.
- quantitative sensory testing (QST) through the use of devices that generate specific physical vibratory or thermal stimuli and those that deliver electrical impulses at specific frequencies.

TREATMENT (see also Chs 4 and 5)

Facial hypoaesthesia or anaesthesia result in the loss of protective reflexes and a trigeminal trophic syndrome with facial ulceration can follow. If the cornea is anaesthetic or hypoaesthetic, an eye pad must be worn over the closed eyelids, since the protective corneal reflex is lost and the cornea may be damaged.

If there has been neurotmesis, early surgical correction can achieve good results. In benign, potentially reversible causes of sensory loss, the underlying cause should be corrected,

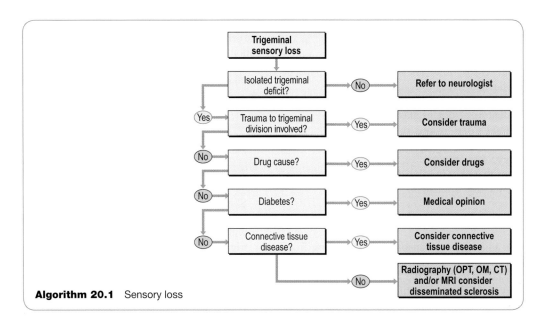

Algorithm 20.1 Sensory loss

and the patient reassured that there should be some if not full return of sensation over the subsequent 18 months.

MOTOR CHANGES

Facial paralysis (palsy) is discussed here. Abnormal facial movements are described in Ch. 20.

The facial nerve (seventh cranial) is the motor nerve to the muscles of facial expression, and facial nerve lesions cause paralysis of the muscles of facial expression, including the:

- orbicularis oculi
- orbicularis oris
- buccinator
- platysma
- scalp and auricle muscles.

The facial nerve supplies the stylohyoid and stapedius muscles and has, besides these motor components:

- secretomotor fibres – tearing – lacrimal gland
- saliva production – sublingual, submandibular, nasal and palatine glands
- nervus intermedius, associated with taste perception in anterior two-thirds of the tongue
- sensory component to the external ear.

Facial paralysis (palsy) can be very disfiguring, since the ability to smile is impaired, the eye cannot close, and the patient may drool.

AETIOLOGY AND PATHOGENESIS

Lesions of the facial nerve central connections (supranuclear or upper motor neurone lesions) or the facial nerve itself (nuclear and infranuclear or lower motor neurone lesions), or muscle disease, can lead to facial weakness.

UPPER MOTOR NEURONE (UMN) LESIONS (SUPRANUCLEAR LESIONS)

UMN lesions may be due to (**Boxes 20.3** and **20.4, Fig. 20.2**):

- stroke (cerebrovascular events), commonly due to haemorrhage or thrombosis in or around the brain internal capsule
- a focal brain lesion which may be moderately selective or cause a cerebral palsy
- rarely, a brain cortical lesion affecting the cerebral hemispheres.

BOX 20.3   Main causes of facial palsy (paralysis)

- Upper motor neurone lesion:
  - cerebrovascular event (stroke)
  - other cerebral disease
- Lower motor neurone lesion:
  - Bell palsy (herpes simplex virus usually)
  - tumour affecting facial nerve
  - middle ear disease
  - parotid lesion
  - trauma to facial nerve
  - disseminated sclerosis

BOX 20.4   Advanced list of causes of facial palsy (paralysis)

- Upper motor neurone lesion:
  - cerebrovascular event
  - trauma
  - tumour
  - infection
  - disseminated sclerosis
  - Moebius syndrome (Ch. 56)
  - connective tissue disease
- Lower motor neurone lesion:
  - systemic infection
    - Bell palsy (herpes simplex virus usually)
    - HIV infection
    - HTLV-1 infection
    - Lyme disease (*Borrelia burgdorferi*)
    - Varicella-zoster virus infection (± Ramsay–Hunt syndrome)
    - cytomegalovirus, Epstein–Barr virus and influenza viruses
  - Other:
    - other infections, e.g. leprosy, Guillain–Barré syndrome, Kawasaki disease (Ch. 56)
    - diabetes
    - middle-ear disease: otitis media, cholesteatoma
    - lesion of skull base: fracture, infection, sarcoidosis
    - parotid lesion: tumour
    - trauma to branch of facial nerve
    - inferior dental regional anaesthetic affecting the facial nerve
    - barotrauma
    - Melkersson–Rosenthal syndrome/Crohn disease/OFG
    - Drugs (e.g. Vinca alkaloids)

LOWER MOTOR NEURONE (LMN) LESIONS (INFRANUCLEAR LESIONS)

LMN-related palsy may be due to lesions at various levels, including:

- Facial nucleus; such as poliomyelitis, rarely.
- Pontine or posterior cranial fossa. As there are a large number of tracts in close approximation in the pons, the features may be diffuse with frequent bilateral or contralateral involvement. The sixth and eighth cranial nerves are often involved along with the seventh nerve and serve as a good localizing feature in facial palsy. The causes may include:
  - disseminated sclerosis
  - pseudobulbar palsy
  - neoplasm (acoustic neuroma, metastases, glioma or even more rarely a meningioma)
  - vascular disease (basilar artery aneurysm)
  - meningitis
  - intrathecal drug injections (e.g. methotrexate for leukaemia).
- Temporal bony canal. The level of involvement can be estimated in three ways: (1) below the geniculate ganglion where lacrimation will be spared; (2) below the chorda tympani where taste from the anterior two-thirds of the tongue is spared; or (3) below the nerve to stapedius which, if involved, may give rise to hyperacusis due to fixation of the stapedius muscle. The causes can be from ganglion peripherally:

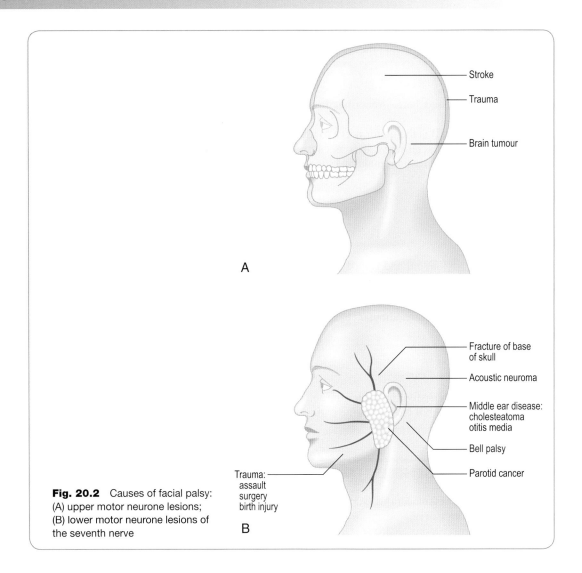

Fig. 20.2 Causes of facial palsy: (A) upper motor neurone lesions; (B) lower motor neurone lesions of the seventh nerve

- acute infective polyneuritis (Guillain–Barré syndrome) a peripheral nervous system affliction often following a viral infection and manifesting mainly with weakness or tingling sensations in the legs. In many instances, the weakness and abnormal sensations spread to the arms and upper body
- Ramsay–Hunt syndrome, caused by varicella-zoster virus infection, which allegedly involves the facial nerve at the geniculate ganglion
- fracture of the temporal bone can involve the nerve anywhere in the bony canal
- haemorrhage may occur into the canal in hypertension
- glomus tumour, leukaemic and other malignant deposits or sarcoidosis are rare causes.
- Middle-ear, which include:
  - chronic otitis media
  - cholesteatoma
  - ear surgery, especially mastoidectomy
  - Bell palsy (can involve the nerve anywhere in the bony stylomastoid canal)
  - damage caused to the facial nerve after leaving the stylomastoid canal.
- Trauma: barotrauma or use of forceps in delivery, stab wounds and facial lacerations can cause facial paralysis.

- Parotid lesions: benign tumours in the main displace the facial nerve, but malignant tumours infiltrate the nerve and cause paralysis.
- Sarcoidosis of the parotid gland (as part of uveoparotitis), Crohn disease and related conditions are rare causes.
- Leprosy. It may be possible to palpate the nerve as a cord which can be rolled under the skin.

However, the most common causes of facial paralysis are:

- Strokes, seen mainly in older males and usually caused by a cerebrovascular event.
- Bell palsy, seen mainly in younger patients and mainly related to infection and swelling within the confines of the stylomastoid canal, usually due to herpes simplex virus.
- Lesions affecting the distal facial nerve (e.g. assault with a knife or bottle, malignant tumours in, or surgery to, the parotid or submandibular region).
- Occasionally, a temporary facial palsy follows the (mal) administration of an inferior alveolar local analgesic, if the anaesthetic diffuses from the pterygomandibular space distally through the parotid gland, when it can reach and temporarily paralyse the facial nerve.

CLINICAL FEATURES

- In facial palsy, the patient typically complains of impaired:
  - smile
  - speech
  - ability to whistle.
- In addition, on the affected side:
  - the forehead is unfurrowed
  - the patient is unable to close the eye
  - the eye rolls upward (Bell sign) on attempted closure
  - tears tend to overflow onto the cheek (epiphora)
  - the nasolabial fold is obliterated
  - the corner of the mouth droops
  - saliva may drool from the commissure
  - food collects in the vestibule
  - plaque accumulates on the teeth.
- Lesion laterality and level are important in determining the specific clinical features.
- Upper motor neurone lesions produce lower facial weakness and hemiparesis. The neurological lesion is contralateral to the lower facial weakness. The facial weakness does not affect the forehead, since the neurones to the upper face receive bilateral UMN innervation. UMN facial palsy is usually caused by damage in the middle capsule of the brain. Damage thus extends to include hemiplegia and sometimes affects speech, but extrapyramidal influences remain and thus there can still be involuntary facial movements, for example, on laughing because of the bilateral cortical representation. A UMN lesion, therefore, is characterized by:
  - contralateral facial palsy
  - some sparing of the frontalis and orbicularis oculi muscles
  - spontaneous facial movements with emotional responses.
- There may also be aphasia and, on the side of facial palsy:
  - paresis of the arm (monoparesis)
  - paresis of the arm and leg (hemiparesis).
- Lower motor neurone lesions produce full ipsilateral hemifacial weakness, including the forehead. The facial nucleus itself is affected unilaterally or bilaterally in poliomyelitis and in motor neurone disease – the latter usually bilaterally. Lesions at lower levels than the facial nucleus are recognized by the association of LMN facial weakness with other signs.
- Pontine lesions. The sixth (abducens) nerve nucleus is often also involved, manifesting with a convergent squint (lateral rectus palsy) as well as the unilateral facial weakness. When the neighbouring paramedian pontine reticular formation and corticospinal tracts are involved, there is a combination of:
  - LMN facial weakness
  - failure of conjugate lateral gaze (towards the lesion)
  - contralateral hemiparesis.
- Cerebellopontine angle lesions. The fifth, sixth and eighth nerves are affected along with the seventh.
- Petrous temporal lesions. Facial nerve lesions within the petrous temporal bone result in a combination of loss of taste on the anterior two-thirds of the tongue and hyperacusis (unpleasantly loud noise distortion) caused by paralysis of the nerve to stapedius.
- Skull base, parotid gland and in the face itself. This produces a lower motor neurone facial palsy characterized only by:
  - total unilateral paralysis of all muscles of facial expression
  - absence of voluntary and emotional facial responses
  - no hemiparesis or aphasia.

DIAGNOSIS

The history should be directed to elicit features suggestive of stroke, trauma, including underwater diving (barotrauma), camping or walking in areas that may contain ticks (Lyme disease), the possibility of HIV infection and, in Afro-Caribbeans, the possibility of HTLV-1 infection. A facial paresis, which is slowly evolving, associated with other focal neurology, facial twitching, multiple cranial nerve deficits or with chronic Eustachian tube dysfunction suggests a possible malignant cause. A neck or parotid mass or history of previous head or neck malignancy is suspicious (**Algorithm 20.2**).

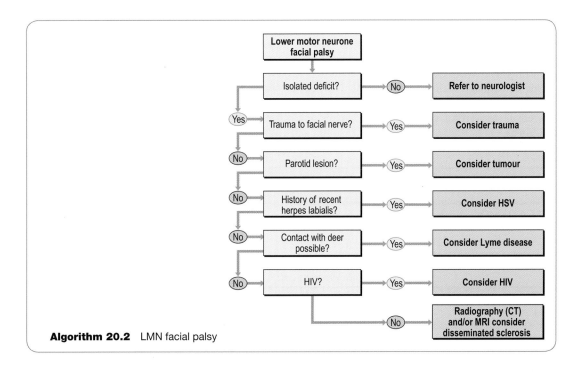

Algorithm 20.2 LMN facial palsy

- Differentiating supranuclear from infranuclear lesions depends on the presence of other neurological signs.
- Contralateral limb weakness suggests a pontine level lesion and therefore a nuclear facial nerve lesion.
- Cerebellopontine angle lesions typically affect multiple cranial nerves as well as producing hyperacusis and disturbances of lacrimation, taste and salivation.
- Salivation and taste are affected by all facial canal lesions. Lacrimation is affected in a proximal lesion of the facial canal, but is spared in a more distal lesion.
- Facial level lesions affect only muscle function, leaving lacrimation, salivation and taste intact.

The examination should include the following:

- Ear and mouth examination to exclude Ramsay–Hunt syndrome (herpes zoster of the facial nerve ganglion which causes lesions in the palate and ipsilateral ear, and facial palsy).
- Ear examination to look for discharge and other signs of middle-ear disease.
- A full neurological examination, especially to exclude lesions of other cranial nerves, and to exclude a stroke. Test for the facial nerve weakness by asking the patient to:
  - close the eyes against resistance
  - raise the eyebrows
  - raise the lips to show the teeth
  - try to whistle.
- A test for loss of hearing should be carried out.
- A test for taste loss should be carried out.

Investigations that may be indicated include the following (**Table 20.3**):

- A study of evoked potentials to assess the degree of nerve damage. Facial nerve stimulation or needle electromyography may be useful, as may electrogustometry.
- Imaging with CT/MRI, and chest and skull radiography to look particularly for central lesions.
- Blood pressure measurement to exclude hypertension.
- Fasting blood sugar levels to exclude diabetes.
- Test for Lyme disease (tick-borne infection with *Borrelia burgdorferi*) by enzyme-linked immunosorbent assay (ELISA) or C6 peptide antibodies, confirming equivocal and positive results with Western blot.
- Tests for virus infections, such as HSV, VZV, HIV or HTLV-1.
- Serum angiotensin converting enzyme (ACE) levels to exclude sarcoidosis.
- Lumbar puncture is needed occasionally.

Table 20.3 Aids that might be helpful in diagnosis/prognosis/management in some patients with motor changes*

In most cases	In some cases
Neurological testing	Blood pressure
	Full blood picture
	Serum ferritin, vitamin B_{12} and corrected whole blood folate levels
	ESR
	Blood glucose
	SACE
	Serology (HIV, HTLV-1, HSV, VZV, HCV, Lyme disease, syphilis)
	ANA
	RF
	Nasendoscopy
	Audiometry
	Radiography (panoral, occipitomental, lateral and postero-anterior skull)
	MRI
	Lumbar puncture

*See text for details and glossary for abbreviations.

TREATMENT (see also Chs 4 and 5)

Management is of the underlying condition. Most patients with Bell palsy are otherwise healthy and present no other management difficulties, but there are occasional (possibly coincidental) associations with diabetes mellitus, hypertension and lymphoma.

AUTONOMIC NEUROPATHIES

Autonomic neuropathies are uncommon, diverse and rarely affect the orofacial region. Autonomic cephalgias and sialosis are attributed to autonomic dysfunction. Autonomic neuropathies may cause insensitivity to pain, resulting in oral self-mutilation, such as biting injuries and scarring (of tongue, lip, and buccal mucosa). Familial dysautonomia (Riley–Day syndrome) may manifest with self-mutilation (Ch. 56) and also sialorrhoea, while cholinergic dysautonomia may cause hyposalivation. Hereditary sensory and autonomic neuropathy type IV causes congenital insensitivity to pain plus anhidrosis (inability to sweat normally, which may cause heat intolerance). Other autonomic neuropathies can also cause loss of bladder control; and postural or orthostatic hypotension. Gastrointestinal symptoms frequently accompany autonomic neuropathy.

Autonomic neuropathies may become life- threatening as they can affect cardiorespiratory function.

FURTHER READING

Alvarez, F.K., de Siqueira, S.R., Okada, M., et al., 2007. Evaluation of the sensation in patients with trigeminal post-herpetic neuralgia. J. Oral. Pathol. Med. 36 (6), 347–350.

Benatar, M., Edlow, J., 2004. The spectrum of cranial neuropathy in patients with Bell's palsy. Arch. Intern. Med. 164 (21), 2383–2385.

Blanchet, P.S., Rompre, P.H., Lavigne, G.S., Lamorche, C., 2005. Oral dyskinesia: a clinical overview. Int. J. Prosthodont. 18, 190–199.

Bodner, L., Woldenberg, Y., Pinsk, V., Levy, J., 2002. Orofacial manifestations of congenital insensitivity to pain with anhidrosis: a report of 24 cases. ASDC J. Dent. Child. 69 (3), 293–296.

Critchley, E.P., 2004. Multiple sclerosis initially presenting as facial palsy. Aviat. Space Environ. Med. 75 (11), 1001–1004.

Elloumi-Jellouli, A., Ben Ammar, S., Fenniche, S., et al., 2003. Trigeminal trophic syndrome: a report of two cases with review of literature. Dermatol. Online J. 9 (5), 26.

Kim, H.K., Lee, Y.S., Kho, H.S., et al., 2003. Facial and glossal distribution of anaesthesia after inferior alveolar nerve block. J. Oral. Rehabil. 30 (2), 189–193.

Lobbezzo, F., Naeije, M., 2007. Dental implications of some common movement disorders; a concise review. Arch. Oral. Biol. 52, 395–398.

Lyu, R.K., Chen, S.T., 2004. Acute multiple cranial neuropathy: a variant of Guillain–Barré syndrome? Muscle Nerve 30 (4), 433–436.

Peñarrocha, M., Cervelló, M., Martí, E., Bagán, J., 2007. Trigeminal neuropathy. Oral. Dis. 13, 141–150.

Pickett, G.E., Bisnaire, D., Ferguson, G.G., 2005. Percutaneous retrogasserian glycerol rhizotomy in the treatment of tic douloureux associated with multiple sclerosis. Neurosurgery 56 (3), 537–545.

Scardina, G.A., Mazzullo, M., Messina, P., 2002. Early diagnosis of progressive systemic sclerosis: the role of oro-facial phenomena. Minerva Stomatol. 51 (7–8), 311–317.

Scully, C., Felix, D.H., 2005. Oral medicine – Update for the dental practitioner. 7. Disorders of orofacial sensation and movement. Br. Dent. J. 199, 703–709.

Vicic, S., Tian, D., Chong, P.S., et al., 2006. Facial onset sensory and motor neuronopathy (FOSMN syndrome): a novel syndrome in neurology. Brain 129, 3884–3890.

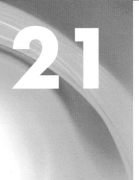

21 Soreness and ulcers

INTRODUCTION

The mouth can be sore for a number of reasons, especially where there are distinct conditions, such as:

- Dry mouth – this predisposes to soreness, since the lubricating and protective functions of saliva are reduced and infections, such as candidosis, are more common. It is especially a problem after irradiation to the head and neck.
- Epithelial thinning or breaches can also result in soreness. This occurs in:
  - mucosal inflammation: any inflammatory lesion can cause soreness; candidosis is one example (antibiotic sore tongue)
  - mucosal atrophy: this is the term often used for thinning of the epithelium, which has a red appearance since the underlying lamina propria shows through. Most commonly seen in geographic tongue (erythema migrans, benign migratory glossitis), atrophy may also be seen in lichen planus or systemic disorders, such as deficiency states (of iron, folic acid or B vitamins)
  - mucosal erosions: this is the term used for superficial breaches of the epithelium, which often initially have a red appearance, since there is little damage to the underlying lamina propria. If a breach penetrates the full thickness of the epithelium, however, it typically becomes covered by a fibrinous exudate and then has a yellowish appearance. Erosions are common in radiation-induced mucositis and in lichen planus
  - mucosal ulcers: this is the term used usually where there is damage to both epithelium and lamina propria, and then a crater forms, sometimes made more obvious clinically by oedema or proliferation causing swelling of the surrounding tissue (**Fig. 21.1**). An inflammatory halo, if present, also highlights the ulcer with a red halo, around the yellow or grey ulcer. Ulcers are common in recurrent aphthous stomatitis. Most other ulcers/erosions are due to local causes, such as trauma or burns, but neoplasms and systemic disorders must always be considered
- Soreness may also be encountered in an apparently normal mouth with no clinical signs of any of the above. This can be due to:
  - subclinical mucosal disease, such as a haematinic deficiency state, particularly of vitamin B_{12}, or even anaemia
  - neuropathies, such as in diabetes mellitus
  - psychogenic causes, which can underlie a sore tongue or sore mouth (often described as a burning sensation) – sometimes known as oral dysaesthesia.

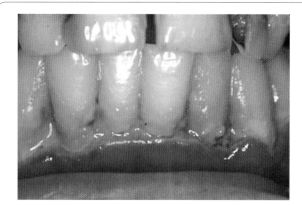

Fig. 21.1 Ulceration in acute necrotizing gingivitis destroys the interdental papillae particularly

ULCERS

- Ulcers and erosions can be the final common manifestation of a spectrum of conditions ranging from epithelial damage resulting from an immunological attack (as in pemphigus, pemphigoid or lichen planus) to damage because of an immune defect as in HIV disease and leukaemia, infections as in herpesviruses, tuberculosis and syphilis, or nutritional defects, such as in vitamin deficiencies and some intestinal disease (**Box 21.1**). A useful pneumonic to remember the main causes is 'So many laws and directives' (systemic; malignant; local; aphthae; drugs), and the systemic causes are mainly blood; infections; gastrointestinal and skin diseases ('bigs').
- The most important feature of ulceration is whether the ulcer is persistent, since this may indicate that the ulcer is caused by a chronic condition such as:
  - neoplasia, such as carcinoma

BOX 21.1 Main causes of mouth ulcers

- **S**ystemic disease:
  - **b**lood disorders
  - **i**nfections
  - **g**astrointestinal disease
  - **s**kin diseases
- **M**alignant neoplasms
- **L**ocal causes
- **A**phthae
- **D**rugs

- chronic trauma, such as from a rough restoration, appliance or tooth
- systemic disease, such as a blood disorder (e.g. leukaemia); infection, such as syphilis, tuberculosis or a mycosis; gastrointestinal disease such as Crohn disease or ulcerative colitis; or skin disease such as lichen planus, pemphigoid or pemphigus.

- An important feature is whether one or more than one ulcer is present, since malignant tumours usually cause a single lesion. A single ulcer persisting for >3 weeks without signs of obvious healing must be taken very seriously, as it could be a neoplasm or chronic infection.
- Multiple persistent ulcers are mainly caused by:
  - **b**lood diseases
  - **i**nfection or immune defect
  - **g**astrointestinal disease
  - **s**kin diseases.
- Multiple non-persistent ulcers can be caused by aphthae, when the ulcers heal spontaneously, usually within 1 week to 1 month. If this is not the case, an alternative diagnosis should be considered.
- Erosions or ulcers on both sides at the commissures of the lips are usually angular stomatitis (cheilitis), but sores are also sometimes caused at the angles by trauma (such as dental treatment) or infection (such as recurrent herpes labialis).

SYSTEMIC DISEASE

A wide range of systemic diseases, especially blood, infectious, gut and skin disorders ('bigs'), may cause oral lesions,

which, because of the moisture, trauma and infection in the mouth, tend to break down to leave ulcers or erosions (**Box 21.2**). If the oral ulcers clinically resemble RAS, they are termed aphthous-like ulcers (ALU).

- Blood (haematological) disease can cause ALU. Deficiency anaemia may underlie some cases. Mouth ulcers may be seen in leukaemias and myelodysplastic syndromes, associated with cytotoxic therapy, with viral, bacterial or fungal infection, or be non-specific. Other oral features may include purpura, gingival bleeding, lymphadenopathy, recurrent herpes labialis and candidosis. Hypereosinophilic syndrome may also present with ulcers.
- Infective causes of mouth ulcers include mainly viral infections, especially the herpesviruses. Other viruses that may cause mouth ulcers include Coxsackie, ECHO and HIV viruses. Bacterial causes of mouth ulcers are less common, apart from acute necrotizing (ulcerative) gingivitis. Syphilis, either the primary or secondary stages, and tuberculosis have been uncommon in the developed world, but are increasing, especially in HIV/AIDS. Fungal causes of ulcers are also uncommon in the developed world, but are increasingly seen in immunocompromised persons and travellers. Protozoal causes of ulcers, such as leishmaniasis, are rare in the developed world, but are appearing in HIV/AIDS. Other causes are shown in **Table 21.1**.
- Gastrointestinal disorders may result in soreness or mouth ulcers. Some patients with aphthae have intestinal disease, such as coeliac disease, causing malabsorption and deficiencies of haematinics, when they may also develop

---

BOX 21.2 More advanced list of causes of mouth ulcers

Systemic disease

Blood disorders:
- Anaemia
- Gammopathies
- Haematinic deficiencies
- Hypereosinophilic syndrome
- Leukaemias
- Myelodysplastic syndromes
- Neutropenia
- Other white cell dyscrasias

Infections:
- Viruses:
  - chickenpox
  - hand, foot and mouth disease
  - herpangina
  - herpetic stomatitis
  - HIV
  - infectious mononucleosis
- Bacteria:
  - acute necrotizing gingivitis
  - syphilis
  - tuberculosis
- Fungi:
  - blastomycosis
  - cryptococcosis
  - histoplasmosis
  - paracoccidioidomycosis
- Parasites:
  - leishmaniasis

Gastrointestinal disease:
- Coeliac disease
- Crohn disease (and orofacial granulomatosis)
- Ulcerative colitis

Skin disease:
- Chronic ulcerative stomatitis
- Dermatitis herpetiformis
- Epidermolysis bullosa
- Erythema multiforme
- Lichen planus and lichenoid lesions
- Linear IgA disease
- Pemphigoid and variants
- Pemphigus vulgaris
- Other dermatoses

Others:
- Rheumatic diseases:
  - lupus erythematosus
  - Sweet syndrome
  - Reiter syndrome (reactive arthritis)
- Vasculitides:
  - Behçet syndrome
  - Wegener granulomatosis
  - periarteritis nodosa
  - giant cell arteritis
- Endocrine disorders:
  - diabetes
  - glucagonoma
- Disorders of uncertain pathogenesis:
  - eosinophilic ulcer
  - necrotizing sialometaplasia

BOX 21.2 **More advanced list of causes of mouth ulcers—cont'd**

Malignant neoplasms
Oral or encroaching from antrum, salivary glands, nose or skin:
- Carcinomas
- Lymphomas
- Sarcomas
- Others

Local causes
Trauma:
- Sharp teeth or restorations
- Appliances
- Non-accidental injury
- Self-inflicted
- Iatrogenic

Burns:
- Heat
- Cold

- Chemical
- Radiation
- Electric

Aphthae
Recurrent aphthous stomatitis and autoinflammatory disorders

Drugs
- Bisphosphonates
- Cytotoxics
- NSAIDs
- Nicorandil
- Propylthiouracil
- Many others (Table 54.9)

Table 21.1 Infectious diseases that may produce oral ulceration

Disease	Causal agent	Major manifestations
AIDS (HIV infection)	HIV	Pneumonia, Kaposi sarcoma, lymphomas, general lymphadenopathy, candidosis, herpes simplex virus, hairy leukoplakia, periodontal disease, ulcers, cervical lymph node enlargement
Chickenpox (varicella)*	VZV	Rash evolves through macule, papule, vesicle and pustule; rash crops and is most dense on trunk General lymphadenopathy, oral ulcers, cervical lymph node enlargement
Cytomegalovirus*	CMV	Glandular-fever-type syndrome (Paul–Bunell negative), general lymphadenopathy, ulcers in immunocompromised people
Gonorrhoea	*Neisseria gonorrhoea*	Urethritis, pharyngitis
Hand, foot and mouth disease	Coxsackie viruses	Rash, minor malaise, oral ulceration (usually mild)
Herpangina	Coxsackie viruses	Fever, sore throat, vesicles and ulcers on soft palate, cervical lymph node enlargement
Herpes simplex*	HSV	Fever, oral ulceration, gingivitis, gingivostomatitis, herpes labialis (secondary infection), cervical lymph node enlargement
Herpes zoster* (shingles)	VZV	Rash like chickenpox, but limited to dermatome Severe pain Oral ulceration in zoster of maxillary or mandibular division of trigeminal nerve Ulcers on palate and in pinna of ear in Ramsay–Hunt syndrome
Infectious mononucleosis	EBV	Fever, pharyngitis, general lymphadenopathy, tonsillar exudate, palatal petechiae, oral ulceration
Mucocutaneous lymph node syndrome (Kawasaki disease)	?	Rash, hands and feet desquamation, general lymphadenopathy, myocarditis, strawberry tongue, labial oedema, pharyngitis
Mycoplasmal pneumonia (atypical pneumonia)	Mycoplasma	Sore throat, fever, pneumonia, erythema multiforme occasionally
Pertussis† (whooping cough)	*Bordetella pertussis*	Cough, fever, occasionally ulceration of lingual fraenum
Syphilis	*Treponema pallidum*	Chancre, lymphadenopathy, rash, ulceration, mucous patches, gumma
Toxoplasmosis*	*Toxoplasma gondii*	Glandular-fever-type syndrome (Paul–Bunell negative), general lymphadenopathy, cough, sore throat
Tuberculosis*	*Mycobacterium tuberculosis*	Ulceration, fever, weight loss, general lymphadenopathy

*Prevalent and often widespread infections in the immunocompromised, high-risk patients such as organ transplant, HIV or leukaemic patients.
†Some cases are caused by *Bordetella parapertussis* or by viruses.

angular stomatitis or glossitis. Crohn disease and pyostomatitis vegetans may cause ulcers. Orofacial granulomatosis (OFG), which has many features reminiscent of Crohn disease, may also cause ulceration.

- Skin (mucocutaneous) disorders that may cause oral erosions or ulceration (or occasionally blisters) include particularly lichen planus, occasionally pemphigoid, and rarely pemphigus, erythema multiforme and epidermolysis bullosa.
- Other causes can include the following:
  - rheumatic diseases: lupus erythematosus, rheumatoid disease and Reiter syndrome
  - vasculitides: Behçet syndrome, periarteritis nodosa, Wegener granulomatosis and giant cell arteritis
  - endocrine causes: diabetes or glucagonoma
  - disorders whose pathogenesis is uncertain: eosinophilic ulcer (traumatic ulcerative granuloma with stromal eosinophilia; TUGSE), necrotizing sialometaplasia (see Ch. 57), sarcoidosis, autoinflammatory syndromes such as periodic fever, aphthae, pharyngitis and adenitis (PFAPA) (see Ch. 34).

MALIGNANT ULCERS

A range of neoplasms may present with ulcers, most commonly these are carcinomas, but Kaposi sarcoma, lymphomas and other neoplasms may be seen (see Ch. 31).

LOCAL CAUSES

- At any age there may be factitious ulceration, especially of the maxillary gingivae, or burns with chemicals of various kinds, heat, cold, or ionizing radiation.
- In children, they are usually caused by accidental biting, or following dental treatment or other trauma, hard foods or appliance (**Fig. 21.2**). In child abuse (non-accidental injury), ulceration of the upper labial fraenum may follow a traumatic fraenal tear. Bruised and swollen lips, and even subluxed teeth or fractured mandible, can be other features of child abuse. The lingual fraenum may be traumatized by repeated rubbing over the lower incisor teeth in children with recurrent bouts of coughing as in whooping cough (termed Riga–Fedes disease) or in self-mutilating conditions. Chronic trauma may produce an ulcer with a keratotic margin.
- Trauma can produce ulceration in adults. Sometimes the lingual fraenum is damaged by trauma in cunnilingus, or the palate in fellatio.

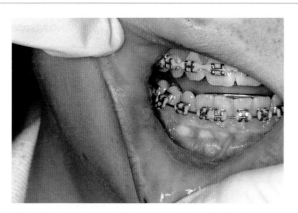

Fig. 21.2 Traumatic ulcer induced by orthodontic appliance

APHTHAE (RECURRENT APHTHOUS STOMATITIS; RAS) (Ch. 34)

Ulcers are commonly aphthae (**Fig. 21.3**), in persons who are otherwise well or at least, no systemic disease is evidently causal, though occasionally they are associated with haematinic deficiencies.

Rarely, similar ulcers are seen in patients with systemic disease such as Behçet syndrome (see Ch. 36), PFAPA (see Ch. 34), HIV infection (see Ch. 53) or Crohn disease – when they are best termed aphthous-like ulcers (ALU), rather than RAS.

DRUG-INDUCED ULCERATION (see Ch. 54)

Drugs may induce ulcers by producing a local burn or by a variety of mechanisms. Cytotoxic drugs (e.g. methotrexate), NSAIDs, sirolimus, everolimus and nicorandil (a potassium channel activator used in cardiac disorders) or others may be the cause.

DIAGNOSIS

Making a diagnosis of the cause for oral soreness or ulceration is based mainly on the history and clinical features. The number, persistence, shape, character of the edge of the ulcer and the appearance of the ulcer base should also be noted.

Acute multiple ulcers are often viral in origin; chronic multiple ulcers may be RAS if recurrent, or vesiculobullous diseases if persistent – when biopsy may be indicated.

A chronic single ulcer may be traumatic, drug-induced, a chronic infection (e.g. tuberculosis, syphilis or mycosis), or a neoplasm (**Table 21.2**)

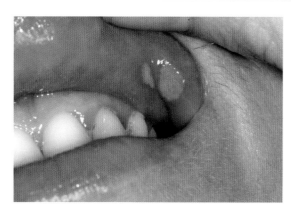

Fig. 21.3 Aphthous ulceration

Table 21.2 Differentiation of mouth ulcers (main causes)

	Single ulcer	Multiple ulcers
Recurrent	Trauma	RAS Aphthous-like ulcers Erythema multiforme Recurrent herpes
Persistent	Neoplasm Trauma Chronic infection (syphilis, TB, fungal) Drugs	Lichen planus Pemphigoid Pemphigus Drugs

Ulcers should always be examined for induration (firmness on palpation), which may be indicative of malignancy. Unless the cause is undoubtedly local, general physical examination is also indicated, looking especially for mucocutaneous lesions, lymphadenopathy or fever (**Algorithms 21.1–21.6**).

Features that might suggest a systemic background to mouth ulcers include:

- Extraoral features such as:
  - skin lesions
  - ocular lesions
  - anogenital lesions
  - purpura
  - fever
  - lymphadenopathy
  - hepatomegaly
  - splenomegaly
  - chronic cough
  - gastrointestinal complaints (e.g. pain, altered bowel habits, blood in faeces)
  - loss of weight or, in children, a failure to thrive
  - weakness.
- An atypical history or ulcer behaviour such as:
  - onset of ulcers in later adult life
  - exacerbation of ulcers
  - severe aphthae
  - aphthae unresponsive to topical hydrocortisone or triamcinolone.
- Other oral lesions, especially:
  - candidosis
  - herpetic lesions
  - glossitis

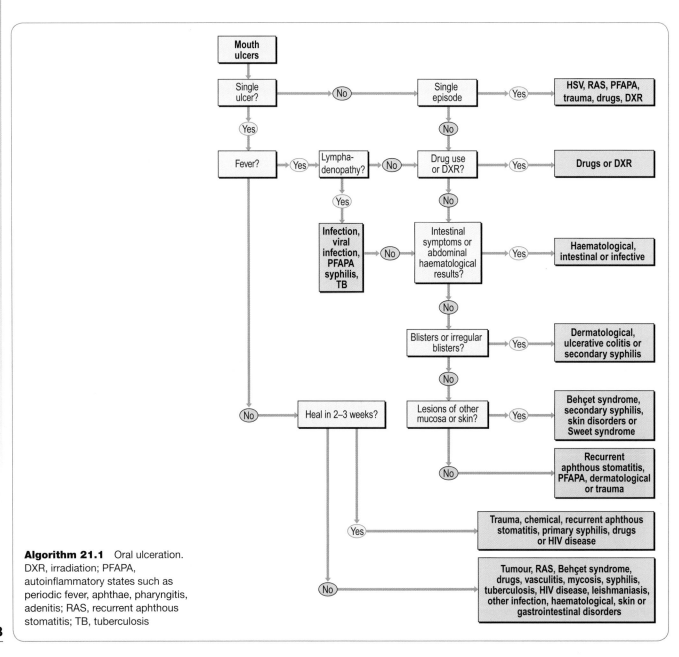

Algorithm 21.1 Oral ulceration. DXR, irradiation; PFAPA, autoinflammatory states such as periodic fever, aphthae, pharyngitis, adenitis; RAS, recurrent aphthous stomatitis; TB, tuberculosis

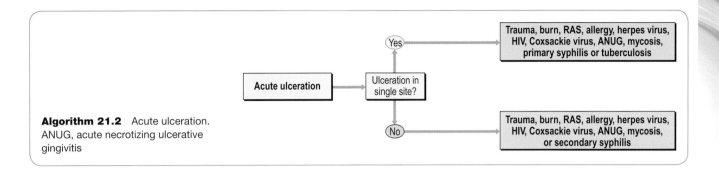

Algorithm 21.2 Acute ulceration. ANUG, acute necrotizing ulcerative gingivitis

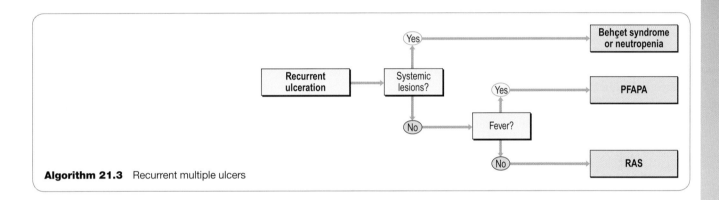

Algorithm 21.3 Recurrent multiple ulcers

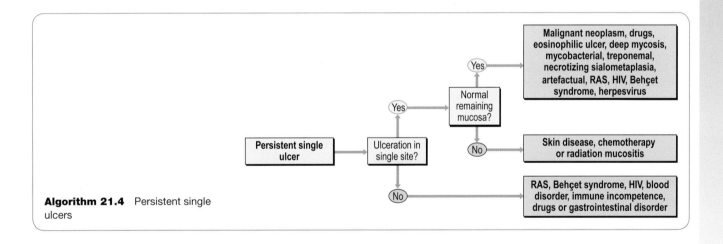

Algorithm 21.4 Persistent single ulcers

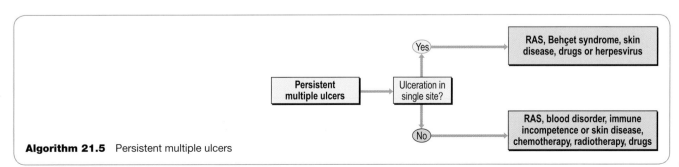

Algorithm 21.5 Persistent multiple ulcers

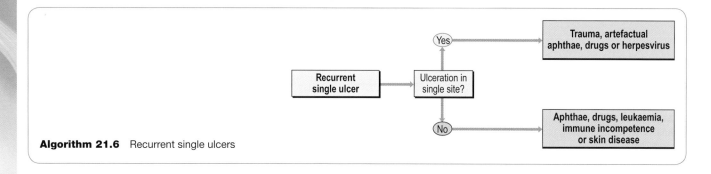

Algorithm 21.6   Recurrent single ulcers

- petechiae
- gingival bleeding
- gingival swelling
- necrotizing gingivitis or periodontitis
- hairy leukoplakia
- Kaposi sarcoma.

Investigations that may sometimes be indicated include the following (**Table 21.3**):

- Blood tests: may be useful for excluding possible haematinic deficiencies or other conditions when a systemic cause, such as leukaemia, EBV or HIV infection, is suspected.
- Microbiological and serological investigations: may be needed, especially if microbial causes are suspected.
- Glucose assays (urine and blood): may occasionally be needed to exclude diabetes.
- Biopsy: may be needed, especially where there:
  - is a single ulcer persisting for >3 weeks
  - is an ulcer that might have been traumatic in aetiology, but persists for >3 weeks after relief from the trauma
  - is induration
  - are skin lesions
  - are lesions in other mucosae
  - are other related systemic lesions, signs or symptoms.
- Imaging and other special investigations: may be indicated where there are possible lesions, such as tuberculosis, the deep mycoses, carcinoma or sarcoidosis.

TREATMENT (see also Chs 4 and 5) (Fig. 21.4)

- Treat the underlying cause.
- Remove aetiological factors.
- Ensure any possible traumatic element is removed (e.g. a denture flange).
- Prescribe a chlorhexidine 0.2% aqueous mouthwash.
- Maintain good oral hygiene.

Table 21.3   Aids that might be helpful in diagnosis/prognosis/management in some patients with soreness and ulcers*

In most cases	In some cases
Full blood picture	Blood glucose
Serum ferritin, vitamin	Transglutaminase
B$_{12}$ and corrected whole	ESR
blood folate	Serum immunoglobulins
levels	Urinalysis for immunoglobulin light chains
	Serology (HIV, HTLV-1, HSV, VZV, EBV, syphilis, mycoplasma)
	ANA
	ANCA
	Culture and sensitivity
	Biopsy
	ELISA for desmoglein
	Chest radiography

*See text for details and glossary for abbreviations.

- A benzydamine mouthwash or spray, or silver nitrate application to an ulcer may help ease discomfort.
- Topical corticosteroids are useful in the management of many oral ulcerative conditions where there is no systemic involvement, such as recurrent aphthous stomatitis and oral lichen planus (see **Table 21.3**).
- Corticosteroid creams, gels and inhalers are better than ointments since the latter adhere poorly to the mucosa. However, creams can be bitter and gels can irritate.
- Patients should not eat or drink for 30 min after using the corticosteroid, in order to prolong contact with the lesion.
- Adverse effects are important mainly with systemic corticosteroids. With many topical corticosteroids there is little systemic absorption and thus no significant adrenocortical suppression. In patients using potent topical corticosteroids for more than a month it is prudent to add an antifungal, since candidosis may arise.

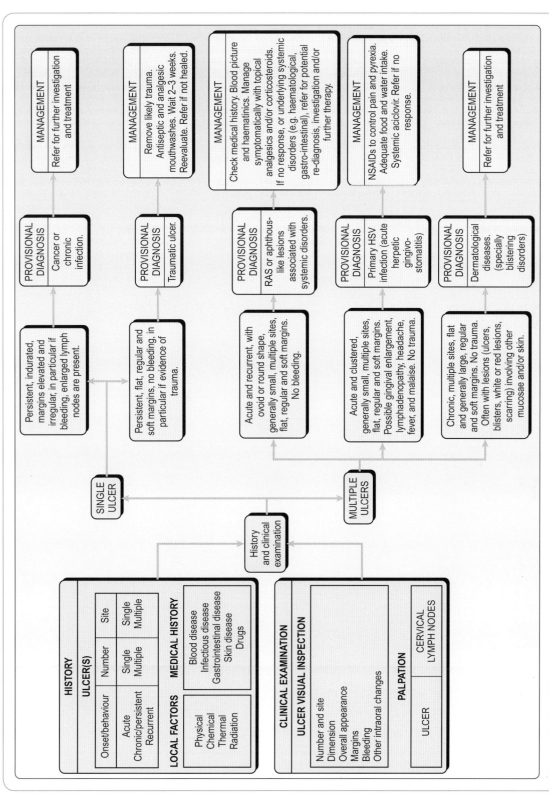

Fig. 21.4 Overall flow diagram for ulcer management (Courtesy of Scully, Fedele, Porter and Mignogna BMJ 2013 in press).

FURTHER READING

Al Attia, H.M., 2006. Borderline systemic lupus erythematosus (SLE): a separate entity or a forerunner to SLE? Int. J. Dermatol. 45 (4), 366–369.

Baroni, A., Capristo, C., Rossiello, L., et al., 2006. Lingual traumatic ulceration (Riga–Fede disease). Int. J. Dermatol. 45 (9), 1096–1097.

Bruce, A.J., Subtil, A., Rogers 3rd, R.S., Castro, L.A., 2006. Monomorphic Epstein–Barr virus (EBV)-associated large B-cell post-transplant lymphoproliferative disorder presenting as a tongue ulcer in a pancreatic transplant patient. Oral. Surg. Oral. Med. Oral. Pathol. Oral. Radiol. Endod. 102 (4), e24–e28.

Chi, A.C., Ravenel, M.C., Neville, B.W., Bass Jr., E.B., 2006. A patient with painful oral ulcers. J. Am. Dent. Assoc. 137 (5), 626–629.

Ebenezer, J., Samuel, R., Mathew, G.C., et al., 2006. Primary oral tuberculosis: report of two cases. Indian J. Dent. Res. 17 (1), 41–44.

Ganesh, R., Suresh, N., Ezhilarasi, S., et al., 2006. Crohn's disease presenting as palatal ulcer. Indian J. Pediatr. 73 (3), 229–231.

Ionescu, M., Murata, H., Janin, A., 2008. Oral mucosa lesions in hypereosinophilic syndrome – an update. Oral. Dis. 14, 115–122.

Karincaoglu, Y., Esrefoglu, M., Aki, T., Mizrak, B., 2006. Propylthiouracil-induced vasculitic oral ulcers with anti-neutrophil cytoplasmic antibody. J. Eur. Acad. Dermatol. Venereol. 20 (1), 120–122.

Kolokotronis, A., Doumas, S., 2006. Herpes simplex virus infection, with particular reference to the progression and complications of primary herpetic gingivostomatitis. Clin. Microbiol. Infect. 12 (3), 202–211.

Mansur, A.T., Kocaayan, N., Serdar, Z.A., Alptekin, F., 2005. Giant oral ulcers of Behçet's disease mimicking squamous cell carcinoma. Acta Derm. Venereol. 85 (6), 532–534.

Pereira, C.M., Gasparetto, P.F., Aires, M.P., 2006. Pemphigus vulgaris in a juvenile patient: case report. Gen. Dent. 54 (4), 262–264.

Scully, C., 2002. Oral Medicine for the general practitioner: part two: sore mouth and ulcers. Independent Dent. 7 (9), 19–26.

Scully, C., Azul, A., Crighton, A., et al., 2001. Nicorandil can induce severe oral ulceration. Oral. Surg. Oral. Med. Oral. Pathol. 91, 189–193.

Scully, C., Felix, D.H., 2005. Oral medicine – Update for the dental practitioner. 1. Aphthous and other common ulcers. Br. Dent. J. 199, 259–264.

Scully, C., Felix, D.H., 2005. Oral medicine – Update for the dental practitioner. 2. Mouth ulcers of more serious connotation. Br. Dent. J. 199, 339–343.

Scully, C., Hodgson, T., 2008. Recurrent oral ulceration: aphthous-like ulcers in periodic syndromes. Oral. Surg. Oral. Med. Oral. Pathol. Oral. Radiol. Endod. 106 (6), 845–852.

Scully, C., Hodgson, T., Lachmann, H., 2008. Auto-inflammatory syndromes and oral health. Oral. Dis. 14 (8), 690–699.

Scully, C., Shotts, R., 2000. ABC of Oral Health. 5. Mouth ulcers, and other causes of orofacial soreness and pain. Student BMJ. 8, 411–414.

Segura, S., Pujol, R., 2008. Eosinophilic ulcer of the oral mucosa: a distinct entity or a non-specific reactive pattern? Oral. Dis. 14, 287–295.

Van Damme, P.A., Bierenbroodspot, F., Telgtt, D.S., et al., 2006. A case of imported paracoccidioidomycosis: an awkward infection in The Netherlands. Med. Mycol. 44 (1), 13–18.

Verstappen, M.C., Mattijssen, V., van der Reijden, B.A., et al., 2006. A man with oral ulcers caused by hypereosinophilic syndrome and a good response to the tyrosine-kinase inhibitor imatinib. Ned. Tijdschr. Geneeskd. 150 (21), 1188–1192.

Taste abnormalities 22

INTRODUCTION

Taste drives appetite and protects people from ingesting poisons. What is called taste in fact is often flavour – a combination of taste with smell (aroma), with texture and other features (e.g. temperature and spiciness).

The sense of taste is mediated by specialized taste buds – oval bodies made up of groups of neuroepithelial and supporting cells (**Fig. 22.1**). The neuroepithelial cells are rod-shaped with a peripheral hair-like process projecting into the taste pores at the surface of the overlying mucous membrane (**Fig. 22.2**). There are five basic tastes but they do not appear to be detected by structurally different taste buds:

- Salt taste: mediated via sodium chloride (NaCl) ions. Na^+ ions enter the receptor cells via Na^+ channels, cause a depolarization, calcium ions enter through voltage-sensitive Ca^{2+} channels, transmitter release occurs and results in increased firing in the primary afferent nerve.
- Sour taste: mediated by protons (H^+), which block potassium channels causing depolarization, Ca^{2+} entry, transmitter release and increased firing in the primary afferent nerve.

- Sweet taste: receptors bind glucose, which activates adenyl cyclase, thereby increasing cyclic adenosine monophosphate (cAMP), causing phosphorylation of K^+ channels, inhibiting them. Depolarization occurs, Ca^{2+} enters and transmitter is released, increasing firing in the primary afferent nerve.
- Bitter taste: bitter substances cause a second messenger (inositol trisphosphate (IP3)) mediated release of Ca^{2+} resulting in transmitter release and firing of the primary afferent nerve.
- Umami taste: certain amino acids (e.g. glutamate, aspartate) bind to a glutamate receptor (mGluR4) activating a G-protein, raising intracellular Ca^{2+}. Glutamate may also stimulate the NMDA (N-methyl-D-aspartate)-receptor, when non-selective cation channels open, and Ca^{2+} enters, causing transmitter release and increased firing in the primary afferent nerve.

The terminal branches of the nerve fibres subserving taste end in close relationship to these special neuroepithelial cells. Taste buds are found in the mucous membrane of the tongue, soft palate, fauces and pharynx, and, in the newborn, on the lips and cheeks. Taste buds on the tongue are on the fungiform, circumvallate and foliate, but not on the filiform, papillae (**Fig. 22.2**). Papillae at the front of the tongue have more taste buds

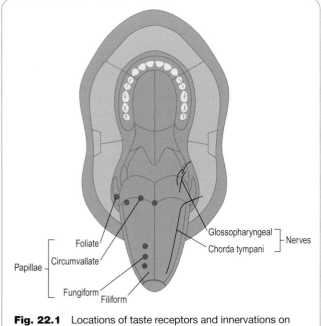

Fig. 22.1 Locations of taste receptors and innervations on tongue

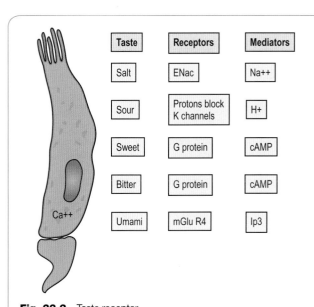

Fig. 22.2 Taste receptor.
Ca, calcium; Na, sodium; H, hydrogen; AMP, adenosine monophosphate; K, potassium; Ip3, inositol triphosphate; ENac, epithelial sodium channels; mGluR4, G protein coupled receptor

compared to the mid-region. Taste buds are also located throughout the oral cavity, in the pharynx, the laryngeal epiglottis and at the entrance of the oesophagus. Sensitivity to all tastes is distributed across the whole tongue and to other regions where there are taste buds (epiglottis, soft palate), but some areas are more responsive to certain tastes than others:

- Fungiform papillae are innervated by the chorda tympani branch of the facial (VIIth cranial) nerve, responding mainly to sodium chloride and/or to sucrose.
- Foliate papillae are predominantly sensitive to sour tastes. Innervated by the glossopharyngeal (IXth cranial) nerve, responding mainly to bitter.
- Circumvallate papillae confer a sour/bitter sensitivity to the posterior two-thirds of the tongue. Innervated by the glossopharyngeal (IXth cranial) nerve, they respond mainly to bitter.

Electrical signals generated in the taste cells transmit information via sensory nerves, which arise from the ganglion cells of branches of cranial nerves:

- chorda tympani nerve: via the lingual nerve (cranial nerve V) from the tongue (anterior two thirds and lateral).
- glossopharyngeal nerve: from the tongue (posterior third).
- vagus nerve: from pharynx and larynx.

All three nerves connect in the brainstem in the nucleus solitarius, before proceeding to the thalamus and then to the brain frontal lobe (the insula and the frontal operculum cortex) for the conscious perception of taste, and the hypothalamus, amygdala and insula for the 'affective' component of taste – responsible for the behavioural response (e.g. feeding behaviour).

TASTE CHANGES

Taste and olfaction are susceptible to the general sensory phenomenon known as adaptation, i.e. the progressive reduction in the appreciation of a stimulus during the course of continual exposure to that stimulus. Taste exhibits almost complete adaptation to a stimulus – perception of a substance fades to almost nothing in seconds. Both taste and olfaction are also susceptible to genetic, hormonal, age and other factors. The cells of the taste buds undergo continual renewal, with a life span of about 10 days, renewal being modulated by nutrition, hormones, and age, and other factors such as drugs and radiation.

- Genetics are important to taste. For example, sensitivity to the bitter taste of phenylthiourea is genetically determined and some patients are genetically unable, for example, to smell fish. In contrast, people who have more than the normal number of taste papillae (and taste buds and increased density of fungiform papillae) have extreme sensitivity to n-propylthiouracil (PROP), are called supertasters and account for 25% of the population (more women than men) – they tend not to like green vegetables and fatty foods.
- Hormones may also influence taste: the sense of taste may vary through the menstrual cycle and may be distorted during pregnancy, often with the appearance of cravings for unusual foods.
- Age affects taste sense; the number of taste buds declines and there are changes in taste cell membranes involving altered function of ion channels and receptors with age.
- Drugs can influence taste (Ch. 54). For example, taste can be suppressed by local anaesthetics applied to the tongue. Amiloride blocks Na^+ channels and reduces the ability to taste salt. Adenosine monophosphate (AMP) may block bitterness. Gymnemic acid (from the Indian tree/shrub *Gymnema sylvestre*) decreases sweet perception. The active compounds of artichokes, chlorogenic acid and cynarin, by suppressing sour and bitter taste receptors, enhance sweet taste. Miracle fruit via an active ingredient, 'miraculin' makes sour substances taste sweet.

TASTE ABNORMALITIES (DYSGEUSIA)

Frequently, when individuals say they cannot taste, the problem is that they cannot appreciate the flavour of food. As the aroma of food contributes to about 75% of its flavour, these individuals have often suffered a loss of smell ability only.

True taste disorders are uncommon, but may present as a loss of taste, or as an abnormal taste in the mouth, an unpleasant taste, or even an electrical sensation. Taste impairment ranges from distorted taste to a complete loss of taste – ageusia, hypogeusia (partial taste loss), and dysgeusia (persistent abnormal taste). Some have termed the phantom sensation of bitterness as 'phantogeusia' (**Table 22.1**). Disorders of taste sense can be distressing and sometimes incapacitating, and can even cause anorexia and depression.

Taste abnormalities can be caused by anything that interrupts the taste pathways from the mucosa, taste buds, non-myelinated nerves, or cranial nerves to the brainstem and brain, or conditions that affect the way the brain interprets taste stimuli (**Table 22.2**).

The most common causes of loss of sense of taste are viral upper respiratory tract infections and head injury, both of which affect olfaction but also, thereby, decrease the appreciation of food and may be perceived as taste loss.

Normal aging produces taste loss.

Surgical procedures affecting cranial nerves V, VII, IX or X may alter taste. These include:

- lingual nerve damage as a result of surgery or even dental injections
- lingual resections
- otological surgery which damages the chorda tympani nerve.

Abnormal tastes may be caused by injury to or disease affecting the taste buds, the nerves responsible for taste, or to a variety of other conditions such as:

- Familial dysautonomia (i.e. Riley–Day syndrome): causes absence of taste buds.
- Radiation and chemotherapy: damage taste receptors and decrease salivary flow altering taste perception.
- Drugs: such as antithyroid drugs, captopril, cytotoxic agents, griseofulvin, histone deacetylase inhibitors (e.g. valproic acid and some cytotxic agents), lithium, penicillamine, procarbazine, rifampin, vinblastine, or vincristine.

Table 22.1 Terminology of taste disorders

Dysfunction	Sense of taste
Absence	Ageusia
Diminished	Hypogeusia
Distorted	Dysgeusia
Heightened	Hypergeusia

Table 22.2 Causes of dysgeusia

Mechanism	Main causes	Examples	
		Common	Less common
Drugs (various effects)	Those causing hyposalivation histone deacetylase inhibitors (e.g. valproic acid Ch. 54)	See Table 54.8	
Olfaction impaired	Nasopharyngeal pathology	Common cold Influenza Nasal infection Nasal polyps Sinusitis Viral pharyngitis	Head injuries, due to tearing of olfactory fibres, and aging
Sensory receptor disorders or environment changes	Oral Hyposalivation Sepsis Smoking Aging (taste bud numbers diminish)	Gastric regurgitation Vitamin (B_{12}) or mineral (zinc) deficiency	Chemotherapy Radiation Salivary gland infections
Cranial nerve disorders	Trauma Neuropathies	Trauma to mouth, nose, or head, or to lingual, chorda tympani or facial nerves, e.g. oral or middle ear surgery	Bell palsy Disseminated sclerosis
Cerebral disorders	Demyelinating disease Cancer Psychogenic disorders Trauma	Hypochondriasis Lung cancer	Frontal lobe tumours Leukaemia or other brain metastases Parkinson disease

- Decreased zinc, copper, and nickel levels.
- Hormonal fluctuations: in menstruation and pregnancy or diabetes, hypogonadism, pseudohypoparathyroidism, hypothyroidism and adrenal cortical insufficiency.
- CNS or nerve damage: as in disseminated sclerosis, facial paralysis, and thalamic or uncal lesions.

DIAGNOSIS

Taste detection can be measured by applying the selected solution to precise regions of the oral mucosa. The tongue is most sensitive for salt and sweet tastes. Sour and bitter tastes can also be recognized on the tongue, but not as well as by the palatal mucosa. Salt and sweet tastes can be appreciated on the palate also, but higher solution concentrations are required. Taste function in the various areas of the tongue and oral cavity can be measured using a spatial test. Four standardized sizes of filter paper are soaked with strong concentrations of the 4 basic tastes. The papers are randomly placed on the 4 quadrants of the tongue and on both sides of the soft palate. Patients then identify the quality of the taste and rate its intensity using the same scale as in whole mouth assessment. Tastes used are:

- sucrose for sweet taste
- vinegar or citric acid to produce sour taste
- sodium chloride for the taste of salt
- quinine for bitter.

Saccharose, aspartame, acetic acid, citric acid, caffeine, monosodium glutamate (MSG) and inosine 5′-monophosphate (IMP) have also been used.

Electrogustometric testing is also available using, for example, TR-06 (Rion Co. Tokyo, Japan).

TREATMENT (see also Chs 4 and 5)

- Treat the cause, if possible (**Table 22.3**): supplements of zinc or vitamin D have been successful in some patients.
- Treat any nasal pathology causing impaired olfaction.
- Treat any dry mouth, oral mucosal disorders or haematinic deficiency.

Table 22.3 Aids that might be helpful in diagnosis/prognosis/management in some patients with taste abnormalities*

In most cases	In some cases
Neurological testing	Blood pressure Full blood picture Serum ferritin, vitamin B_{12} and corrected whole blood folate levels Serum zinc levels ESR Blood glucose SACE Serology (HIV, HTLV-1, HSV, VZV, HCV, Lyme disease, syphilis) ANA RF Nasendoscopy Audiometry Radiography (panoral, occipitomental, lateral and postero-anterior skull) MRI Lumbar puncture Psychological assessment

*See text for details and glossary for abbreviations.

- Consider eliminating any suspect drugs.
- Advise patients to chew food well to increase the release of tastants and saliva production, and drink well. Switching different foods during the meal can decrease the phenomenon of adaptation and can improve taste appreciation.

- In the rare case of familial dysautonomia, in which there is a complete lack of taste buds, methacholine subcutaneously may help.
- Refer for a medical opinion if there are any endocrine or neuropsychiatric disorders.

FURTHER READING

Cowart, B., 2011. Taste dysfunction: a practical guide for oral medicine. Oral. Dis. 17, 2–6.

Gromysz-Kalkowska, K., Wojcik, K., Szubartowska, E., Unkiewicz-Winiarczyk, A., 2002. Taste perception of cigarette smokers. Ann. Univ. Mariae Curie Sklodowska [Med.] 57 (2), 143–154.

Henkin, R.I., Velicu, I., 2010. Differences between and within human parotid saliva and nasal mucus cAMP and cGMP in normal subjects and in patients with taste and smell dysfunction. J. Oral. Pathol. Med. 40 (6), 504–509.

Kanemaru, N., Harada, S., Kasahara, Y., 2002. Enhancement of sucrose sweetness with soluble starch in humans. Chem. Senses 27 (1), 67–72.

Kinnamon, S.C., 2000. A plethora of taste receptors. Neuron 25, 507–510.

Mojet, J., Christ-Hazelhof, E., Heidema, J., 2001. Taste perception with age: generic or specific losses in threshold sensitivity to the five basic tastes? Chem. Senses 26 (7), 845–860.

Nelson, G., Chandrashekar, J., Hoon, M.A., et al., 2002. An amino-acid taste receptor. Nature 416, 199–204.

Nelson, G., Hoon, M.A., Chandrashekar, J., et al., 2001. Mammalian sweet taste receptors. Cell 106, 381–390.

Roberts, D., 2002. Signals and perception.Open University – Palgrave Macmillan. Basingstoke.

Sako, N., Harada, S., Yamamoto, T., 2000. Gustatory information of umami substances in three major taste nerves. Physiol. Behav. 71 (1–2), 193–198.

Tomita, H., Ikeda, M., Okuda, Y., 1986. Basic and practice of clinical taste examinations. Auris Nasus Larynx 13 (Suppl. 1) S1-S1S15.

Yackinous, C.A., Guinard, J.X., 2000. Relationship between PROP (6-n-propylthiouracil) taster status, taste anatomy and dietary intake measures for young men and women. Appetite 38, 201–209.

INTRODUCTION

Normal mouth opening in an adult ranges from 35–55 mm inter-incisally. Trismus (lockjaw) (from the Greek *Trimos* = 'grating', 'grinding) is the inability to open the mouth normally usually due to muscle spasm. Trismus can have consequences including impaired mastication, difficulty in speaking, in achieving adequate oral hygiene and in access for oral care. If left untreated, degenerative processes in the masticatory muscles, with disuse atrophy, may ensue.

In some people, such as persons who have received radiation to the head and neck, trismus is often seen in conjunction with difficulty in swallowing. In trismus caused by radiation treatment, hyposalivation and mucositis are also common associated challenges. Occasionally in temporomandibular joint trauma or infection, and rarely in pain-dysfunction syndrome, the joint may become fibrotic, or even ankylosed.

AETIOLOGY AND PATHOGENESIS

Limited opening of the jaw is usually due to extra-articular disease with masticatory muscle spasm secondary to stress, trauma or local infection (e.g. pericoronitis around a partially erupted mandibular third molar). Occasionally trismus is caused by joint (intra-articular and intra-capsular) disease, or conditions affecting the adjacent soft (peri-capsular) tissues such as scarring, infiltrating neoplasms or oral submucous fibrosis.

Trismus is usually caused by inflammation and masticatory muscle spasm, or inflexible scarring or other tissues (**Boxes 23.1** and **23.2**). Life-threatening causes include tetanus, malignant neoplasms and fascial space infections. In stroke patients, trismus may appear as a sequel to the CNS dysfunction. Some psychotomimetics (e.g. amphetamines and ecstasy (methylenedioxymethamphetamine; MDMA)) can cause masticatory muscle spasm which forcibly causes bruxism and difficulty in mouth opening, which can be reduced by sucking on a pacifier or lollipop. In some mental states such as hysteria, it may appear that the patient has trismus.

BOX 23.1 Main causes of trismus

- Infections
- Trauma
- Submucous fibrosis
- Neoplasms

BOX 23.2 Advanced list of causes of trismus

Acute trismus
- Infection:
  - pericoronitis
  - odontogenic infection with spread involving masticatory muscles, TMJ, bone or fascial spaces
  - TMJ or bone infections
  - tonsillar or pharyngeal infections
  - parotitis
  - otitis
  - tetanus
- Trauma:
  - jaws
  - facial soft tissues
- Postoperative:
  - third molar teeth removal
  - other jaw and oral surgery
  - associated with haematoma
  - local anaesthetic injection trauma to pterygoid muscles
- Drug related: (see Table 54.25)
  - psychotomimetics such as ecstasy
  - extra-pyramidal reaction to anti-emetics (e.g. metoclopramide)
- Malignant hyperthermia
- Temporomandibular joint disease (e.g. gout, rheumatoid arthritis) and pain-dysfunction syndrome

Sub-acute trismus
- Tumour infiltration of muscles or joint
- Chronic infection
- Temporomandibular joint disease and pain-dysfunction syndrome

Chronic trismus
- Soft tissue scar formation or TMJ damage after surgery, trauma, radiation or burns
- Submucous fibrosis (Ch. 30)
- Scleroderma
- Rheumatoid arthritis
- Temporomandibular joint disease and pain-dysfunction syndrome
- TMJ ankylosis
- Masticatory muscle disorders (e.g. myotonia, myositis ossificans, fibrodysplasia ossificans, fibrosclerosis)
- Suprabulbar palsy

DIAGNOSIS

Except for those cases caused by acute trauma and tetanus, trismus tends to develop slowly and some patients may not be aware until they can only open their mouth to 20 mm or less (**Fig. 23.1**). A simple diagnostic test is the 'three finger test'. Ask the patient to insert three of their fingers into the mouth. If all three fingers can fit between the incisors, mouth opening is considered normal but if less than three can be inserted, trismus is likely.

The cause should be sought (**Algorithm 23.1**; **Table 23.1**) and a thorough clinical and imaging examination must be performed to rule out neoplasms in the pharynx and infratemporal regions as well as the TMJ, jaws and parotid salivary glands.

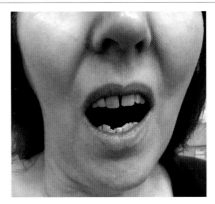

Fig. 23.1   Trismus in severe temporomandibular pain-dysfunction syndrome

TREATMENT (see also Chs 4 and 5)

The underlying condition should be treated where possible. Tetanus is a medical emergency and should be treated with antimicrobials (penicillin or metronidazole), tetanus immunoglobulin, and muscle relaxants (e.g. diazepam).

Trismus treatment should begin early in the progression of the trismus since it then is likely to be more effective, and easier on the patient. If treatment is delayed, the difficulty in reversing trismus increases.

If local infection is the cause, appropriate antimicrobials are indicated early on. In most cases, a soft diet is indicated. Symptomatic relief may include antiinflammatory analgesics such as NSAIDs, muscle relaxants such as benzodiazepines, warmth, physical therapy, and 'range of motion' devices. Warmth is best applied with moist hot towels placed on the affected area for 15 min every hour. Use of sugar-free chewing gum may help. Soft lasers, splints and botulinum toxoid have also occasionally been employed.

'Range of motion' devices provide passive motion which, applied several times per day, provides significant improvement in opening and reduction in inflammation and pain. It is important to record the initial opening (inter-incisal distance) before starting therapy and keep a patient log-book. Then the patient should open and close the mouth with assisted opening 5 times, holding the open position to the maximum opening that can be sustained *without pain* for 5 s. They should do this 5 times per day. The most common way to achieve such passive motion is by using tongue spatulas (depressors) which can be stacked, forced and held between the teeth in an attempt to lever the mouth open slowly over time. One simple modification has been reported – the Pat-Bite device (Patient-Bite). The Therabite (Platon Medical Ltd., Eastbourne, UK; (http://www.atosmedical.com)) functions similarly to the spatula

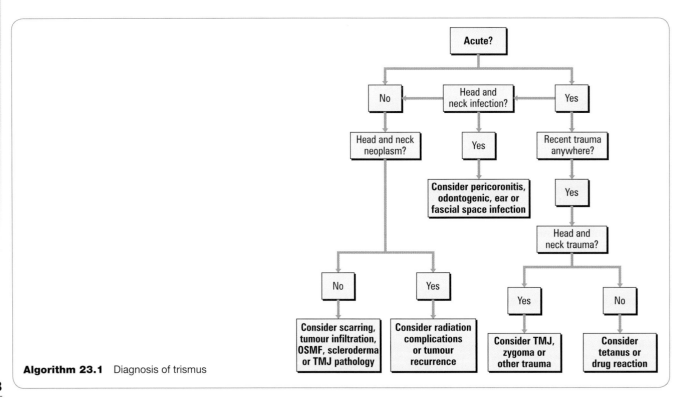

Algorithm 23.1   Diagnosis of trismus

Table 23.1 Aids that might be helpful in diagnosis/prognosis/management in some patients with trismus*

In most cases	In some cases
Radiography of jaw, TMJ	CT/MRI
	Nasendoscopy
	Ultrasound
	Biopsy
	Culture and sensitivity
	Full blood picture
	ESR
	Serum uric acid
	Antinuclear antibodies (ANA)
	Anti-topoisomerase 1 antibodies (ATA or anti-Scl-70)
	Anticentromere, antibodies (ACA)
	Rheumatoid factor (RF)
	Psychological assessment

*See text for details and glossary for abbreviations.

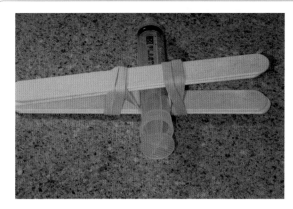

Fig. 23.2 Homemade trismus reliever

systems. Patients using spatulas or the Therabite may gain up to 1.5 mm of sustainable opening gains per week, and thus may need to exercise for up to 10 weeks to achieve useful oral opening. Many patients will need to continue to mobilize and stretch daily at least once each day, for life (**Fig. 23.2**).

Continuous passive motion devices are also commercially available (e.g. Dynasplint; Stevensville, Maryland, USA; (http://www.dynasplint.com/divisions/jaw/)). More sophisticated and expensive devices can be custom made for each patient. Microcurrent electrotherapy and pentoxifylline may also increase mouth opening significantly. In rare cases, persons with severe limitation to opening may need cricothyrotomy or intubation.

FURTHER READING

Albertin, A., Kerppers, I.I., Amorim, C.F., et al., 2010. The effect of manual therapy on masseter muscle pain and spasm. Electromyogr. Clin. Neurophysiol. 50 (2), 107–112.

Angadi, P.V., Rao, S., 2010. Management of oral submucous fibrosis: an overview. Oral. Maxillofac. Surg. 14 (3), 133–142.

Angadi, P.V., Rekha, K.P., 2011. Oral submucous fibrosis: a clinicopathologic review of 205 cases in Indians. Oral. Maxillofac. Surg. 15 (1), 15–19.

Aras, M.H., Güngörmüş, M., 2010. Placebo-controlled randomized clinical trial of the effect two different low-level laser therapies (LLLT) – intraoral and extraoral – on trismus and facial swelling following surgical extraction of the lower third molar. Lasers Med. Sci. 25 (5), 641–645.

Chen, P.Y., Lin, P.Y., Tien, S.C., et al., 2010. Duloxetine-related tardive dystonia and tardive dyskinesia: a case report. Gen. Hosp. Psychiatry 32 (6), 646.e9–646.e11.

Conner, G.A., Duffy, M., 2009. Myositis ossificans: a case report of multiple recurrences following third molar extractions and review of the literature. J. Oral. Maxillofac. Surg. 67 (4), 920–926.

Cox, S., Zoellner, H., 2009. Physiotherapeutic treatment improves oral opening in oral submucous fibrosis. J. Oral. Pathol. Med. 38 (2), 220–226.

Dhanrajani, P.J., Jonaidel, O., 2002. Trismus aetiology, differential diagnosis and treatment. Dent. Update 29, 88–94.

Hassan, B., Popoola, A., Olokoba, A., Salawu, F.K., 2011. A survey of neonatal tetanus at a district general hospital in north-east Nigeria. Trop. Doct. 41 (1), 18–20.

Holle, J., 2009. Lockjaw treatment after noma in the third world. J. Craniofac. Surg. 20 (Suppl. 2), 1910–1912.

Hoole, J., Jenkins, G.W., Kanatas, A.N., Mitchell, D.A., 2011. Reliability and validity of a new method of nurse-led assessment of trismus. Br. J. Oral. Maxillofac. Surg. 49 (6), 430–437.

Kwong, Y.L., Leung, A.Y., Cheung, R.T., 2011. Pregabalin-induced trismus in a leukemia patient. J. Hosp. Med. 6 (2), 103–104.

Lee, J.H., Jung, K.Y., 2012. Emergency cricothyrotomy for trismus caused by instantaneous rigor in cardiac arrest patients. Am. J. Emerg. Med. 30 (6), 1014.e1–2.

Mehanna, P., 2010. Battling trismus: the 'Pat-Bite' device. Br. J. Oral. Maxillofac. Surg. 48 (4), 316.

Melchers, L.J., Van Weert, E., Beurskens, C.H., et al., 2009. Exercise adherence in patients with trismus due to head and neck oncology: a qualitative study into the use of the Therabite. Int. J. Oral. Maxillofac. Surg. 38 (9), 947–954.

Mubeen, K., Kumar, C.N., Puja, R., et al., 2010. Psychiatric morbidity among patients with oral sub-mucous fibrosis: a preliminary study. J. Oral. Pathol. Med. 39 (10), 761–764.

Nussbaum, B.L., 2009. Dental care for patients who are unable to open their mouths. Dent. Clin. North Am. 53 (2), 323–328.

Paliwal, V.K., 2010. Neuromyotonia masquerading as tetanus. J. Clin. Neurosci. 17 (6), 814–815.

Shulman, D.H., Shipman, B., Willis, F.B., 2008. Treating trismus with dynamic splinting: A cohort, case series. Adv. Ther. 25 (1), 9–16.

Stubblefield, M.D., Manfield, L., Riedel, E.R., 2010. A preliminary report on the efficacy of a dynamic jaw opening device (dynasplint trismus system) as part of the multimodal treatment of trismus in patients with head and neck cancer. Arch. Phys. Med. Rehabil. 91 (8), 1278–1282.

Wetsch, W.A., Böttiger, B.W., Padosch, S.A., 2010. Masseter spasm after induction of general anaesthesia using propofol and remifentanil. Eur. J. Anaesthesiol. 27 (12), 1069–1070.

Wilson, M.C., Laskin, D.M., 2009. Surgical management of limited mouth opening associated with congenital suprabulbar paresis: report of a case. J. Oral. Maxillofac. Surg. 67 (3), 650–652.

Wright, E.F., 2011. Medial pterygoid trismus (myospasm) following inferior alveolar nerve block: Case report and literature review. Gen. Dent. 59 (1), 64–67.

Xue, F.S., He, N., Liao, X., et al., 2011. Further observations on retromolar fibreoptic orotracheal intubation in patients with severe trismus. Can. J. Anaesth. 58 (9), 868–869.

24 White lesions

INTRODUCTION

Lesions in the mouth may be white because there is material (e.g. candidosis or material alba (debris from poor oral hygiene)) on the epithelial surface, or the epithelium is thickened (e.g. in keratosis, lichen planus or leukoplakia).

An acronym by which to remember the causes is CLINK (congenital (e.g. leukoedema and white sponge naevus); lichen planus; infections (e.g. candidosis or hairy leukoplakia); neoplastic and preneoplastic (leukoplakia or carcinoma); keratosis). Some other common conditions are yellowish rather than white in colour, such as Fordyce spots/granules and geographic tongue but they may cause diagnostic confusion. Fordyce spots are therefore discussed here; geographic tongue is in Ch. 41.

Burn, scars, grafts and furred or hairy tongue may also be white.

FORDYCE SPOTS

Fordyce spots, also known as Fordyce granules, are creamy yellowish soft granules beneath the oral mucosa, usually seen along the border between the vermilion and the oral mucosa of the upper lip (**Fig. 24.1**) and in the buccal mucosa particularly inside the commissures, and also in the retromolar regions and lips. They are sebaceous glands containing neutral lipids similar to those found in skin sebaceous glands, but they are not associated with hair follicles.

Probably 80% of the population have Fordyce spots but they are not usually evident in infants (though they are present histologically), appearing clinically in children after the age of 3 years, increasing during puberty and then again in later adult life. They are noticeable mainly in adults, more prominent in men and seem to be more obvious:

- with advancing age
- in patients with a greasy skin
- in some rheumatic disorders
- in hereditary non-polyposis colorectal cancer syndrome: the most common site then is the lower gingiva and vestibular oral mucosa.

Fordyce spots are totally benign, though the occasional patient or physician becomes concerned about them or misdiagnoses them as, for example, thrush or lichen planus. No treatment is reliable or indicated, other than reassurance.

LEUKOEDEMA

Leukoedema is not a mucosal disease – simply the description of very faint whitish lines in some normal buccal mucosae, seen very often in people of African heritage. The whitish lines are bilateral and disappear if the mucosa is stretched (a diagnostic test).

OTHER WHITE LESIONS

White lesions can be due to materia alba (debris from poor oral hygiene), but are mainly traumatic or inflammatory in cause such as candidosis or hairy leukoplakia. Some may be due to potentially malignant disorders such as lichen planus and leukoplakia (**Boxes 24.1** and **24.2**).

Linea alba (occlusal line) is a simple line of frictional keratosis seen in the buccal mucosae, horizontally aligned with the occlusal surfaces of the teeth, sometimes with small vertical lines coincident with the interdental areas. More prominent

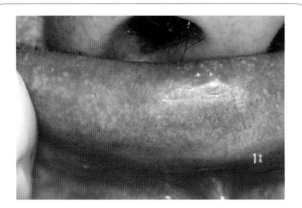
Fig. 24.1 Fordyce spots in the upper lip

> **BOX 24.1   Main causes of white oral lesions**
>
> - Congenital (e.g. leukoedema, Fordyce spots, white sponge naevus):
> - Lichen planus
> - Infections:
>   - candidosis (thrush: candidal leukoplakia)
>   - hairy leukoplakia
> - Neoplasms and preneoplastic diseases:
>   - carcinoma
>   - leukoplakia
> - Keratoses (e.g. frictional keratosis (and cheek/lip biting), smoker's keratosis and snuff-dipper's keratosis)

BOX 24.2 More advanced list of causes of oral white lesions

Congenital
- Leukoedema
- Fordyce spots
- White sponge naevus
- Focal palmoplantar and oral mucosa hyperkeratosis syndrome
- Darier disease
- Pachyonychia congenita
- Dyskeratosis congenita

Lichen planus and other mucocutaneous disorders
- Lupus erythematosus
- Darier disease

Infections
- Candidosis
- Hairy leukoplakia
- Syphilitic mucous patches and keratosis
- Koplik spots (measles)
- Some papillomas
- Reiter syndrome
- Koilocytic dysplasia (papilloma virus)

Neoplastic and possibly pre-neoplastic
- Leukoplakia:
  - homogeneous
  - non-homogeneous, either nodular (verrucous) or speckled (erythroleukoplakia)
- Carcinoma
- Verruciform xanthoma

Keratoses
- Frictional
- Smokers
- Snuff
- Betel

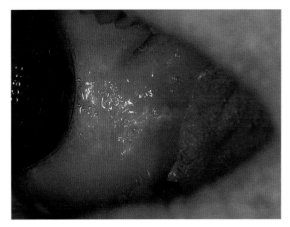

Fig. 24.2 Cheek biting (morsicatio buccarum) is seen mainly around the occlusal area

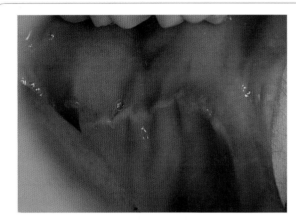

Fig. 24.3 Linea alba (occlusal line) – a keratosis

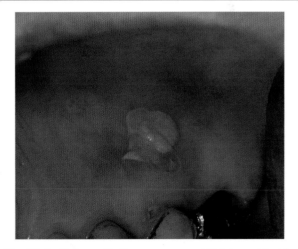

Fig. 24.4 Collapsed bullae can appear whitish (pemphigoid)

where there is bruxism or clenching. No treatment is required. The tongue is often scalloped also.

DIAGNOSIS

Collections of debris (materia alba) or fungi (candidosis) may look white, but these can usually easily be wiped off with a dry sterile gauze swab. Other lesions appear white usually because they are composed of thickened keratin, which looks white when wet, and these lesions, being inherent in the mucosa, will not wipe away with a gauze swab.

White lesions are usually painless, but can be focal, multifocal, striated or diffuse, and these features may give a guide to the diagnosis. For example:

- Focal lesions are often caused by cheek-biting (**Fig. 24.2**), at the occlusal line (**Fig. 24.3**), where there are collapsed bullae (**Fig. 24.4**) or keratosis (**Fig. 24.5**).
- Multifocal lesions are common in thrush (pseudomembranous candidosis) and lichen planus.
- Striated lesions are typical of lichen planus.
- Diffuse white areas are seen in the buccal mucosa in leukoedema, and in the palate in stomatitis nicotina.

Diagnosis of white lesions is mainly clinical; lesions should also be sought on the skin or other mucosae. Haematological tests and/or biopsy or imaging or other investigation may be indicated (**Algorithm 24.1**; **Table 24.1**).

TREATMENT (see also Chs 4 and 5)

Treatment is usually of the underlying cause.

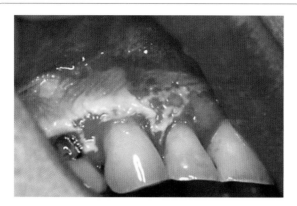

Fig. 24.5 Leukoplakia on the gingivae

Table 24.1 Aids that might be helpful in diagnosis/prognosis/management in some patients with persistent white lesions*

In most cases where the lesion does not wipe off with a gauze swab	In some cases
Biopsy	Full blood picture
	Serum ferritin, vitamin B_{12} and corrected whole blood folate levels
	ESR
	Chest radiography
	Microbiological swabs
	Viral serology (HCV, HIV)
	Syphilis serology
	Blood CD4 counts
	Immunologist opinion
	Dermatological opinion
	Genetic opinion

*See text for details and glossary for abbreviations.

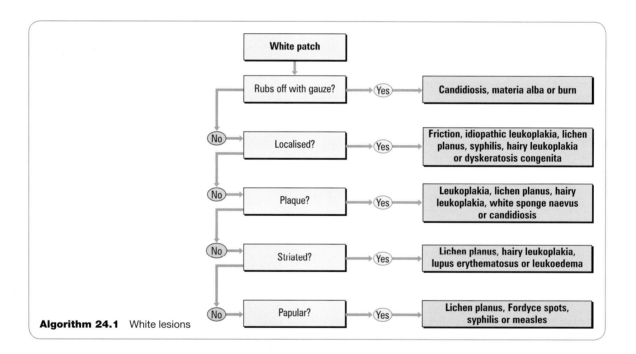

Algorithm 24.1 White lesions

FURTHER READING

De Felice, C., Parrini, S., Chitano, G., et al., 2005. Fordyce granules and hereditary non-polyposis colorectal cancer syndrome. Gut 54 (9), 1279–1282.

Elston, D.M., Meffert, J., 2001. Photo quiz. What is your diagnosis? Fordyce spots. Cutis 68 (1), 24–49.

Flaitz, C.M., Baker, K.A., 2000. Treatment approaches to common symptomatic oral lesions in children. Dent. Clin. North Am. 44, 671–696.

Freitas, M.D., Blanco-Carrion, A., Gandara-Vila, P., et al., 2006. Clinicopathologic aspects of oral leukoplakia in smokers and nonsmokers. Oral. Surg. Oral. Med. Oral. Pathol. Oral. Radiol. Endod. 102 (2), 199–203.

Gillenwater, A.M., Chambers, M.S., 2006. Diagnosis of premalignant lesions and early cancers of the oral cavity. Tex. Dent. J. 123 (6), 512–520.

Huber, M.A., 2010. White oral lesions, actinic cheilitis, and leukoplakia: confusions in terminology and

definition: facts and controversies. Clin. Dermatol. 28 (3), 262–268.

Noonan, V.L., Kabani, S., 2005. Diagnosis and management of suspicious lesions of the oral cavity. Otolaryngol. Clin. North Am. 38 (1), 21–35.

Ocampo-Candiani, J., Villarreal-Rodriguez, A., Quinones-Fernandez, A.G., et al., 2003. Treatment of Fordyce spots with CO_2 laser. Dermatol. Surg. 29 (8), 869–871.

Reichart, P.A., 2000. Oral mucosal lesions in a representative cross-sectional study of aging Germans. Community Dent. Oral. Epidemiol. 28 (5), 390–398.

Roosaar, A., Yin, L., Sandborgh-Englund, G., et al., 2006. On the natural course of oral lichen lesions in a Swedish population-based sample. J. Oral. Pathol. Med. 35 (5), 257–261.

Scully, C., 2003. Oral medicine for the general practitioner: part four: red, white and coloured lesions. Independent Dent. 8, 87–94.

Scully, C., Felix, D.H., 2005. Oral medicine – update for the dental practitioner. 6. Red and pigmented lesions. Br. Dent. J. 199, 639–645.

Scully, C., Felix, D.H., 2005. Oral medicine – update for the dental practitioner. 5. Oral white patches. Br. Dent. J. 199, 565–572.

Scully, C., Newman, L., Bagan, J.V., 2005. The role of the dental team in preventing and diagnosing cancer: 3. Oral cancer diagnosis and screening. Dent. Update 32 (6), 326–328 331–332, 335–337.

Warnakulasuriya, K.A., Ralhan, R., 2007. Clinical, pathological, cellular and molecular lesions caused by oral smokeless tobacco – a review. J. Oral. Pathol. Med. 36 (2), 63–77.

CANCER AND POTENTIALLY MALIGNANT DISORDERS

There is no medicine like hope, no incentive so great, and no tonic so powerful as expectation of something better tomorrow.

Orison Swett Marden

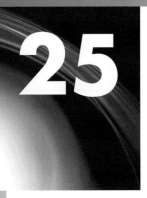

25 Potentially malignant disorders

INTRODUCTION

Most mouth cancers are oral squamous cell carcinomas (OSCC) and appear to arise in apparently normal mucosa, in apparently otherwise healthy people but some are preceded by clinically obvious potentially malignant (sometimes termed premalignant) disorders (PMD) and OSCC is also increased in patients who:

- have had previous oral malignancy
- have had previous malignancy in the upper aerodigestive tract (nose, pharynx, trachea, lungs, oesophagus)
- are immune incompetent.

PMD include (**Table 25.1**) mainly:

- Actinic cheilitis (solar elastosis) (Ch. 26).
- Erythroplakia (erythroplasia – red patch; **Fig. 25.1**) (Ch. 27): defined by the World Health Organization (WHO) as 'any lesion of the oral mucosa that presents as bright red velvety plaques which cannot be characterized clinically or pathologically as any other recognizable condition'. This is rare but has a very high malignant potential and many cases are already a carcinoma on microscopic examination.
- Leukoplakia (white patch; **Figs 25.2–25.6**) (Ch. 28): defined by the WHO as 'clinical white patches that cannot be wiped off the mucosa and cannot be classified clinically or microscopically as another specific disease entity (such as lichen planus)'. Leukoplakia is, thus, a clinical diagnosis only and can only be made by exclusion. A workshop

coordinated by the WHO Collaborating Centre for Oral Cancer and Precancer agreed that the term leukoplakia should be used to recognize 'white plaques of questionable risk having excluded (other) known diseases or disorders that carry no increased risk for cancer'.
- Lichen planus/lichenoid lesions (Ch. 29): in many geographic areas these are the most common PMDs.
- Submucous fibrosis (Ch. 30).
- Palatal lesions in reverse smokers.

Apart from the conditions noted above, rare conditions that predispose to OSCC include:

- discoid lupus erythematosus (Ch. 57)
- dyskeratosis congenita (Ch. 57)
- epidermolysis bullosa (Ch. 57)
- Fanconi anaemia (Ch. 56)
- Paterson–Kelly syndrome (sideropenic dysphagia; Plummer–Vinson syndrome) (Ch. 56)
- Xeroderma pigmentosum (Ch. 57).

There are also occasional associations of OSCC with:

- diabetes, and the metabolic syndrome
- scleroderma.

Erythroplakia has a very high malignant potential. Leukoplakia can have a malignant potential – particularly high in the following types (**Table 25.2**):

- speckled leukoplakia (red and white patch – erythroleukoplakia)
- nodular or verrucous leukoplakia.

AETIOLOGY AND PATHOGENESIS

Although genetics clearly predispose to PMD in some cases (such as in dyskeratosis congenita, Fanconi anaemia and xeroderma pigmentosum), lifestyle habits are often implicated, and most of these have psychotropic actions and are habit-forming or addictive. Those habits that are known to predispose to potential malignancy include:

- tobacco use (**Fig. 25.6**)
- alcohol use
- betel nut chewing and possibly other chewing habits.
- sunlight exposure.

Marijuana use, and oro-genital or oro-anal sex (via human papillomavirus (HPV) transmission) may also be implicated as discussed below and in Ch. 31.

Table 25.1 Potentially malignant oral disorders

Disorder		Aetiological factors	Features
Actinic cheilitis (solar elastosis)		Sunlight	White plaque/erosions
Erythroplasia		Tobacco/alcohol/betel	Flat red plaque
Leukoplakia	Homogeneous	Tobacco/alcohol/betel, human papilloma virus	White plaque
Leukoplakia	Speckled (erythroleukoplakia)	Tobacco/alcohol/betel, human papilloma virus	Speckled plaque
	Nodular/verrucous	Tobacco/alcohol/betel, human papilloma virus	Nodular white plaque
	Proliferative verrucous leukoplakia	Tobacco/alcohol	White or speckled nodular plaque
	Sublingual leukoplakia	Tobacco/alcohol	White plaque
	Candidal leukoplakia	Candida albicans	White or speckled plaque
	Syphilitic leukoplakia	Syphilis	White plaque
Lichen planus		Idiopathic	White plaque/erosions
Submucous fibrosis		Areca nut/betel	Immobile mucosa, white plaque
Palatal lesions in reverse smokers		Tobacco	White or speckled plaque
Immunocompromised patients		Papilloma viruses Candidosis	White or speckled plaques
Discoid lupus erythematosus		Idiopathic	White plaque/erosions
Dyskeratosis congenita		Genetic	White plaques
Epidermolysis bullosa		Genetic	Scarring
Fanconi anaemia		Genetic	White plaques Periodontal disease
Paterson–Kelly syndrome (sideropenic dysphagia; Plummer–Vinson syndrome)		Iron deficiency	Postcricoid web
Xeroderma pigmentosum		Genetic	White plaque/erosions

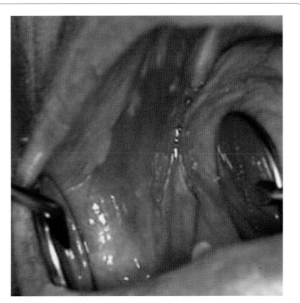

Fig. 25.1 Erythroplakia: usually a potentially malignant disorder, or carcinoma

RISK FACTORS: TOBACCO

Many studies have shown an association between tobacco use and oral PMD and OSCC. The relative risk of having an oral dysplastic lesion for smokers compared with non-smokers was estimated at 7.0. Oral leukoplakia can be related to tobacco use. Tobacco users are also predisposed to a number of other cancers and potentially malignant conditions (oesophageal, breast, stomach, colorectal, bladder, lung and hepatocellular cancer), and other systemic and oral health issues.

Tobacco contains at least 50 compounds including polycyclic aromatic hydrocarbons such as benzpyrene, nitrosamines, aldehydes and aromatic amines. The precise role of tobacco however, is surprisingly difficult to define, not least because many heavy smokers also drink alcohol – which is carcinogenic. However, studies of those who are teetotal and abstain from such habits (e.g. Mormons, Seventh Day Adventists) have shown a very low incidence of OSCC.

Different tobacco habits have varied effects:

- Cigarette smokers appear about five times more likely to develop OSCC than do non-smokers and, in contrast, those who abstain have had a lower incidence. In one recent study, the odds ratio for consumption of >20 cigarettes/day

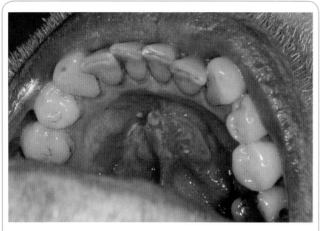

Fig. 25.2 Speckled leukoplakia: often a potentially malignant lesion

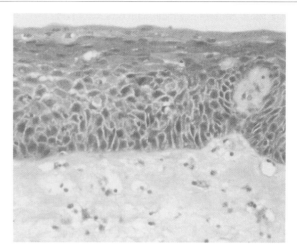

Fig. 25.4 Dysplasia: moderate

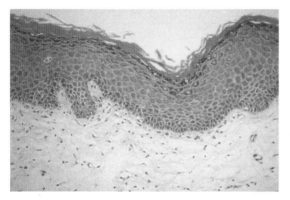

Fig. 25.3 No dysplasia detectable from this biopsy and thus the lesion is presumed benign

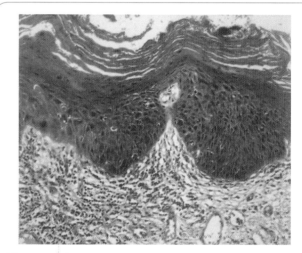

Fig. 25.5 Dysplasia: severe, and suggestive of a potentially malignant disorder

was double that of smokers consuming <20 cigarettes/day. Compared to non-smokers, the risk of OSCC to low/medium cigarette smokers was 8.5 and for high tar cigarette smokers was significantly greater at 16.4 in one European study. Black tobacco seems more carcinogenic than blonde.

- Bidi smoking (reverse smoking) is strongly associated with leukoplakia and oral cancer. Palatal or other oral carcinoma can result. Bidi (unfiltered cigarettes containing a small amount of flaked tobacco), widely prevalent in south Asia (mainly India, Taiwan and the Philippines) and in South America, are smoked with the lit end within the mouth.
- Cigar smoking may predispose to OSCC, and some studies have shown an association with floor of mouth leukoplakia in women smokers.
- Pipe smoking is most often associated with nicotinic stomatitis, a non-premalignant condition, but there is evidence from some countries that pipe smoking may be associated with a predisposition to OSCC.
- Smokeless tobacco (ST), for example, snuff-dipping (placing snuff in the buccal sulcus) in women in south-eastern USA, has been shown to predispose to gingival and alveolar carcinoma close to the area snuff is placed.

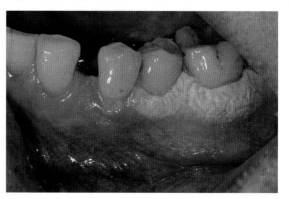

Fig. 25.6 Leukoplakia in a person who for most of his adult life drank a bottle of vodka and smoked 20 cigarettes daily; he also incidentally developed myeloma

Table 25.2 Malignant potential in the most important oral potentially malignant disorders

	Malignant potential		
	High (>60%)	**Medium (<30%)**	**Low (<10%)**
Main entities	Erythroplakia	Leukoplakia (non-homogeneous) Candidal leukoplakia	Leukoplakia (homogeneous) Lichen planus/lichenoid lesions
Uncommon entities		Actinic cheilitis Submucous fibrosis	Discoid lupus erythematosus
Rare entities	Dyskeratosis congenita*	Fanconi anaemia*	

*Malignant potential unclear but involves OSCC (mainly tongue) and other neoplasms, especially acute myeloid leukaemia.

ST predisposes to OSCC and the products include paan, chaalia, gutka and naswar, and are used in all sections of South Asian society. In India, different forms of chewing tobacco are used such as betel (**Table 25.3**), khaini, pattiwala tobacco, maiwpuri tobacco, zarda, kiwam and gadakhu. Tobacco-chewing, along with a variety of ingredients in a 'betel quid' (betel vine leaf, betel (areca) nut, catechu, and slaked lime, often together with tobacco) appears to predispose to OSCC, particularly when started early in life and used frequently and for prolonged periods (see below). It is common in peoples from parts of Asia.

- Many migrants to the West and other countries also continue to use ST products even several decades after migration. Asian ethnic migrants to the UK have a significantly higher incidence of oral cancer compared with the native UK populations presumably related to ST use. Bangladeshis in particular are likely to retain the habit of betel use.

The combined effect of alcohol and tobacco is far greater than the sum of the two effects and is multiplicative.

RISK FACTORS: ALCOHOL

Increased consumption of any alcohol-containing beverages is associated with a risk of PMD and OSCC. The risk is greatest among the heaviest drinkers of alcohol (ethanol). The type of alcoholic beverage also appears to influence the risk – spirits confer higher risks than wine or beer. Ecological studies suggest that the impact of alcohol on oral cancer deaths has increased in recent years. Alcoholic beverages may contain carcinogens or procarcinogens, including ethanol; this is

Table 25.3 Main forms of smokeless tobacco use

Name	Constituents	Used mainly in populations from
Betel (paan)	3 basic types: Areca nut no tobacco e.g. sweet pan (Gutkha; or Gutaka) Tobacco no areca nut Areca nut plus tobacco products	South Asia, Papua New Guinea
Chewing tobacco	Tobacco	Western Europe, North America
Gudakhu	Tobacco, molasses, other ingredients	Southeast Asia
Khaini	Tobacco powdered mixed with slake lime paste, sometimes used with areca nut; placed inside the mouth	Southeast Asia
Kiwam	Tobacco leaf, boiled in rose water and spices added	Southeast Asia
Maiwpuri	Tobacco, slaked lime, areca nut and spices	Southeast Asia
Mishri	Tobacco dark roasted powdered, used as tooth cleaning agents	Southeast Asia
Nass	Tobacco, cotton ash or sesame oil, lime and gum	Iran, Central Asia, Afghanistan and Pakistan
Naswar	Tobacco powdered, slaked lime and indigo	Afghanistan, Pakistan
Pattiwala	Tobacco leaf, with or without lime	South Asia
Shammah	Tobacco leaf powdered, ash, lime	Saudi Arabia
Toombak	Tobacco and sodium bicarbonate	Sudan
Zarda	Tobacco leaf boiled with spices and lime	India and Middle East

metabolized by alcohol dehydrogenase (ADH) and to some extent by cytochrome p450 (CYP) to acetaldehyde, which may be carcinogenic. Acetaldehyde is degraded by aldehyde dehydrogenses (ALDH) to acetic acid. Genetic variations in the activities of ADH and ALDH (and other enzymes) may influence the outcome of exposure to alcohol, and thus its carcinogenicity in any individual. Many alcoholic drinks also contain congeners and some local brews may contain carcinogens such as nitrosamines or urethane contaminants. For example, in parts of France, such as Brittany, there is a close relationship between consumption of Calvados, a pot-stilled spirit, and cancer of the mouth and oesophagus. Furthermore, alcohol users are also predisposed to a number of other cancers and potentially malignant conditions, and other systemic and oral health issues.

The risk of OSCC decreases after stopping alcohol use but the effects appear to persist for several years.

The carcinogenic potential of proprietary alcohol-containing mouthwashes remains controversial.

RISK FACTORS: CHEWING HABITS

Betel quid is widely used across the world, in south Asian communities particularly, though contents vary in different parts of the world and cultures. The betel quid contents are betel leaf, tobacco, areca nut, spices, and sometimes slaked lime. A large variety of additives may be incorporated. Betel (paan; the leaf, stem or inflorescence of *Piper betel*) leaves are from the betel vine, a relative of the pepper family. The leaf contains allylbenzene compounds such as chavibetol, chavicol, estragole, eugenol and methyl eugenol. Areca nut, sometimes referred to as betel nut (although it is from a different plant than the betel leaf) is the seed of *Areca catechu* – the areca palm. Betel quid can be made up at home or purchased as ready to chew.

The betel quid is placed in the mouth, usually the cheek, and gently chewed and sucked sometimes for hours. Betel use not only causes discolouration of the oral mucosa and teeth, but can also predispose to PMD such as submucous fibrosis, erythroplakia and leukoplakia, and also to OSCC. CYP genes may play a role in betel-induced OSCC.

Furthermore, betel users are also predisposed to a number of other cancers and potentially malignant conditions (oesophageal, pancreatic and hepatocellular cancer), and other systemic health issues, including;

- Cancers:
  - oral
  - oesophageal
  - pancreatic
  - hepatocellular.

- Other conditions:
  - hypertension
  - metabolic syndrome
  - adverse birth outcomes
  - liver cirrhosis
  - chronic kidney disease
  - contact dermatitis
  - periodontitis.

Other chewing habits, usually involving tobacco and stimulants, are used in different cultures (e.g. Qat (Khat), Shammah, Toombak).

RISK FACTORS: SUNLIGHT AND TANNING BEDS

Actinic radiation may predispose to lip cancer. Facts that support such a relationship include:

- lip cancer involves the more exposed lower lip, rather than the upper lip
- there is a higher incidence of lip cancer in outdoor workers and rural populations than in office workers or urban populations
- fair-skinned people in sunny climates tend to develop lip cancer more than dark-skinned people (as well as skin cancer and melanoma).

Sunlight contains:

- visible light
- infrared radiation
- ultraviolet (UV) radiation.

It is the ultraviolet (UV) radiation that can cause harmful effects to the skin and lip. There are three basic types of UV:

- UVA (long-wave UV)
- UVB (sunburn UV)
- UVC (short-wave UV).

The effects of UV are shown in **Table 25.4**; UVB appears to be most carcinogenic. Tanning beds typically emit about 97% UVA and 3% UVB, and there is no available reliable evidence that these cause oral or lip cancer.

RISK FACTORS: OTHERS

The carcinogenicity of other psychotropic products such as marijuana remains controversial.

Immune defects may predispose to OSCC, especially lip cancer. This is increased in, for example, immunosuppressed renal transplant recipients – possibly due to human papillomavirus (HPV) infection and patients with chronic mucocutaneous candidosis.

Table 25.4 Types of ultraviolet radiation

UV type	Filtered out in atmosphere by ozone layer	Effects on skin	Other features
UVA	No	Some tan and harmful long-term	Passes through glass: levels relatively constant through the day
UVB	Partially	Burns, tans, wrinkling, aging and cancer	Some does not pass through glass: highest intensity at noon
UVC	Yes	Burns and cancer	Major artificial sources are germicidal lamps

HPV is increasingly linked to the rise in oropharyngeal cancer in young people.

Diet

Charcoal-grilled red meat and fried foods have been implicated as risk factors. An increased consumption of fruits and vegetables is associated with lower risk of oral cancer.

NATURAL HISTORY AND MALIGNANT TRANSFORMATION

The natural history of PMDs is not absolutely clear but cessation of smoking habits appears to result in some lesions regressing or resolving. The risk of malignant development does not seem to be predictable but is greatest in:

- older patients
- females
- never-users of tobacco
- non-homogenous PMD
- PMD on the lateral and ventral tongue, floor of mouth and retromolar/soft palate complex
- large lesions covering several intraoral subsites
- PMD of long duration.

Factors predictive of future malignant transformation may also include:

- epithelial dysplasia
- history of cancer in the upper aerodigestive tract
- expression of P53 tumour suppressor protein
- changes involving chromosomes 3p or 9p; these are termed ' loss of heterozygosity,' or LOH
- chromosomal polysomy.

Epithelial dysplasia (from Greek dys = poor and plasia = a moulding) is a term describing the combination of disorderly maturation and disturbed cell proliferation (**Box 25.1**) seen in OSCC and some PMD.

Although not all clinically PMD show dysplasia on biopsy examination (**Fig. 25.3**), most do show dysplasia, and this is one of the main histological features that appears to precede the onset of malignancy and it appears to be the most predictive marker for malignant potential in current use. Cellular atypia is the main feature of dysplasia.

Dysplasia is in general, graded as:

- Mild dysplasia: atypical and immature basal cells extend above the basal layers into the lower third of the epithelium.

- Moderate dysplasia: atypical and immature basal cells extend above the basal layers into the middle third of the epithelium.
- Severe dysplasia: atypical and immature basal cells extend throughout the epithelium.
- Carcinoma: atypical and immature basal cells extend throughout the epithelium together with invasion of the lamina propria.

Dysplasia thus varies in severity from mild to moderate dysplasia – where few of the features of dysplasia are present and the epithelium is reasonably well organized (**Fig. 25.4**), to the more severe grades where epithelial organization is disrupted and many cellular abnormalities present (**Fig. 25.5**), the epithelial basement membrane is not seen to be breached but there is a malignant potential. Dysplasia however, does not always indicate a malignant potential, since it can also be seen in regenerating tissue and some non-precancerous lesions such as some:

- ulcers
- viral infections
- candidal infections
- granular cell tumours.

Nevertheless, many now believe that seeing severe dysplasia is often tantamount to a diagnosis of early carcinoma – since the epithelial basement membrane may well be breached though not detected in the biopsy specimen.

DIAGNOSIS

Most PMD mandate biopsy; the specimen should be taken from the most clinically suspicious area, such as redness, an area of surface thickening or a symptomatic area. To improve the sensitivity and specificity of identification of an area to biopsy, vital tissue staining may be used, with a dye, such as toluidine (tolonium) blue – an acidophilic metachromatic thiazine dye that selectively stains tissue acids, particularly DNA and RNA. Staining is based on the fact that dysplastic cells usually contain more nucleic acid than normal cells. Vital staining is not totally specific or sensitive, but can assist in deciding where to perform a biopsy.

Nevertheless, despite the assistance of vital staining, a negative biopsy cannot reliably exclude the presence of carcinoma or dysplastic foci within a lesion. Biomarkers with potential predictive value and which may prove to be clinically relevant include DNA ploidy, computerized nuclear image analysis and microsatellite instability at chromosomes 3p and 9p.

BOX 25.1 Features of epithelial dysplasia

- Drop-shaped rete processes
- Basal cell hyperplasia
- Irregular epithelial stratification
- Nuclear hyperchromatism
- Increased nuclear-cytoplasmic ratio
- Increased normal and abnormal mitosis
- Enlarged nucleoli
- Individual cell keratinization
- Loss or reduction of cellular cohesion
- Cellular pleomorphism
- Loss of basal cell polarity

TREATMENT (see also Chs 4 and 5)

Management of patients with PMD is a controversial issue (**Algorithm 25.1**), discussed in more depth in relation to the specific entities. A specialist opinion is advised. Fully informed consent is crucial, all the uncertainties being discussed with the patient.

Surgery may have a beneficial effect, but there is no evidence that this will reliably reduce the risk of later recurrence, nor malignant transformation of PMD, at the same or another site.

Medical measures that lessen the size, extent or histopathological features of dysplasia within PMD are associated with a risk of adverse effects, particularly with systemic agents (which themselves may be contra-indicated in some individuals), and relapse or later malignant transformation can still occur.

FOLLOW-UP OF PATIENTS

There is neither evidence base nor absolute consensus as to the optimum review interval or protocol. Since there is no hard evidence as to the ideal frequency of follow-up, it has been suggested that patients with PMD be re-examined by a health professional:

- within 1 month
- at 3 months
- at 6 months
- at 12 months
- annually thereafter.

Any changes in clinical features, especially the appearance of a lump or ulcer, merit a specialist opinion and usually a biopsy.

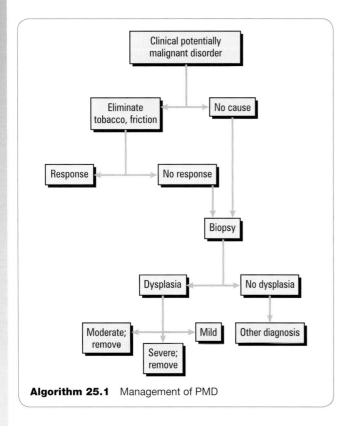

Algorithm 25.1 Management of PMD

PREVENTION AND DETECTION OF POTENTIALLY MALIGNANT DISORDERS AND CANCER

Unfortunately, many of the population – especially those at highest risk, such as older men who smoke and drink – rarely seek regular dental care or examination. In a recent study, risk factors in patients with tongue OSCC were being: age >80, widowed, social marginalized, a current smoker, or a smoker-heavy drinker. Risk factors in people with floor of mouth cancer were being: age >70, and socially marginalized. Having a regular dentist was protective.

Patients thus often present late to physicians and with advanced cancers, and furthermore, physicians and surgeons have often received little or no training in the examination of the mouth.

It should be noted also that clinically differentiating PMD and OSCC from lesions that are benign can be difficult even for highly trained professionals, because these lesions do not always display well-defined clinical features. Not uncommonly, PMD and OSCC are asymptomatic, appear innocuous and can be overlooked.

Clinicians should be aware that single ulcers, lumps, red patches or white patches, particularly if any of these are persisting for >3 weeks, may also be manifestations of frank malignancy: biopsy is invariably indicated. Even common, benign-looking oral lesions attributed to friction or trauma require evaluation when they persist. Despite this fewer than 27% of leukoplakias, a common PMD, are ever subjected to biopsy. As a result, many are left to progress to more advanced stages or cancer.

Late cancer diagnosis results in treatment that is usually more mutilating, with higher morbidity and costs, and a worse prognosis.

USEFUL WEBSITES

Medscape, Premalignant Conditions of the Oral
  Cavity: http://emedicine.medscape.com/
  article/1491418-overview

FURTHER READING

Alexander, R.E., Wright, J.M., Thiebaud, S., 2001.
  Evaluating, documenting and following up oral
  pathological conditions. A suggested protocol. J. Am.
  Dent. Assoc. 132, 329–335.
Chen, P.H., Lee, K.W., Chen, C.H., et al., 2011.
  CYP26B1 is a novel candidate gene for betel
  quid-related oral squamous cell carcinoma.
  Oral. Oncol. 47 (7), 594–600.

Gallagher, R.P., Lee, T.K., 2006. Adverse effects of
  ultraviolet radiation: a brief review. Prog. Biophys.
  Mol. Biol. 92 (1), 119–131.
Gandolfo, S., Pentenero, M., Broccoletti, R., et al.,
  2006. Toluidine blue uptake in potentially
  malignant oral lesions in vivo: clinical
  and histological assessment. Oral. Oncol.
  42, 89–95.

Groome, P.A., Rohland, S.L., Hall, S.F., et al., 2011.
  A population-based study of factors associated with
  early versus late stage oral cavity cancer diagnoses.
  Oral. Oncol. 47 (7), 642–647.
Hashibe, M., Jacob, B.J., Thomas, G., et al., 2003.
  Socioeconomic status, lifestyle factors and
  oral premalignant lesions. Oral. Oncol. 39 (7),
  664–671.

Holmstrup, P., Vedtofte, P., Reibel, J., Stoltze, K., 2006. Long-term treatment outcome of oral premalignant lesions. Oral. Oncol. 42 (5), 461–474.

Holmstrup, P., Vedtofte, P., Reibel, J., Stoltze, K., 2007. Oral premalignant lesions: is a biopsy reliable? J. Oral. Pathol. Med. 36 (5), 262–266.

Hsue, S.S., Wang, W.C., Chen, C.H., et al., 2007. Malignant transformation in 1458 patients with potentially malignant oral mucosal disorders: A follow-up study based in a Taiwanese hospital. J. Oral. Pathol. Med. 36, 25–29.

Jaber, M.A., Porter, S.R., Speight, P., et al., 2003. Oral epithelial dysplasia: clinical characteristics of western European residents. Oral. Oncol. 39, 589–596.

Kim, J., Shin, D.M., El-Naggar, A., et al., 2001. Chromosome polysomy and histological characteristics in oral premalignant lesions. Cancer Epidem. 10, 319–325.

Lippman, S.M., Hong, W.K., 2001. Molecular markers of the risk of oral cancer. N. Engl. J. Med. 344, 1323–1326.

Lodi, G., Porter, S., 2008. Management of potentially malignant disorders: evidence and critique. J. Oral. Pathol. Med. 37 (2), 63–69.

Napier, S.S., Speight, P.M., 2008. Natural history of potentially malignant oral lesions and conditions: an overview of the literature. J. Oral. Pathol. Med. 37 (1), 1–10.

Pentenero, M., Carrozzo, M., Pagano, M., et al., 2003. Oral mucosal dysplastic lesions and early squamous cell carcinomas: underdiagnosis from incisional biopsy. Oral. Dis. 9, 68–72.

Scully, C., Sudbo, J., Speight, P.M., 2003. Progress in determining the malignant potential of oral lesions. J. Oral. Pathol. Med. 32 (5), 251–256.

Thomas, G., Hashibe, M., Jacob, B.J., et al., 2003. Risk factors for multiple oral premalignant lesions. Int. J. Cancer 107 (2), 285–291.

Warnakulasuriya, S., Kovacevic, T., Madden, P., et al., 2011. Factors predicting malignant transformation in oral potentially malignant disorders among patients accrued over a 10-year period in South East England. J. Oral. Pathol. Med. 40, 665–732.

Yen, A.M., Chen, S.L., Chiu, S.Y., Chen, H.H., 2011. Association between metabolic syndrome and oral pre-malignancy: A community- and population-based study (KCIS No. 28). Oral. Oncol. 47 (7), 625–630.

Actinic cheilitis (solar cheilosis)

INTRODUCTION

This chapter should be read along with Ch. 25.

INCIDENCE

Actinic cheilitis (actinic keratosis of lip, solar keratosis, solar cheilosis; from the Greek *aktino* = rays and *cheili* = lips) is common in sun-overexposed individuals, and is essentially a burn. This chapter discusses chronic actinic cheilitis (solar cheilosis) – a potentially malignant disorder (~ 6% risk of squamous carcinoma).

AGE

Occurs mainly in older adults.

GENDER

Most prevalent in men.

GEOGRAPHIC

Mainly seen in persons from the tropics and less in black people.

PREDISPOSING FACTORS

Ultraviolet light from the sun can damage the lips and skin, particularly the vermilion of the lower lip. Commonly seen in Caucasians in the tropics, less in people with coloured skins. Particularly at risk are people whose lifestyles include much time spent outdoors, especially farmers, sailors, fishermen, windsurfers, skiers, mountaineers, golfers, etc.

Other forms of radiation including arc-welding can occasionally cause similar damage. Actinic cheilitis rarely may be an early manifestation of a genetic susceptibility to light damage as in xeroderma pigmentosum or part of the syndrome of actinic prurigo. Immune defects (including immunosuppression in organ transplant recipients) also predispose to malignant transformation.

CLINICAL FEATURES

Actinic cheilitis is most common on the lower lip, with sparing of the oral commissures. In the early, acute stages, the lip may be red and oedematous, but after months or years (chronic cheilitis) may become dry and scaly and wrinkled with grey to white

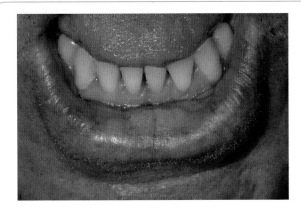

Fig. 26.1 Chronic actinic chelitis (solar cheilosis).

changes. Lesions may appear as a smooth or scaly, friable patch or can involve the entire lip later, becoming palpably thickened with small greyish white plaques (**Fig. 26.1**). Eventually, warty nodules may form, which may evolve into OSCC.

DIAGNOSIS

A careful history and a biopsy are indicated (**Table 26.1**). Lupus erythematosus and lichen planus must also be considered in the differential diagnosis.

TREATMENT (see also Chs 4 and 5)

Prevention is advised, especially in high-risk individuals (patients with photosensitivity disorders, xeroderma pigmentosum, transplant recipients), and those whose exposure to UVB is high by wearing broad-brimmed hats, and using adequate UV-protective sunscreens and avoiding mid-day sun exposure.

Table 26.1 Aids that might be helpful in diagnosis/prognosis/management in some patients suspected of having solar cheilosis*

In most cases	In some cases
Biopsy	Dermatological opinion

*See text for details and glossary for abbreviations.

Management of established solar cheilosis is required both to relieve symptoms and to endeavour to prevent development of OSCC. This is best achieved by the removal of the premalignant epithelium by topical chemoexfoliants (e.g. trichloroacetic acid, 5-fluorouracil, bleomycin, 3% diclofenac in 2.5% hyaluronic acid gel, 5% imiquimod), or by photodynamic therapy, or laser or scalpel surgery (**Table 26.2**).

Trichloroacetic acid application is easy and convenient, but the least efficacious treatment. Vermilionectomy using the W-plasty technique appears to give the best cosmetic results and remains the gold standard.

EMERGENT TREATMENTS

Toll-like receptor 9 agonists (synthetic oligodeoxynucleotides containing immune stimulatory 'CpG motifs' which induce activation and maturation of plasmacytoid dendritic cells and enhance differentiation of B cells into antibody-secreting plasma cells), and ingenol mebutate (the active ingredient from the plant *Euphorbia peplus*) may have a therapeutic role in the future.

FOLLOW-UP OF PATIENTS

Solar cheilosis carries a potential for malignant development, necessitating regular monitoring, perhaps every six months, which can be carried out by the general practitioner. If there is any change causing concern, particularly the development of a lump, a specialist opinion should best be obtained.

Table 26.2 Regimens that might be helpful in management of patient suspected of having solar cheilosis

Regimen	Use in primary care	Use in secondary care
Likely to be beneficial	Topical chemoexfoliants (e.g. trichloroacetic acid or diclofenac 3% gel)	Topical chemoexfoliants (trichloroacetic acid, diclofenac, 5 fluorouracil, bleomycin or tretinoin) Photodynamic therapy (PDT) Surgery: cryosurgery, laser or surgical excision with advancement of a mucosal flap (vermilionectomy; lip shave), electrodesiccation, curettage, carbon dioxide laser vaporization
Unproven effectiveness		Imiquimod 5% cream
Emergent treatments		Ingenol mebutate Toll 9 receptor agonists
Supportive	Sunscreens	Sunscreens

USEFUL WEBSITES

Dermnet, N.Z., Solar cheilitis. http://dermnetnz.org/site-age-specific/solar-cheilitis.html

Wikipedia, Actinic cheilitis. http://en.wikipedia.org/wiki/Actinic_cheilitis

FURTHER READING

Armenores, P., James, C.L., Walker, P.C., Huilgol, S.C., 2010. Treatment of actinic cheilitis with the Er:YAG laser. J. Am. Acad. Dermatol. 63 (4), 642–646.

Castiñeiras, I., Del Pozo, J., Mazaira, M., et al., 2010. Actinic cheilitis: evolution to squamous cell carcinoma after carbon dioxide laser vaporization. A study of 43 cases. J. Dermatolog. Treat 21 (1), 49–53.

Cavalcante, A.S., Anbinder, A.L., Carvalho, Y.R., 2008. Actinic cheilitis: clinical and histological features. J. Oral. Maxillofac. Surg. 66 (3), 498–503.

Grossberg, A.L., Gaspari, A.A., 2011. Topical antineoplastic agents in the treatment of mucocutaneous diseases. Curr. Probl. Dermatol. 40, 71–82.

Güleç, A.T., Haberal, M., 2010. Lip and oral mucosal lesions in 100 renal transplant recipients. J. Am. Acad. Dermatol. 62 (1), 96–101.

Huber, M.A., 2010. White oral lesions, actinic cheilitis, and leukoplakia: confusions in terminology and definition: facts and controversies. Clin. Dermatol. 28 (3), 262–268.

Junqueira, J.L., Bönecker, M., Furuse, C., 2011. Actinic cheilitis among agricultural workers in Campinas, Brazil. Community Dent. Health 28 (1), 60–63.

Kodama, M., Watanabe, D., Akita, Y., et al., 2007. Photodynamic therapy for the treatment of actinic cheilitis. Photodermatol. Photoimmunol. Photomed. 23 (5), 209–210.

Lima Gda, S., Silva, G.F., Gomes, A.P., 2010. Diclofenac in hyaluronic acid gel: an alternative treatment for actinic cheilitis. J. Appl. Oral. Sci. 18 (5), 533–537.

McDonald, C., Laverick, S., Fleming, C.J., White, S.J., 2010. Treatment of actinic cheilitis with imiquimod 5% and a retractor on the lower lip: clinical and histological outcomes in 5 patients. Br. J. Oral. Maxillofac. Surg. 48 (6), 473–476.

Markopoulos, A., Albanidou-Farmaki, E., Kayavis, I., 2004. Actinic cheilitis: clinical and pathologic characteristics in 65 cases. Oral. Dis. 10 (4), 212–216.

Rossi, R., Assad, G.B., Buggiani, G., Lotti, T., 2008. Photodynamic therapy: treatment of choice for actinic cheilitis? Dermatol. Ther. 21 (5), 412–415.

Rossoe, E.W., Tebcherani, A.J., Sittart, J.A., Pires, M.C., 2011. Actinic cheilitis: aesthetic and functional comparative evaluation of vermilionectomy using the classic and W-plasty techniques. An. Bras. Dermatol. 86 (1), 65–73.

Sand, M., Altmeyer, P., Bechara, F.G., 2010. Mucosal advancement flap versus primary closure after vermilionectomy of the lower lip. Dermatol. Surg. 36 (12), 1987–1992.

Savage, N.W., McKay, C., Faulkner, C., 2010. Actinic cheilitis in dental practice. Aust. Dent. J. 55 (Suppl. 1), 78–84.

Shah, A.Y., Doherty, S.D., Rosen, T., 2010. Actinic cheilitis: a treatment review. Int. J. Dermatol. 49 (11), 1225–1234.

Siller, G., Gebauer, K., Welburn, P., et al., 2009. PEP005 (ingenol mebutate) gel, a novel agent for the treatment of actinic keratosis: results of a randomized, double-blind, vehicle-controlled, multicentre, phase IIa study. Australas. J. Dermatol. 50 (1), 16–22.

Smith, K.J., Germain, M., Yeager, J., Skelton, H., 2002. Topical 5% imiquimod for the therapy of actinic cheilitis. J. Am. Acad. Dermatol. 47 (4), 497–501.

Sotiriou, E., Apalla, Z., Chovarda, E., et al., 2010. Photodynamic therapy with 5-aminolevulinic acid in actinic cheilitis: an 18-month clinical and histological follow-up. J. Eur. Acad. Dermatol. Venereol. 24 (8), 916–920.

Sotiriou, E., Apalla, Z., Koussidou-Erremonti, T., Ioannides, D., 2008. Actinic cheilitis treated with one cycle of 5-aminolaevulinic acid-based photodynamic therapy: report of 10 cases. Br. J. Dermatol. 159 (1), 261–262.

Ulrich, C., Forschner, T., Ulrich, M., 2007. Management of actinic cheilitis using diclofenac 3% gel: a report of six cases. Br. J. Dermatol. 156 (Suppl. 3), 43–46.

Ulrich, M., González, S., Lange-Asschenfeldt, B., et al., 2011. Non-invasive diagnosis and monitoring of actinic cheilitis with reflectance confocal microscopy. J. Eur. Acad. Dermatol. Venereol. 25 (3), 276–284.

27 Erythroplakia (erythroplasia)

INTRODUCTION

This chapter should be read along with Ch. 25.

Erythroplakia (from the Greek *erythros* = red and *plakia* = patch) is defined by the World Health Organization as 'any lesion of the oral mucosa that presents as bright red velvety plaques which cannot be characterized clinically or pathologically as any other recognizable condition'. Erythroplastic lesions are well-defined velvety red plaques and are the oral lesions with the most severe dysplasia and greatest predilection to develop to carcinoma: at least 80% are severely dysplastic or frankly malignant.

INCIDENCE

Rare: mainly seen in older men. Erythroplakia is much less common than leukoplakia.

AGE

Occurs in the middle aged and the older patient.

GENDER

Occurs mostly in men.

GEOGRAPHIC

There is no known geographic incidence.

AETIOLOGY AND PATHOGENESIS

Unknown, but tobacco and alcohol or betel use may be involved (Ch. 25).

CLINICAL FEATURES

Red velvety patch of variable configuration, usually level with or depressed below surrounding mucosa, commonly seen on:

- soft palate
- floor of mouth
- buccal mucosa (**Fig. 27.1**).

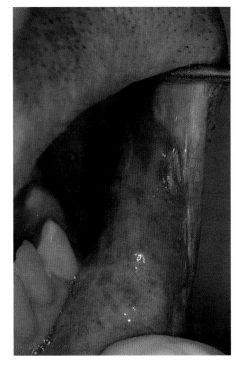

Fig. 27.1 Erythroplakia: usually a potentially malignant lesion. Carcinoma developed in this patient, who actually had long-standing lichen planus with lichenoid dysplasia

Some erythroplakias are associated with white patches, and are then termed speckled leukoplakia or erythroleukoplakia (**Table 27.1**).

DIAGNOSIS

A biopsy should be done to examine for epithelial dysplasia and carcinoma. The lesion should be differentiated from inflammatory and atrophic lesions (e.g. in deficiency anaemias, geographic tongue, lichen planus).

TREATMENT (see also Chs 4 and 5)

Patient information is an important aspect in management. Any causal factor, such as tobacco use should be stopped and the lesions removed (**Table 27.1**).

Table 27.1 Regimens that might be helpful in managementof patient suspected of having erythroplakia

Regimen	Use in secondary care (severe oral involvement and/or extraoral involvement)
Likely to be beneficial	Excision
Unproven effectiveness	Photodynamic therapy Chemotherapy
Supportive	Cease tobacco, alcohol or betel use

FOLLOW-UP OF PATIENTS

Erythroplakia or erythroleukoplakia carries a very high potential for malignant development, necessitating regular monitoring, which is best carried out by the specialist. If there is any change causing concern, particularly the development of a lump, a further biopsy should best be obtained.

There is no hard evidence as to the ideal frequency of follow-up, but it has been suggested that patients with such mucosal potentially malignant lesions be re-examined:

- within 1 month
- at 3 months
- at 6 months
- at 12 months
- annually thereafter.

USEFUL WEBSITES

Maxillofacial Center, Erythroplakia of the Head & Neck. http://www.maxillofacialcenter.com/BondBook/mucosa/erythroplakia.htm

Wikipedia, Erythroplakia. http://en.wikipedia.org/wiki/Erythroplakia

FURTHER READING

Alexander, R.E., Wright, J.M., Thiebaud, S., 2001. Evaluating, documenting and following up oral pathological conditions. A suggested protocol. J. Am. Dent. Assoc 132, 329–335.

Arduino, P.G., Surace, A., Carbone, M., et al., 2009. Outcome of oral dysplasia: a retrospective hospital-based study of 207 patients with a long follow-up. J. Oral. Pathol. Med. 38 (6), 540–544.

Awan, K.H., Morgan, P.R., Warnakulasuriya, S., 2011. Utility of chemiluminescence (ViziLite™) in the detection of oral potentially malignant disorders and benign keratoses. J. Oral. Pathol. Med. 40 (7), 541–544.

Brennan, M., Migliorati, C.A., Lockhart, P.B., Wray, D., 2007. Management of oral epithelial dysplasia: a review. Oral. Surg. Oral. Med. Oral. Pathol. Oral. Radiol. Endod 103, S19.e1–S19.e12.

Cantarelli Morosolli, A.R., Schubert, M.M., Niccoli-Filho, W., 2006. Surgical treatment of erythroleukoplakia in lower lip with carbon dioxide laser radiation. Lasers Med. Sci. 21 (3), 181–184.

Epstein, J.B., Gorsky, M., Fischer, D., et al., 2007. A survey of the current approaches to diagnosis and management of oral premalignant lesions. J. Am. Dent. Assoc 138 (12), 1555–1562; quiz 1614.

Eversole, L.R., 2009. Dysplasia of the upper aerodigestive tract squamous epithelium. Head Neck Pathol. 3 (1), 63–68.

Hosni, E.S., Salum, F.G., Cherubini, K., et al., 2009. Oral erythroplakia and speckled leukoplakia: retrospective analysis of 13 cases. Braz. J. Otorhinolaryngol. 75 (2), 295–299.

Lin, H.P., Chen, H.M., Yu, C.H., et al., 2010. Topical photodynamic therapy is very effective for oral verrucous hyperplasia and oral erythroleukoplakia. J. Oral. Pathol. Med. 39 (8), 624–630.

O'Sullivan, E.M., 2011. Prevalence of oral mucosal abnormalities in addiction treatment centre residents in Southern Ireland. Oral. Oncol. 47 (5), 395–399.

Pentenero, M., Carrozzo, M., Pagano, M., et al., 2003. Oral mucosal dysplastic lesions and early squamous cell carcinomas: underdiagnosis from incisional biopsy. Oral. Dis. 9, 68–72.

Pentenero, M., Giaretti, W., Navone, R., et al., 2011. Evidence for a possible anatomical subsite-mediated effect of tobacco in oral potentially malignant disorders and carcinoma. J. Oral. Pathol. Med. 40 (3), 214–217.

Pitiyage, G., Tilakaratne, W.M., Tavassoli, M., Warnakulasuriya, S., 2009. Molecular markers in oral epithelial dysplasia: review. J. Oral. Pathol. Med. 38 (10), 737–752.

Reichart, P.A., Philipsen, H.P., 2005. Oral erythroplakia – a review. Oral. Oncol. 41 (6), 551–561.

Scully, C., Sudbo, J., Speight, P.M., 2003. Progress in determining the malignant potential of oral lesions. J. Oral. Pathol. Med. 32 (5), 251–256.

Tan, N.C., Mellor, T., Brennan, P.A., Puxeddu, R., 2010. Use of narrow band imaging guidance in the management of oral erythroplakia. Br. J. Oral. Maxillofac. Surg. 49 (6), 488–490.

Thomas, G., Hashibe, M., Jacob, B.J., et al., 2003. Risk factors for multiple oral premalignant lesions. Int. J. Cancer 107 (2), 285–291.

Tilakaratne, W.M., Sherriff, M., Morgan, P.R., Odell, E.W., 2011. Grading oral epithelial dysplasia: analysis of individual features. J. Oral. Pathol. Med. 40 (7), 533–540.

van der Waal, I., 2009. Potentially malignant disorders of the oral and oropharyngeal mucosa; terminology, classification and present concepts of management. Oral. Oncol. 45 (4–5), 317–323.

van der Waal, I., 2010. Potentially malignant disorders of the oral and oropharyngeal mucosa; present concepts of management. Oral. Oncol. 46 (6), 423–425.

van der Waal, I., Scully, C., 2011. Oral cancer: comprehending the condition, causes, controversies, control and consequences. 4. Potentially malignant disorders of the oral and oropharyngeal mucosa. Dent. Update 38 (2), 138–140.

Vladimirov, B.S., Schiodt, M., 2009. The effect of quitting smoking on the risk of unfavorable events after surgical treatment of oral potentially malignant lesions. Int. J. Oral. Maxillofac. Surg. 38 (11), 1188–1193.

Warnakulasuriya, S., Johnson, N.W., van der Waal, I., 2007. Nomenclature and classification of potentially malignant disorders of the oral mucosa. J. Oral. Pathol. Med. 36 (10), 575–580.

Warnakulasuriya, S., Reibel, J., Bouquot, J., Dabelsteen, E., 2008. Oral epithelial dysplasia classification systems: predictive value, utility, weaknesses and scope for improvement. J. Oral. Pathol. Med. 37 (3), 127–133.

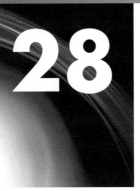

28 Leukoplakia

INTRODUCTION

This chapter should be read along with Ch. 25.

Many white lesions were formerly known as 'leukoplakia' (from the Greek *leukos* = white and *plakia* = patch), a term causing misunderstanding and confusion.

Leukoplakia was then defined by the World Health Organization as 'clinical white patches that cannot be wiped off the mucosa and cannot be classified clinically or microscopically as another specific disease entity (such as lichen planus)'. A subsequent International Seminar defined leukoplakia more precisely as 'a whitish patch or plaque that cannot be characterized clinically or pathologically as any other disease and which is not associated with any physical or chemical causative agent except the use of tobacco'. Leukoplakias are 'white plaques of questionable risk having excluded (other) known diseases or disorders that carry no increased risk for cancer'.

Leukoplakia is, thus, a clinical diagnosis only, can only be made by exclusion, can be precancerous or a marker for cancer elsewhere in the upper aerodigestive tract, or is sometimes totally benign.

Frictional keratosis and specific tobacco-induced lesions, such as smoker's keratosis, are now termed 'keratoses' (*not* 'leukoplakias') and are not considered as PMDs.

INCIDENCE

Occurs in about 0.1% of the population.

AGE

Occurs predominantly in the middle-aged and older patient.

GENDER

Occurs more in men than women.

GEOGRAPHIC

It has no known special geographic incidence.

AETIOLOGY AND PATHOGENESIS

Predisposing factors include habits such as (Ch. 25):

- tobacco use
- alcohol use
- betel use
- sanguinarine (pseudochelerythrine) use. This is a quaternary benzophenanthridine alkaloid extracted from some plants, including Bloodroot (*Sanguinaria canadensis*), Mexican Prickly Poppy (*Argemone mexicana*), *Chelidonium majus*, and *Macleaya cordata* and is used in some oral health-care products. Sanguinarine is a potent suppressor of NF-β activation and induces a rapid apoptotic response by glutathione-depletion.

Leukoplakias show, to a varying degree, three main microscopic features:

- Increased keratin production: increased keratin produces the white clinical appearance of keratoses. If nuclei persist into the superficial cell layers the term 'hyperparakeratosis' is used, whereas if there is excessive mature keratin, with a prominent granular cell layer, the term 'hyperorthokeratosis' is applied. Any leukoplakia can show either or both types of change, neither of which are an index of premalignancy.
- Change in epithelial thickness: thinning (hypoplasia) or thickening (hyperplasia) may be present and, although neither are indices of premalignancy, malignant change is more likely in a hypoplastic epithelium.
- Disordered epithelial maturation: although clinical features, such as the admixture of red lesions, may suggest the degree of malignant potential of a lesion, histological assessment of the degree of disordered proliferation, maturation and organization of the epithelium (i.e. the degree of dysplasia) continues to provide the best guide.

Leukoplakias, even when clinically homogeneous may be histologically inhomogeneous and may contains areas of dysplasia, and some studies have even shown carcinoma *in situ*, or invasive carcinoma in up to 5–10% of leukoplakias *that on biopsy had shown little or no dysplasia.*

CLINICAL FEATURES

Leukoplakias vary in size: some are small and focal, others more widespread – occasionally involving very large areas of the oral mucosa – and in other patients several discrete separate areas of leukoplakia can be seen. Leukoplakia has a wide range of clinical presentations, from homogeneous white plaques, which can be faintly white or very thick and opaque, to nodular white lesions, or lesions admixed with red lesions (see **Box 28.1**).

It is clear that only a minority of leukoplakias are premalignant, but the problem is to identify those which are.

Leukoplakia: homogeneous
- Flat
- Corrugated
- Pumice-like
- Wrinkled

Leukoplakia: non-homogeneous
- Verrucous
- Proliferative and verrucous
- Nodular
- Erythroleukoplakia (speckled)

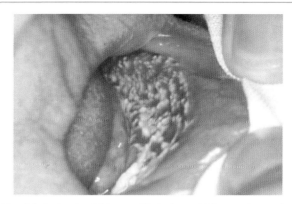

Fig. 28.3 Leukoplakia: speckled – has a high prevalence of malignant change

MALIGNANT POTENTIAL

The malignant potential of leukoplakia overall is in the region of 3% over 10 years but in some can be as high as 30%. The malignant potential can be estimated from the clinical appearance, site, histology and some aetiological factors.

Appearance

- Homogeneous leukoplakias: the most common type, are uniformly white plaques – common in the buccal (cheek) mucosa and usually of *low* malignant potential (**Fig. 28.1**). Sometimes lesions are widespread, suggesting there are widespread molecular changes in the mucosa (**Fig. 28.2**).

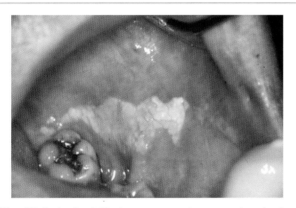

Fig. 28.1 Leukoplakia: homogeneous type – most are benign

- Non-homogeneous or heterogeneous leukoplakias: nodular, verrucous and speckled leukoplakias, which consist of white patches or nodules in a red, often eroded, area of mucosa (**Fig. 28.3**) have a *high* risk of malignant transformation and, therefore, are far more serious.

Site

High-risk sites for malignant transformation include the soft palate complex and possibly the ventrolateral tongue and floor of the mouth (where sublingual leukoplakia has been suggested to have a particularly high risk of malignant change but this is controversial). Sublingual leukoplakia (**Fig. 28.4**) is more common in women than men, and has a typical 'ebbing-tide' appearance clinically.

Histology

It is generally accepted that dysplasia may precede malignant change – the connotation of severe dysplasia being that malignant change is likely (Ch. 25). DNA ploidy studies may become useful in this respect. Histopathology and the detection of dysplasia alone clearly cannot always reliably identify early malignant changes, since it:

- is subjective; there is wide inter-examiner variability
- is subject to considerable intra-examiner variability; studies have shown pathologists to disagree with their previous diagnosis in up to 50% of cases

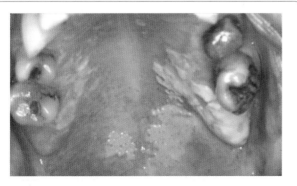

Fig. 28.2 Leukoplakia: proliferative verrucous leukoplakia with widespread field change over, at least, the palate

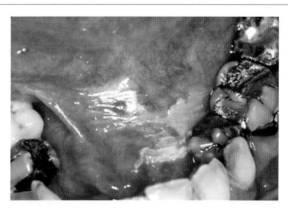

Fig. 28.4 Leukoplakia: floor of mouth or sublingual type

- samples are representative of only a small area and, thus, absence of dysplasia in a biopsy specimen does not necessarily mean that the whole lesion lacks dysplasia.

Aetiological factors

- Proliferative verrucous leukoplakia is a diffuse white and/or papillary lesion seen in older patients, often associated with human papilloma viruses, which has an inexorably slow progression over one or two decades, to verrucous or squamous cell carcinoma.
- Candidal leukoplakias may be associated with an increased risk of malignant change (Ch. 39). *C. albicans* can cause or colonize other keratoses, particularly in smokers, and is especially likely to form speckled leukoplakias at commissures. They may be dysplastic and have higher malignant potential than some other keratoses. Candidal leukoplakias may respond to antifungals and stopping smoking.
- Syphilitic leukoplakia, especially of the dorsum of the tongue, is a feature of tertiary syphilis rarely seen now, but the malignant potential is high.
- Hairy leukoplakia is caused by Epstein–Barr virus (EBV). It usually has a corrugated surface and affects margins of the tongue almost exclusively. It is seen in the immunocompromised and is a complication of HIV infection. It is seen in all groups at risk of HIV infection. The condition appears to be benign and self-limiting.

DIAGNOSIS

There are no clinical signs or symptoms that reliably predict whether a leukoplakia will undergo malignant change (**Algorithm 28.1**). The prevalence of malignant transformation in leukoplakias ranges from 3–30% over 10 years and is highest in lesions with severe dysplasia. Biopsy is, therefore, generally indicated, and is mandatory for leukoplakias that are:

- in patients with previous or concurrent head and neck cancer
- non-homogeneous, i.e. have red areas, are verrucous or are indurated
- in a high-risk site such as the floor of the mouth or the tongue
- focal
- with symptoms
- without obvious aetiological factors.

Biopsy is not always completely diagnostic, partly because dysplastic changes are not always demonstrable in the specimen obtained and there may be skip areas within dysplastic epithelium characterized by normal or hyperplastic epithelium. Serial sectioning of removed leukoplakic lesions may reveal a wide range of grades of dysplasia in different parts of a lesion and previously unsuspected carcinoma in up to 5–10%.

Overall:

- 2–5% of all leukoplakias become malignant in 10 years
- 5–20% of leukoplakias are dysplastic
- 10–35% of leukoplakias showing dysplasia proceed to carcinoma in 10 years.

Since it is not at present possible to reliably predict which leukoplakias will progress to carcinoma, much effort has gone into identifying the genetic and other changes that underlie progression to OSCC, and currently, the most predictive markers of transformation are leukoplakias that are:

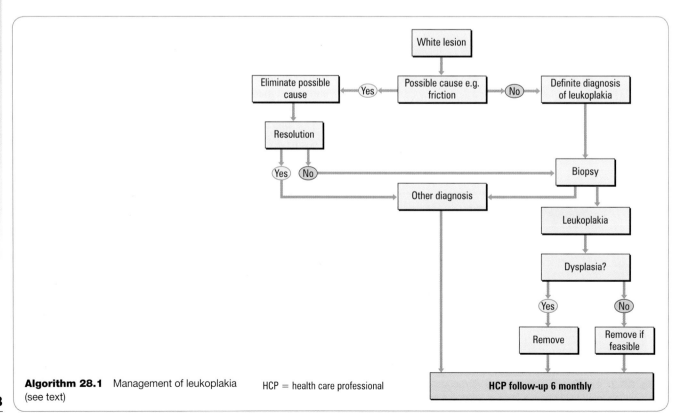

Algorithm 28.1 Management of leukoplakia (see text)   HCP = health care professional

Table 28.1 Aids that might be helpful in diagnosis/prognosis/management in some patients suspected of having leukoplakia*

In most cases	In some cases
Biopsy	Full blood picture
	Serum ferritin, vitamin B_{12} and corrected whole blood folate levels
	ESR
	Serology (syphilis)
	Renal function tests

*See text for details and glossary for abbreviations.

- speckled (erythroleukoplakia)
- verrucous
- from high-risk sites, including the soft palate/fauces and possibly floor of the mouth/ventrum of the tongue
- in a patient with previous cancer in the upper aerodigestive tract
- in non-smoking female
- dysplastic
- DNA polysomic (aneuploidy or tetraploidy)
- positive for genetic markers such as mutated tumour suppressor factor p53, or loss of heterozygosity on chromosomes 3p or 9p.

Occasionally in a patient with leukoplakia, other investigations are also indicated (**Table 28.1**).

TREATMENT (see also Chs 4 and 5)

Leukoplakia may be potentially malignant (or in a small number may already be carcinomatous) and, thus, both behaviour (lifestyle) modification to eliminate risk factors, and active treatment of the lesion are indicated (**Table 28.2**):

- Patient information is an important aspect in management.
- Removal of known risk factors (tobacco, alcohol, betel and trauma) is a mandatory step. Up to 45% of leukoplakias may regress or totally disappear if tobacco use is stopped. Leukoplakias induced by smokeless tobacco may resolve if the habit is stopped. Success is difficult to achieve,

Table 28.2 Regimens that might be helpful in management of patient suspected of having leukoplakia

Regimen	Use in secondary care
Likely to be beneficial	Excise
Unproven effectiveness	Photodynamic therapy
	Retinoids
	Vitamins A, C, and E
	Carotenes
	Lycopene
	Attenuated adenovirus
	Radiotherapy
	Chemotherapy
Supportive	Cease tobacco, betel or alcohol use

however: in one series of 145 patients operated on for oral leukoplakias, only 20 gave up smoking and only five stopped drinking alcohol. Many patients with leukoplakias belong to resource-poor groups and do not always accept or understand the need to stop the habit or to re-attend.

- The former practice of 'watchful waiting' and excision only when signs of cancerization arise appears unacceptable since even leukoplakias that show only dysplasia on prior biopsy if excised may still contain carcinomatous foci. Even when surgical specimens of excised leukoplakias showed no dysplasia but only orthokeratosis, or parakeratosis with epithelial hyperplasia and minimal inflammation, in some 5% of such patients there were OSCC.
- Thus, a reasonable initial approach to the management of leukoplakias is the removal of aetiological factors coupled with simultaneous antifungal therapy. If this does not produce good results within 3 weeks, surgical excision and histopathological examination of the whole specimen seems to be the most rational next step (**Table 28.3**) (despite there being no evidence that this will reliably prevent recurrence or even progression to carcinoma).

SURGERY

Surgery is the obvious option for the management of leukoplakia, certainly for patients with high predisposition to malignant transformation. Resection with a scalpel or CO_2 laser is probably the most effective and safe means of removing pathologic tissue since – unlike the case with cryosurgery, coagulation or laser vaporization – a specimen for pathologic evaluation (of histology and margins) is produced, and the pain and postoperative scarring are less with these techniques than with coagulation. Finally, laser excision (usually with the carbon dioxide laser) seems to have advantage over the use of a scalpel, as intraoperative bleeding and the need for mucosal or dermoepidermal flaps are reduced.

FOLLOW-UP OF PATIENTS

Reported recurrence rates range up to more than 30%, largely depending on the selection of leukoplakias and the duration of the follow-up. Therefore, regular monitoring, perhaps every six months, which can be carried out by the general dental practitioner is indicated for the lower risk lesions. If there is any change causing concern, particularly the development of a lump, a specialist opinion should best be obtained.

Patients should be regularly checked at 3, 6, and 12 months, and then annually for any:

- size change
- appearance of red lesions
- ulceration
- recurrences
- new lesions.

Other leukoplakias are best monitored by the specialist.

MEDICAL THERAPIES

- Since leukoplakias are only potentially malignant, it is generally accepted that radiotherapy or systemic chemotherapy are inappropriate treatments.

Table 28.3 Minimal treatment for leukoplakias

Location	No dysplasia	Mild dysplasia	Moderate or severe dysplasia
Buccal	Watchful waiting	Watchful waiting or remove	Remove
Hard palate	Watchful waiting	Watchful waiting or remove	Remove
Dorsum of tongue	Watchful waiting	Watchful waiting or remove	Remove
Ventrum of tongue/floor of mouth	Watchful waiting	Remove	Remove
Lateral border of tongue	Watchful waiting	Remove	Remove
Fauces	Watchful waiting	Remove	Remove
Vermilion	Watchful waiting	Remove	Remove

- Topical anticancer drugs or retinoids however can induce regression of leukoplakia and are generally well-tolerated and effective, but their efficacy is only temporary, and perhaps their best indication is when the location or extent of the lesion render surgical removal difficult.
- Topical treatment of leukoplakia with podophyllin solution or bleomycin has induced some regression or even total resolution of dysplasia and clinical lesions, and lesions recur more slowly than after surgery.
- Treatment with photodynamic therapy, in which a light-sensitizing dye is given to the patients, and light shone on the lesion to activate the dye and cause necrosis of the pathological tissue, is still in its infancy.

CHEMOPREVENTION

Two different approaches have been proposed for clinical chemoprevention trials:

- Chemoprevention by treatment of leukoplakias to prevent malignant transformation. 13-*cis*-Retinoic acid can result in lesions regressing, but adverse effects are severe and many patients do not complete the planned treatment. Moreover, lesions recur a few months after the end of the intervention.
- Chemoprevention in patients following removal of leukoplakias. Fenretinide used in patients with negative

histology for cancer following laser excision of leukoplakias is well tolerated and preliminary results show a significant protective effect. Unfortunately, the drug is not readily available.

Chemoprevention with retinoids is not a definitive treatment since:

- after the treatment has stopped, lesions recur in a large number of cases
- adverse effects are common and most retinoids are teratogenic.

PATIENT INFORMATION SHEET
Leukoplakia

▼ Please read this information sheet. If you have any questions, particularly about the treatment or potential side-effects, please ask your doctor.
- This is an uncommon condition.
- Sometimes it is caused by friction or tobacco.
- It is not inherited.
- It is not known to be infectious.
- In a very small number, and after years, it may lead to a tumour. You should get yourself checked regularly.
- Blood tests and biopsy may be required.
- There is no universally agreed management and this can be by simple observation, drugs or surgery. You should avoid alcohol or tobacco in future.

USEFUL WEBSITES

MedlinePlus, Oral Cancer. http://www.nlm.nih.gov/
medlineplus/oralcancer.html
http://www.oralcancerfoundation.com/

FURTHER READING

Alexander, R.E., Wright, J.M., Thiebaud, S., 2001. Evaluating, documenting and following up oral pathological conditions. A suggested protocol. J. Am. Dent. Assoc. 132, 329–335.

Arduino, P.G., Surace, A., Carbone, M., et al., 2009. Outcome of oral dysplasia: a retrospective hospital-based study of 207 patients with a long follow-up. J. Oral. Pathol. Med. 38 (6), 540–544.

Awan, K.H., Morgan, P.R., Warnakulasuriya, S., 2011. Utility of chemiluminescence (ViziLite™) in the detection of oral potentially malignant disorders and benign keratoses. J. Oral. Pathol. Med. 40 (7), 541–544.

Bagan, J., Scully, C., Jimenez, Y., Martorell, M., 2010. Proliferative verrucous leukoplakia: a concise update. Oral. Dis. 16, 328–332.

Bagan, J.V., Jimenez, Y., Sanchis, J.M., et al., 2003. Proliferative verrucous leukoplakia; high incidence of gingival squamous cell carcinoma. J. Oral. Pathol. Med. 32, 379–382.

Bagán, J.V., Murillo, J., Poveda, R., et al., 2004. Proliferative verrucous leukoplakia (PVL); unusual locations of oral squamous cell carcinomas (OSCC), and field cancerization as shown by the appearance of multiple OSCCs. Oral. Oncol. 40, 440–443.

Boyle, P., Autier, P., Bartelink, H., et al., 2003. European Code Against Cancer and Scientific Justification: Third Version. Annals Oncol. 14, 973–1005.

Brennan, M., Migliorati, C.A., Lockhart, P.B., Wray, D., 2007. Management of oral epithelial dysplasia: a review. Oral. Surg. Oral. Med. Oral. Pathol. Oral. Radiol. Endod. 103, S19.e1–S19.e12.

Cantarelli Morosolli, A.R., Schubert, M.M., Niccoli-Filho, W., 2006. Surgical treatment of erythroleukoplakia in lower lip with carbon dioxide laser radiation. Lasers Med. Sci. 21 (3), 181–184.

Femiano, F., Gombos, F., Scully, C., 2001. Oral proliferative verrucous leukoplakia; open trial of surgery compared with combined therapy using surgery and methisoprinol. Int. J. Oral. Maxillofac. Surg. 30, 318–322.

Femiano, F., Gombos, F., Scully, C., et al., 2001. Oral leukoplakia; open trial of topical therapy with calcipotriol compared with tretinoin. Int. J. Oral. Maxillofac. Surg. 30, 402–406.

Freitas, M.D., Blanco-Carrion, A., Gandara-Vila, P., et al., 2006. Clinicopathologic aspects of oral leukoplakia in smokers and nonsmokers. Oral. Surg. Oral. Med. Oral. Pathol. Oral. Radiol. Endod. 102 (2), 199–203.

Gandolfo, S., Pentenero, M., Broccoletti, R., et al., 2006. Toluidine blue uptake in potentially malignant oral lesions in vivo: clinical and histological assessment. Oral. Oncol. 42, 89–95.

Hashibe, M., Jacob, B.J., Thomas, G., et al., 2003. Socioeconomic status, lifestyle factors and oral premalignant lesions. Oral. Oncol. 39 (7), 664–671.

Holmstrup, P., Vedtofte, P., Reibel, J., Stoltze, K., 2006. Long-term treatment outcome of oral premalignant lesions. Oral. Oncol. 42 (5), 461–474.

Holmstrup, P., Vedtofte, P., Reibel, J., Stoltze, K., 2007. Oral premalignant lesions: is a biopsy reliable? J. Oral. Pathol. Med. 36 (5), 262–266.

Jaber, M.A., Porter, S.R., Bain, L., Scully, C., 2003. Lack of association between hepatitis C virus and oral epithelial dysplasia in British patients. Int. J. Oral. Maxillofac. Surg. 32 (2), 181–183.

Jaber, M.A., Porter, S.R., Speight, P., et al., 2003. Oral epithelial dysplasia: clinical characteristics of western European residents. Oral. Oncol. 39, 589–596.

Kim, J., Shin, D.M., El-Naggar, A., et al., 2001. Chromosome polysomy and histological characteristics in oral premalignant lesions. Cancer Epidemiol. 10, 319–325.

Kondoh, N., Ohkura, S., Arai, M., et al., 2007. Gene expression signatures that can discriminate oral leukoplakia subtypes and squamous cell carcinoma. Oral. Oncol. 43, 455–462.

Lalli, A., Tilakaratne, W.M., Ariyawardana, A., et al., 2008. An altered keratinocyte phenotype in oral submucous fibrosis: correlation of keratin K17 expression with disease severity. J. Oral. Pathol. Med. 37 (4), 211–220.

Lee, J.J., Hong, W.K., Hittelman, W.N., et al., 2000. Predicting cancer development in oral leukoplakia: ten years of translational research. Clin. Cancer Res. 6, 1702–1710.

Lippman, S.M., Hong, W.K., 2001. Molecular markers of the risk of oral cancer. N. Engl. J. Med. 344, 1323–1326.

Lodi, G., Porter, S., 2008. Management of potentially malignant disorders: evidence and critique. J. Oral. Pathol. Med. 37 (2), 63–69.

Lodi, G., Sardella, A., Bez, C., et al., 2006. Interventions for treating oral leukoplakia. Cochrane Database Syst. Rev. (4): CD001829.

Napier, S.S., Speight, P.M., 2008. Natural history of potentially malignant oral lesions and conditions: an overview of the literature. J. Oral. Pathol. Med. 37 (1), 1–10.

Pentenero, M., Carrozzo, M., Pagano, M., et al., 2003. Oral mucosal dysplastic lesions and early squamous cell carcinomas: underdiagnosis from incisional biopsy. Oral. Dis. 9, 68–72.

Pentenero, M., Giaretti, W., Navone, R., et al., 2011. Evidence for a possible anatomical subsite-mediated effect of tobacco in oral potentially malignant disorders and carcinoma. J. Oral. Pathol. Med. 40 (3), 214–217.

Petti, S., Scully, C., 2005. The role of the dental team in preventing and diagnosing cancer: 5. Alcohol and the role of the dentist in alcohol cessation. Dent. Update 32 (8), 454–455, 458–460, 462.

Petti, S., Scully, C., 2006. Association between different alcoholic beverages and leukoplakia among non- to moderate-drinking adults: a matched case-control study. Eur. J. Cancer 42, 521–527.

Pitiyage, G., Tilakaratne, W.M., Tavassoli, M., Warnakulasuriya, S., 2009. Molecular markers in oral epithelial dysplasia: review. J. Oral. Pathol. Med. 38 (10), 737–752.

Poate, T.W.J., Buchanan, J.A.G., Hodgson, T.A., et al., 2004. An audit of the efficacy of the oral brush biopsy technique in a specialist oral medicine unit. Oral. Oncol. 40, 829–834.

Poh, C.F., Zhang, L., Anderson, D.W., et al., 2006. Fluorescence visualization detection of field alterations in tumor margins of oral cancer patients. Clin. Cancer Res. 12 (22), 6716–6722.

Reichart, P.A., Philipsen, H.P., 2005. Oral erythroplakia – a review. Oral. Oncol. 41 (6), 551–561.

Ribeiro, A.S., Salles, P.R., da Silva, T.A., Mesquita, R.A., 2010. A review of the nonsurgical treatment of oral leukoplakia. Int. J. Dent. 2010, 186018.

Roosaar, A., Yin, L., Johansson, A.L., et al., 2007. A long-term follow-up study on the natural course of oral leukoplakia in a Swedish population-based sample. J. Oral. Pathol. Med. 36 (2), 78–82.

Scardina, G.A., Carini, F., Maresi, E., et al., 2006. Evaluation of the clinical and histological effectiveness of isotretinoin in the therapy of oral leukoplakia: ten years of experience: is management still up to date and effective? Methods Find. Exp. Clin. Pharmacol. 28 (2), 115–119.

Scully, C., Felix, D.H., 2005. Oral medicine – update for the dental practitioner: red and pigmented lesions. Br. Dent. J. 199 (10), 639–645.

Scully, C., Sudbo, J., Speight, P.M., 2003. Progress in determining the malignant potential of oral lesions. J. Oral. Pathol. Med. 32 (5), 251–256.

Thomas, G., Hashibe, M., Jacob, B.J., et al., 2003. Risk factors for multiple oral premalignant lesions. Int. J. Cancer 107 (2), 285–291.

Tilakaratne, W.M., Sherriff, M., Morgan, P.R., Odell, E.W., 2011. Grading oral epithelial dysplasia: analysis of individual features. J. Oral. Pathol. Med. 40 (7), 533–540.

van der Waal, L., Schepman, K.P., van der Meij, E.H., 2000. A modified classification and staging system for oral leukoplakia. Oral. Oncol. 36, 264–266.

Warnakulasuriya, S., Johnson, N.W., van der Waal, I., 2007. Nomenclature and classification of potentially malignant disorders of the oral mucosa. J. Oral. Pathol. Med. 36 (10), 575–580.

Warnakulasuriya, S., Reibel, J., Bouquot, J., Dabelsteen, E., 2008. Oral epithelial dysplasia classification systems: predictive value, utility, weaknesses and scope for improvement. J. Oral. Pathol. Med. 37 (3), 127–133.

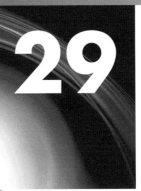

29 Lichen planus

Key Points

- Lichen planus is a common immunologically mediated mucocutaneous disorder
- Lichenoid reaction is a term used when a putative aetiological factor can be identified
- Aetiological factors include drugs, dental materials, graft-versus-host disease hepatitis C and other factors
- Lesions of lichen planus are typically bilateral and affect the buccal mucosae mainly
- Diagnosis is clinical supported by biopsy
- Management usually includes topical corticosteroids
- The malignant potential matches that of leukoplakias overall

INTRODUCTION

This chapter should be read along with Ch. 25.

Lichen planus (LP) is an inflammatory autoimmune-type of mucocutaneous disease that can affect stratified squamous epithelia – the skin, oral mucosa and genitalia (**Fig. 29.1**).

INCIDENCE

Lichen planus is not uncommon and has a prevalence of the order of 1%.

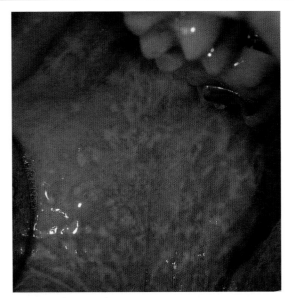

Fig. 29.1 Papuloreticular lichen planus in the most common site

AGE

It usually affects persons between the ages of 30–65 years.

GENDER

There is a slight female predisposition to LP.

GEOGRAPHIC

LP is seen worldwide.

PREDISPOSING FACTORS (Fig. 29.2)

- A genetic basis for oral LP (OLP) is supported by the fact that there are occasional familial cases; IL-6 and TNF-alpha homozygous genotypes are significantly more often detected in OLP patients and these genotypes are associated with an increased risk of OLP development. TNF polymorphisms may contribute to the development of additional cutaneous lesions. IL-1-beta and IL-10 gene polymorphisms however, are not related to OLP development.
- There is no definitive immunogenetic basis yet established for LP, but studies have reported various HLA associations:
  - in OLP, an increase in HLA B15, Bw57, B5, B7, BX, DR2 and HLA-te22, and a decrease in the frequency of HLA-DQ1, DR4 and B18
  - in patients with hepatitis C virus-associated OLP, an increased frequency of HLA-DR6
  - in patients with carbohydrate metabolism disorders and OLP, an increased frequency of HLA B16, B2 and B40
  - in cutaneous LP, an increase in HLA-DR1 (mainly HLA-DRB1*0101), DQ1, DR3 or DR9.
- Stress has been widely held to be an important aetiological factor in LP, but, of the remarkably few studies, most have not objectively examined stress. A statistically significant difference was, indeed, found in the psychological profiles of patients affected by LP – who have a tendency to be depressed and anxious, but the chronic discomfort that can afflict patients with LP can of course itself be a stressing factor.
- Lesions clinically and histologically similar to LP, termed 'lichenoid lesions', are sometimes caused by:
  - dental restorative materials (mainly amalgam and gold)
  - chronic graft-versus-host disease, seen in bone marrow (haemopoietic stem cell) transplant patients
  - infection with hepatitis C virus in some populations, such as those from southern Europe and Japan
  - a variety of other systemic disorders, such as hypertension and diabetes, but this is probably a manifestation of a reaction to the drugs used

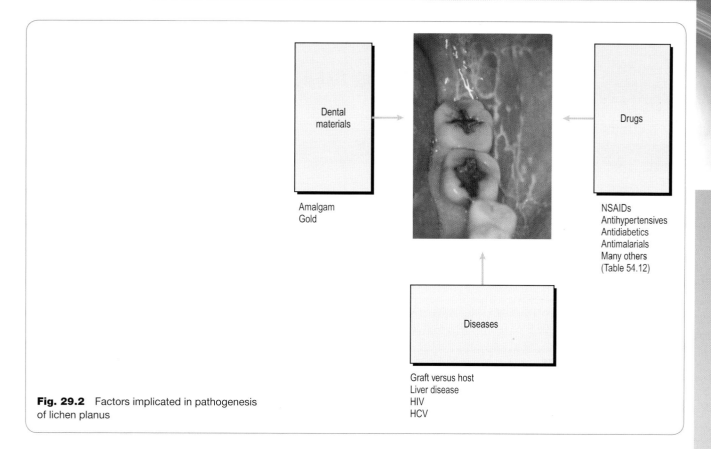

Fig. 29.2 Factors implicated in pathogenesis of lichen planus

- drug and vaccine use: antidiabetic drugs; antirheumatic drugs (NSAIDs mainly, but also others); antihypertensive agents, such as beta-blockers, thiazides and diuretics; antimalarials, such as quinacrine; many other drugs; occasionally, hepatitis B vaccine, omalizumab or TNF-alpha antagonists.

AETIOLOGY AND PATHOGENESIS

LP involves epithelial damage (**Fig. 29.3**) immunologically mediated by cytotoxic T cells directed against basilar keratinocytes and resulting in vacuolar degeneration and lysis of basal cells. However, it is not a classical autoimmune disorder.

- The antigen(s) responsible for LP are unknown, but studies have revealed a LP-specific epidermal antigen. Studies looking for any causal bacteria, fungi and viruses have proved negative.
- The earliest features of LP are changes in, and close to, the basal epithelium. The appearance of antigen-processing cells (Langerhans cells) is one of the first observable changes.
- A band-like dense mononuclear inflammatory cell infiltrate, mainly of T CD8+ cells, then appears in the upper lamina propria, representing a local cell-mediated immunological response (**Fig. 29.4**).
- The NF-κB path is thereby activated with a change of NF-κB-dependent pro-inflammatory cytokines, including tumour necrosis factor-α (TNF-α), and interleukins IL-8, and IL-6.
- T-cell cytokines such as TNF-α and interferon-γ (IFN-γ) then cause apoptosis (controlled cell death) in the epithelial basal keratinocytes. There are also changes in the TGF-β pathway and IL-4.

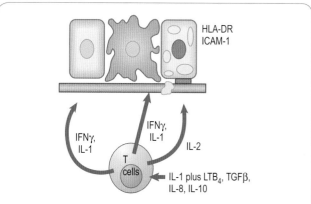

Fig. 29.3 Aetiopathogenesis of lichen planus (see text). IL, interleukin; IFN, interferon; LTB, leukotriene; TGF, transforming growth factor

- The basal keratinocytes degenerate and die, undergoing flattening and hydropic changes causing intercellular spaces to appear, with splitting of epithelium away from the basement membrane – termed basal cell liquefaction.
- Round or ovoid 'colloid bodies' (also termed cytoid, globular, hyaline, Civatte and Sabouraud bodies) appear mainly in the epithelial spinous layer and in the lamina propria.
- Immune deposits (typically fibrin and sometimes IgM) are seen in the colloid bodies and at the basement membrane zone, and probably represent non-specific exudation, not autoantibodies.
- The rest of the epithelium appears to react with thickening of the spinous (acanthosis) and granular cell layers (hyperparakeratosis) or hyperorthokeratosis – which accounts for the clinical white lesions.

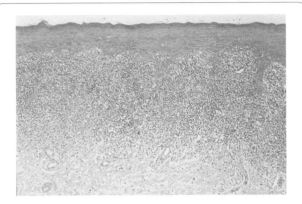

Fig. 29.4 Histopathology of lichen planus showing the subepithelial Tc cell infiltrate

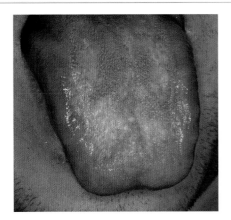

Fig. 29.6 Lichen planus of the plaque type, resembling leukoplakia

- The rete ridges adopt a 'saw tooth' configuration (more commonly than in skin lesions).
- Epithelial atrophy and even erosions can appear – leading to discomfort and the appearance of red lesions and/or ulceration.

CLINICAL FEATURES

- Oral LP may occur in isolation, or oral lesions may precede, accompany or follow lichen planus affecting other stratified squamous epithelia or appendages (see below) but there are no known predictive factors for this involvement.
- The clinical picture is mainly of white lesions but is often mixed; six clinical types of OLP lesions have been described:
  - reticular, a network of raised white lines termed striae (reticular pattern)
  - papular, white papules (**Fig. 29.5**)
  - plaque-like, white patches simulating leukoplakia (**Fig. 29.6**)
  - red atrophic areas – LP is one of the most common causes of desquamative gingivitis (**Fig. 29.7**).
- Erosive/ulcerative – persistent, irregular, and painful erosions with a yellowish slough (this type is less common) (**Fig. 29.8**).
- Bullous (possibly caused by superficial mucoceles).
- LP typically presents as lesions which are:
  - mostly white
  - reticular, but may be papular or plaque-like and associated with red atrophic areas in the posterior buccal mucosa bilaterally

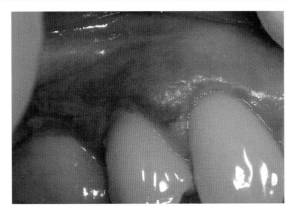

Fig. 29.7 Atrophic lichen planus causing desquamative gingivitis

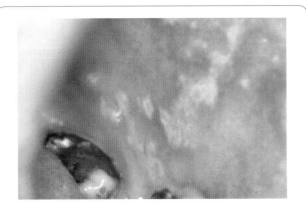

Fig. 29.5 Papuloreticular lichen planus

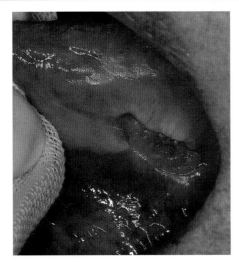

Fig. 29.8 Erosive lichen planus resembling lupus erythematosus

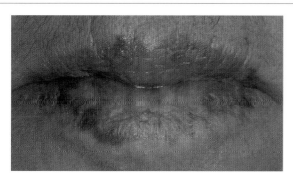

Fig. 29.9 Lichen planus on lips

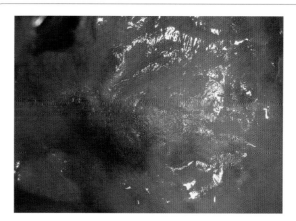

Fig. 29.10 Pigmentary incontinence in lichen planus

- occasionally on the dorsum of the tongue where they may be reticular, papular or plaque-like and associated with red atrophic or erosive areas
- occasionally on the gingiva, as a white lacework of white striae and papules, or as 'desquamative gingivitis' (may also develop in about 25% of patients with erosive LP and can be the initial or the only sign of oral involvement)
- rarely on the lips – usually a white lacework of white striae and papules (**Fig. 29.9**)
- rarely on the palate – usually a white lacework of white striae and papules.
- LP is often asymptomatic, especially when there are only white lesions but there may be soreness from atrophic areas of thin, red mucosa or erosions, especially when eating or drinking substances which are acidic or spicy. Mild oral discomfort or burning sensations are the common complaints in most symptomatic cases but in some the discomfort can be severe.

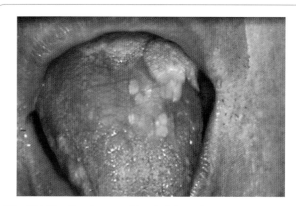

Fig. 29.11 Carcinoma arising in lichen planus

PROGNOSIS

Often the onset of lichen planus is slow, taking months to reach its peak. It often clears from the skin within 18 months, but in a few people persists for many years. Oral lesions are often persistent. In people with dark skin there may be pigmentary incontinence with dark areas appearing (**Fig. 29.10**). Extraoral lesions may be present at, or follow the onset of, oral LP but a careful history and examination may reveal latent lesions or lesions previously considered due to another disorder. For example, genital LP is not uncommon in patients who complain only of gingival lesions (vulvo-vaginal-gingival syndrome of Pelisse).

LP and especially lichenoid lesions have a small malignant potential – probably of the order of <1–3%, and predominantly in non-reticular lesions (**Fig. 29.11**).

EXTRAORAL LESIONS

Lichen planus may also cause lesions elsewhere, including:

- Skin: rash characterized by lesions, which are:
  - **p**urple
  - **p**olygonal
  - **p**ruritic (itchy)
  - **p**apules – often crossed by fine white lines (Wickham striae) (**Fig. 29.12**).

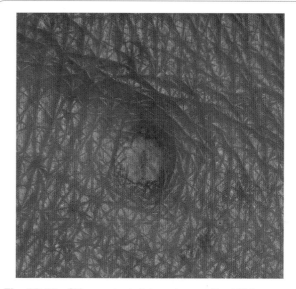

Fig. 29.12 Skin papules in lichen planus with whitish Wickham striae

It is most often seen on the:

- front (flexor surface) of the wrists
- lower back
- ankles and shins.

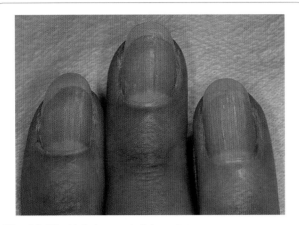

Fig. 29.13 Nail changes in lichen planus

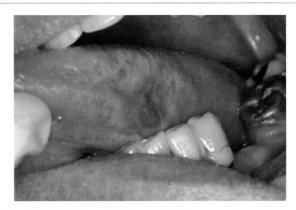

Fig. 29.14 Lichenoid lesions related to an amalgam restoration on the molar tooth

Trauma may induce new skin lesions (Koebner phenomenon):

- Skin appendages: in 10% of cases there is nail involvement, usually a minor change (**Fig. 29.13**), but occasionally resulting in shedding or destruction of the nail. The scalp is uncommonly affected, but permanently bald patches may develop.
- Ano-genital mucosae:
  - the 'vulvo-vaginal-gingival syndrome' is fairly common and involves coincident onset of gingival and genital lesions in about half the reported patients, the remainder developing lesions at both sites within 2 years. The oral lesions mainly affect the labial gingivae
  - the peno-gingival syndrome and anal LP are less common and less incapacitating.
- Ocular mucosae: conjunctival involvement with scarring is a recognized complication of LP.

DIAGNOSIS

Lichen planus is often fairly obviously diagnosed from the clinical features, but it can sometimes closely simulate other conditions, such as:

- lupus erythematosus (see **Fig. 29.8**)
- chronic ulcerative stomatitis
- keratosis
- carcinoma.

Lichenoid lesions that may need to be excluded include:

- drug-induced lesions
- dental-material-induced lesions (**Fig. 29.14**)
- diabetes mellitus
- graft-versus-host disease
- hepatic disease or hepatitis C virus infection
- HIV.

Lichenoid lesions clinically resemble LP, but may:

- be unilateral
- be associated with erosions
- resolve on discontinuation of any offending drug.

Skin testing for hypersensitivity to drugs or dental materials is only rarely of clinical value.

Lichenoid lesions histopathologically are more likely than LP to be associated with:

- a mixed cellular infiltrate including plasma cells and eosinophils
- a deeper infiltrate
- a perivascular infiltrate
- parakeratosis
- colloid bodies in the epithelium
- basal cell autoantibodies.

The firm diagnosis of LP, therefore, relies upon biopsy and histopathological examination of lesional tissue, occasionally aided by direct immunostaining. However, often the histological and immunological findings revealed are no more than 'consistent with lichen planus', but this at least serves to exclude the more dangerous conditions. Other investigations may sometimes be indicated (**Table 29.1**). *Lichenoid and granulomatous stomatitis* is a rare entity presenting with mucosal lesions of the upper lip characterized by lichenoid with concomitant granulomatous inflammation. This may be plaque-related and respond to chlorhexidine.

Table 29.1 Aids that might be helpful in diagnosis/prognosis/management in some patients suspected of having lichen planus*

In most cases	In some cases
Biopsy ± immunofluorescence	Dermatological/gynaecological/ophthalmic opinions Full blood picture Serum ferritin, vitamin B$_{12}$ and corrected whole blood folate levels Smear and culture for candida ssp ESR ANA Serology (HCV, HIV) Patch testing G6PD and TPMT levels Blood pressure Blood glucose

*See text for details and glossary for abbreviations.

TREATMENT (see also Chs 4 and 5)

Patient information is an important aspect in management. Unfortunately, although the natural history of cutaneous LP is one often of remission, oral LP remits completely only in a few if any patients, and there are no cures currently available. Treatment is indicated for the discomfort of symptomatic LP (**Algorithm 29.1**), i.e. mainly for atrophic or erosive LP.

Predisposing factors should be corrected:

- It may be wise to consider removal of dental amalgams or other materials if the lesions are clearly closely related to these, or unilateral. Unfortunately, no tests, such as patch tests, will reliably indicate which patients might benefit.
- A physician should be consulted if there is HCV infection or other systemic background, or if drugs are implicated, and a relevant specialist if skin, genital or ocular involvement is possible.

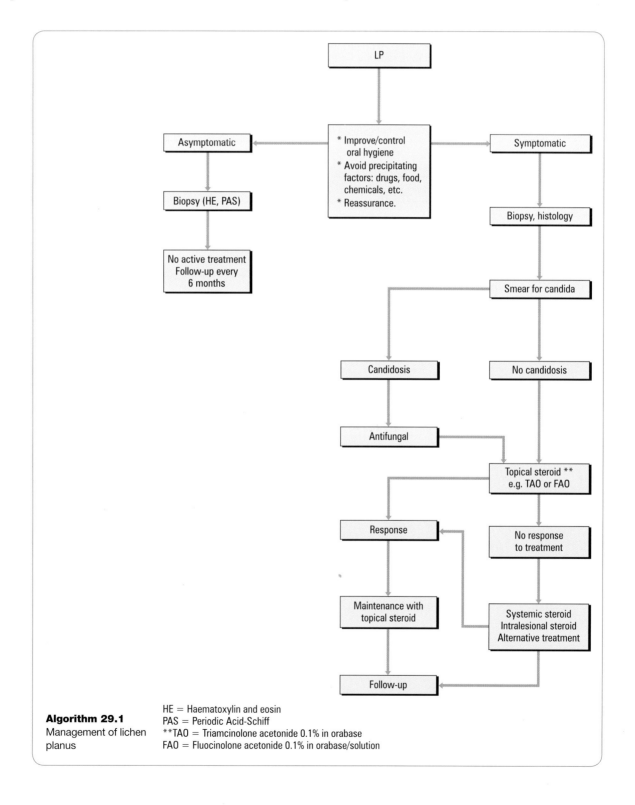

Algorithm 29.1
Management of lichen planus

HE = Haematoxylin and eosin
PAS = Periodic Acid-Schiff
**TAO = Triamcinolone acetonide 0.1% in orabase
FAO = Fluocinolone acetonide 0.1% in orabase/solution

- Improvement in oral hygiene may result in some subjective benefit. Chlorhexidine or triclosan mouthwashes may help.
- Symptoms can often be controlled with topical medication. Benzydamine hydrochloride (0.15%) spray or mouthrinse or 2% lidocaine gel applied to painful areas can be helpful.

There are many therapies suggested but few with a reliable evidence base (**Table 29.2**).

Topical corticosteroids can often control LP (Ch. 5). Topical corticosteroids are the primary therapeutic agents used to treat ulcerative mucosal lesions which have an immunologically-based aetiology such as lichen planus. A mild potency agent such as hydrocortisone may be effective but more typically a medium potency corticosteroid such as betamethasone or a higher potency one such as fluocinonide or beclomethasone are required , moving to a super-potent topical corticosteroid, e.g. clobetasol, if the benefit is inadequate (see **Table 5.5**). Patients should be instructed to apply a small quantity of the agent three times daily, refraining from speaking, eating and drinking for the subsequent 0.5 h. A theoretical concern is that long-term immunosuppression might predispose to neoplastic change. In long-term use, candidosis can arise and thus topical antifungal medication such as miconazole may be prudent. The more major concern – of adrenal suppression with long-term and/or repeated application – has rarely been addressed, although the topical preparations noted in Ch. 5 (apart from super potent halogenated corticosteroids when used several times a day) appear not to cause a significant problem.

Topical tacrolimus, pimecrolimus and even thalidomide, may also be effective (Ch. 5). There have been cases reported

Table 29.2 Regimens that might be helpful in management of patient suspected of having lichen planus

Regimen	Use in primary care	Use in secondary care (severe oral involvement and/or extraoral involvement)
Beneficial	Topical corticosteroids (Ch. 5)	Systemic corticosteroids (Ch. 5)
Likely to be beneficial	Aloe vera Hyaluronic acid Topical tacrolimus (but FDA advisory: see p. 52) Topical pimecrolimus	Acitretin Azathioprine Ciclosporin Cyclophosphamide Dapsone Hydroxychloroquine Interferon Mycophenolate Thalidomide
Unproven effectiveness		Ciclosporin Diethyldithiocarbamate Dapsone Doxycycline Enoxaparin Glycyrrhizin Griseofulvin Hydroxychloroquine Interferon Laser Levamisole Magnetism Mesalazine Methotrexate mofetil Pentoxifylline Phenytoin Photopheresis Psychotherapy Psoralen plus UVA Reflexotherapy Retinoids Sirolimus Sulodexide Surgery Thalidomide
Emergent treatments		Alefacept Basiliximab Etanercept
Supportive	Benzydamine Diet with little acidic, spicy or citrus content Smoking cessation	

of carcinoma developing in LP treated with tacrolimus, though a causal relationship is not established and the FDA have therefore produced an Advisory Note (Ch. 5).

Alternative therapies that have been employed include aloe vera, and calendula officinalis.

SEVERITY-DEPENDENT TREATMENT
Mild LP

Topical aloe vera may help symptomatically but topical corticosteroids are the mainstay of therapy, although erosive and gingival lesions are often recalcitrant. High potency corticosteroids, such as clobetasol, fluocinonide or fluticasone, may initially be employed and should then be changed to a lower potency drug (e.g. hydrocortisone hemisuccinate, triamcinolone acetate or fluocinolone). Topical creams or pastes can be applied in a suitable customized tray or veneer to be worn at night.

Moderate LP

If there is severe or extensive oral involvement, topical ciclosporin may be of significant benefit, often being used along with a high or super potent topical corticosteroid. This regimen is useful in the management of LP-related desquamative gingivitis recalcitrant to other therapies.

Severe LP

In severe LP in multiple sites, patients may require systemic corticosteroids (prednisolone, deflazacort), or other immunomodulatory agents such as mycophenolate mofetil (Ch. 5; **Table 29.2**).

EMERGENT TREATMENTS
New biologicals used in management of LP include:

- alefacept
- basiliximab
- etanercept.

FOLLOW-UP OF PATIENTS

Oral lichen planus carries a small potential for malignant development, of the order of 1–3% or so over 10 years, necessitating regular monitoring, perhaps every six months, which can be carried out by the general dental practitioner. NICE guidelines clearly state that patients with oral lichen planus should be monitored for oral cancer as part of the routine dental examination (Referral guidelines for suspected cancer. Clinical Guideline 27 NICE June 2005).

If there is any change causing concern, particularly the development of a lump, a specialist opinion should best be obtained.

PATIENT INFORMATION SHEET
Lichen planus

▼ Please read this information sheet. If you have any questions, particularly about the treatment or potential side-effects, please ask your doctor.
- This is a common condition.
- The cause is unknown.
- Children do not usually inherit it from parents.
- It is not thought to be infectious.
- Lichen planus is sometimes related to drugs, dental fillings or other conditions.
- Some patients have the condition on the skin or elsewhere.
- Blood tests and biopsy may be required.
- The condition tends to persist in the mouth.
- Lichen planus can be controlled, but rarely cured.
- Most lichen planus is benign.
- Some forms of lichen planus may rarely, after years, lead to a tumour. In this case, you should get yourself checked regularly if the specialist advises.

USEFUL WEBSITES

American Academy of Dermatology, Lichen planus:
http://www.aad.org/pamphlets/lichen.html

The International Oral Lichen Planus Support Group:
http://bcdwp.web.tamhsc.edu/iolpdallas/

FURTHER READING

Al-Hashimi, I., Schifter, M., Lockhart, P.B., et al., 2007. Oral lichen planus and oral lichenoid lesions: diagnostic and therapeutic considerations. Oral Surg. Oral Med. Oral Pathol. Oral Radiol. Endod 103, (Suppl.) S25.e1–S25.e12.

Asarch, A., Gottlieb, A.B., Lee, J., et al., 2009. Lichen planus-like eruptions: an emerging side effect of tumor necrosis factor-alpha antagonists. J. Am. Acad. Dermatol. 61 (1), 104–111.

Bäckman, K., Jontell, M., 2007. Microbial-associated oral lichenoid reactions. Oral Dis. 13 (4), 402–406.

Belfiore, P., Di Fede, O., Cabibi, D., et al., 2006. Prevalence of vulval lichen planus in a cohort of women with oral lichen planus: an interdisciplinary study. Br. J. Dermatol. 155 (5), 994–998.

Bermejo-Fenoll, A., Lopez-Jornet, P., 2006. Familial oral lichen planus: presentation of six families. Oral Surg.

Oral Med. Oral Pathol. Oral Radiol. Endod. 102 (2), e12–e15.

Bez, C., Hallet, R., Carrozzo, M., et al., 2001. Lack of association between hepatotropic transfusion transmitted virus infection and oral lichen planus in British and Italian populations. Br. J. Dermatol. 145, 990–993.

Bidarra, M., Buchanan, J.A., Scully, C., 2008. Oral lichen planus: a condition with more persistence and extra-oral involvement than suspected? J. Oral Pathol. Med. 37 (10), 582–586.

Brewer, J.D., Ekdawi, N.S., Torgerson, R.R., et al., 2011. Lichen planus and cicatricial conjunctivitis: disease course and response to therapy of 11 patients. J. Eur. Acad. Dermatol. Venereol. 25 (1), 100–104.

Carbone, M., Arduino, P., Carrozzo, M., et al., 2009. Course of oral lichen planus: a retrospective study

of 808 northern Italian patients. Oral Dis. 15, 235–243.

Carbone, M., Arduino, P.G., Carrozzo, M., et al., 2009. Topical clobetasol in the treatment of atrophic-erosive oral lichen planus: a randomized controlled trial to compare two preparations with different concentrations. J. Oral Pathol. Med. 38 (2), 227–233.

Carrozzo, M., Brancatello, F., Dametto, E., et al., 2005. Hepatitis C virus-associated oral lichen planus: is the geographical heterogeneity related to HLA-DR6? J. Oral Pathol. Med. 34, 204–208.

Carrozzo, M., Francia Di Celle, P., Gandolfo, S., et al., 2001. Increased frequency of HLA-DR6 allele in Italian patients with hepatitis C virus-associated oral lichen planus. Br. J. Dermatol. 144, 803–808.

Carrozzo, M., Thorpe, R., 2009. Oral lichen planus: a review. Minerva Stomatol. 58 (10), 519–537.

Cheng, A., Mann, C., 2006. Oral erosive lichen planus treated with efalizumab. Arch. Dermatol. 142 (6), 680–682.

Choonhakarn, C., Busaracome, P., Sripanidkulchai, B., Sarakarn, P., 2008. The efficacy of aloe vera gel in the treatment of oral lichen planus: a randomized controlled trial. Br. J. Dermatol. 158 (3), 573.

Clayton, R., Chaudhry, S., Ali, I., et al., 2010. Mucosal (oral and vulval) lichen planus in women:are angiotensin-converting enzyme inhibitors protective, and beta-blockers and non-steroidal anti-inflammatory drugs associated with the condition? Clin. Exp. Dermatol. 35 (4), 384–387.

Cleach, L.L., Chosidow, O., 2012. Lichen planus. N Engl J Med. 366, 723–732.

Crincoli, V., Di Bisceglie, M.B., Scivetti, M., et al., 2011. Oral lichen planus: update on etiopathogenesis, diagnosis and treatment. Immunopharmacol. Immunotoxicol. 33 (1), 11–20.

Danielsson, K., Wahlin, Y.B., Coates, P.J., Nylander, K., 2010. Increased expression of Smad proteins, and in particular Smad3, in oral lichen planus compared to normal oral mucosa. J. Oral Pathol. Med. 39 (8), 639–644.

Di Fede, O., Belfiore, P., Cabibi, D., et al., 2006. Unexpectedly high frequency of genital involvement in women with clinical and histological features of oral lichen planus. Acta Derm. Venereol. 86 (5), 433–438.

Femiano, F., Gombos, F., Scully, C., 2003. Oral erosive/ulcerative lichen planus: preliminary findings in an open trial of sulodexide compared with cyclosporine (ciclosporin) therapy. Int. J. Dermatol. 42, 308–311.

Femiano, F., Scully, C., 2006. Oral lichen planus: clinical and histological evaluation in an open trial using a low molecular weight heparinoid (sulodexide). Int. J. Dermatol. 45 (8), 986–989.

Gonzalez-Garcia, A., Diniz-Freitas, M., Gandara-Vila, P., et al., 2006. Triamcinolone acetonide mouth rinses for treatment of erosive oral lichen planus: efficacy and risk of fungal over-infection. Oral Dis. 12 (6), 559–565.

Gonzalez-Moles, M.A., Bascones-Ilundain, C., Gil Montoya, J.A., et al., 2006. Cell cycle regulating mechanisms in oral lichen planus: molecular bases in epithelium predisposed to malignant transformation. Arch. Oral Biol. 51 (12), 1093–1103.

Gonzalez-Moles, M.A., Scully, C., Gil-Montoya, J., 2008. Oral lichen planus: controversies surrounding malignant transformation. Oral Dis. 14, 229–243.

Heffernan, M.P., Smith, D.I., Bentley, D., et al., 2007. A single-center, open-label, prospective pilot study of subcutaneous efalizumab for oral erosive lichen planus. J. Drugs Dermatol. 6, 310–314.

Ingafou, M., Leao, J.C., Porter, S.R., Scully, C., 2006. Oral lichen planus: a retrospective study of 690 British patients. Oral Dis. 12 (5), 463–468.

Kimkong, I., Hirankarn, N., Nakkuntod, J., Kitkumthorn, N., 2011. Tumour necrosis factor-alpha gene polymorphisms and susceptibility to oral lichen planus. Oral Dis. 17, 206–209.

Laeijendecker, R., Tank, B., Dekker, S.K., Neumann, H.A., 2006. A comparison of treatment of oral lichen planus with topical tacrolimus and triamcinolone acetonide ointment. Acta Derm. Venereol. 86 (3), 227–229.

Lodi, G., Carrozzo, M., Harris, K., et al., 2000. Hepatitis G virus-associated oral lichen planus; no influence from hepatitis G virus co-infection. J. Oral Pathol. Med. 29, 39–42.

Lodi, G., Scully, C., Carrozzo, M., et al., 2005. Current controversies in oral lichen planus: report of an international consensus meeting. Part 1. Viral infections and etiopathogenesis. Oral Surg. Oral Med. Oral Pathol. Oral Radiol. Endod. 100, 40–51.

Lodi, G., Scully, C., Carrozzo, M., et al., 2005. Current controversies in oral lichen planus: report of an international consensus meeting. Part 2. Clinical

management and malignant transformation. Oral Surg. Oral Med. Oral Pathol. Oral Radiol. Endod 100, 164–178.

Lodi, G., Pellicano, R., Carrozzo, M., 2010. Hepatitis C virus infection and lichen planus: a systematic review with meta-analysis. Oral Dis. 16, 601–612.

López-Jornet, P., Camacho-Alonso, F., Salazar-Sanchez, N., 2010. Topical tacrolimus and pimecrolimus in the treatment of oral lichen planus: an update. J. Oral Pathol. Med. 39 (3), 201–205.

Lozada-Nur, F.I., Sroussi, H.Y., 2006. Tacrolimus powder in Orabase 0.1% for the treatment of oral lichen planus and oral lichenoid lesions: an open clinical trial. Oral Surg. Oral Med. Oral Pathol. Oral Radiol. Endod. 102 (6), 744–749.

Mansourian, A., Momen-Heravi, F., Saheb-Jamee, M., et al., 2011. Comparison of Treatment Efficacy of Daily Use of Aloe Vera Mouthwash With Triamcinolone Acetonide 0.1% on Oral Lichen Planus: A Randomized Double-Blinded Clinical Trial. Am. J. Med. Sci. 342 (6), 447–451.

Mattsson, U., Jontell, M., Holmstrup, P., 2002. Oral lichen planus and malignant transformation: Is a recall of patients justified? Crit. Rev. Oral Biol. Med. 13, 390–396.

Mattsson, U., Magnusson, B., Jontell, M., 2010. Squamous cell carcinoma in a patient with oral lichen planus treated with topical application of tacrolimus. Oral Surg. Oral Med. Oral Pathol. Oral Radiol. Endod. 110 (1), e19–e25.

Mignogna, M.D., Fedele, S., Lo Russo, L., 2006. Dysplasia/neoplasia surveillance in oral lichen planus patients: a description of clinical criteria adopted at a single centre and their impact on prognosis. Oral Oncol. 42 (8), 819–824.

Mignogna, M.D., Fedele, S., Lo Russo, L., et al., 2006. Field cancerization in oral lichen planus. Eur. J. Surg. Oncol. 33, 383–389.

Nolan, A., Badminton, J., Maguire, J., Seymour, R.A., 2009. The efficacy of topical hyaluronic acid in the management of oral lichen planus. J. Oral Pathol. Med. 38 (3), 299–303.

O'Neill I Scully C., 2012. Biologics in oral medicine: ulcerative disorders, oral Diseases Mar 15 [Epub ahead of print]

Poomsawat S., Buajeeb, W., Khovidhunkit, S.O., Punyasingh, J., 2011. Overexpression of cdk4 and p16 in oral lichen planus supports the concept of premalignancy. J. Oral Pathol. Med. 40 (4), 294–299.

Robinson, C.M., Oxley, J.D., Weir, J., Eveson, J.W., 2006. Lichenoid and granulomatous stomatitis: an entity or a non-specific inflammatory process? J. Oral Pathol. Med. 35 (5), 262–267.

Robinson, N.A., 2000. Lichenoid tissue reactions of the oral mucosa. Singapore Dent. J. 23 (Suppl. 1), 56–63.

Roopashree, M.R., Gondhalekar, R.V., Shashikanth, M.C., et al., 2010. Pathogenesis of oral lichen planus – a review. J. Oral Pathol. Med. 39 (10), 729–734.

Roosaar, A., Yin, L., Sandborgh-Englund, G., et al., 2006. On the natural course of oral lichen lesions in a Swedish population-based sample. J. Oral Pathol. Med. 35 (5), 257–261.

Salazar-Sánchez, N., López-Jornet, P., Camacho-Alonso, F., Sánchez-Siles, M., 2010. Efficacy of topical Aloe vera in patients with oral lichen planus: a randomized double-blind study. J. Oral Pathol. Med. 39 (10), 735–744.

Scully, C., Carrozzo, M., 2008. Oral mucosal disease: Lichen planus. Br. J. Oral Maxillofac. Surg. 46 (1), 15–21.

Scully, C., Eisen, D., Bagan, J.V., 2004. The diagnosis and management of oral lichen planus; a consensus approach. Oral Biosci. Med. 1, 21–28.

Scully, C., Eisen, D., Carrozzo, M., 2000. Management of oral lichen planus. Am. J. Clin. Dermatol. 1, 287–306.

Seeborg, F.O., Rihal, P.S., Czelusta, A., et al., 2009. Lichen planus associated with omalizumab administration in an adult with allergic asthma. Ann. Allergy Asthma Immunol. 102 (4), 349–351.

Stojanovic, L., Lunder, T., Rener-Sitar, K., et al., 2011. Thorough clinical evaluation of skin, as well as oral, genital and anal mucosa is beneficial in lichen planus patients. Coll. Antropol. 35 (1), 15–20.

Sun, A., Wu, Y.C., Wang, J.T., 2000. Association of HLA-te22 antigen with antinuclear antibodies in Chinese patients with erosive oral lichen planus. Proc. Natl. Sci. Counc. Repub. China B 24, 63–69.

Tao, X.A., Li, C.Y., Rhodus, N.L., et al., 2008. Simultaneous detection of IFN-gamma and IL-4 in lesional tissues and whole unstimulated saliva from patients with oral lichen planus. J. Oral Pathol. Med. 37 (2), 83–87.

Thongprasom, K., Carrozzo, M., Furness, S., Lodi, G., 2011. Interventions for treating oral lichen planus (Review). Cochrane Database Syst. Rev. (7) CD001168.

Thongprasom, K., Chaimusig, M., Korkij, W., et al., 2007. A randomized-controlled trial to compare topical cyclosporin with triamcinolone acetonide for the treatment of oral lichen planus. J. Oral Pathol. Med. 36 (3), 142–146.

Thongprasom, K., Dhanuthai, K., 2008. Steriods in the treatment of lichen planus: a review. J. Oral Sci. 50 (4), 377–385.

Thornhill, M.H., Sankar, V., Xu, X.J., et al., 2006. The role of histopathological characteristics in distinguishing amalgam-associated oral lichenoid reactions and oral lichen planus. J. Oral Pathol. Med. 35 (4), 233–240.

van der Meij, E.H., Mast, H., van der Waal, I., 2007. The possible premalignant character of oral lichen planus and oral lichenoid lesions: A prospective five-year follow-up study of 192 patients. Oral Oncol. 43, 742–748.

van der Meij, E.H., Schepman, K.P., Smeele, L.E., et al., 1999. A review of the recent literature regarding malignant transformation of oral lichen planus. Oral Surg. Oral Med. Oral Pathol. Oral Radiol. Endod. 88, 307–310.

Won, T.H., Park, S.Y., Kim, B.S., et al., 2009. Levamisole monotherapy for oral lichen planus. Ann. Dermatol. 21 (3), 250–254.

Wongwatana, S., Leao, J.C., Porter, S.R., Scully, C., 2005. Oxpentifylline is not effective for symptomatic oral lichen planus. J. Oral Pathol. Med. 34, 106–108.

Wu, Y., Zhou, G., Zeng, H., et al., 2010. A randomized double-blind,positive-control trial of topical thalidomide in erosive oral lichen planus. Oral Surg. Oral Med. Oral Pathol. Oral Radiol. Endod. 110 (2), 188–195.

Xavier, G.M., de Sá, A.R., Guimarães, A.L., et al., 2007. Investigation of functional gene polymorphisms interleukin-1beta, interleukin-6, interleukin-10 and tumor necrosis factor in individuals with oral lichen planus. J. Oral Pathol. Med. 36 (8), 476–481.

Xia, J., Li, C., Hong, Y., et al., 2006. Short-term clinical evaluation of intralesional triamcinolone acetonide injection for ulcerative oral lichen planus. J. Oral Pathol. Med. 35 (6), 327–331.

Yoke, P.C., Tin, G.B., Kim, M.J., et al., 2006. Asian Lichen Planus Study Group. A randomized controlled trial to compare steroid with cyclosporine for the topical treatment of oral lichen planus. Oral Surg. Oral Med. Oral Pathol. Oral Radiol. Endod 102 (1), 47–55.

Zakrzewska, J.M., Chan, E.S., Thornhill, M.H., 2005. A systematic review of placebo-controlled randomized clinical trials of treatments used in oral lichen planus. Br. J. Dermatol. 153 (2), 336–341.

Submucous fibrosis **30**

Key Points

- Submucous fibrosis is caused by betel use
- It is a potentially malignant disorder
- Treatment is mainly by physiotherapy

INTRODUCTION

This chapter should be read along with Ch. 25.

Oral submucous fibrosis (OSMF) is a chronic disorder seen only in persons who chew betel (*Areca catechu*) nuts, pan masala or gutkha – and is characterized by tightening of the buccal, and sometimes palatal and lingual mucosae, causing trismus.

INCIDENCE

4/1 000 adults in rural India.

AGE

It usually affects persons between the ages of 30–65 years.

GENDER

There is a slight female predisposition to OSMF.

GEOGRAPHIC

OSMF is seen worldwide but it is extremely rare in people not of Asian extraction.

PREDISPOSING FACTORS

Betel chewing.

AETIOLOGY AND PATHOGENESIS

The basic issue in OMSF appears to be an increase in submucosal collagen, for which there may be some genetic predisposition. Patients have an increased frequency of HLA-A10, HLA-B7, and HLA-DR3. Further, the HLA class I chain-related gene A (MICA), particularly the phenotype frequency of allele A6 of MICA is increased in OSMF, expressed by keratinocytes and other epithelial cells and interacts with gamma/delta T cells in the submucosa. Increased levels of pro-inflammatory cytokines and reduced antifibrotic interferon gamma may be central to the pathogenesis.

The lesions of OSMF appear to arise due to exposure to areca nut constituents which act by increasing collagen cross-linking or other effects. One betel nut alkaloid, arecoline, stimulates production of:

- collagen
- interleukin 6
- keratinocyte growth factor-1
- insulin-like growth factor-1
- cystatin C (a protein up-regulated in a variety of fibrotic diseases)
- tissue inhibitor of matrix metalloproteinases (TIMP).

Arecoline inhibits matrix metalloproteinases (MMPs – particularly MMP-2), and chewing areca quid may also activate NF-κB expression, thereby further stimulating collagen fibroblasts. Flavonoids, catechin, tannin and possibly copper in betel nuts may cause collagen fibres to cross-link, making them less susceptible to collagenase degradation.

CLINICAL FEATURES

OSMF can affect the oral and sometimes pharyngeal mucosa, and develops insidiously, usually diffusely, often initially presenting with oral burning sensations, and a non-specific vesicular stomatitis. Later symmetrical fibrosis of the cheeks, lips, tongue or palate appears as vertical bands running through the mucosa, and oral opening becomes restricted (**Table 30.1**). The fibrosis can become so severe that the affected site appears white and becomes firm, and severely

Table 30.1 Grading of OMSF severity

Grade	Features
1	Oral opening >35 mm
2	Oral opening 20–35 mm
3	Oral opening <20 mm
4	Oral opening <20 mm + PMD
5	Oral opening <20 mm + OSCC

After Kerr et al 2011.
PMD, potentially malignant disorder; OSCC, oral squamous cell carcinoma.

201

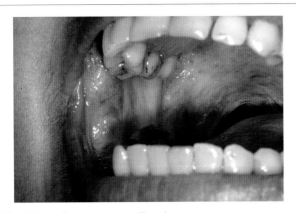

Fig. 30.1 Oral submucous fibrosis

restricts mouth opening and tongue and/or palate mobility (**Fig. 30.1**).

There is epithelial atrophy and sometimes frank erythroplakia or leukoplakia, and carcinoma may eventually develop – possibly in up to 8%. There can be oesophageal fibrosis and, if the palatal and paratubal muscles are involved, conductive hearing loss may appear because of functional stenosis of the Eustachian tube.

Betel use may also predispose to other conditions (Ch. 25).

PROGNOSIS

OSMF produces epithelial atrophy, and there is a malignant potential – carcinoma develops possibly in up to 8%.

DIAGNOSIS

OSMF is often fairly obviously diagnosed from the clinical features, and exclusively seen in people of Asian extraction. There is a history of betel chewing and often of slowly increasing trismus. Diagnosis can be confirmed if necessary by biopsy, and haematology often reveals coexistent anaemia (**Table 30.2**).

TREATMENT (see also Chs 4 and 5)

Patient information is an important aspect in management.

Management is first to stop areca nut use (**Table 30.3**). Correct any nutritional deficiencies, such as iron and vitamin B complex deficiencies. Asymptomatic cases should be observed only.

Table 30.2 Aids that might be helpful in diagnosis/prognosis/management in some patients suspected of having submucous fibrosis*

In most cases	In some cases
Biopsy	Full blood count and haemoglobin Oesophagoscopy

*See text for details and glossary for abbreviations.

Table 30.3 Regimens that might be helpful in management of patient suspected of having submucous fibrosis

Regimen	Use in primary care	Use in secondary care (severe oral involvement)
Beneficial	Physiotherapy	
Likely to be beneficial	Cox-2 inhibitors Hyaluronidase Intralesional corticosteroids	
Unproven effectiveness	Lycopene Human placental extract Interferon gamma Pentoxifylline	Surgery
Supportive	Physiotherapy (jaw opening exercises) Correct any nutritional deficiencies, such as iron and vitamin B complex deficiencies	

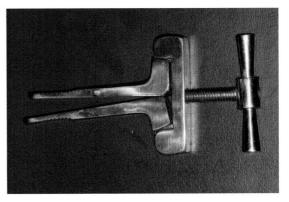

Fig. 30.2 Device used by a patient with OSFM to increase oral opening

There is no reliably effective treatment, and the condition is typically irreversible though some believe it may reverse if seen early and the betel habit stopped. Symptomatic cases with restricted opening respond best to physiotherapy to stretch the fibrous bands (Ch. 23; **Fig. 30.2**). Devices to help are described in Ch. 23.

Medical therapies range from topical medication (e.g. with COX-2 inhibitors); to intralesionally injected medicaments such as corticosteroids, collagenase, or hyaluronidase; to systemic medication with lycopene or pentoxifylline.

Surgical therapies range from laser release to excision of the bands and split skin, radial forearm or other flap repair.

FOLLOW-UP OF PATIENTS

Patients should be seen regularly by a health professional in view of the malignant potential.

USEFUL WEBSITES

Wikipedia, Oral submucous fibrosis. http://en.wikipedia. org/wiki/Oral_submucous_fibrosis

FURTHER READING

Ahmad, M.S., Ali, S.A., Ali, A.S., Chaubey, K.K., 2006. Epidemiological and etiological study of oral submucous fibrosis among gutkha chewers of Patna, Bihar, India. J. Indian Soc. Pedod. Prev. Dent. 24 (2), 84–89.

Ariyawardana, A., Athukorala, A.D., Arulanandam, A., 2006. Effect of betel chewing, tobacco smoking and alcohol consumption on oral submucous fibrosis: a case-control study in Sri Lanka. J. Oral. Pathol. Med. 35 (4), 197–201.

Chung-Hung, T., Shun-Fa, Y., Yu-Chao, C., 2007. The upregulation of cystatin C in oral submucous fibrosis. Oral. Oncol. 43 (7), 680–685.

Cox, S., Zoellner, H., 2009. Physiotherapeutic treatment improves oral opening in oral submucous fibrosis. J. Oral. Pathol. 38, 220–226.

Eipe, N., 2005. The chewing of betel quid and oral submucous fibrosis and anesthesia. Anesth. Analg. 100 (4), 1210–1213.

Fedorowicz, Z., Chan Shih-Yen, E., Dorri, M., 2008. Interventions for the management of oral submucous fibrosis. Cochrane Database Syst. Rev. (4): CD007156.

Gupta, S.C., Khanna, S., Singh, M., Singh, P.A., 2000. Histological changes to palatal and paratubal muscles in oral submucous fibrosis. J. Laryngol. Otol. 114 (12), 947–950.

Jacob, B.J., Straif, K., Thomas, G., et al., 2004. Betel quid without tobacco as a risk factor for oral precancers. Oral. Oncol. 40 (7), 697–704.

Kerr, A.R., Warnakulasuriya, S., Mighell, A.J., et al., 2011. A systematic review of medical interventions for oral submucous fibrosis and future research opportunities. Oral. Dis. 17 (Suppl. 1), 42–57.

Kumar, A., Bagewadi, A., Keluskar, V., Singh, M., 2007. Efficacy of lycopene in the management of oral submucous fibrosis. Oral. Surg. Oral. Med. Oral. Pathol. Oral. Radiol. Endod. 103 (2), 207–213.

Lin, S.C., Chung, M.Y., Huang, J.W., et al., 2004. Correlation between functional genotypes in the matrix metalloproteinases-1 promoter and risk of oral squamous cell carcinomas. J. Oral. Pathol. Med. 33 (6), 323–326.

Liu, C.J., Lee, Y.J., Chang, K.W., et al., 2004. Polymorphism of the MICA gene and risk for oral submucous fibrosis. J. Oral. Pathol. Med. 33 (1), 1–6.

Nayak, D.R., Mahesh, S.G., Aggarwal, D., et al., 2009. Role of KTP-532 laser in management of oral submucous fibrosis. J. Laryngol. Otol. 123 (4), 418–421.

Ni, W.F., Tsai, C.H., Yang, S.F., Chang, Y.C., 2007. Elevated expression of NF-κB in oral submucous fibrosis – evidence for NF-κB induction by safrole in human buccal mucosal fibroblasts. Oral. Oncol. 43 (6), 557–562.

Pandya, S., Chaudhary, A.K., Singh, M., et al., 2009. Correlation of histopathological diagnosis with habits and clinical findings in oral submucous fibrosis. Head Neck Oncol. 1 (1), 10.

Rajendran, R., Rani, V., Shaikh, S., 2006. Pentoxifylline therapy: a new adjunct in the treatment of oral submucous fibrosis. Indian J. Dent. Res. 17 (4), 190–198.

Reichart, P.A., Nguyen, X.H., 2008. Betel quid chewing, oral cancer and other oral mucosal diseases in Vietnam: a review. J. Oral. Pathol. Med. 37 (9), 511–514.

Reichart, P.A., Phillipsen, H.P., 1998. Betel chewer's mucosa – a review. J. Oral. Pathol. Med. 27 (6), 239–242.

Sur, T.K., Biswas, T.K., Ali, L., Mukherjee, B., 2003. Anti-inflammatory and anti-platelet aggregation activity of human placental extract. Acta Pharmacol. Sin. 24 (2), 187–192.

Tilakaratne, W.M., Klinikowski, M.F., Saku, T., et al., 2006. Oral submucous fibrosis: review on aetiology and pathogenesis. Oral. Oncol. 42 (6), 561–568.

Trivedy, C.R., Craig, G., Warnakulasuriya, S., 2002. The oral health consequences of chewing areca nut. Addict. Biol. 7 (1), 115–125.

Trivedy, C.R., Warnakulasuriya, K.A., Peters, T.J., et al., 2000. Raised tissue copper levels in oral submucous fibrosis. J. Oral. Pathol. Med. 29 (6), 241–248.

Tsai, C.H., Yang, S.F., Chen, Y.J., et al., 2004. Regulation of interleukin-6 expression by arecoline in human buccal mucosal fibroblasts is related to intracellular glutathione levels. Oral. Dis. 10 (6), 360–364.

Tsai, C.H., Yang, S.F., Chen, Y.J., et al., 2005. Raised keratinocyte growth factor-1 expression in oral submucous fibrosis in vivo and upregulated by arecoline in human buccal mucosal fibroblasts in vitro. J. Oral. Pathol. Med. 34 (2), 100–105.

Tsai, C.H., Yang, S.F., Chen, Y.J., et al., 2005. The upregulation of insulin-like growth factor-1 in oral submucous fibrosis. Oral. Oncol. 41 (9), 940–946.

Tu, H.F., Liu, C.J., Chang, C.S., et al., 2006. The functional (1171 5A>6A) polymorphisms of matrix metalloproteinase 3 gene as a risk factor for oral submucous fibrosis among male areca users. J. Oral. Pathol. Med. 35 (2), 99–103.

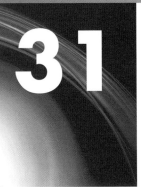

31 Cancer

Key Points

- Oral cancer is mostly squamous cell carcinoma (OSCC)
- OSCC is seen mainly in older men
- Risk factors include sun exposure (lips), tobacco, alcohol and betel use
- Most OSCC affects the lower lip, or margin of tongue
- OSCC usually manifests as a chronic mucosal lesion
- Oropharyngeal carcinoma is increasingly seen in younger people, and related to human papillomaviruses
- Diagnosis needs biopsy confirmation
- Treatment is with radiotherapy and/or surgery

INTRODUCTION

This is a potentially lethal condition; the chapter should be read along with Ch. 25.

Oral cancer accounts for a large proportion of cancers in the head and neck. Oral cancer affects mainly the lip or tongue but is classified according to site by the International Classification of Diseases (ICD):

- lip (ICD-10, C00)
- tongue (ICD-10, C01, C02) (**Fig. 31.1**)
- gum (ICD-10, C03)
- floor of the mouth (ICD-10, C04)
- unspecified parts of the mouth (ICD-10, C06), tonsil (ICD-10, C09), oropharynx (ICD-10, C10), and other ill-defined sites (ICD-10, C14).

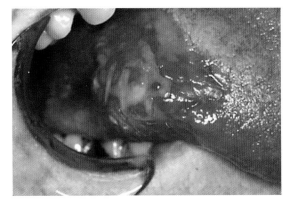

Fig. 31.1 Cancer of the tongue (squamous cell carcinoma) in a typical site

More than 90% of oral cancer is oral squamous cell carcinoma (OSCC) (**Box 31.1**) but other malignant oral neoplasms include:

- Epithelial malignancies:
  - other carcinomas
  - arising from a surface (e.g. melanoma)
  - maxillary antral carcinoma (or other neoplasms)
  - glandular (e.g. salivary gland malignant neoplasms)
  - intrabony epithelial (e.g. malignant odontogenic tumours).
- Lymphoreticular neoplasms: lymphomas rank second only to carcinoma in frequency in the head and neck region. The upper jaw, mandible, palate, vestibule and gingiva are, respectively, the most common locations. Swelling, ulceration, and radiographic demonstration of bone destruction are the most common signs.
- Sarcomas: rare but present at any age, have a rapid growth with extensive and ulcerated tumours, and may arise:
  - in bone (e.g. osteosarcoma)
  - in connective tissue (e.g. sarcoma)
  - in muscle (e.g. rhabdomyosarcoma)
  - from blood vessels (e.g. Kaposi sarcoma).
- Metastatic tumours:
  - within a lymph node (e.g. metastases from the mouth)
  - within bone (e.g. metastases from lung, breast, kidney, stomach, liver cancer), when most patients complain of swelling, pain and paraesthesia which develops in a relatively short period
  - in the oral soft tissues rarely. Early manifestation of gingival metastases may resemble a hyperplastic or reactive lesion.

ORAL SQUAMOUS CELL CARCINOMA (OSCC)

INTRODUCTION

Carcinoma (**Fig. 31.1**) is an epithelial lesion out of growth control, as shown by severe dysplasia extending through the full thickness of the epithelium with extension of the rete pegs into the underlying lamina propria (i.e. invasion across the epithelial basement membrane), with local invasion and eventual lymphatic and blood spread, leading ultimately to metastasis to lymph nodes, and organs (mainly liver, brain and bones).

INCIDENCE

OSCC is among the 10 most common cancers worldwide: around 300 000 new cases worldwide annually, amounting to around 3% of total cancers.

BOX 31.1 WHO classification of oral tumours

Malignant tumours
Odontogenic carcinomas
- Metastasizing (malignant) ameloblastoma 9310/3
- Ameloblastic carcinoma:
  - primary type 9270/3
  - secondary type (dedifferentiated), intraosseous 9270/3
  - secondary type (dedifferentiated), peripheral 9270/3
- Primary intraosseous squamous cell carcinoma:
  - solid type 9270/3
  - derived from keratocystic odontogenic tumour 9270/3
  - derived from odontogenic cysts 9270/3
- Clear cell odontogenic carcinoma 9341/3
- Ghost cell odontogenic carcinoma 9302/3

Odontogenic sarcomas
- Ameloblastoma fibrosarcoma 9330/3
- Ameloblastic fibrodentino- and fibro-odontosarcoma 9290/3

Benign tumours
Odontogenic epithelium with mature, fibrous stroma without odontogenic ectomesenchyme
- Ameloblastoma:
  - solid/multicystic type 9310/0
  - extraosseous/peripheral type 9310/0
  - desmoplastic type 9310/0
  - unicystic type 9310/0
- Squamous odontogenic tumour 9312/0
- Calcifying epithelial odontogenic tumour 9340/0
- Adenomatoid odontogenic tumour 9300/0
- Keratocystic odontogenic tumour 9270/0

Odontogenic epithelium with odontogenic ectomesenchyme, with or without hard tissue formation
- Ameloblastic:
  - fibroma 9330/0
  - fibrodentinoma 9271/0
  - fibro-odontoma 9290/0
- Odontoma: 9280/0
  - complex type 9282/0
  - compound type 9281/0
- Odontoameloblastoma 9311/0
- Calcifying cystic odontogenic tumour 9301/0
- Dentinogenic ghost cell tumour 9302/0

Mesenchyme and/or odontogenic ectomesenchyme with or without odontogenic epithelium
- Odontogenic:
  - fibroma 9321/0
  - myxoma/myxofibroma 9320/0
- Cementoblastoma 9273/0

Bone-related lesions
- Ossifying fibroma 9262/0
- Fibrous dysplasia
- Osseous dysplasia
- Central giant cell lesion (granuloma)
- Cherubism
- Aneurysmal bone cyst
- Simple bone cyst

Other tumours
- Melanotic neuroectodermal tumour of infancy 9363/0

Morphology code of the International Classification of Diseases for Oncology (ICD-O) (821) and the Systematized Nomenclature of Medicine (http://snomed.org). Behaviour is coded /0 for benign tumours, /3 for malignant tumours and /1 for borderline or uncertain behaviour.

Age

OSCC is seen predominantly in older patients (over 65 years), but intraoral cancer is increasing, especially in younger adults (under 45 years) and particularly in the oropharynx.

Gender

OSCC is seen predominantly in males, but the male/female differential is decreasing.

Geographic

There is marked inter-country variation in both the incidence of and mortality from OSCC.

There is growing evidence of intra-country differences in OSCC including ethnic differences in incidence and mortality.

- In the developing world, particularly South-East Asia and Brazil, the incidence of oral cancer is the highest in the world, but varies widely in different areas.
- In the developed world, the incidence of OSCC varies between countries and between different regions of the same country. For example, OSCC is more than twice as common in Scotland than in England and Wales and, even within Scotland, there are regional differences.

- In the Western world, parts of France and Newfoundland have the highest incidences, with about 10 times the incidence of OSCC in the UK.
- In Europe, OSCC is uncommon except in Eastern Europe and northern France where it is amongst the highest in the world.

PREDISPOSING FACTORS (RISK FACTORS) FOR OSCC

See Ch. 25 for a fuller discussion of risk factors. Lifestyle, environment and genetics may play a role but OSCC appears related mainly to a number of lifestyle factors (**Box 31.2**) which are adopted for their stimulant effects. OSCC is seen especially in the following groups (Ch. 25):

- tobacco users
- alcohol users
- betel quid users (some 20% of the world's population use betel)
- resource-poor groups
- ethnic minority groups.

Dietary, genetic and immunological factors may also play a part, since neither do all tobacco/alcohol users develop cancer, and equally nor do all patients with cancer have these habits.

Infections in the oral cavity such as herpesviruses, chronic candidosis, syphilis and poor oral hygiene, and periodontal disease, also link statistically with cancer. Human papillomaviruses (HPV), especially HPV-16, are implicated mainly in oropharyngeal cancer (tongue base: fauces). HPV-associated cancers are:

- often basaloid carcinomas
- associated with HPV-16 (90%): also types 18, 31, 33
- associated with reduced tumour suppressor gene expression (p53 and Rb genes)
- not linked to alcohol or tobacco use or poor oral health status
- possibly associated with a genetic element
- associated with a better prognosis than other OSCC.

HPV can be transmitted between the mouth and ano-genital region, and there are associations demonstrated between oral and ano-genital cancers. It seems irrefutable therefore, that at least some forms of oral cancer can be sexually shared. A vaccine against HPV is now administered to young people in an effort to prevent cervical cancer but the evidence however, as to any protective effect against OSCC, is not yet available.

Social deprivation is associated with an increased risk for oral cancer.

Diets rich in fresh fruits and vegetables and of vitamin A may have a protective effect on oral cancer and pre-cancer. No single dietary factor alone appears responsible: antioxidants may be anti-carcinogenic e.g. in green tea, but a Cochrane review concluded that the evidence is insufficient and conflicting. Similarly, any role of polyphenols abundant in vegetarian diets and recent reports of a protective effect of coffee, call for more investigation.

Genetics typically plays a minor role in OSCC but rare patients have a predisposition to develop multiple tumours because they have an inherited condition such as:

- Fanconi anaemia: a recessively inherited disease, characterized by congenital anomalies and bone marrow failure, and a predisposition to develop cancer, particularly squamous cell carcinomas in the head and neck and anogenital regions, and leukaemia.
- Dyskeratosis congenital: a disease of defective telomere maintenance, characterized by mucocutaneous abnormalities, bone marrow failure and cancer predisposition. Leukoplakias occur in approximately 80% of patients and typically involve the buccal mucosa, tongue, and oropharynx. Other sites may be involved (e.g. oesophagus, urethra, lacrimal duct, conjunctiva, anogenital). Patients have an increased prevalence of malignant disease, often squamous cell carcinoma within sites of leukoplakia (especially the tongue), or of the skin, Hodgkin lymphoma, gastrointestinal adenocarcinoma, bronchial and laryngeal carcinoma and leukaemia.
- Xeroderma pigmentosum: a rare disease of defective DNA repair mechanisms, predisposing to cancer in light-exposed areas such as skin and lips.
- Rare patients with a mutation in one allele of the tumour suppressor gene p53 locus (Li Fraumeni syndrome) have a predisposition not to OSCC but to breast cancer, brain tumours, leukaemia, and sarcomas – sometimes in the jaw.

Primary prevention

Possibly 75% of OSCC could be prevented by eliminating tobacco and alcohol use: smoking cessation reduces the increased risk by 35% within 5 years and by 80% by 20 years of quitting. Treatment of tobacco dependence is therefore important and can be addressed in primary care and smoking cessation clinics.

Protection against solar irradiation and photosensitisers could further reduce lip cancers.

Secondary prevention

A recent Cochrane review concluded that there is insufficient evidence to recommend screening of the general population for OSCC either by using visual examination or adjunctive tools (e.g. toluidine blue, brush biopsy, fluorescence imaging) to decrease mortality. The authors recommend regular screening by visual inspection by qualified healthcare providers for *high-risk* groups.

AETIOLOGY AND PATHOGENESIS

Potentially malignant (precancerous) disorders that can progress to OSCC are discussed in Ch. 25 and include, especially:

- actinic cheilitis (Ch. 26)
- erythroplasia (erythroplakia) (Ch. 27)
- leukoplakia (Ch. 28)
- lichenoid lesions (Ch. 29)
- submucous fibrosis (Ch. 30).

OSCC arises as a consequence of DNA mutations caused mainly by free radicals and oxidants, DNA mutations change various crucial genes and other nucleic acid components involved in cell growth and control (and are potential targets for anti-cancer therapies), such as:

- Tumour suppressor genes: such as p16 and p53 – control the fate of chromosomally damaged cells and the cell growth cycle.
- Oncogenes: such as the epidermal growth factor receptor (*EGFR*) gene, PRAD-1, Int-2, hst-1, bcl-1 and H-*ras* – involved in cell signalling.
- Telomerase genes: control telomerases – enzymes involved in chromosome shortening.
- MicroRNAs: non-coding pieces of RNA which are incorporated into the RNA-induced silencing complex which binds to mRNA to mediate gene expression.

The accumulation of genetic changes can lead to cell dysregulation to the extent that growth becomes autonomous and invasive mechanisms develop – this is carcinoma.

The neoplastic process manifests first intraepithelially (oral intraepithelial neoplasia) near the basement membrane as a focal, clonal overgrowth of altered keratinocyte stem cells, which expand upward and laterally, replacing normal epithelium.

After some time (sometimes years), invasion of the epithelial basement membrane signifies the start of invasive cancer (**Box 31.3**). Epithelial cells then proliferate into and invade the underlying tissues (**Fig. 31.2**). Cancer spread locally may cause pain and other symptoms (dysarthria, dysphagia, tooth mobility and halitosis) and, in many instances, leads ultimately to death. However, many people survive and many succumb from other diseases, or die after living with undetected (latent) cancer which has not impaired their lifespan.

Ultimately, cancer spreads (metastasizes) via lymphatics to regional lymph nodes, later by the blood stream to vital organs such as the lungs, brain, and liver and to bone and elsewhere.

CLINICAL FEATURES

OSCC usually presents as a single lesion persisting for >3 weeks but may present assuming a range of guises (**Table 31.1**, **Fig. 31.3**). PMD precedes some carcinomas (Ch. 25).

Lip cancer

- In the developed world, nearly 30% of all OSCC affects the lip: in some ways this can be regarded as a somewhat different disease to intraoral carcinoma.
- Lip cancer may follow chronic actinic cheilitis, induced by sunlight irradiation (Ch. 26). Photosensitisers such as antihypertensives may predispose.
- Lip cancer affects mainly the lower lip and has a far better prognosis than intraoral cancers.

Intraoral cancer

Most OSCC involve the lateral border of the tongue (**Fig. 31.4**) and/or the floor of the mouth, but the very invasive nature of these tumours can make it difficult to precisely define the site

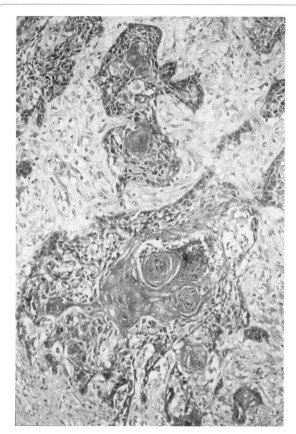

Fig. 31.2 Histopathology of squamous cell carcinoma showing islets of dysplastic epithelium and cell nests in lamina propria

---

BOX 31.3 Microscopic features of carcinoma

Disordered cell maturation
- Irregular hyperplasia and/or atrophy
- Keratosis/parakeratosis
- Drop-shaped rete processes
- Irregular stratification
- Disturbed cell polarity
- Premature and individual cell keratinization
- Reduced cell cohesion
- Cell pleomorphism

Disturbed cell proliferation
- Loss of basal cell polarity
- Basal cell hyperplasia
- Increased nuclear/cytoplasmic ratio
- Enlarged nucleoli
- Nuclear hyperchromatism
- Increased mitoses
- Anisonucleosis
- Abnormal mitoses
- Mitoses in stratum spinosum

Tissue changes
- Loss of regular epithelial stratification
- Reduced cell-to-cell cohesion
- Bullous or drop-shaped rete pegs
- Keratin or epithelial pearls

Invasion of the basement membrane

---

of origin. Nevertheless, most arise from the lower part of the mouth (**Figs 31.5** and **31.6**, **Table 31.2**) raising questions as to why this site appears predisposed to tumour development. Perhaps carcinogens pool in saliva in this so-called 'graveyard' or 'coffin' area?

Unfortunately, most OSCC are detected only when present for some weeks or months: most intraoral tumours are larger than 2 cm in diameter at presentation.

Carcinomas in the anterior mouth are usually detected at an earlier stage than are OSCC of the posterior oral cavity. In the developed world, some 25% of OSCC affects the tongue, and appears related largely to tobacco and/or alcohol use.

In the developing world, OSCC is most common in the buccal mucosa and arises mainly from betel use.

Second primary tumours

Although a primary OSCC usually presents as a single persistent lesion, patients with OSCC may develop other primary cancers in the upper aerodigestive tract (this includes the mouth, nose, pharynx, larynx, bronchi and lungs, and the oesophagus). These second primary tumours (SPTs) arise usually because smoking tobacco exposes the whole of the aerodigestive tract to carcinogens. SPTs appear either at the same time (synchronously – actually within 6 months of the diagnosis of the primary tumour), or later (metachronously, i.e. at least six months after the primary tumour) (**Table 31.3**). SPTs may be seen over 3 years in 15–25% (overall about 3% per year), of patients, and in up to 40% of those who continue to smoke.

Table 31.1 Features suggestive of OSCC

Features	Comment
Red lesion	Erythroplasia or erythroplakia may be associated
Mixed red/white lesion	Erythroleukoplakia may be associated
Irregular white lesion	Verrucous or nodular leukoplakia may be associated
Lump	Especially if enlarging and/or hard
Ulcer	Especially if persistent, or with fissuring or raised exophytic margins
Pain or numbness	May be a late feature
Abnormal blood vessels supplying a lump	
Tooth mobility	Or abnormal 'periodontal disease'
Extraction socket not healing	
Induration beneath a lesion	Firm infiltration beneath the mucosa
Fixation of lesion	To deeper tissues or to overlying skin or mucosa
Lymph node enlargement	Especially if there is hardness in a lymph node or fixation Enlarged cervical nodes in a patient with OSCC may be caused by infection, reactive hyperplasia secondary, or metastatic disease
Dysphagia	
Weight loss	

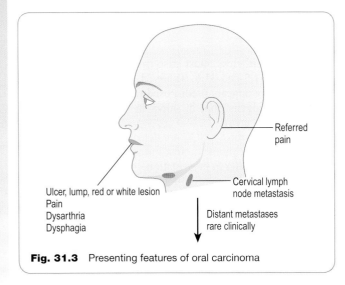

Fig. 31.3 Presenting features of oral carcinoma

Referred pain

Cervical lymph node metastasis

Distant metastases rare clinically

Ulcer, lump, red or white lesion
Pain
Dysarthria
Dysphagia

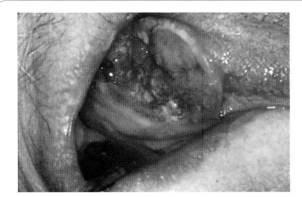

Fig. 31.4 Cancer of the tongue – an ulcerated indurated swelling

The carcinogens also circulate throughout the body to be excreted in urine and bile and thus, not surprisingly, can also lead to bladder cancer.

Other medical problems

Most patients with OSCC are older adults, many have been exposed to tobacco, betel, alcohol or a combination, and they are often also of resource-poor groupings, sometimes malnourished. Co-morbidities are therefore common, such as cardiovascular (e.g. hypertension and ischaemic heart disease), respiratory (e.g. obstructive airways disease) and hepatic (e.g. cirrhosis).

DIAGNOSIS

Early diagnosis is important, since it is generally accepted that prognosis is best in early carcinomas, especially those that are well-differentiated (**Box 31.4**); and treatment of an early OSCC is likely to be less invasive.

Single ulcers, lumps, red patches or white patches, particularly if any of these persist for >3 weeks, may be manifestations of frank malignancy and thus biopsy is invariably indicated. There should thus always be a high index of suspicion. The whole oral mucosa should be examined as there may be widespread dysplastic mucosa ('field change'), or SPTs, and the cervical lymph nodes must always be examined.

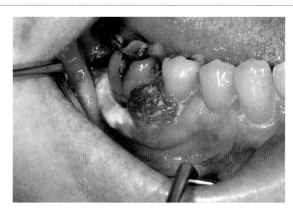

Fig. 31.5 Carcinoma on the gingiva

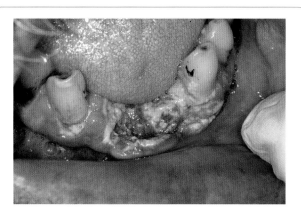

Fig. 31.6 Carcinoma on the alveolus

Table 31.2 Frequency of carcinoma at different sites

Location	Approximate % of all OSCC	Approximate % of intraoral OSCC
Lip	30	–
Tongue	25	45
Soft palate/trigone area	15	30
Hard palate	5	10
Gingiva	5	10
Buccal mucosa	2	5

Frank tumours should be inspected and palpated to determine the extent of spread.

Examination under general anaesthetic (EUA) may be indicated, particularly for patients with:

- tumours in the posterior tongue
- tumours where the margins cannot be readily defined
- an enlarged cervical node but no visible primary neoplasm. Positron emission tomography (PET) may be helpful to identify latent primary neoplasms. Biopsy of the tonsil or fossa of Rosenmuller may also be indicated.

Table 31.3 Location of second primary tumours in patients with oral squamous cell carcinoma

Within upper aerodigestive tract	Outwith upper aerodigestive tract
Larynx	Bladder
Lung	Breast
Oesophagus	Colon
Oral cavity	Lymphomas
Pharynx	Ovary
Trachea	Pancreas
	Skeletal bone
	Stomach
	Vulva

BOX 31.4 Grades of carcinoma

Well-differentiated
- Elongated rete pegs invading lamina propria, with keratin pearls

Moderately differentiated
- Irregular invading rete pegs; loss of cellular cohesion

Poorly differentiated
- Sheets of invading epithelium with no obvious architecture, but severe cellular abnormalities such as pleomorphism and hyperchromatism

- any suggestion of a SPT, as patients may then need panendoscopy of larynx, pharynx and oesophagus, and/or PET. Fluorodeoxyglucose PET (FDG-PET) will also help detect distant metastases.

OSCC should be staged according to the TNM (tumour, node, metastases) classification of the International Union against Cancer (UICC) – according to tumour size, nodal metastases and distant metastases (**Box 31.5**; **Table 31.4**) – since this classification relates well to overall survival rate (i.e. the earlier the stage of tumour, the better the prognosis and the less complicated and mutilating is the treatment).

Clinical palpation of the cervical lymph nodes is necessary but generally regarded as inaccurate (sensitivity and specificity 60–70%), and impalpable micrometastases may be present. Memorial Sloan-Kettering Cancer Center, USA developed the lymph node regional definitions most widely used today. To describe the lymph nodes of the neck (for neck dissection to remove nodes with metastases), the neck is divided into 6 areas called levels, identified by Roman numerals, increasing towards the chest (**Table 31.5**).

Investigations are indicated, the principles being to:

- Confirm the cancer diagnosis histopathologically.
- Determine if there is malignant disease elsewhere:
  - local invasion (e.g. bone, muscles or cervical regional lymph nodes)
  - metastases, which initially are to lymph nodes and later to liver, bone and brain. Imaging may detect abnormalities that escape clinical examination.
- SPTs: there is controversy as to the cost-effectiveness for endoscopy in all cases.

BOX 31.5   TNM classification*

Primary tumour size (T)
Tx No available information
   T0 No evidence of primary tumour
   Tis Only carcinoma in situ
   T1, T2, T3, T4 Increasing size of tumour[†]

Regional lymph node involvement (N)
Nx Nodes could not be or were not assessed
   N0 No clinically positive nodes
   N1 Single clinically positive homolateral node <3 cm in diameter
   N2 Single clinically positive homolateral node 3–6 cm in diameter, or multiple clinically positive homolateral nodes, none >6 cm in diameter
   N2a Single clinically positive homolateral node 3–6 cm in diameter

N2b Multiple clinically positive homolateral nodes, none >6 cm in diameter
   N3 Massive homolateral node(s), bilateral nodes or contralateral node(s)
   N3a Clinically positive homolateral node(s), one >6 cm in diameter
   N3b Bilateral clinically positive nodes
   N3c Contralateral clinically positive node(s)

Involvement by distant metastases (M)
Mx Distant metastasis was not assessed
   M0 No evidence of distant metastasis
   M1, M2, M3 Distant metastasis is present. Increasing degrees of metastatic involvement, including distant nodes

*Several other classifications are available, e.g. STNM (S, site).
[†]T1, maximum diameter 2 cm; T2, maximum diameter 4 cm; T3, maximum diameter >4 cm; T4, massive tumour >4 cm diameter, with involvement of antrum, pterygoid muscles, base of tongue or skin.

Table 31.4   Stage grouping and prognosis (see Box 31.5)

Stage		TNM		Approximate survival at 5 years (%)
0	Tis	N0	M0	>85
I	T1	N0	M0	85
II	T2	N0	M0	65
III	T1, T2	N1	M0	40
	T3	N0, N1	M0	
IVa	T1, T2, T3	N2	M0	10
	T4a	N0, N1, N2	M0	
IVb	Any T	N3	M0	
	T4b	Any N	M0	
IVc	Any T	Any N	M1	

Adapted from Sciubba (2001).

Ensure the patient is as prepared for major surgery, particularly in terms of their understanding and informed consent, general anaesthesia, potential blood loss and ability to metabolize drugs.

Address potential dental or oral problems pre-operatively, to minimize or avoid later complications.

These principles almost invariably mandate the following investigations (**Table 31.6**).

Lesional biopsy

An incisional biopsy is invariably required. An excisional biopsy should be avoided, since this is unlikely to have excised an adequately wide margin of tissue if the lesion is malignant, but will have destroyed clinical evidence of the site and character of the lesion.

The biopsy should be sufficiently large to include enough suspect and apparently normal tissue to give the pathologist a chance to make a diagnosis and not to have to request a further specimen. Most patients tolerate (physically and psychologically) one biopsy session, although it is never a particularly pleasant experience. Most biopsy wounds, whether 0.5 cm (too small) or 1.5 cm long (usually adequate) heal within 7–10 days. Therefore, it is better to take at least one ample specimen. Some authorities always take several biopsies at the first visit in order to avoid the delay and aggravation resulting from a negative pathology report in a patient who is strongly suspected to be suffering from a malignant neoplasm. If the pathology report denies malignancy, and yet clinically cancer is still the diagnosis, then the pathology should be re-checked and a re-biopsy may be indicated.

Table 31.5 Nomenclature of anatomical site of cervical lymph nodes

Level	Contents
I	Submental and submandibular triangles bounded by the posterior belly of the digastric muscle, the hyoid bone inferiorly and the body of the mandible superiorly
II	Upper jugular lymph nodes and extends from the level of the hyoid bone inferiorly to the skull base superiorly
III	Middle jugular lymph nodes from the hyoid bone superiorly to the cricothyroid membrane inferiorly
IV	Lower jugular lymph nodes from the cricothyroid membrane superiorly to the claviole inferiorly
V	Posterior triangle lymph nodes bounded by the anterior border of the trapezius posteriorly, the posterior border of the sternocleidomastoid muscle anteriorly and the clavicle inferiorly
VI	Anterior compartment lymph nodes from the hyoid bone superiorly to the suprasternal notch inferiorly. On each side the lateral border is formed by the medial border of the carotid sheath

Table 31.6 Aids that might be helpful in diagnosis/prognosis/management in some patients suspected of having cancer*

In most cases	In some cases
Biopsy	Angiography
Full blood picture	Doppler
Cervical node biopsy	Liver function tests
Jaw radiography	Panendoscopy
MRI head and neck	Psychological assessment
Ultrasound	Urea and electrolytes
Chest radiography or CT	
Blood pressure	
ECG	

*See text for details and glossary for abbreviations.

Radiography

- Jaw (often rotating pantomography or CT), which might demonstrate bone invasion
- Chest plain radiography or CT as a pre-anaesthetic check, especially in patients with known respiratory disease, and to demonstrate SPTs or metastases to lungs or hilar lymph nodes, ribs or vertebrae.
- MRI of the primary tumour site, of the head and neck, and of suspected sites of distant metastases, and of the neck to delineate the extent of cervical node metastases. Some units also routinely examine the chest and abdomen by MRI.
- PET/CT scans combine the advantages of CT for anatomy and PET for function, potentially producing an earlier diagnosis and more accurate staging. FDG-PET scan uses fluorodeoxyglucose, a modified sugar, that is absorbed by cancer cells which shows as a dark area on the scan.

- Ultrasound and biopsy or fine needle aspiration of neck lymph nodes that may contain metastases. Ultrasound guided fine needle aspiration cytology (US-guided FNAC) requires particular expertise and experience, but can have a sensitivity of 76% and a specificity of 100%.
- CT of the neck has a higher sensitivity in detecting metastatic disease in lymph nodes (69–93%) than physical examination. MRI is even better than CT but less readily available. PET/CT scanning is currently under evaluation.

In selected cases other investigations that may be indicated include:

- Bronchoscopy, if chest radiography reveals any lesions.
- Endoscopy of the upper aerodigestive tract, especially if there is a history of tobacco use.
- Gastroscopy, if a PEG (per-endoscopic gastrostomy) is to be used for feeding.
- Liver ultrasound, if there is hepatomegaly or abnormal liver function.
- Doppler duplex flow studies, in planning radial free forearm flaps.
- Angiography, in planning lower limb free flaps.
- Electrocardiography.
- Blood tests:
  - full blood picture and haemoglobin
  - blood for grouping and cross-matching
  - urea and electrolytes
  - liver function tests.

TREATMENT (see also Chs 4 and 5)
Patient communication

Patient communication and information are crucial aspects in management. One of the most difficult clinical situations in which clinicians find themselves is with the patient in whom serious disease, such as cancer, is suspected. If the patient is to be referred for a diagnosis and insists (rightly) on a full explanation as to why you need to refer for a second opinion, it is unwise for you to suggest a serious diagnosis to the patient. Better that you admit ignorance about the field and say that you are trained more to be suspicious, but doubt the lesion is anything to worry about, though you would be failing in your duty if you did not ask for a second opinion. That is what you would do for a member of your family – why should the patient be treated any the less?

Communication, especially breaking bad news such as about cancer well, can help all involved, and reduce the inevitable distress experienced. Hope is all-important and management must include especial attention to psychological reactions. Denial is common. Patients may or may not know, or may not want to know, that they have cancer and, even if they are aware of it, may not appreciate, or be willing to accept, the prognosis. Communication with partners, family and friends can be essential and, provided the patient consents, all close to the patient should be kept aware of:

- the intended outcomes
- prognosis
- how much the patient understands about their disease
- psychological reactions of the patient to cancer
- potential adverse effects of treatment.

Quality of life issues

Cancer survival rates have been, and are improving so more patients are living with cancer but also having to cope with the adverse effects of cancer and its treatment. OSCC and its management are associated with more physical, emotional and psychosocial disruption than is the case with some other tumours. This affects patients' 'quality of life' (QoL) and, while the aims of cancer treatment must ideally be to remove or destroy the tumour entirely, the outcome is a balance between this and adverse effects (of treatment and psychological sequelae).

Patients with OSCC may be aware they almost certainly face pain and swelling and at least some difficulties in eating, chewing, drinking, breathing, speaking, as well as possible changes in appearance and a common concern is fear of the cancer recurring. HRQoL is thus significantly affected. Psychosocial dysfunction is virtually invariably to be anticipated, and interventions needed. The main factors influencing HRQoL are radiotherapy, advanced clinical stage, socioeconomic status, patient age and access to oral healthcare.

Cancer to many, if not most, patients is a term that forebodes disaster – not unreasonably, since most have had relatives or friends who have died of the disease. The prognosis, at least of intraoral carcinoma, is not especially good, but little is gained by expressing this to the patient or relative. On the other hand, early lesions in otherwise healthy patients, especially those in sites such as the lip, have such a good prognosis that they can be said to be 'curable'. You must leave discussion of actual treatment and prognosis to the surgeon/oncologist concerned, as only they are in a position to give accurate facts to the patient concerned. If you are concerned, phone a specialist or fax, e-mail or write for an urgent opinion. If a cancer diagnosis has been established, it is reasonable to discuss with the patient, their partner and relatives that:

- tumours differ in their degree of malignancy
- their tumour has been detected at an early stage (hopefully)
- treatment is continually improving
- you have referred them to the best possible centre for treatment
- the oncological multidisciplinary team (MDT) will provide fuller details of treatment options.

Multidisciplinary cancer care

Cancer care planning is based upon an MDT offering:

- Medicine, cardiology, respiratory, dental, psychological, anaesthetic and, sometimes, palliative advice.
- Speech and language therapy advice: for pre-operative counselling regarding potential speech and swallowing rehabilitation.
- Dietary advice: to assess nutritional status and need for feeding by percutaneous gastrostomy (PEG).

The MDT plans the cancer treatment, including avoidance of postoperative complications – this includes planned oral and dental care such as discussions regarding restorative and surgical interventions required before cancer treatment, including osseointegrated implants and jaw reconstruction. Oral care is especially important when radiotherapy is to be given or bisphosphonates are used, since there is a liability complications, and a risk of osteonecrosis – the initiating factor for which is often trauma, such as tooth extraction, or ulceration from an appliance, or oral infection. As much as possible of dental treatment should be completed before starting cancer treatment.

Cancer treatment planning is based on:

- tumour size, nodal status and metastases
- balance of benefit of a particular treatment and its potential adverse reactions
- co-existent medical conditions
- social circumstances
- most importantly, the wishes of the patient.

Generally speaking, surgery alone or with post-operative radiotherapy remains the main treatment for OSCC since the adverse effects of therapeutic radiotherapy (RT) and chemotherapy (CTX), are generally greater (**Table 31.7**; **Box 31.6**) though targeted CTX is improving rapidly. OSCC is thus treated largely by surgery and/or RT to control the primary tumour and metastases in the draining cervical lymph nodes with a considered balance between length of survival and the quality of remaining life.

Table 31.7 Treatments for oral cancer

Regimen	Use in secondary care
Beneficial	Surgery
	Radiotherapy
Likely to be beneficial	Chemotherapy
	Robotic surgery
	Conformal radiotherapy
Emergent treatments	Targeted therapies (Table 31.9)
Supportive	Speech therapy
	Dietetics

BOX 31.6 Management of oral cancer

- Lip cancer: treated mainly surgically
- Intraoral cancers <4 cm in diameter: treated equally effectively by surgery or radiotherapy
  - T1 tumours: generally managed surgically
  - T2 tumours: generally managed surgically. However, tumours of the lateral margin of tongue may be treated by radiotherapy using external beam (40 Gy) plus radioactive iridium implants (25–30 Gy). For many patients, the treatment must include treatment of the lymph nodes in the neck and thus often the treatment of choice is surgery (tumour excision with radical neck dissection), together with radiotherapy
  - T3 tumours: generally treated by surgery followed by radiotherapy if there is extracapsular spread or multiple lymph node involvement. For many patients, the treatment must include treatment of the lymph nodes in the neck and thus often the treatment of choice is surgery (tumour excision with radical neck dissection), together with radiotherapy
  - T4 tumours: may be treated with chemo-radiotherapy. Drugs used include cisplatin, fluorouracil (5-Fu) taxanes and methotrexate. TPF is a common regimen (taxane platinum, 5-Fu)

Surgery

Advantages of surgery include the possibilities of:

- complete tumour and lymph node excision with full histological examination
- removal of involved bone
- use for radio-resistant tumours.

Disadvantages of surgery are mainly that it is mutilating for very large tumours and there is, in any event, perioperative mortality and morbidity, but modern techniques have significantly decreased these and the aesthetic and functional defects.

Surgery attempts to achieve more than one of the following goals:

- Cure: the excision of a tumour confined to one area. Surgery may be used along with RT and/or CTX given before, during or after surgery. Transoral laser microsurgery is an innovation for complete resection of tumours with preservation of function (organ preservation). Neck dissection to clear the neck of cancer containing lymph nodes is often also needed in addition to the excision of the primary tumour. Initially radical and leading to complications such as pain and damage to the spinal accessory nerve, currently neck dissection is function-preserving, resulting in less frequent and less severe neck and shoulder pain, less disability, less depression and with less pain and better QoL. The types of neck dissection are:
  - radical neck dissection (RND): removal of all ipsilateral cervical lymph node groups from levels I through V, together with spinal accessory nerve (SAN), sternocleidomastoid muscle (SCM), and internal jugular vein (IJV)
  - modified radical neck dissection (MRND): removal of all lymph node groups routinely removed in a RND, but with preservation of one or more nonlymphatic structures (SAN, SCM and IJV)
  - selective neck dissection (SND) (together with the use of parentheses to denote the levels or sublevels removed): cervical lymphadenectomy with preservation of one or more lymph node groups that are routinely removed in a RND. Thus for OSCC, SND (I–III) is commonly performed
  - extended neck dissection: removal of one or more additional lymph node groups or nonlymphatic structures, or both, not encompassed by the RND.
- The concept of sentinel lymph node (SLN) biopsy has gradually been established in the management of early oral cancer to establish whether neck dissection is required (Ch. 3).
- Reconstruction: crucially important to restore appearance and/or the function (e.g. the use of tissue flaps, bone grafts, or prosthetic materials).
- Debulking: used when removing a tumour entirely would cause too much damage to an organ or vital structures.
- Palliation: used to treat complications of advanced disease, not to cure.

PRINCIPLES

The principles of most cancer surgery are to:

- Remove the whole tumour:
  - ablative surgery excises the cancer with at least a 2 cm margin of clinically normal tissue, to try and ensure no tumour remains. Radical neck dissection, for the same reason, removes also the internal jugular vein, lymphatics

and accessory nerve, as well as the cervical sensory nerves and the sternomastoid, omohyoid and, often, digastric muscles.

- Retain as much normal anatomy and function as possible. 'Functional' neck dissection, preserving the above vital structures is gaining popularity; moderate-dose radiotherapy is, therefore, sometimes used to 'sterilize' such necks of residual cancer cells.
- Permit normal breathing – tracheostomy (**Fig. 31.7**) may be necessary.
- Support alimentation (feeding) – often via nasogastric tube or a PEG (**Fig. 31.8**).

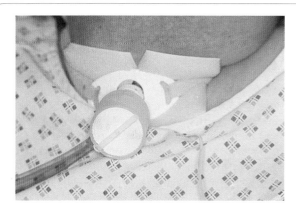

Fig. 31.7 Tracheostomy

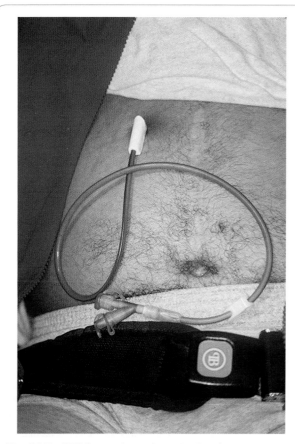

Fig. 31.8 PEG (per-endoscopic gastrostomy)

- Reconstruct to achieve acceptable function and cosmetics. From both the operator's and the patient's and family's viewpoint, reconstruction is best performed at the time of initial surgery, but must be tailored to the patient's ability to cope with a long operation (up to 10h or more) and the risk of significant morbidity. For soft tissue reconstruction, local flaps (e.g. nasolabial flaps) can repair small defects. Distant flaps are required to repair larger defects; these include:
  - free flaps: microvascular surgery facilitates excellent reconstruction at a single operation using, for example, forearm flaps based on radial vessels which are particularly useful to replace soft tissue, or those based on the fibula where bone is required
  - pedicle flaps: myocutaneous or osteomyocutaneous flaps based on a feeding vessel to muscle and perforators to the skin paddle, e.g. flaps based on the pectoralis major, latissimus dorsi or trapezius are now used in a one-stage operation to replace skin and, since they also contain muscle, they have adequate bulk to repair defects and may also be used to import bone (usually rib)
  - hard tissue: mandibular defects are reconstructed with implants to maintain aesthetics and anatomy temporarily until the patient is tumour free and bone grafting possible. Bone is traditionally taken as free non-vascularized bone grafts from the iliac crest or rib, but these often show poor survival in a contaminated area like the mouth, or in a relatively avascular field after irradiation. An osteomyocutaneous flap, such as a fibula graft, greatly improves the vascular bed for the graft, but is time consuming and requires considerable expertise. Maxillary defects are reconstructed with an obturator (bung), which has the advantage that the cavity can be readily inspected.

COMPLICATIONS OF SURGERY

See Ch. 54.

Radiotherapy

Advantages of RT include the facts that:

- normal anatomy and function are maintained
- general anaesthesia is not needed
- salvage surgery is still available if radiotherapy fails.

Disadvantages of RT may include mainly that:

- subsequent surgery is more difficult and hazardous and survival further reduced
- failure is probably because of cancer cell repopulation and hypoxia
- cure is uncommon for large cancers
- adverse effects are common with conventional RT which causes significant acute (during and up to 3 months post-radiation), and late, toxicities (Ch. 54).

PRINCIPLES

RT is an extremely effective treatment for OSCC, sometimes as a primary modality or as an adjuvant following surgery. RT may be used as the sole treatment modality for primary oral cancers without obvious lymph node involvement and also for inoperable tumours.

X-rays were the first form of photon radiation to be used to treat cancer. The higher the energy of the X-ray beam, the deeper X-rays penetrate the target. The daily dose must be enough to destroy cancer cells while sparing normal tissues of excessive radiation: typically 2 Gy is delivered daily to a 64–70 Gy total dose (Gray (Gy) = energy absorption of 1 joule/kg (1 Gy = 100 rads)).

Planning before RT includes CT scan and measurements of the area to be treated, as well as skin markings to help treatment positioning. A mask immobilizes the patients' head so that RT will only be delivered to specifically designated areas. Most of this time is spent ensuring that blocking devices, which restrict the RT to the appropriate area, are properly located, and patient and machine properly positioned. RT can be given by different techniques (**Table 31.8**).

INTENSITY MODULATED RADIOTHERAPY (IMRT, CONFORMATIONAL OR 3D RADIATION)

IMRT uses 3D computerized treatment planning and conformal therapy with X-ray accelerators to deliver radical RT to the target while sparing most normal tissue, thereby reducing toxicities and improving outcomes in patients with OSCC, and their QoL. IMRT irradiates irregularly-shaped volumes and can produce concavities in treatment volumes, thus permitting more precision and greater sparing of normal structures including;

- salivary glands, showing a significant reduction in hyposalivation
- pharyngeal constrictor muscles, therefore potentially reducing radiation-induced dysphagia.

Table 31.8 Types of radiation treatment

Type	Definition	Sub-types
External beam	Focus radiation (e.g. X-rays) on cancer Gamma rays are another form of photon radiation produced as elements (such as radium, uranium, and cobalt 60) decay	Linear accelerators produce X-rays of increasingly greater energy Intensity modulated radiotherapy (IMRT) Intensity graded radiotherapy (IGRT)
Particle beam radiation therapy	Fast-moving subatomic particles (neutrons, pions, and heavy ions) deposit more energy (high linear energy transfer or high LET) than do X-rays or gamma rays, causing more damage to targeted cells	Intensity modulated proton therapy (IMPT)
Internal radiotherapy	Radioactive implants placed directly into tumour (less radiation exposure to other body parts)	Brachytherapy, interstitial irradiation

- mucosa, thus reducing mucositis
- cochlea, with potential to reduce radiation-induced hearing loss
- optic nerves, brain stem, and spinal cord

IMRT can be optimized further using advances in the imaging techniques, i.e. image-guided radiotherapy.

IMAGE GUIDED RADIOTHERAPY (IGRT)

IGRT uses adaptive RT based on regular scanning and planning to reduce dosimetric uncertainties associated with the volume changes in tumours and organs at risk. FDG-PET is used to highlight proliferating areas of a tumour, and can guide dose escalation using IMRT. PET using two tracers (fluorine-18-labelled fluoromisonidazole (F-MISO) and copper (II)-diacetyl-bis(N(4)-methylthiosemicarbazone (Cu-ATSM)) can highlight hypoxic areas where the RT dose can be escalated without additional acute toxicity.

VOLUMATED INTENSITY MODULATED ARC THERAPY (VMAT)

VMAT delivers IMRT-like distributions in a single rotation of the gantry (e.g. RapidArc), potentially offering shorter planning and treatment time, better dose homogeneity and better sparing of normal tissue.

INTENSITY MODULATED PROTON THERAPY (IMPT)

IMPT permits 3D dose distributions using charged particles like protons, which deposit little energy until they reach the end of their range –when most of their energy is deposited in a small area. The advantages are of low radiation dose to normal tissue with tissue sparing, and better dose homogeneity.

COMPLICATIONS OF RADIOTHERAPY

See Ch. 54.

Chemotherapy

CTX use in OSCC has been restricted by adverse effects (toxicities). If the cancer is advanced (advanced stage III or stage IV) however, RT schedules sometimes include CTX, most commonly using cisplatin and cetuximab (a monoclonal antibody against epidermal growth factor receptor). Occasionally, other drugs used may include fluorouracil (5-FU), carboplatin, and paclitaxel.

Systemic CTX administered with radiotherapy (termed chemoradiotherapy; CRT) is given either:

- before (induction or neo-adjuvant chemotherapy),
- during (concomitant chemotherapy) or
- after (adjuvant chemotherapy).

Induction CTX using combinations of cisplatin and 5-fluorouracil (PF) is the most common regimen and gives a 5% improvement in 5-year survival.

COMPLICATIONS OF CHEMOTHERAPY

See Ch. 54.

Concomitant chemoradiotherapy

CRT has emerged as the 'standard of care' for organ preservation. CRT using single agent cisplatin improves locoregional control rates, and organ conservation. Most centres use a schedule of 2 cisplatin cycles, weekly low dose cisplatin or single agent carboplatin. Combinations of paclitaxel and carboplatin weekly, 5-fluouracil (5-FU) and carboplatin and 5-FU and mitomycin-C are other choices.

High-dose intra-arterial cisplatin and CRT (RADPLAT) may minimize drug toxicity by using simultaneous intravenous infusion of the neutralizing agent sodium thiosulphate.

Drugs may act as radiosensitizers however, and increase the mucositis produced by RT, and this is seen especially with regimens involving:

- cisplatin and fluorouracil
- cisplatin, epirubicin and bleomycin
- carboplatin.

Newer targeted cancer therapies

Therapies being developed to target specific molecules and pathways in carcinogenesis are shown in **Table 31.9**. Generally speaking, targeted therapies have less severe adverse effects than does conventional CTX but if combined with conventional CTX, adverse effects (such as oral ulceration) may actually be increased.

Epidermal growth factor receptor (EGFR) inhibitors (EGFRI) affect signal transduction pathways, thereby inhibiting cell proliferation. The main EGFRI are cetuximab and panitumumab (**Table 31.9**). Erlotinib and gefitinib are small molecule tyrosine kinase inhibitors (TKIs) of EGFR. Lapatinib is a TKI active against EGFR and Her-2. Cetuximab combined with RT versus RT alone, showed comparable toxicities except for higher incidences of acneiform rashes, mucosal toxicity and infusion reactions. Panitumumab can induce stomatitis. Combining CTX with TKIs makes scientific sense as both agents are active in head and cancer and have different mechanisms of action, but gefitinib in combination with CTX (docetaxel and carboplatin), produces mucositis and myelosuppression in many patients.

Anti-angiogenic approaches with mTOR (mammalian target of rapamycin (sirolimus)) inhibitors such as everolimus, temsirolimus and deforolimus or anti-vascular endothelial growth factor (VEGF) antibodies, which inhibit VEGF, also show some promise. Aphthous-like ulcers are their most common adverse effects. Bevacizumab is a monoclonal antibody against VEGF, which can cause stomatitis and impaired wound healing. Sunitinib maleate is a TKI of VEGF and platelet derived growth factor (PDGF), which may induce stomatitis or dysguesia, or dry mouth. Trastuzumab, a MAb against HER2 can cause mucositis and neuropathy. Imatinib and sorafenib can cause pigmentation or taste changes.

Table 31.9 Targeted therapies for oral cancer*

Therapies	Examples
EGFR inhibitors	Cetuximab, panitumumab, erlotinib in combination with gemcitabine
mTOR inhibitors	Deforolimus, rapamycin (sirolimus) and temsirolimus
TKIs of PDGF	Imatinib
Raf multi-kinase inhibitors	Sorafenib
TKIs of VEGF and PDGF	Sunitinib

*See text for explanation of abbreviations.

REHABILITATION

Cancer patients are understandably concerned primarily with ridding themselves of the tumour, but QoL, aesthetics and restoration of dignity and function are also extremely important. Feeding can be a problem and it may be necessary to feed via perendoscopic gastrostomy (PEG) or an indwelling central venous (Hickmann) line. Attention is also required to speech, swallowing, oral hygiene and appearance, with prostheses, implants or camouflage in some cases. Physiotherapy is often required.

PROGNOSIS

Intraoral cancer should be one of the most readily detected neoplasms because of the easy access for clinical and biopsy examination, yet the prognosis is still little better than for lung cancer, i.e. an overall 5-year survival of only about 30%. Factors influencing prognosis include the following:

- Tumour factors:
  - grade: well-differentiated OSCC have better prognosis
  - stage: and depth of infiltration, size of tumour and presence of metastases adversely affect prognosis. Thus the prognosis for stage I tumours is around 85% 5-year survival, but this figure plummets to 10% in stage IV tumours. Patients still present for treatment after inordinate delays. Most present at a stage (stage II) when tumours are relatively advanced in size (T2 or more), but when there is little clinical evidence of local metastases to lymph nodes and only rarely are distant metastases detectable
  - thickness: deep tumours have a worse prognosis
  - site: prognosis is better where the cancer does not involve the floor of mouth, posterior tongue or maxilla.
- Lymph node factors (invasion, capsular rupture, nodal site, number of involved nodes). Nodal involvement decreases cure rates by around 50%.
- Patient factors. The prognosis is usually worse for:
  - male gender: possibly because of the somewhat later presentation of males for treatment, or because of associated medical problems. Many male patients with oral cancer are heavy smokers and drinkers, and some have cirrhosis and nutritional defects
  - age: the poor general health of some aged patients may limit their resistance to the disease or its treatment.
- Treatment factors:
  - quality of surgical margins: if excision margins are tumour-free, prognosis is better.

The major impact treatment has had on the prognosis of oral cancer has been in relation to improved anaesthetic and medical care. Apart from the general improved expertise of surgical care, planning, reconstructive surgery, RT and aftercare have also significantly improved.

USEFUL WEBSITES

PubMed Health, Oral cancer. http://www.ncbi.nlm.nih.gov/pubmedhealth/PMH0002030/

FURTHER READING

Anantharaman, D., Marron, M., Lagiou, P., et al., 2011. Population attributable risk of tobacco and alcohol for upperaerodigestive tract cancer. Oral Oncol. 47 (8), 725–731.

Bagan, J.V., Scully, C., 2011. Cancer of the mouth for the dental team; comprehending the condition, causes, controversies, control and consequences 5. Clinical features and diagnosis. Dent. Update 38, 209–211.

Barnes, L., Eveson, J.W., Reichart, P., Sidransky, D., 2005. WHO classification of tumours; pathology and genetics – head and neck tumours. IARC, Lyon.

Bradley, P.J., Ferlito, A., Genden, E.M., et al., 2006. Referral Guidelines for Suspected Cancer of the Head and Neck. Auris Nasus Larynx 33, 1–5.

Cancela-Rodríguez, P., Cerero-Lapiedra, R., Esparza-Gómez, G., et al., 2011. The use of toluidine blue in the detection of pre-malignant and malignant oral lesions. J. Oral Pathol. Med. 40 (4), 300–304.

Chen, Y.W., Lin, J.S., Fong, J.H., et al., 2007. Use of methylene blue as a diagnostic aid in early detection of oral cancer and precancerous lesions. Br. J Oral Maxillofac. Surg. 45 (7), 590–591.

Clark, J.R., Naranjo, N., Franklin, J.H., et al., 2006. Established prognostic variables in N0 oral carcinoma. Otolaryngol. Head Neck Surg. 135 (5), 748–753.

Colella, G., Cappabianca, S., Giudice, A., Scully, C., 2004. Liver ultrasound in oral squamous cell carcinoma. Oral Bioscience Med. 1, 55–60.

Conway, D.I., 2006. To screen or not to screen? Is it worth it for oral cancer? Evid. Based Dent 7 (3), 81–82.

Diz Dios, P., Scully, C., 2011. Cancer of the mouth for the dental team; comprehending the condition, causes, controversies, control and consequences 7. Staging and diagnostic clinical aids. Dent. Update 38, 354–356.

Friedman, G.D., Asgari, M.M., Warton, E.M., et al., 2012. Antihypertensive drugs and lip cancer in non-hispanic whites. Arch. Intern. Med. Aug 6 [Epub ahead of print].

Galeone, C., Tavani, A., Pelucchi, C., et al., 2010. Coffee and tea intake and risk of head and neck cancer: pooled analysis in the international head and neck cancer epidemiology consortium. Cancer Epidemiol. Biomarkers Prev. 19 (7), 1723–1736.

Genden, E.M., Ferlito, A., Bradley, P.J., et al., 2003. Neck disease and distant metastases. Oral Oncol. 39, 207–212.

Hashibe, M., Morgenstern, H., Cui, Y., et al., 2006. Marijuana use and the risk of lung and upper aerodigestive tract cancers:results of a population-based case-control study. Cancer Epidemiol. Biomarkers Prev. 15 (10), 1829–1834.

Heck, J.E., Berthiller, J., Vaccarella, S., et al., 2010. Sexual behaviours and the risk of head and neck cancers: a pooledanalysis in the International Head and Neck Cancer Epidemiology (INHANCE) consortium. Int. J. Epidemiol. 39 (1), 166–181.

Kerr, A.R., Sirois, D.A., Epstein, J.B., 2006. Clinical evaluation of chemiluminescent lighting: an adjunct for oral mucosal examinations. J. Clin. Dent. 17 (3), 59–63.

Kim, H.Y., Elter, J.R., Francis, T.G., Patton, L.L., 2006. Prevention and early detection of oral and pharyngeal cancer in veterans. Oral Surg. Oral Med. Oral Pathol. Oral Radiol. Endod. 102 (5), 625–631.

Kujan, O., Glenny, A.M., Oliver, R.J., et al., 2006. Screening programmes for the early detection and prevention of oral cancer. Cochrane Database Syst. Rev. CD004150.

Lavelle, C.L.B., Scully, C., 2005. The criteria to rationalize the control of oral cancer by population screening. Oral Oncol. 41, 11–16.

Lee, C.H., Lee, K.W., Fang, F.M., et al., 2011. The use of tobacco-free betel-quid in conjunction with alcohol/tobacco impacts early-onset age and carcinoma distribution for upper aerodigestive tract cancer. J. Oral Pathol. Med. Mar 8 [Epub ahead of print].

Lingen, M., Pinto, A., Mendes, R., et al., 2011. Genetics/epigenetics of oral premalignancy: current status and future research. Oral Dis. 17, 7–22.

Lubin, J.H., Muscat, J., Gaudet, M.M., et al., 2011. An examination of male and female odds ratios by BMI, cigarette smoking, and alcohol consumption for cancers of the oral cavity, pharynx, and larynx in pooled data from 15 case-control studies. Cancer Causes Control 22 (9), 1217–1231.

Macfarlane, T.V., Macfarlane, G.J., Oliver, R.J., et al., 2010. The aetiology of upper aerodigestive tract cancers among young adults in Europe: the ARCAGE study. Cancer Causes Control 21 (12), 2213–2221.

Mackenzie, J., Ah-See, K., Thakker, N., et al., 2000. Increasing incidence of oral cancer amongst young persons: what is the aetiology? Oral Oncol. 36, 387–389.

Martinez, E.M., Bagan, J.V., Scully, C., 2004. Evaluation of dental health and the need for dental treatment prior to radiotherapy in 83 patients with head and neck cancer. Oral Biosci. Med. 1, 181–185.

McKay, J.D., Truong, T., Gaborieau, V., et al., 2011. A genome-wide association study of upper aerodigestive tract cancers conducted within the INHANCE consortium. PLoS Genet. 7 (3), e1001333.

Meurman, J.H., Scully, C., 2011. Cancer of the mouth for the dental team; comprehending the condition, causes, controversies, control and consequences 3. Other risk factors. Dent. Update 38, 66–68.

Newton, J.T., Scully, C., 2011. Cancer of the mouth for the dental team; comprehending the condition, causes, controversies, control and consequences 8. Communicating about cancer. Dent. Update 38, 426–428.

Park, S.L., Lee, Y.C., Marron, M., et al., 2011. The association between change in body mass index and upper aerodigestive tract cancers in the ARCAGE project: multicenter case-control study. Int. J. Cancer 128 (6), 1449–1461.

Pastore, L., Fiorella, M.L., Fiorella, R., Lo Muzio, L., 2008. Multiple Masses on the Tongue of a Patient with Generalized Mucocutaneous Lesions. PLoS Med. 5 (11), e212.

Petti, S., Scully, C., 2005. Oral cancer: the association between nation-based alcohol-drinking profiles and oral cancer mortality. Oral Oncol. 41, 828–834.

Petti, S., Scully, C., 2005. The role of the dental team in preventing and diagnosing cancer; 5. risk factor reduction –alcohol cessation. Dent. Update 32, 454–455, 458–460, 462.

Porter, S.R., Scully, C., 2001. Oral malignancy and potential malignancy; good referrals benefit patients. Dent. Pract. 39, 15–16.

Renaud-Salis, J.L., Blanc-Vincent, M.P., Brugere, J., et al., 2001. Epidermoid cancers of the oropharynx. Br. J. Cancer 84 (Suppl. 2), 37–41.

Richiardi, L., Corbin, M., Marron, M., et al., 2012. Occupation and risk of upper aerodigestive tract cancer: The ARCAGE study. Int. J. Cancer 130 (10), 2397–2406.

Sciubba, J.J., 2001. Oral cancer. The importance of early diagnosis and treatment. Am. J. Clin. Dermatol. 2, 239–251.

Scully, C., 2001. Aetiopathogenesis of intraoral squamous cell oral carcinoma. Continuing Professional Development in Dentistry 2, 9–13.

Scully, C., 2005. Oral cancer; the evidence for sexual transmission. Br. Dent. J. 199, 203–207.

Scully, C., Bagan, J., 2009. Oral squamous cell carcinoma: overview of current understanding of aetiopathogenesis and clinical implications. Oral Dis. 15, 388–399.

Scully, C., Bagan, J.V., Newman, L.N., 2005. The role of the dental team in preventing and diagnosing cancer. 3. Oral cancer diagnosis and screening. Dent. Update 32, 326–337.

Scully, C., Bedi, R., 2000. Ethnicity and oral cancer. Lancet Oncol. 1, 37–42.

Scully, C., Boyle, P., 2005. The role of the dental team in preventing and diagnosing cancer; 1. Cancer in general. Dent. Update 32, 204–212.

Scully, C., Epstein, J., Sonis, S., 2003. Oral mucositis: A challenging complication of radiotherapy, chemotherapy, and radiochemotherapy: Part 1, pathogenesis and prophylaxis of mucositis. Head Neck 25, 1057–1070.

Scully, C., Epstein, J., Sonis, S., 2004. Oral mucositis; A challenging complication of radiotherapy, chemotherapy, and radiochemotherapy: Part 2, diagnosis and management of mucositis. Head Neck 26, 77–84.

Scully, C., Field, J.K., Tanezawa, H., 2000. Genetic aberrations in oral or head and neck squamous cell carcinoma (SCCHN). 1. Carcinogen metabolism, DNA repair and cell cycle control. Oral Oncol. 36, 256–263.

Scully, C., Field, J.K., Tanezawa, H., 2000. Genetic aberrations in oral or head and neck squamous cell carcinoma (SCCHN). 2. Chromosomal aberrations. Oral Oncol. 36, 311–327.

Scully, C., Field, J.K., Tanezawa, H., 2000. Genetic aberrations in oral or head and neck squamous cell carcinoma (SCCHN). 3. Clinico-pathological applications. Oral Oncol 36, 404–413.

Scully, C., Newman, L.N., Bagan, J.V., 2005. The role of the dental team in preventing and diagnosing cancer; 2. Oral cancer risk factors. Dent. Update 32, 261–274.

Scully, C., Warnakulasuriya, S., 2005. The role of the dental team in preventing and diagnosing cancer; 4. Risk factor reduction – tobacco cessation. Dent. Update 32, 394–401.

Scully, C., Warnakulasuriya, S., 2010. Cancer of the mouth for the dental team; comprehending the condition, causes, controversies, control and consequences 1. General Principles. Dent. Update 37, 638–640.

Scully, C., 2002. Oral squamous cell carcinoma; from an hypothesis about a virus, to concern about possible sexual transmission. Oral Oncol. 38, 227–234.

van der Waal, I., Scully, C., 2011. Cancer of the mouth for the dental team; comprehending the condition, causes, controversies, control and consequences. 4. Potentially malignant disorders of the oral and oropharyngeal mucosa. Dent. Update 38, 138–140.

van der Waal, I., Scully, C., 2011. Cancer of the mouth for the dental team; comprehending the condition, causes, controversies, control and consequences. 6. Co-morbidities. Dent.Update 38, 283–284.

Warnakulasuriya, S., Scully, C., 2010. Cancer of the mouth for the dental team; comprehending the condition, causes, controversies, control and consequences. 2. Main risk factors and epidemiology. Dent. Update 37, 710–712.

Warnakulasuriya, S., Sutherland, G., Scully, C., 2005. Tobacco, oral cancer, and treatment of dependence. Oral Oncol. 41, 244–260.

Watters, A.L., Epstein, J.B., Agulnik, M., 2011. Oral complications of targeted cancer therapies; a narrative literature review. Oral Oncol 47, 441–448.

Xu, G.Z., Guan, D.J., He, Z.Y., 2011. (18)FDG-PET/CT for detecting distant metastases and second primary cancers in patients with head and neck cancer. A meta-analysis. Oral Oncol. 47 (7), 560–565.

Xu, G.Z., Zhu, X.D., Li, M.Y., 2011. Accuracy of whole-body PET and PET-CT in initial M staging of head and neck cancer: a meta-analysis. Head Neck 33 (1), 87–94.

COMMON AND IMPORTANT OROFACIAL CONDITIONS

Body and soul cannot be separated for purposes of treatment, for they are one and indivisible.
Sick minds must be healed as well as sick bodies.

C. Jeff Miller

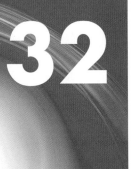

32 Angioedema

Key Points

- Angioedema is acute oral or facial swelling
- Neck oedema may hazard the airway
- Most cases are allergic
- Emergency treatment is with intramuscular adrenaline (epinephrine)

INTRODUCTION

This is a potentially lethal condition. Angioedema manifests with rapid development of oedematous swelling of the lip(s), tongue and oral or facial swelling (**Fig. 32.1**). This can be life-threatening as oedema may also involve the neck and hazard the airway. The swelling in angioedema is usually relatively transient and the skin does not scale.

Angioedema is usually allergic (a type 1 hypersensitivity response seen mainly in those with an atopic tendency) but can rarely be drug-induced, hereditary (hereditary angio-neurotic oedema or HANE; caused by a deficiency of the complement component C1 esterase inhibitor – C1-INH) or C1-INH deficiency can be acquired.

All types of angioedema may be aggravated by the oral contraceptive pill or hormone replacement therapy.

ALLERGIC ANGIOEDEMA

INCIDENCE

Allergic angioedema is common – far more common than HANE.

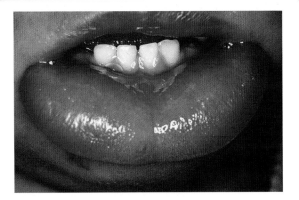

Fig. 32.1 Lip swelling in angioedema

Age

It occurs mainly in adults.

Gender

It is most prevalent in females.

Geographic

No known geographic incidence.

AETIOLOGY AND PATHOGENESIS

Allergic angioedema is a type 1 hypersensitivity reaction that may be induced by:

- Foods: nuts are a well-known cause but many other foods (e.g. shellfish, eggs, milk) may be implicated
- Latex
- Drugs (Table 54.20), especially:
  - antibiotics
  - aspirin
- Other allergens – such as radiocontrast media, hepatitis B immunization, and insect bites/stings.

It is IgE mediated and causes mast cell activation and degranulation, with release of histamine and bradykinin, causing vasodilatation and increased vascular permeability. The C4 complement component is consumed and thus plasma levels fall, but the levels of C1 and C3 are usually normal.

CLINICAL FEATURES

- The acute oedema, which appears < 2 h of antigen exposure, can cause pronounced itchy labial and periorbital swelling, and can involve any oral site, but when oedema involves the tongue and neck and extends to the larynx, it can cause rapidly fatal respiratory obstruction.
- Acute allergic oedema usually develops along with urticaria ('hives') and may be associated with anaphylactic reactions.

DIAGNOSIS

Angioedema is diagnosed clinically and from a history of atopic disease and/or exposure to allergen, and sometimes by allergy testing (prick test), but only where there are appropriate resuscitation facilities and an emergency kit containing injectable adrenaline at hand. Mast cell tryptase levels may be raised. Hereditary angioedema (HANE) may need to be excluded – HANE has low C4, but normal C3 levels, and absence of C1-INH activity (**Table 32.1**).

Table 32.1 Aids that might be helpful in diagnosis/prognosis/management in some patients suspected of having angioedema*

In most cases	In some cases
Serum complement C3 and C4 levels	Full blood picture
C1 esterase Inhibitor activity	ESR

*See text for details and glossary for abbreviations.

TREATMENT (see also Chs 4 and 5)

Although the swelling is of acute onset and often only mild and transient, there is always the potential of obstruction of the airway, and thus urgent treatment is indicated (**Table 32.2**). If the airway is threatened, urgent hospital care is required and intubation may be needed.

- In severe cases, especially if there is any potential or real threat to the airway, the emergency should be managed with intramuscular adrenaline (epinephrine), and with systemic corticosteroids and/or antihistamines, such as chlorphenamine or loratidine.
- Mild angioedema may respond to antihistamines, or to a sympathomimetic agent, such as ephedrine, by mouth.
- The rare intractable chronic cases may respond to systemic corticosteroids.

DRUG-INDUCED (NON-ALLERGIC) ANGIOEDEMA

Non-allergic orofacial swelling can arise in response to drug exposure – especially to angiotensin converting enzyme (ACE) inhibitors – due to a rise in levels of bradykinins and/or altered levels or function of C1 esterase inhibitor. The reaction may manifest first only after many weeks of drug treatment. Other drugs that may also be responsible can include antidepressants, bupropion and NSAIDs (Table 54.20). People of African heritage may be at particular risk of this adverse drug reaction.

The swelling usually affects the lips, although it can be localized to the tongue, and is occasionally fatal. The causal drug should be immediately discontinued.

Management is to ensure a patent airway. Adrenaline, antihistamines, and corticosteroids may be indicated. Endotracheal intubation or tracheostomy is required in severe cases.

Table 32.2 Regimens that might be helpful in management of patient suspected of having allergic angioedema

Regimen	Use in primary and secondary care
Beneficial	Epinephrine (adrenaline)
Likely to be beneficial	Corticosteroids Antihistamines
Supportive	Avoid allergens

HEREDITARY ANGIOEDEMA (HANE: C1 ESTERASE INHIBITOR DEFICIENCY)

HANE mimics the other types of angioedema, but is usually a more severe reaction. Despite its hereditary nature, usually as an autosomal dominant trait, the disease may not present until later childhood or adolescence, and nearly 20% of cases are caused by spontaneous mutation.

INCIDENCE

It is uncommon.

Age

It can occur at any age.

Gender

It occurs equally in both sexes.

Geographic

No known geographic incidence.

PREDISPOSING FACTORS

A genetically determined mutation in the SERPING1 gene results in deficiency of an inhibitor of the enzyme C1 esterase (C1-INH) (Type I), or C1-INH is dysfunctional (Type II). Type III is X-linked and seen in women in relation to pregnancy or oral contraceptive pill (OCP) use linked with F12 gene mutations which encodes blood coagulation factor XII. Autoimmune C1-INH deficiency most commonly arises in B-cell lymphoproliferative disorders. In all these types of angioedema, there is continued complement activation after trauma, and activation of kinin-like substances that cause a sudden increase in capillary permeability (**Fig. 32.2**).

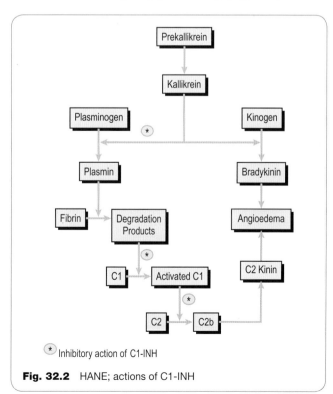

* Inhibitory action of C1-INH

Fig. 32.2 HANE; actions of C1-INH

Alcohol or cinnamon, which are vasodilators, may increase the likelihood of an attack in susceptible patients, as may NSAIDs. Some attacks follow emotional stress.

CLINICAL FEATURES OF C1-INH DEFICIENCY

- Blunt injury is the most consistent precipitating event: the trauma of dental treatment is a potent trigger.
- Abdominal pain, nausea or vomiting, diarrhoea, rashes and peripheral oedema sometimes herald an attack.
- There is an acute onset of non-itchy or painful oedema affecting the lips, tongue, mouth, face and neck region, the extremities and the gastrointestinal tract – with abdominal pain and sometimes diarrhoea. There may be a leukocytosis.
- Angioedema may persist for many hours and even up to 4 days and, throughout, involvement of the airway is a constant threat.
- The mortality may be as high as 30% in some families, but the disease is compatible with prolonged survival if emergencies are avoided or effectively treated.

DIAGNOSIS

Diagnosis of HANE is made from (**Table 32.1**):

- family history
- clinical features with a history of oedema after trauma
- blood tests: low C4, but normal C3 levels, and absence of C1-INH activity. In 85% of cases C1-INH levels are reduced (type I HANE), but in 15% C1-INH is present though dysfunctional (type II HANE).

TREATMENT (see also Chs 4 and 5)

Precipitants should be avoided where possible.

There is no beneficial response to corticosteroids or antihistamines. Management is by avoiding precipitants, and with C1-INH replacement with concentrates. Other treatments include fresh plasma; plasminogen inhibitors, such as tranexamic acid; or androgenic steroids, such as danazol or stanazolol (**Table 32.3**).

EMERGENT TREATMENTS

Emerging treatments include a kallikrein inhibitor (ecallantide) or a bradykinin B2 receptor antagonist (icatibant).

FOLLOW-UP OF PATIENTS

Patients with HANE should be under specialist care.

Table 32.3 Regimens that might be helpful in management of patient suspected of having hereditary angioedema

Regimen	Use in secondary care (severe oral involvement and/or extraoral involvement)
Beneficial	C1-INH concentrates
Likely to be beneficial	Danazol Stanazolol Fresh plasma
Emergent treatments	Ecallantide Icatibant
Supportive	Avoid trauma, stress, alcohol and NSAIDs

USEFUL WEBSITES

US Hereditary Angioedema Association: http://www.haea.org/

FURTHER READING

Bouillet, L., 2011. Icatibant in hereditary angioedema: news and challenges. Expert Rev. Clin. Immunol. 7 (3), 267–272.

Bowen, T., Cicardi, M., Farkas, H., et al., 2010. International consensus algorithm for the diagnosis, therapy and management of hereditary angioedema. Allergy Asthma Clin. Immunol. 6 (1), 24.

Chiu, A.G., Newkirk, K.A., Davidson, B.J., et al., 2001. Angiotensin-converting enzyme inhibitor-induced angioedema: a multicenter review and an algorithm for airway management. Ann. Otol. Rhinol. Laryngol. 110, 834–840.

Dean, D.E., Schultz, D.L., Powers, R.H., 2001. Asphyxia due to angiotensin converting enzyme (ACE) inhibitor mediated angioedema of the tongue during the treatment of hypertensive heart disease. J. Forensic Sci. 46, 1239–1243.

Kandala, V., Playfor, S., 2003. Massive tongue swelling following the use of synthetic saliva. Paediatr. Anaesth. 13 (9), 827–828.

Kyrmizakis, D.E., Papadakis, C.E., Liolios, A.D., et al., 2004. Angiotensin-converting enzyme inhibitors and angiotensin II receptor antagonists. Arch. Otolaryngol. Head Neck Surg. 130 (12), 1416–1419.

Sinclair, D., Smith, A., Cranfield, T., Lock, R.J., 2004. Acquired C1 esterase inhibitor deficiency or serendipity? The chance finding of a paraprotein after an apparently low C1 esterase inhibitor concentration. J. Clin. Pathol. 57 (4), 445–447.

Sondhi, D., Lippmann, M., Murali, G., 2004. Airway compromise due to angiotensin-converting enzyme inhibitor-induced angioedema: clinical experience at a large community teaching hospital. Chest 126 (2), 400–404.

Angular cheilitis (angular stomatitis)

33

INTRODUCTION

Angular cheilitis is inflammation typically seen at both commissures (angles) of the lips (**Fig. 33.1**).

INCIDENCE

Angular cheilitis is common.

AGE

It occurs mostly in adults, particularly the older age group.

GENDER

It occurs in both males and females.

GEOGRAPHIC

No known geographic incidence.

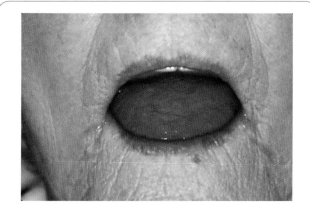

Fig. 33.1 Angular cheilitis – typical bilateral lesions

PREDISPOSING FACTORS

Angular cheilitis is most often chronic, seen in the older, and due to infective and/or mechanical causes. It is predisposed by what are known as the '3Ds' (**Fig. 33.2**):

- Dental appliance or denture-wearing, denture-related stomatitis and disorders that predispose to candidosis:
  - dry mouth
  - tobacco smoking.
- Deficiency states, such as:
  - deficiency anaemias
  - iron deficiency
  - hypovitaminoses (especially B)
  - malabsorption states (e.g. Crohn disease) or eating disorders
  - possibly zinc deficiency, but only rarely
  - immune defects, such as in Down syndrome, HIV infection, diabetes (**Figs 33.3** and **33.4**), cancer, immunosuppressed people, eating disorders and others.
- Disorders where the lip anatomical relationships are changed – such as when the vertical dimension of occlusion is reduced – or where lips are enlarged, such as in orofacial granulomatosis, Crohn disease and Down syndrome.

AETIOLOGY

A number of factors (infective, mechanical, nutritional or immunological) may be implicated alone or in combination.

- Most angular cheilitis is seen in older patients who are wearing a complete maxillary denture beneath which is denture-related stomatitis. Infective agents, mainly *Candida albicans* or *Staphylococcus aureus*, can be isolated in up to 54% of lesions. *Candida albicans* is the most commonly isolated and is typically carried in the saliva, and was probably responsible for some cases of cheilitis attributed

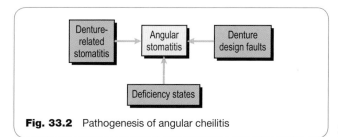

Fig. 33.2 Pathogenesis of angular cheilitis

223

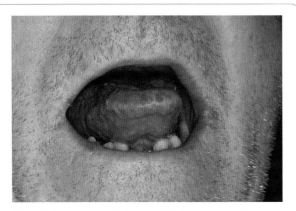

Fig. 33.3 Angular cheilitis in diabetes, same patient as shown in Fig. 33.4

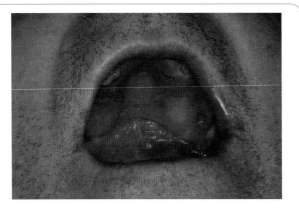

Fig. 33.4 Angular cheilitis in diabetes, same patient as shown in Fig. 33.3 showing denture stomatitis

to allergy to denture materials – since contamination of denture-material by *Candida* may cause false-positive patch-test reactions.

- Mechanical factors may play a part. As a consequence of ageing, the upper lip overhangs the lower at the angles of the mouth, producing a fold that keeps a small area of skin macerated. Infective agents are probably the major cause.
- Nutritional deficiencies that may underlie some cases include deficiency of haematinics (factors required for blood formation) or of immunity (which can lead to proliferation of *Candida* species and other micro-organisms). Dry mouth also predisposes to candidosis. Angular cheilitis is, very occasionally, an isolated initial sign of anaemia or iron or vitamin deficiency, but then more often there is also ulceration and glossitis.
- Immune deficiency such as in diabetes, Down syndrome, HIV disease or immunosuppressed patients may result in angular cheilitis associated with candidosis.

CLINICAL FEATURES

- The common complaints are of soreness, erythema and fissuring affecting the angles of the mouth symmetrically. Typically the condition persists or recurs. Angular cheilitis most commonly presents as roughly triangular areas of

erythema and oedema at both commissures. Atrophy, erythema, ulceration, crusting, and scaling may be seen. Lesions occasionally extend beyond the vermilion border onto the skin in the form of linear furrows or fissures radiating from the angle of the mouth (rhagades), mainly in the more severe forms, especially in denture wearers. An eczematous dermatitis may extend some distance onto the cheek or chin as an infective eczematoid reaction or as a reaction to topical medicaments. In long-standing lesions, suppuration and granulation tissue may develop.

- Commonly, there is also associated denture-related stomatitis.
- Rarely, there is also commissural candida-related leukoplakia intraorally.

DIAGNOSIS

- This is usually a clinical diagnosis, made by clinical examination. Maceration of the commissural epithelium can also be brought about by habitual licking as a nervous tic, or by sucking on objects (perleche), but this is not true angular cheilitis and the erythema usually extends well beyond the commissural areas and vermilion. Intraoral inspection in angular cheilitis may reveal palatal erythema caused by associated denture-related stomatitis, usually due to candidosis. An underlying nutritional deficiency may be revealed by a depapillated tongue (glossitis) in iron deficiency, a depapillated glossy red tongue in folate deficiency or a reddish-purple depapillated tongue in vitamin B deficiency. Angular cheilitis if accompanied by systemic features such as diarrhoea and non-specific oral ulcerations, most commonly of the tongue and buccal mucosa, may suggest Crohn disease, HIV infection or zinc deficiency. If the cheilitis is unilateral, a local cause (such as trauma), or a systemic problem (such as a split papule of syphilis), may be identifiable.
- In all cases of angular cheilitis in wearers of dental appliances, Candida should be sought not only in the lesions, but also from the appliance-fitting surface. The skin lesions should also be swabbed. Microbial cultures and a haematological workup (blood picture, and assays of levels of serum iron/ferritin, serum vitamin B_{12} and corrected red blood cell folate) are indicated when systemic involvement is suspected. Diagnosis is often supported by investigations, especially if there are associated lesions such as ulceration and/or glossitis (**Table 33.1**).

Table 33.1 Aids that might be helpful in diagnosis/prognosis/management in some patients suspected of having angular cheilitis (angular stomatitis)*

In most cases	In some cases
Full blood picture	Culture and sensitivity
Serum ferritin, vitamin B_{12} and corrected whole blood folate levels	CD4 counts
ESR	Serum zinc
Blood glucose	Serology for infections (HIV, syphilis)

*See text for details and glossary for abbreviations.

TREATMENT (see also Chs 4 and 5)

Management of angular cheilitis is sometimes difficult and therapy may need to be prolonged (**Table 33.2**):

- Tobacco habits should be stopped.
- Underlying systemic disease must be sought and treated: a course of oral iron and vitamin B supplements may be helpful in indolent cases.
- If infection is the cause of angular cheilitis, treatment will only be effective if the infection is also treated. Permanent cure can be achieved only by eliminating candidosis as well as the growth of Candida beneath, and in, the denture-fitting surface. Recurrence of angular cheilitis must be prevented, by eliminating organisms from their reservoir on the denture, so the dentures should be kept out of the mouth at night and disinfected in a candidacidal solution, such as hypochlorite. Denture-related stomatitis should be treated with an antifungal. Miconazole may be preferable (muco-adhesive buccal tablets applied locally, together with the oral gel) as it has some Gram-positive bacteriostatic action, but there is a high relapse rate unless treatment is prolonged. Miconazole is absorbed systemically and may occasionally potentiate the action of warfarin, phenytoin and the sulphonylureas. In patients taking these drugs, nystatin (as oral suspension) should, therefore, be tried first.
- Angular cheilitis should be treated with a topical antifungal (e.g. miconazole). Staphylococcus infection can be cleared with topical antibiotics, such as fusidic acid (fucidin) ointment or cream used at least four times daily. Mixed infections of Candida and Staphylococcus respond best to topical miconazole. Miconazole plus hydrocortisone cream, fucidin plus hydrocortisone cream, clotrimazole plus hydrocortisone cream, nystatin plus hydrocortisone cream, or clioquinol plus betamethasone cream, are other choices.
- Mechanical predisposing factors should be corrected. A change in dentures may be necessary; new dentures that restore facial contour may help. In rare intractable cases, surgery or, occasionally, collagen or silicone or other filler injections may be useful in trying to restore normal lip commissural anatomy.

Table 33.2 Regimens that might be helpful in management of patient suspected of having angular cheilitis

Regimen	Use in primary and secondary care
Beneficial	Miconazole Fucidin
Likely to be beneficial	Clioquinol
Supportive	Treat related denture stomatitis

USEFUL WEBSITES

Wikipedia, Angular cheilitis. http://en.wikipedia.org/wiki/Angular_cheilitis

FURTHER READING

Figueiral, M.H., Azul, A., Pinto, E., et al., 2007. Denture–related stomatitis: identification and characterisation of aetiological and predisposing factors – a large cohort. J. Oral Rehabil. 34, 448–455.

Golecka, M., Oldakowska-Jedynak, U., Mierzwinska-Nastalska, E., Adamczyk-Sosinska, E., 2006. Candida-associated denture stomatitis in patients after immuno-suppression therapy. Transplant. Proc. 38 (1), 155–156.

Jainkittivong, A., Aneksuk, V., Langlais, R.P., 2002. Oral mucosal conditions in older dental patients. Oral Dis. 8 (4), 218–223.

Lu, S.Y., Wu, H.C., 2004. Initial diagnosis of anemia from sore mouth and improved classification of anemias by MCV and RDW in 30 patients. Oral Surg. Oral Med. Oral Pathol. Oral Radiol. Endod. 98 (6), 679–685.

Ogunbodede, E.O., Fatusi, O.A., Akintomide, A., et al., 2005. Oral health status in a population of Nigerian diabetics. J. Contemp. Dent. Pract. 6 (4), 75–84.

Scully, C., Bagan, J.V., Eisen, D., et al., 2000. Dermatology of the lips. Isis Medical Media, Oxford.

Strumia, R., 2005. Dermatologic signs in patients with eating disorders. Am. J. Clin. Dermatol. 6 (3), 165–173.

34

Aphthae (recurrent aphthous stomatitis)

Key Points

- Aphthae are multiple recurrent small, round or ovoid ulcers which have circumscribed margins, erythematous haloes, and yellow or grey floors, appearing first in childhood or adolescence
- A minor degree of immunological dysregulation underlies aphthae
- A family history of aphthae is common
- Most patients appear otherwise well and predisposing factors are unclear
- Ulcers similar to aphthae (aphthous-like ulcers) may be seen in some immune disorders
- Topical corticosteroids control most aphthae

INTRODUCTION

Recurrent aphthous stomatitis (RAS), is a common condition which is characterized by presenting typically:

- With multiple recurrent, round or ovoid ulcers known as aphthae or canker sores, which have circumscribed margins, erythematous haloes, and yellow or grey floors (**Fig. 34.1**):
  - on non-keratinized and mobile mucosae – they are rare on gingivae or palate.
- With first onset in childhood or adolescence.
- With no systemic disease.

It is important to note that individual aphthae last only a limited period of time, before they heal spontaneously. This is quite a different history from ulcers that persist without healing, such as malignant ulcers and those associated with vesiculobullous disorders such as pemphigoid and pemphigus.

INCIDENCE

RAS affects at least 10% of the population, and the highest prevalence (up to 25%) is in resource-rich groups.

AGE

RAS typically starts in childhood or adolescence.

GENDER

There is a slight female predisposition to RAS.

GEOGRAPHIC

RAS occurs worldwide though it appears to be most common in the developed world.

PREDISPOSING FACTORS

There is a genetic predisposition shown by a positive family history in about one-third of patients and by an increased frequency of HLA types (HLA-A2, A11, B12 and DR2). There is an association between RAS and inheritance of a single-nucleotide polymorphism of the NOS2 gene (encoding inducible nitric oxide synthase). Inheritance of the G/G genotype of both interleukins IL-1B and IL-6 is a particularly strong predictor for RAS:

- Stress underlies RAS in some cases and ulcers appear to exacerbate during school or university examination times.
- Trauma from biting the mucosa or from dental appliances may lead to aphthae in some people.
- Cessation of smoking may precipitate or exacerbate RAS in some cases, but the reason is unclear.
- Haematinic deficiency may be relevant in a minority. In up to 20% of patients, deficiencies of iron, folic acid (folate) or vitamin B are found and sometimes the correction of this may relieve the ulceration. Iron deficiency is usually due to chronic haemorrhage (e.g. from the gastrointestinal or genitourinary tract). Folic acid is found in green leafy vegetables especially, and body stores are small; deficiencies may be dietary, or related to malabsorption or drugs (alcohol, anticonvulsants, carbamazepine, and some cytotoxic drugs). Vitamin B_{12} is found especially in meat, is absorbed via intrinsic factor from the gastric parietal cells in the ileum and stored in the liver for about 3 years. Dietary B_{12} deficiency can arise particularly in vegans, in pernicious anaemia and after gastrectomy, and in ileal disease (e.g. Crohn disease). Histamine H2 receptor antagonists (cimetidine, ranitidine, omeprazole) can also impede vitamin B_{12} absorption.
- Endocrine factors are relevant in some women where RAS are related to the fall in progestogen level in the luteal phase of the menstrual cycle, or to the contraceptive pill, and then RAS may regress temporarily in pregnancy.
- Allergies to food occasionally underlie RAS, and there is a high incidence of atopy.
- Sodium lauryl sulphate (SLS), a detergent in some toothpastes and other oral healthcare products, may produce oral ulceration.

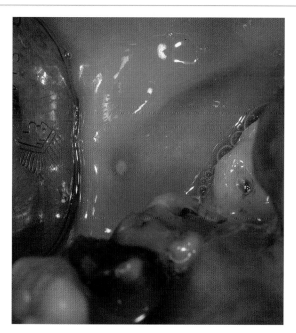

Fig. 34.1 Minor aphthae; typical round shape, yellow sunken ulcer floor and erythematous halo

APHTHOUS-LIKE ULCERS (ALU)

(see Table 34.3)

The diagnosis of RAS is not infrequently misapplied to the similar ulcers (aphthous-like ulcers), which may be seen in a range of systemic conditions. The history and examination should be directed to eliciting any cutaneous, gastrointestinal, genital, ocular, joint problems or history of fever, which might point to these conditions. They include conditions such as:

- Immune deficiencies such as HIV (Ch. 53), cyclical neutropenia and other immune defects.
- Behçet syndrome, where mouth ulcers are seen along with ulcers of the genitals (Ch. 36).
- Coeliac disease: in about 3% of patients with recurrent mouth ulcers, coeliac disease (gluten-sensitive enteropathy) – an allergic reaction to gluten in wheat – is seen.
- Crohn disease, where ulcers are seen with an enteropathy (Ch. 46).
- Autoinflammatory conditions such as periodic fever, aphthous stomatitis, pharyngitis and cervical adenitis (PFAPA) syndrome, which is seen in children, appears related to a disorder of innate immunity with complement activation and IL-1β/-18, resolves spontaneously and rarely has long-term sequelae. Corticosteroids are highly effective symptomatically; tonsillectomy and cimetidine treatment have been effective in a few patients.
- Sweet syndrome, in which mouth ulcers are found with conjunctivitis, episcleritis and inflamed tender skin papules or nodules.
- Drug use, especially NSAIDs and nicorandil.

AETIOLOGY AND PATHOGENESIS

The aetiology of RAS is not entirely clear, and therefore aphthae are termed 'idiopathic'. Indeed, RAS may not be a single condition, but rather may be the manifestation of a group of disorders of quite different aetiology.

Many studies have explored an infectious aetiology, but there is no evidence of transmissibility and RAS does not at present appear to be infectious, contagious, or sexually shared.

It seems likely that a minor degree of immunological dysregulation underlies aphthae, and a genetic tendency to ulceration, and cross-reacting antigens between the oral mucosa and microorganisms may be involved. Reactions to heat shock proteins (HSP) are one possibility. Patients with RAS have circulating lymphocytes reactive with peptide 91-105 of HSP 65-60. HSP27 is a powerful inductor of interleukin IL-10, a major inhibitor of Th1 response and in RAS, there is a reduced cellular expression of HSP27 and IL-10. Decreased IL-10 suggests a failure of the immune system to suppress inflammation.

Immune mechanisms that appear to play a role in a people with a genetic predisposition to oral ulceration include the following (**Fig. 34.2**):

- A local cell-mediated immune response involving cytotoxic CD8+ T-cells, natural killer (NK) cells, macrophages and mast cells.
- T-helper cells (gamma-delta cells), predominate in the early RAS lesions, along with some natural killer (NK) cells.
- Cytotoxic cells then appear in the lesions and there is evidence for an antibody-dependent cellular cytotoxicity (ADCC) reaction, and neutrophils and NK cells may be involved.
- HSP can block the production of pro-inflammatory cytokines (e.g. tumour necrosis factors (TNFs) and interleukins (IL-1β, IL-6 and IL-8)) through inhibition of NF-κB and mitogen-activated protein kinase (MAPK) pathways, or activate antiinflammatory cytokines (e.g. transforming growth factor-β1), and therefore control the magnitude of the immune response.
- IL-1β and IL-6 gene polymorphisms are associated with an increased risk for RAS. Systemic immunological abnormalities in RAS include increased plasma levels of IL-8 and IL-6. Serum IL-6 (via IL-1β over-production) typically fluctuates in auto-inflammatory syndromes, which also manifest with recurrent ulceration.
- There is increased intra-lesional expression of TNF-α and IL-2. Systemic immunological abnormalities in RAS include increased plasma levels of TNF-α and IL-2,
- There is an overly exuberant inflammation reaction which may be caused by derangement of toll-like receptor (TLR) gene expression.

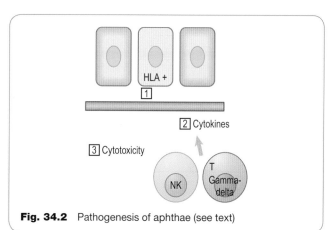

Fig. 34.2 Pathogenesis of aphthae (see text)

- Regulatory T cells (TReg) CD4($^+$)CD25($^+$), crucial in regulating immune responses, are both functionally and quantitatively compromised in RAS.
- There is decreased constitutive expression of indoleamine 2,3-dioxygenase (IDO) in the oral mucosa in RAS which may lead to the loss of local immune tolerance.
- NOS2 (nitric oxide synthase) gene polymorphisms implicate a role of inducible nitric oxide synthase.

CLINICAL FEATURES

Patients with RAS have no clinically detectable systemic symptoms or signs; if ulceration affects the genitals or other mucosae, the diagnosis cannot be of RAS alone – rather of aphthous-like ulceration.

There are three main clinical types of RAS (**Table 34.1**), though any significance of these distinctions is unclear (they could be three distinct disorders):

- minor aphthous ulcers (~ 80% of all RAS)
- major aphthous ulcers
- herpetiform ulcers.

MINOR APHTHOUS ULCERS (MiAU; MIKULICZ ULCER)

This type of RAS:

- occurs mainly in the 10–40 year age group
- often causes minimal symptoms
- consists of small round or ovoid ulcers 2–4 mm in diameter (**Fig. 34.3**), in groups of only a few ulcers (1–6) at a time, with initially yellowish floors surrounded by an erythematous halo and some oedema, but the floors assume a greyish hue as healing and epithelialization proceeds
- affects mainly the non-keratinized mobile mucosae of the lips, cheeks, floor of the mouth, sulci or ventrum of the tongue
- heals in 7–10 days
- recurs at intervals of 1–4 months
- leaves little or no evidence of scarring.

MAJOR APHTHOUS ULCERS (MjAU)

This type of RAS, also known as Sutton's ulcers or periadenitis mucosa necrotica recurrens (PMNR):

- are round or ovoid
- reach a large size, usually about 1 cm in diameter or even larger
- are found on any area of the oral mucosa, including the keratinized dorsum of the tongue or palate (**Fig. 34.4**)
- occur in groups of only a few ulcers (1–6) at one time
- heal slowly over 10–40 days
- recur extremely frequently
- may heal with scarring
- occasionally are found with a raised ESR, CRP or PV.

HERPETIFORM ULCERATION (HU)

This type of RAS:

- are found in a slightly older age group than the other RAS
- are found mainly in females
- begin with vesiculation, which passes rapidly into multiple minute pinhead-sized discrete ulcers (**Fig. 34.5**)

Table 34.1 Clinical characteristics of the different clinical types of aphthae

	Minor	Major	Herpetiform
Percentage of all aphthae	75–85	10–15	5–10
Size (mm)	2–5	>10	<5
Duration (days)	10–14	>14	10–14
Scarring	No	Yes	No

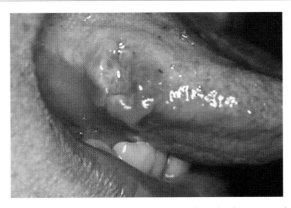

Fig. 34.4 Major aphthae; large ulcer healing slowly over weeks

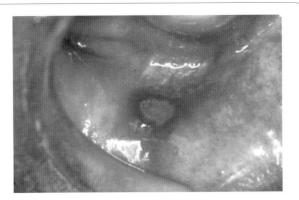

Fig. 34.3 Minor aphthae; small ulcers healing within 7–10 days

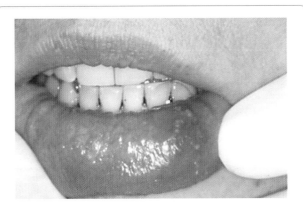

Fig. 34.5 Herpetiform ulcers; many minute ulcers

- increase in size and coalesce to leave large, round, ragged ulcers
- involve any oral site, including the keratinized mucosa
- heal in 10 days or longer
- are often extremely painful
- recur so frequently that ulceration may be virtually continuous.

DIAGNOSIS

Diagnosis of RAS is based on the history and clinical features, as no specific tests are available (**Algorithm 34.1**). The diagnosis of RAS is not infrequently misapplied to the similar ulcers (aphthous-like ulcers), which may be seen in a range of systemic conditions. The history and examination should be directed to eliciting any cutaneous, gastrointestinal, genital, ocular, joint problems or history of fever, which might point to these conditions. Biopsy is rarely indicated, and is only usually needed where a different diagnosis is suspected but even vesicullobullous disorders can on occasion present with recurring ulcers. Therefore, to exclude a number of systemic disorders, it is often useful to undertake investigations (**Table 34.2**) on:

- blood
- ESR, CRP or PV
- a full blood picture
- haemoglobin
- white cell count and differential
- red cell indices
- red cell folate assay
- serum
- ferritin levels (or other iron studies)
- vitamin B_{12} measurements
- calcium measurements (low in coeliac disease)
- tissue transglutaminase and IgA anti-endomysial antibody assays (positive in coeliac disease).

TREATMENT (see also Chs 4 and 5)

Disorders where aphthous-like ulcers are also seen (**Table 34.3**) should be excluded and RAS managed as follows:

- Predisposing factors should be corrected (**Algorithm 34.2**):
  - trauma: patients should avoid hard or sharp foods (e.g. toast, potato crisps) and brush their teeth atraumatically (e.g. by using a small-headed, soft toothbrush)

Table 34.2 Aids that might be helpful in diagnosis/prognosis/management in some patients suspected of having aphthae (recurrent aphthous stomatitis) or aphthous-like ulcers*

In most cases	In some cases
Full blood picture	Biopsy rarely
Serum ferritin, vitamin B_{12}, corrected whole blood folate and calcium levels	G6PD and TPMT levels**
ESR	Blood glucose
Serum immunoglobulins	Blood pressure**
IgA antiendomysial antibodies	DEXA (dual-emission X-ray absorptiometry) scan**
Antibodies to tissue transglutaminase (anti-tGt)	Endoscopy/gastroscopy and jejunal biopsy

*See text for details and glossary for abbreviations.
**If systemic immunomodulation considered.

- if SLS is implicated, this should be avoided; a number of SLS-free toothpastes is available (e.g. AloeDent; Biotene; CloSYS; Green People's organic toothpastes; Kingfisher; Kiss my face; Natural toothpaste; Radiance toothpaste; Sensodyne; Squigle; Therabreath; White kiss)
- any iron or vitamin deficiency should be corrected, once the cause of that deficiency has been established. There is some evidence of benefit from vitamin B_{12}, even in the absence of any deficiency
- if there is an obvious relationship to certain foods, these should be excluded from the diet; patch-testing to reveal allergies may be indicated
- the occasional patient who relates ulcers to the menstrual cycle or to an oral contraceptive may benefit from suppression of ovulation with a progestogen, or a change in the oral contraceptive.
- Relief of pain and reduction of ulcer duration.
  - Good oral hygiene should be maintained; chlorhexidine or triclosan mouthwashes may help. An SLS-free toothpaste such as Sensodyne Pro-enamel may help.

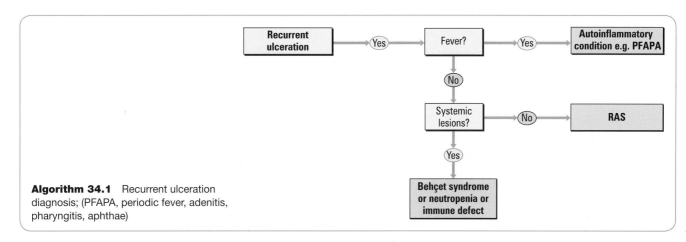

Algorithm 34.1 Recurrent ulceration diagnosis; (PFAPA, periodic fever, adenitis, pharyngitis, aphthae)

Table 34.3 Some disorders with aphthous-like ulceration

Disease	Comment
Autoinflammatory diseases	e.g. PFAPA syndrome (Periodic fever, aphthae like ulceration, pharyngitis and cervical adenitis). Rare, tends to occur in young children, self-limiting, and non-recurrent. May respond to cimetidine (via suppression of T lymphocyte function)
Behçet syndrome	ALU may be more severe than typical aphthae, and patients also have recurrent genital ulceration, cutaneous and ocular disease and other gastrointestinal, neurological, renal, joint and haematological abnormalities. MAGIC syndrome is a variant (Ch. 36)
Coeliac disease	Ch. 57
Crohn disease	Ch. 56
Cyclic neutropenia	Cyclic reduction in circulating levels of neutrophils about every 21 days Affected patients develop oral ulceration, fever, cutaneous abscesses, upper respiratory tract infections and lymphadenopathy Other oral complications include severe gingivitis and aggressive periodontitis Treated with recombinant granulocyte colony stimulating factor (rG-CSF) Other neutropenias (e.g. chronic neutropenia) can give rise to superficial oral mucosal ulceration without any significant periodicity
Sweet syndrome	Acute neutrophilic dermatosis (Ch. 56)
Viral infections (EBV, HIV or HTLV-1)	Chs 43 and 53

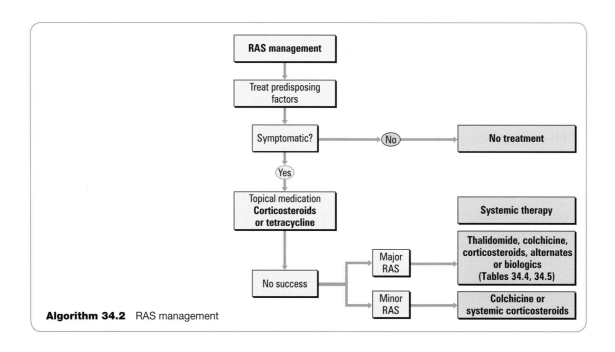

Algorithm 34.2 RAS management

- Antiinflammatory agents: topical agents, such as benzydamine, amlexanox, or diclofenac in hyaluronan may help in the management of discomfort in RAS.
- Active treatment is indicated if the patient has significant discomfort (**Tables 34.4–34.6**): Fortunately, the natural history of RAS is one of eventual remission in most cases, but this may take several years.
- Topical corticosteroids can often control RAS.

Topical corticosteroids are the primary therapeutic agents used to treat ulcerative mucosal lesions, which have an immunologically-based aetiology such as aphthae (**Fig. 34.6**). A mild potency agent such as hydrocortisone may be effective but more typically a medium potency corticosteroid such as betamethasone or a higher potency one such as fluocinonide or beclomethasone are required, moving to a super-potent topical corticosteroid, e.g. clobetasol, if the benefit is inadequate

Table 34.4 Regimens that might be helpful in management of patients suspected of having aphthae (see also Table 34.6)

Regimen	Use in primary care	Use in secondary care (severe oral involvement and/or extraoral involvement)
Beneficial	Chlorhexidine	Corticosteroids (systemically) (e.g. enteric-coated prednisolone) Thalidomide
Likely to be beneficial	Amlexanox if available Corticosteroids (topical) (e.g. hydrocortisone, betamethasone) Diclofenac 3% in hyaluronan Tetracycline 2.5% mouthwash (adults only) Vitamin B$_{12}$	Azathioprine Ciclosporin Chlorambucil Colchicine Cyclophosphamide Interferon-α Levamisole
Unproven effectiveness	Aloe vera Amyloglucosidase and glucose oxidase Laser Licorice extract Myrtus communis Nicotine Rosa damescena Plasma rich in growth factors Poliovirus vaccine Prostaglandin E2 Zinc sulphate	Dapsone Low molecular weight heparin Montelukast Mycophenolate mofetil Pentoxifylline Rebamipide Retinoids
Emergent treatments		Adalimumab Etanercept Infliximab
Supportive	Benzydamine Diet with little acidic, spicy or citrus content Lidocaine paste or gel SLS-free toothpaste	Benzydamine Diet with little acidic, spicy or citrus content Lidocaine paste or gel SLS-free toothpaste

Table 34.5 Treatment regimens for RAS

Treatment*	Examples of preparations available	Particularly suitable for
Covering agents	Orabase	Reducing pain
Topical analgesics/anaesthetics/ antiinflammatory agents	Benzydamine hydrochloride mouthwash or spray Amlexanox 5% paste Lidocaine gel	Reducing pain
Topical antiseptics	Doxycycline 100 mg daily as mouthwash Chlorhexidine gluconate 0.2% mouthwash	Hastening healing
Topical mild potency corticosteroids	Hydrocortisone oromucosal tablets 2.5 mg once daily or triamcinolone 0.1% in carboxymethylcellulose paste if available applied to dried areas with moistened finger	Frequently recurring or severe ulcers
Topical moderate or high potency corticosteroids (Ch. 5)	Beclomethasone dipropionate aerosol 2 puffs (100 μg) spray onto affected area to a maximum of 8 puffs/day Betamethasone sodium phosphate one 0.5 mg tablet dissolved in 10 mL of water used as a mouthwash once daily held in mouth for a minimum of 3 min	Inaccessible sites (e.g. soft palate)
Vitamin B$_{12}$	Cobalamin 50 μg daily	
Systemic immunomodulatory agents	Oral prednisolone (enteric-coated) 40 mg for 5 days, reduce by 5 mg every 2 days to 5 mg, reduce by 1 mg/day until complete Or colchicine 500 μg/day Or pentoxifylline 400 mg three times a day Or azathioprine 50–10 mg daily Or thalidomide 50–200 mg once or twice a day 3–8 weeks	Severe RAS, or aphthous-like ulceration

*Children under 6 cannot be expected to rinse and expectorate effectively; avoid preparations that cannot be safely swallowed. Avoid tetracycline preparations, even as a mouthwash, in children under 12. Systemic agents all have potential significant adverse effects (see **Table 34.6** and Ch. 54).

Table 34.6 Therapies for aphthae shown to have benefit in at least one controlled trial (see Ch. 5 and Tables 34.4 and 34.5)

Agent	Main preparations	Route	Daily dose (adults)	Possible main adverse effects/ contraindications
Mild disease				
Amlexanox	5% in adhesive base	Topical	Applied to ulcers 4 times daily*	Stinging
Chlorhexidine	0.12% or 0.2% aqueous mouthwash or 1% gel	Topical	4 times daily*	Superficial tooth staining (reduce coffee, tea, red wine intake)
Corticosteroids	In adhesive base (carmellose), or as pellet, spray or cream	Topical	Applied to ulcers 4 times daily*	Oral candidosis (recommend adding antifungals to more potent corticosteroids because of this possible risk)
Vitamin B$_{12}$	Tablet	Oral	50 µg	Mild temporary diarrhoea
Severe disease				
Corticosteroids	Tablet or capsule	Systemic	Orally 30–60 mg**	Hypertension Diabetes Weight gain Osteoporosis Peptic ulceration Adrenal suppression
Thalidomide	Tablet	Systemic	Orally 50 mg*	Teratogenic Drowsiness Thromboses

*For 2 or more weeks, repeated if ulcers recur.
**1-week treatment, reducing dose over a further week.

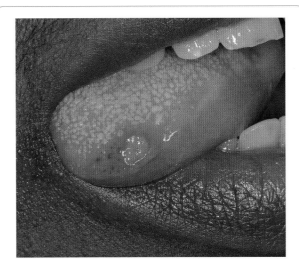

Fig. 34.6 Aphthae on tongue are difficult to manage with pastes

(Tables 5.5 and 34.5). Patients should be instructed to apply a small quantity of the agent three times daily, refraining from speaking, eating and drinking for the subsequent 0.5 h. A theoretical concern is that long-term immunosuppression might predispose to neoplastic change. In long-term use, candidosis can arise and thus topical antifungal medication such as miconazole may be prudent. The more major concern – of adrenal suppression with long-term and/or repeated application – has rarely been addressed, although the topical preparations noted in Ch. 5 (apart from super potent halogenated corticosteroids when used several times a day) appear not to cause a significant problem.

- Topical tetracycline (a capsule of 100 mg doxycycline dissolved in 10 mL water) as a mouth rinse may provide relief and reduce ulcer duration, but must be avoided in children under 12 years old who might ingest the tetracycline and develop tooth staining.
- Among the alternative treatments available, for a few of which there is a reliable evidence base, are amlexanox, amyloglucosidase and glucose oxidase, prostaglandin E2, nicotine tablets, aloe vera, myrtus communis and rosa damescena, licorice extract, poliovirus vaccine, zinc sulphate, laser, plasma rich in growth factors.
- If RAS fails to respond to these measures, systemic immunomodulators may be required, under specialist supervision. These include systemic corticosteroids (e.g. prednisolone (enteric-coated)) (see Ch. 5) and other immunomodulatory agents (e.g. azathioprine, ciclosporin, colchicine, dapsone, interferon or anti-TNF agents - see below). Vitamin B$_{12}$ may have beneficial effect even in the absence of proven deficiency.

FOLLOW-UP OF PATIENTS

Long-term follow-up in primary care is usually adequate for most patients with RAS. Patients with severe RAS or aphthous-like ulcers may need secondary care.

EMERGENT TREATMENTS

If RAS fails to respond to topical measures, systemic immu-nomodulators may be required, under specialist supervision. These include antitumour necrosis factor alpha agents such as pentoxifylline, thalidomide, infliximab, etanercept, adalim-umab, but often either their efficacy has not been well proven or they have unacceptable adverse effects. For example, tha-lidomide can be effective against severe RAS, but is rarely employed since it is teratogenic and can produce neuropathies and thromboses.

PATIENT INFORMATION SHEET
Aphthous ulcers

▼ Please read this information sheet. If you have any questions, particu-larly about the treatment or potential side-effects, please ask your doctor.
- These are common.
- The cause is not known.
- Children may inherit ulcers from parents.
- Aphthous ulcers arc not thought to be infectious.
- Some deficiencies or diseases may predispose to ulcers.
- No long-term consequences are known.
- Blood tests and biopsy may be required.
- Ulcers can be controlled, but rarely cured.

USEFUL WEBSITE

Dermnet, N.Z., Aphthous ulcers. http://dermnetnz.org/site-age-specific/aphthae.html

Medscape, Aphthous Ulcers. http://emedicine.medscape.com/article/867080-overview

FURTHER READING

Altenburg, A., Abdel-Naser, M.B., Seeber, H., et al., 2007. Practical aspects of management of recurrent aphthous stomatitis. J. Eur. Acad. Dermatol. Venereol. 21 (8), 1019–1026.

Aminabadi, N.A., 2008. Plasma rich in growth factors as a potential therapeutic candidate for treatment of recurrent aphthous stomatitis. Med. Hypotheses 70 (3), 529–531.

Barrons, R.W., 2001. Treatment strategies for recurrent aphthous ulcers. Am. J. Health 58, 41–53.

Besu, I., Jankovic, L., Magdu, I., et al., 2009. Humoral immunity to cow's milk proteins and gliadin within the etiology of recurrent aphthous ulcers? Oral Dis. 15, 560–564.

Boulinguez, S., Reix, S., Bedane, C., et al., 2000. Role of drug exposure in aphthous ulcers: a case-control study. Br. J. Dermatol. 143, 1261–1265.

Burgess, J.A., van der Ven, P.F., Martin, M., et al., 2008. Review of over-the-counter treatments for aphthous ulceration and results from use of a dissolving oral patch containing glycyrrhiza complex herbal extract. J. Contemp. Dent. Pract. 9 (3), 88–98.

Femiano, F., Buonaiuto, C., Gombos, F., et al., 2010. Pilot study on recurrent aphthous stomatitis (RAS): a randomized placebo-controlled trial for the comparative therapeutic effects of systemic prednisone and systemic montelukast in subjects unresponsive to topical therapy. Oral Surg. Oral Med. Oral Pathol. Oral Radiol. Endod. 109 (3), 402–407.

Flaitz, C.M., Baker, K.A., 2000. Treatment approaches to common symptomatic oral lesions in children. Dent. Clin. North Am. 44, 671–696.

Fontes, V., Machet, L., Huttenberger, B., et al., 2002. Recurrent aphhous stomatitis: treatment with colchicine. An open trial of 54 cases. Ann. Dermatol. Venereol. 129 (12), 1365–1369.

Gallo, C., Barros, F., Sugaya, N., et al., 2012. Differential expression of toll-like receptor mRNAs in recurrent aphthous ulceration. J. Oral Pathol. Med. 41 (1), 80–85.

Gorsky, M., Epstein, J., Raviv, A., et al., 2008. Topical minocycline for managing symptoms of recurrent aphthous stomatitis. Spec. Care Dentist 28 (1), 27–31.

Guimaraes, A., de Sa, A., Victoria, J., et al., 2006. Association of interleukin-1beta polymorphism with recurrent aphthous stomatitis in Brazilian individuals. Oral Dis. 12 (6), 580–583.

Jaber, L., Weinberger, A., Klein, T., et al., 2001. Close association of HLA-B52 and HLA-B44 antigens in Israeli Arab adolescents with recurrent aphthous stomatitis. Arch. Otolaryngol. Head Neck Surg. 127, 184–187.

Jacobi, A., Debus, D., Schuler, G., Hertl, M., 2008. Infliximab in a patient with refractory mucosal aphthosis. J. Eur. Acad. Dermatol. Venereol. 22 (1), 109–110.

Jurge, S., Kuffer, R., Scully, C., Porter, S.R., 2006. Recurrent aphthous stomatitis. Oral Dis. 12, 1–21.

Karasneh, J.A., Darwazeh, A.M., Hassan, A.F., Thornhill, M., 2011. Association between recurrent aphthous stomatitis and inheritance of a single-nucleotide polymorphism of the NOS2 gene encoding inducible nitric oxide synthase. J. Oral Pathol. Med. Apr 11 [Epub ahead of print].

Koybasi, S., Parlak, A.H., Serin, E., et al., 2006. Recurrent aphthous stomatitis: investigation of possible etiologic factors. Am. J. Otolaryngol. 27 (4), 229–232.

Kozlak, S.T., Walsh, S.J., Lalla, R.V., 2010. Reduced dietary intake of vitamin B12 and folate in patients with recurrent aphthous stomatitis. J. Oral Pathol. Med. 39 (5), 420–423.

Lee, J.H., Jung, J.Y., Bang, D., 2008. The efficacy of topical 0.2% hyaluronic acid gel on recurrent oral ulcers: comparison between recurrent aphthous ulcers and the oral ulcers of Behçet's disease. J. Eur. Acad. Dermatol. Venereol. 22 (5), 590–595.

Leong, S.C., Karkos, P.D., Apostolidou, M.T., 2006. Is there a role for the otolaryngologist in PFAPA syndrome? A systematic review. Int. J. Pediatr. Otorhinolaryngol. 70 (11), 1841–1845.

Lewkowicz, N., Lewkowicz, P., Dzitko, K., et al., 2008. Dysfunction of CD4+CD25high T regulatory cells in patients with recurrent aphthous stomatitis. J. Oral Pathol. Med. 37 (8), 454–461.

Liu, J., Zeng, X., Chen, Q., et al., 2006. An evaluation on the efficacy and safety of amlexanox oral adhesive tablets in the treatment of recurrent minor aphthous ulceration in a Chinese cohort: a randomized, double-blind, vehicle-controlled, unparallel multicenter clinical trial. Oral Surg. Oral Med. Oral Pathol. Oral Radiol. Endod. 102 (4), 475–481.

Martin, M.D., Sherman, J., van der Ven, P., Burgess, J., 2008. A controlled trial of a dissolving oral patch concerning glycyrrhiza (licorice) herbal extract for the treatment of aphthous ulcers. Gen. Dent. 56 (2), 206–210: quiz 211–212, 224.

McBride, D.R., 2000. Management of aphthous ulcers. Am. Fam. Physician 62, 149–154.

McCullough, M.J., Abdel-Hafeth, S., Scully, C., 2007. Recurrent aphthous stomatitis revisited; clinical features, associations, and new association with infant feeding practices? J. Oral Pathol. Med. 36 (10), 615–620.

Miyamoto Jr., N.T., Borra, R.C., Abreu, M., et al., 2008. Immune-expression of HSP27 and IL-10 in recurrent aphthous ulceration. J. Oral Pathol. Med. 37 (8), 462–467.

Moghadamnia, A.A., Motallebnejad, M., Khanian, M., 2008. The efficacy of the bioadhesive patches containing licorice extract in the management of recurrent aphthous stomatitis. Phytother. Res. 23 (2), 246–250.

Mumcu, G., Sur, H., Inanc, N., et al., 2009. A composite index for determining the impact of oral ulcer activity in Behçet's disease and recurrent aphthous stomatitis. J. Oral Pathol. Med. 38 (10), 785–791.

O'Neill I., Scully C., 2012. Biologies in oral medicine ulcerative disorders Oral Diseases, Mar 13 Epub.

Pinto, A., Lindemeyer, R.G., Sollecito, T.P., 2006. The PFAPA syndrome in oral medicine: differential diagnosis and treatment. Oral Surg. Oral Med. Oral Pathol. Oral Radiol. Endod. 102 (1), 35–39.

Popovsky, J.L., Camisa, C., 2000. New and emerging therapies for diseases of the oral cavity. Dermatol. Clin. 18, 113–125.

Porter, S.R., Hegarty, A., Kaliakatsou, F., et al., 2000. Recurrent aphthous stomatitis. Clin. Dermatol. 18, 569–578.

Porter, S.R., Scully, C., 2003. Aphthous ulcers: recurrent. Clinical Evidence Concise 9, 282.

Preshaw, P.M., Grainger, P., Bradshaw, M.H., et al., 2007. Subantimicrobial dose doxycycline in the treatment of recurrent oral aphthous ulceration: a pilot study. J. Oral Pathol. Med. 36 (4), 236–240.

Rodríguez, M., Rubio, J., Sanchez, R., 2007. Effectiveness of two oral pastes for the treatment of recurrent aphthous stomatitis. Oral Dis. 13, 490–494.

Sánchez-Cano, D., Callejas-Rubio, J., Ruiz-Villaverde, R., Ortego-Centeno, N., 2009. Recalcitrant, recurrent aphthous stomatitis successfully treated with adalimumab. J. Eur. Acad. Dermatol. Venereol. 23 (2), 206.

Scully, C., 2006. Clinical practice. Aphthous ulceration. N. Engl. J. Med. 355 (2), 165–172.

Scully, C., Felix, D.H., 2005. Oral medicine – Update for the dental practitioner. 1. Aphthous and other common ulcers. Br. Dent. J. 199, 259–264.

Scully, C., Gorsky, M., Lozada-Nur, F., 2003. The diagnosis and management of recurrent aphthous stomatitis – a consensus approach. J. Am. Dent. Assoc. 134, 200–207.

Scully, C., Hodgson, T., 2008. Recurrent oral ulceration: aphthous-like ulcers in periodic syndromes. Oral Surg. Oral Med. Oral Pathol. Oral Radiol. Endod. 106, 845–852.

Scully, C., Hodgson, T., Lachmann, H., 2008. Auto-inflammatory syndromes and oral health. Oral Dis. 14, 690–699.

Sharquie, K.E., Najim, R.A., Al-Hayani, R.K., 2008. The therapeutic and prophylactic role of oral zinc sulfate in management of recurrent aphthous stomatitis (ras) in comparison with dapsone. Saudi Med. J. 29 (5), 734–738.

Shemer, A., Amichai, B., Trau, H., et al., 2008. Efficacy of a mucoadhesive patch compared with an oral solution for treatment of aphthous stomatitis. Drugs R D 9 (1), 29–35.

Stojanov, S., Lapidus, S., Chitkara, P., et al., 2011. Periodic fever, aphthous stomatitis, pharyngitis, and adenitis (PFAPA) is a disorder of innate immunity and Th1 activation responsive to IL-1 blockade. Proc. Natl. Acad. Sci. U. S. A. 108 (17), 7148–7153.

Veller-Fornasa, C., Gallina, P., 2006. Recurrent aphthous stomatitis as an expression of pathergy in atopics. Acta Dermatovenerol. Alp. Panonica Adriat. 15 (3), 144–147.

Volkov, I., Rudoy, I., Freud, T., et al., 2009. Effectiveness of vitamin B12 in treating recurrent aphthous stomatitis: a randomized, double-blind, placebo-controlled trial. J. Am. Board Fam. Med. 22 (1), 9–16.

Yazdanpanah, M.J., Mokhtari, M.B., Mostofi, K., et al., 2008. Oral poliovirus vaccine in management of recurrent aphthous stomatitis. Acta Microbiol. Immunol. Hung. 55 (3), 343–350.

Zribi, H., Crickx, B., Descamps, V., 2007. Prevention of recurrent aphthous stomatitis by efalizumab (Raptiva). J. Eur. Acad. Dermatol. Venereol. 21 (9), 1286–1287.

Atypical (idiopathic) facial pain

Key Points

- Atypical facial pain (AFP) is a constant chronic orofacial discomfort or pain, for which no organic cause can be found
- Patients are often older women
- The pain is poorly localized; pain persists for much or all of the day, and is often of a deep, dull boring or burning type
- There are often multiple oral and/or other psychogenic related complaints and consultations
- Cognitive behavioural therapy or psychoactive medication may be needed

INTRODUCTION

Atypical or idiopathic facial pain (IFP) is a constant chronic orofacial discomfort or pain, which is defined by the International Headache Society as 'facial pain not fulfilling other criteria'. Therefore, it is a diagnosis that can be difficult to make since it is reached only by the exclusion of organic disease. The organic disease that might cause similar chronic orofacial pain is typically in the local region but may be anywhere in the head and neck, or even in the chest; hence the difficulty in making this diagnosis safely.

IFP falls into the category of medically unexplained symptoms (MUS), most of which appear to have a psychogenic basis. It must be recognized, however, that a patient in pain may well also manifest psychological reactions to the experience.

Characteristics that define IFP are that:

- it is a dull boring or burning continuous type of pain of ill-defined location with few, if any, periods of remission
- objective signs are lacking
- investigations all produce a negative result
- there is no clear explanation as to the cause
- there is poor response to treatment
- there are often multiple consultations.

INCIDENCE

IFP is fairly common, possibly affecting around 1–2% of the population.

AGE

Patients are usually middle-aged or older; IFP is rare in children.

GENDER

Patients are often women (~ 70%).

GEOGRAPHIC

There are no geographic factors implicated.

PREDISPOSING FACTORS

There are often recent adverse life events, such as bereavement or family illness and/or dental or oral interventive procedures.

AETIOLOGY AND PATHOGENESIS

The mouth and para-oral tissues have among the richest sensory innervation in the body. Furthermore, a large part of the sensory homunculus on the cerebral cortex receives information from orofacial structures. Right from infancy the mouth is concerned intimately with the psychological development of the individual, and disorders of structures such as the lips, teeth and oral mucosa can hold enormous emotional significance. It is hardly surprising, therefore, that orofacial disorders can result in considerable stress and that there are a range of psychogenic types of orofacial pain, including IFP.

Most sufferers from IFP are otherwise normal individuals who are, or have been, under extreme stress, such as bereavement or concern about cancer or an infection. Positron emission tomography in persons with IFP shows enhanced cerebral activity, suggesting an enhanced alerting mechanism in response to peripheral stimuli. This may lead to the release of neuropeptides and the production of free radicals, causing cell damage and the release of pain-inducing eicosanoids, such as prostaglandins. There may be a neuromuscular component.

Some patients have personality traits, such as hypochondriasis or neuroses (often depression), and a very few have psychoses.

CLINICAL FEATURES

HISTORY

- The location of the pain is mainly in the upper jaw, unrelated to the anatomical distribution of trigeminal nerve innervation, poorly localized, and sometimes crosses the midline to involve the other side, or moves to another site.

- The pain is chronic and often of a deep, dull boring or burning type, persisting for much or all of the day, but does not waken the patient from sleep.
- Patients only uncommonly use analgesics to try and control the pain.
- Pain is accompanied by altered behaviour, anxiety or depression. Over 50% of such patients are depressed or hypochondriacal, and some have lost or been separated from parents in childhood.
- There are often multiple oral and/or other psychogenic related complaints, such as:
  - dry mouth
  - bad taste
  - headaches
  - chronic back pain
  - irritable bowel syndrome
  - dysmenorrhoea.
- The chronic pain may lead the patients to seek dental intervention, but to little avail. Patients may seek conservative dentistry, but this is rarely helpful – often rather to the contrary. The saga of pain may lead the clinician eventually to undertake endodontics or exodontics.
- There is a high level of utilization of healthcare services: there have often already been multiple consultations and unsuccessful attempts at treatment. Many sufferers persist in blaming organic diseases (or the clinician!) for their pain.

DIAGNOSIS

Making this diagnosis is not simple and follows a process of elimination of other potential causes of orofacial pain (**Table 35.1**). IFP occurs in the trigeminal nerve territory, and the pain may sometimes be as severe as trigeminal neuralgia, but it is usually different in severity, character and distribution. IFP is usually diffuse, persistent, burning, aching, dull, or crushing, whereas trigeminal neuralgia is characterized by quick episodes of jabbing or lancinating pain in a division of the trigeminal nerve. Patients are still reported complaining of such chronic facial pain which proves to be caused by malignant disease – not only in the head and neck but occasionally in the chest; referred pain, due to invasion or compression of the vagus nerve, as well as paraneoplastic syndrome secondary to the production

of circulating humoral factors by the malignant tumour cells, is implicated in the pathophysiology of facial pain associated with non-metastatic lung cancer. An effort should be made to exclude all such pathology but occasionally a lung cancer responsible for facial pain has evaded detection by chest imaging.

Examination of at least the mouth, perioral structures and cranial nerves, and imaging (tooth/jaw/sinus/skull radiography, MRI/CT scan with particular attention to the skull base and chest imaging) to exclude organic disease, such as space-occupying or demyelinating diseases, are important. MRI scan of the head has a better yield than CT because of its better resolution of the brain stem and cranial nerves and has almost completely replaced CT as the diagnostic modality of choice, but CT still plays a role in the assessment of skull base foramina and facial skeleton.

The findings on clinical examination in patients with IFP include:

- no erythema, tenderness or swelling in the area
- no obvious odontogenic or other local cause for the pain
- total lack of objective physical (including neurological) signs.

Investigation findings include:

- all imaging studies are negative
- all blood investigations are negative.

IFP is a clinical diagnosis, only made after careful dental and otolaryngologic evaluation, and thorough neurological scan examination and other tests rule out organic causes for the pain.

TREATMENT (see also Chs 4 and 5)

Few patients with IFP have spontaneous remission and, thus, treatment is indicated (**Algorithm 35.1**; **Table 35.2**).

- Patient information is a very important aspect in management.
- A specialist referral may be appropriate.
- Cognitive–behavioural therapy may be indicated.
- Patients with IFP may be helped by a technique termed 'reattribution' which involves demonstrating an understanding of the complaints by taking a history of related physical, mood and social factors, making the patient feel understood and supported, and widening the agenda – thus making the link between the symptoms and psychological problems. It may help explain that depression/tiredness lower the pain threshold and that muscle overactivity and spasm (being 'uptight') causes pain.

The clinician should:

- clearly acknowledge the reality of the patient's symptoms and distress and never attempt to trivialize or dismiss them
- try and explain the psychosomatic background to the problem, ascribing the symptoms to causes for which the patient cannot be blamed
- set goals, which include helping the patient cope with the symptoms rather than attempting any impossible cure
- avoid repeat examinations or investigations at subsequent appointments, since this only serves to reinforce illness behaviour and health fears
- avoid attempts at relieving pain by operative intervention, such as restorative treatment, endodontia or exodontia, since these are rarely successful; indeed, any active dental

Table 35.1 Aids that might be helpful in diagnosis/prognosis/management in patients suspected of having atypical (idiopathic) facial pain*

In most cases	In some cases
Tooth/jaw/sinus/skull radiography	Neurological opinion
MRI/CT with particular attention to skull base	Chest imaging
	Full blood picture
	Serum ferritin, vitamin B_{12} and corrected whole blood folate levels
	ESR
	Serology (Lyme disease)
	ANA
	Psychological assessment

*See text for details and glossary for abbreviations.

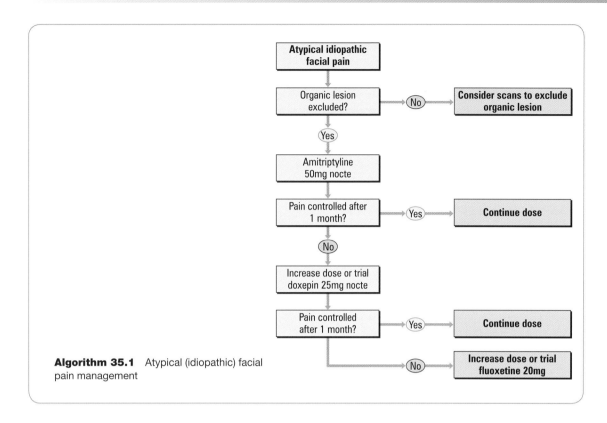

Algorithm 35.1 Atypical (idiopathic) facial pain management

or oral surgical treatment, in the absence of any specific indication, should be avoided

- avoid the patient becoming emotionally dependent.

Pharmacological treatment with antidepressants, antiepileptic or other drugs can also be tried (**Table 35.2**).

Trial of an antidepressant may be appropriate, explaining that this is being used to treat the symptoms rather than any depression and that antidepressants have been shown in controlled trials to be effective for this problem, even in non-depressed persons. The pain reduction achieved with antidepressants exceeds that produced by placebos. Also, although antidepressants must be given for at least 2–3 weeks to achieve any antidepressive effect, many patients with MUS, such as IFP, show benefit within 1 week. Amitryptiline is the primary

choice starting at 10 mg at night, given as tablets or solution, increasing if needed to 75 mg but venlafaxine and fluoxetine treatment can also be considered.

Surgery is rarely appropriate for treatment of IFP but deep brain stimulation of the posterior hypothalamus and pulsed radiofrequency treatment of the pterygopalatine ganglion have been reportedly effective.

FOLLOW-UP OF PATIENTS

Long-term follow-up as shared care is usually appropriate.

ATYPICAL ODONTALGIA

Atypical odontalgia is pain and hypersensitive teeth in the absence of detectable pathology. The pain is typically indistinguishable from pulpitis or periodontitis but is aggravated by dental intervention. It is probably a variant of atypical (idiopathic) facial pain, and should be managed similarly.

PATIENT INFORMATION SHEET
Atypical (IDIOPATHIC) facial pain

▼ Please read this information sheet. If you have any questions, particularly about the treatment or potential side-effects, please ask your doctor.
- This is fairly common.
- The cause is not completely known.
- It is not inherited.
- It may be caused by increased nerve sensitivity.
- There may be a background of stress.
- There are usually no serious long-term consequences.
- X-rays and blood tests may be required.
- Treatment takes time and patience; some nerve-calming drugs can help.

Table 35.2 Regimens that might be helpful in management of patient suspected of having atypical (idiopathic) facial pain

Regimen	Use in primary or secondary care
Beneficial	Cognitive behavioural therapy
Likely to be beneficial	Amitryptiline Venlafaxine Fluoxetine
Unproven effectiveness	Clonazepam Dosulepin Doxepin Gabapentin Milnicipran Nortryptiline Trazodone

USEFUL WEBSITES

Facial Neuralgia Resources, Atypical Facial Pain.
  http://www.facial-neuralgia.org/conditions/atfp.html

FURTHER READING

Abraham, P.J., Capobianco, D.J., Cheshire, W.P., 2003. Facial pain as the presenting symptom of lung carcinoma with normal chest radiograph. Headache 43 (5), 499–504.

Baad-Hansen, L., 2008. Atypical odontalgia – pathophysiology and clinical management. J. Oral Rehabil. 35 (1), 1–11.

Becker, M., Kohler, R., Vargas, M.I., et al., 2008. Pathology of the trigeminal nerve. Neuroimaging Clin. N. Am. 18 (2), 283–307.

Benoliel, R., Eliav, E., 2008. Neuropathic orofacial pain. Oral Maxillofac. Surg. Clin. North Am. 20 (2), 237–254.

Broggi, G., Franzini, A., Leone, M., Bussone, G., 2007. Update on neurosurgical treatment of chronic trigeminal autonomic cephalalgias and atypical facial pain with deep brain stimulation of posterior hypothalamus: results and comments. Neurol. Sci. 28 (Suppl. 2), S138–S245.

Clark, G.T., 2006. Persistent orodental pain, atypical odontalgia, and phantom tooth pain: when are they neuropathic disorders? J. Calif. Dent. Assoc. 34 (8), 599–609.

Cook, R.J., Sharif, I., Escudier, M., 2008. Meningioma as a cause of chronic orofacial pain: case reports. Br. J. Oral Maxillofac. Surg. 46 (6), 487–489.

Cornelissen, P., van Kleef, M., Mekhail, N., Day, M., van Zundert, J., 2009. Evidence-based interventional pain medicine according to clinical diagnoses. 3. Persistent idiopathic facial pain. Pain Pract. 9 (6), 443–448.

Fricton, J.R., 2000. Atypical orofacial pain disorders: a study of diagnostic subtypes. Curr. Rev. Pain 4, 142–147.

Graff-Radford, S.B., 2009. Facial pain. Neurologist 15 (4), 171–177.

Guler, N., Durmus, E., Tuncer, S., 2005. Long-term follow-up of patients with atypical facial pain treated with amitriptyline. N. Y. State Dent. J. 71 (4), 38–42.

Greene, C.S., Murray EM., 2011. Atypical odontalgia: an oral neuropathic pain phenomenon. JADA 142, 1031–1032.

Ito, M., Kimura, H., Yoshida, K., et al., 2010. Effectiveness of milnacipran for the treatment of chronic pain in the orofacial region. Clin. Neuropharmacol. 33 (2), 79–83.

Koratkar, H., Pedersen, J., 2008. Atypical odontalgia: a review. Northwest Dent. 87 (1), 37–38, 62.

List, T., Leijon, G., Helkimo, M., et al., 2006. Effect of local anesthesia on atypical odontalgia – a randomized controlled trial. Pain 122 (3), 306–314.

List, T., Leijon, G., Svensson, P., 2008. Somatosensory abnormalities in atypical odontalgia: A case-control study. Pain 139 (2), 333–341.

Markman, S., Howard, J., Quek, S., 2008. Atypical odontalgia – a form of neuropathic pain that emulates dental pain. J. N. J. Dent. Assoc. 79 (3), 27–31.

Neuman, S.A., Eldrige, J.S., Hoelzer, B.C., 2011. Atypical facial pain treated with upperthoracic dorsal column stimulation. Clin. J. Pain 27 (6), 556–558.

Nóbrega, J.C., Siqueira, S.R., Siqueira, J.T., Teixeira, M.J., 2007. Diferential diagnosis in atypical facial pain: a clinical study. Arq. Neuropsiquiatr. 65 (2A), 256–261.

Quail, G., 2005. Atypical facial pain – a diagnostic challenge. Aust. Fam. Physician 34 (8), 641–645.

Ram, S., Teruel, A., Kumar, S.K., Clark, G., 2009. Clinical characteristics and diagnosis of atypical odontalgia: implications for dentists. J. Am. Dent. Assoc. 140 (2), 223–228.

Ruffatti, S., Zanchin, G., Maggioni, F., 2008. A case of intractable facial pain secondary to metastatic lung cancer. Neurol. Sci. 29 (2), 117–119.

Sardella, A., Demarosi, F., Barbieri, C., Lodi, G., 2009. An up-to-date view on persistent idiopathic facial pain. Minerva Stomatol. 58 (6), 289–299.

Sarlani, E., Schwartz, A.H., Greenspan, J.D., Grace, E.G., 2003. Facial pain as first manifestation of lung cancer: a case of lung cancer-related cluster headache and a review of the literature. J. Orofac. Pain 17 (3), 262–267.

Vickers, E.R., Cousins, M.J., 2000. Neuropathic orofacial pain. Part 1: prevalence and pathophysiology. Aust. Endod. J. 26, 19–26.

Walters, H., Lewis, E., Wolper, R., et al., 2008. Neurotropic melanoma of the trigeminal nerve: a case of atypical facial pain. J. Oral Maxillofac. Surg. 66 (3), 547–550.

Zagury, J.G., Eliav, E., Heir, G.M., et al., 2011. Prolonged gingival cold allodynia: a novel finding in patients withatypical odontalgia. Oral Surg. Oral Med. Oral Pathol. Oral Radiol. Endod. 111 (3), 312–319.

Behçet syndrome

36

Key Points

- Behçet syndrome (BS) is a systemic disease complex manifesting mainly with vasculitis and oral aphthous-like ulcers
- HLA-B5101 underlies many cases
- Diagnosis is on the basis of aphthous-like ulcers plus two or more of recurrent genital ulceration, eye lesions, skin lesions or pathergy
- Patients with BS need specialist advice and systemic immunomodulation

INTRODUCTION

This is a potentially lethal condition. Behçet syndrome (BS), sometimes also known as Adamantiades syndrome and Behçet disease, is a triple symptom complex of aphthous-like ulcers with genital ulceration and eye disease (especially iridocyclitis), though a number of other systemic manifestations may also be seen, characterized by necrotizing vasculitis.

INCIDENCE

BS is rare, with an occurrence of one case per 100 000 in the developed world, but a frequency 10-fold higher in people originating from the eastern Mediterranean countries and Middle East or the 'Silk Road' (between latitudes 30 degrees and 45 degrees north in Asia and Europe).

AGE

Onset of the disease is usually between the ages of 20 and 30 years.

GENDER

BS affects twice as many men as women and has more severe sequelae in men.

GEOGRAPHIC

The disease is found worldwide, but is most common in people from the Mediterranean area and Asia, China, Korea and Japan (along the 'silk road' of Marco Polo). In those countries it is a leading cause of blindness, though this is not often the case in the Western world.

PREDISPOSING FACTORS

There are no proven predisposing factors for BS, though at various times foods, such as pork and walnuts, and oral infections have been suggested as causal. Dental and periodontal therapies may be associated with a flare-up of oral ulcers in the short term, but may decrease their number in longer follow-up. Periodontal status tends to be worse and may be associated with disease severity. CPITN is higher in patients with BS compared with controls and RAS. Mean CPITN was higher in the TNF-alpha-1031C allele CC genotype compared with other genotypes, and the CPITN and CC genotype correlate with the severity of BS. A decline in BS in Japan has been speculated as being related to a decline in oral infections, associated with the improvement in oral health.

AETIOLOGY AND PATHOGENESIS

BS is an immune-related vasculitis that has not been proved to be infectious, contagious, or sexually shared (**Fig. 36.1**):

- There is a genetic predisposition to BS – which is strongly associated with human leukocyte antigen (HLA)-B*51 (HLA-B*5101) and HLA-A*26 (HLA-A*2601). MICA related gene A (MICA) family and MICA6 allele, a polymorphic MHC class I in linkage disequilibrium with HLA-B51, may be associated with BS. HLA-DRB1*14 is significantly increased in patients whose disease appears before age 20 years.

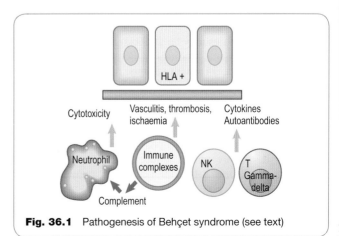

Fig. 36.1 Pathogenesis of Behçet syndrome (see text)

- Associations reported with immune response genes include with:
  - interleukins IL-4, IL-8, IL10, IL12RB2 and IL23R
  - TNF alpha gene polymorphisms at locations -1031C, -238A and the -857T promoter
  - single nucleotide polymorphisms (SNPs) near a ring finger protein (RNF) 39 and on exon 9 of tripartite motif-containing (TRIM) 39.
- An antigen responsible for BS has not been reliably identified though a viral aetiology (possibly herpes simplex virus) has been proposed, and a delayed-type hypersensitivity reaction to the oral bacterium *Streptococcus sanguis* has been implicated. There may be an HLA-independent antibacterial host response toward Th 1 immunity mediated by IL-12. The aetiological factors may have a common denominator in heat shock proteins (HSP), particularly 65kDa microbial HSP, which shows significant homology with the human 60kDa mitochondrial HSP. Indeed, the uncommon serotypes of oral *Streptococcus sanguis* found in BS cross-react with the 65kDa HSP (Hsp-60/65), which also shares antigenicity with an oral mucosal antigen. Although Hsp-60/65 has homologies with the respective T cell epitope, it stimulates peripheral blood mononuclear cells from BS patients. On the other hand, some peptides of Hsp-60/65 reduce IL-8 and IL-12 production from BS patients mononuclear cells during active disease. In BS there are high levels of salivary *S. mutans* colonization associated with oral ulcers and in male patients with a severe disease course and also related to very low levels of serum mannose-binding lectin (MBL). The relationship between increased *S. mutans* and MBL deficiency with active disease may indicate streptococcal hypersensitivity and an impaired innate immune response in BS patients which may predispose to oral infections and a severe disease course. Specific positive signals against human and against streptococcal α-enolase are also common in BS. An HLA-B51 restricted CD8 T cell response is correlated with the target tissues expressing MICA*009 by stress in BS patients with HLA-B51 as the intrinsic factor. Bes-1 gene encodes partial *S. sanguis* genome which is highly homologous with retinal protein Brn3b, and Hsp-60. Hsp-65/60 also has high homologies with the respective T cell epitope of BS patients. Although Hsp-65/60 and peptides of Bes-1 gene were found to stimulate mononuclear from BS patients in the production of pro-inflammatory Th1 type cytokines, some homologous peptides of Hsp-65 with T cell epitopes were found to reduce IL-8, IL-12 and TNF-alpha production. Selenium binding protein may be a target antigen in Behçet uveitis, while anti-*Saccharomyces cerevisiae* antibodies may be implicated in intestinal BS.
- Many immunological findings in BS are similar to those seen in RAS (Ch. 34), with various T lymphocyte abnormalities and increased polymorphonuclear leukocyte motility. There is increased T cell (Th-1) activity, cells infiltrating into lesions expressing interferon (IFN)-gamma. Proinflammatory cytokines IL-12, IL-18 and tumour necrosis factor alpha (TNF-alpha) are increased and some, such as IL-12, are potent inducers of the Th-1 immune reaction. IL-2 and IL-6 cytokines and T regulatory cells (Treg cell) also play a major role, particularly CD4($^+$) CD25(bright) cells. Th17 cells can contribute to the development of the disease with their proinflammatory cytokine IL-17. IL-21 may promote Th17 effectors and suppress

Treg cells. Th2 may also play a role. Interleukin-12B heterozygosity is associated with BS susceptibility and plays an important role in mediating Th1 antistreptococcal immune response.
- Circulating autoantibodies against a number of components, including intermediate filaments found in mucous membranes, cardiolipin and neutrophil cytoplasm, are present. There are raised levels of acute phase proteins and circulating immune complexes and changed levels of complement. There is immunoglobulin and complement deposition within and around blood vessel walls.
- Vasculitis: usually leukocytoclastic vasculitis underlies many of the clinical features (erythema nodosum, arthralgia, uveitis) as in established immune complex diseases/vasculitis. Immunocytes (mostly CD4 cells), B cells, and neutrophils infiltrate perivascularly. Endothelial dysfunction in vasculitis may be detected by assay of a novel autoantigen Sip1 C-ter.
- Hypercoagulability is also a feature: prostanoid synthesis in endothelial cells or vessel walls is impaired, whereas von Willebrand factor, endothelin-1,2, thromboxane and thrombomodulin are increased and factor V Leiden and prothrombin mutations are associated with thromboses in BS.

CLINICAL FEATURES

BS is a chronic multisystem and sometimes life-threatening vasculitis, characterized mainly by:

- Oral aphthous-like ulceration: in 90–100% of cases (**Fig. 36.2**) is the most common and usually the initial manifestation of BS. Oral ulcers precede the diagnosis by 7.5 ± 10 years. However, only few patients with aphthous-like ulceration progress to BS and it is not possible to determine in which patients or when the transition may occur. Recent HLA and immunological findings may eventually help in this respect.
- Recurrent painful genital ulcers that tend to heal with scars: in 64–88% of cases. Genital ulcers are especially common in females with BS, resemble RAS and precede the diagnosis by 1–2 years.
- Ocular lesions: precede the diagnosis by 1–2 years. The most common ocular manifestation is relapsing iridocyclitis, but uveitis with conjunctivitis (early) and hypopyon (late), retinal vasculitis (posterior uveitis), iridocyclitis and optic atrophy can arise.

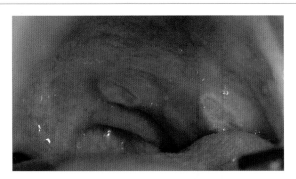

Fig. 36.2 Aphthous-like ulcers in Behçet syndrome: the most common feature

- CNS lesions are predominantly subtentorial (affecting cerebellum, brainstem and spinal cord), with meningoencephalitis, cerebral infarction, psychosis, cranial nerve palsies, and hemi- and quadric-paresis.
- Skin lesions include erythema nodosum-like lesions, papulopustular lesions and acneiform nodules. Venepuncture is, in some patients, followed by pustulation, but this phenomenon (pathergy), is not seen often in UK or US patients.
- Cardiac, or large vein thrombosis (of the inferior vena cava and cranial venous sinuses), can be life-threatening.
- Involvement of the joints, epididymis, heart, intestinal tract, vascular system and most other systems (though not in every case).

A range of non-specific signs and symptoms may precede the onset of the mucosal membrane ulcerations which suggest the diagnosis of BS, by 6 months to 5 years. This includes a history of repeated sore throats, tonsillitis, myalgias, and migratory arthralgias without overt arthritis but features can also include:

- malaise
- anorexia
- weight loss
- generalized weakness
- headache
- sweating
- decreased or elevated temperature
- lymphadenopathy
- pain of the substernal and temporal regions.

DIAGNOSIS

Because BS is rare, early features often non-specific, and the established features overlap those of many other diseases, the condition can be difficult to diagnose. The International Study Group for Behçet's Disease criteria (**Table 36.1**), and newer criteria, suggest the diagnosis should be made on clinical grounds alone – on the basis of oral aphthous-like ulcers plus two or more of:

- recurrent genital ulceration
- eye lesions
- skin lesions

Table 36.1   Features of Behçet syndrome

Major criteria	Minor criteria
Aphthous-like oral ulcers	Arthralgia: large joint arthropathies
Genital ulcers	that are subacute, non-migratory,
Ocular lesions	self-limiting and non-deforming
CNS lesions	Superficial or deep migratory
Skin lesions	thrombophlebitis, especially of
	lower limbs.
	Thromboses of large veins, such
	as the dural sinuses or venae
	cavae
	Intestinal lesions: inflammatory
	bowel disease with discrete
	ulcerations
	Lung disease: pneumonitis
	Renal disease: haematuria and
	proteinuria

Table 36.2   Aids that might be helpful in diagnosis/prognosis/management in some patients suspected of having Behçet syndrome*

In most cases	In some cases
Ophthalmological opinion	Serum immunoglobulins
Rheumatological opinion	Serum complement
Neurological opinion	Cardiolipin antibodies
Full blood picture	
Serum ferritin, vitamin B$_{12}$ and corrected whole blood folate levels	
ESR	
HLA-B5101	
G6PD and TPMT levels	
Blood pressure	
Blood glucose	

*See text for details and glossary for abbreviations.

- pathergy: a >2 mm diameter erythematous nodule or pustule forming 24–48 h after sterile subcutaneous puncture of the forearm skin.

The major limitation of the clinical diagnostic criteria, however, lies in the fact that recurrent oral ulceration is the key for diagnosis of BS. For example, patients with uveitis and genital ulcers, without oral aphthosis, would not be considered to have BS, although this may in fact be a far-advanced form of BS. The differential diagnosis is mainly from other oculomucocutaneous syndromes such as:

- Sweet syndrome: oral ulcers, conjunctivitis, episcleritis, inflamed tender skin papules or nodules
- Erythema multiforme: erosions, target (iris) lesions
- Pemphigoid: bullae, erosions
- Pemphigus: erosions, flaccid skin bullae
- Reiter syndrome: ulcers, conjunctivitis, keratoderma blenorrhagica
- Ulcerative colitis
- Syphilis
- Lupus erythematosus
- Mixed connective tissue disease.

Unfortunately, there are no specific tests for the diagnosis of BS (**Table 36.2**). Findings of HLA-B5101, raised serum IgD and antibodies to cardiolipin are supportive of a diagnosis of BS. Disease activity may be assessed by serum levels of acute-phase proteins (ESR, CRP or PV), α_2-globulins and other acute-phase reactants) and antibodies to intermediate filaments, which are raised in active BS.

TREATMENT (see also Chs 4 and 5)

The effects of BS may be cumulative, especially with neurological, vascular and ocular involvement; one main problem is ophthalmic involvement, which can result in blindness. Mortality though low, but can result from neurological involvement, vascular thromboses, bowel perforation or cardiopulmonary disease, or as a complication of immunosuppressive therapy.

Table 36.3 Regimens that might be helpful in management of patient suspected of having Behçet syndrome (see Ch. 5)

Regimen	Use in primary care – for oral lesions	Use in secondary care (severe oral involvement and/or extraoral involvement)
Beneficial		Prednisolone (enteric-coated) Thalidomide
Likely to be beneficial	Chlorhexidine Tetracycline mouthwash Topical corticosteroids (see Ch. 34)	Azathioprine Ciclosporin Chlorambucil Colchicine Cyclophosphamide Interferon-α Levamisole Mycophenolate sodium
Unproven effectiveness		Dapsone Irsogladine Lasers Lenalidomide Low molecular weight heparin Nicotine patches Mycophenolate mofetil Pentoxifylline Rebamipide Retinoids
Emergent treatments		Adalumimab Efalizumab (now withdrawn) Etanercept Infliximab
Supportive	Benzydamine Diet with little acidic, spicy or citrus content Lidocaine	Benzydamine Diet with little acidic, spicy or citrus content Lidocaine

In the face of such serious potential complications, patients with suspected BS should be referred early for specialist advice and typically require systemic immunomodulation (**Table 36.3**). Patient information is also an important aspect in management:

- Treatment for aphthous-like ulcers in BS includes tetracycline mouthwash and topical corticosteroids (Ch. 5).
- If the ulcers in BS fail to respond to topical measures as used in aphthae (Ch. 34), systemic immunomodulators may be required, under specialist supervision (Ch. 5). The adverse effects of these agents may need to be accepted in such a serious condition (Ch. 5).
- Other therapies for BS include anti-tumour necrosis factor alpha agents such as thalidomide or the biologics. Thalidomide effectively controls ulcers with a dose of 25 mg daily, followed by a median maintenance dose of 100 mg/ week. Adverse events are reported by 85% but are mostly mild (78% of patients), sometimes severe (21%). Nevertheless, after 40 months of follow-up, 60% of patients in some studies were still receiving continuous or intermittent maintenance therapy with favourable efficacy/tolerance ratios.

EMERGENT TREATMENTS

These include adalumimab, etanercept and infliximab.

FOLLOW-UP OF PATIENTS

Long-term follow-up as shared care is usually appropriate.

USEFUL WEBSITES

American Autoimmune Related Diseases Association: http://www.aarda.org/

American Behçet's Disease Association: http://www.behcets.com/

Medscape, Dermatological Aspects of Behçet Disease. http://emedicine.medscape.com/article/1122381

FURTHER READING

Adler, Y.D., Mausmann, U. Zouboulis, C.C, 2001. Mycophenolate mofetil is ineffective in the treatment of mucocutaneons Adamautiadtes- Behcets disease. Dermatology 203, 322–324.

Akman, A., Sallakci, N., Kacaroglu, H., 2008. Relationship between periodontal findings and the TNF-alpha Gene 1031T/C polymorphism in Turkish patients with Behçet's disease. J. Eur. Acad. Dermatol. Venereol. 22 (8), 950–957.

Alexoudi, I., Kapsimali, V., Vaiopoulos, A., et al., 2011. Evaluation of current therapeutic strategies in Behçet's disease. Clin. Rheumatol. 30 (2), 157–163.

Arabaci, T., Kara, C., Ciçek, Y., 2009. Relationship between periodontal parameters and Behçet's disease and evaluation of different treatments for oral recurrent aphthous stomatitis. J. Periodontal Res. 44 (6), 718–725.

B'chir Hamzaoui, S., Harmel, A., Bouslama, K., et al., 2006. Behçet's disease in Tunisia. Clinical study of 519 cases. Rev. Med. Interne 27 (10), 742–750.

Bernabé, E., Marcenes, W., Mather, J., et al., 2010. Impact of Behçet's syndrome on health-related quality of life: influence of the type and number of symptoms. Rheumatology (Oxford) 49 (11), 2165–2171.

Calamia, K.T., Kaklamanis, P.G., 2008. Behçet's disease: recent advances in early diagnosis and effective treatment. Curr. Rheumatol. Rep. 10 (5), 349–355.

Cho, S.B., Lee, J.H., Ahn, K.J., et al., 2010. Identification of streptococcal proteins reacting with sera from Behçet's disease and rheumatic disorders. Clin. Exp. Rheumatol. 28 (Suppl. 4), S31–S38.

Chou, C.T., 2006. The clinical application of etanercept in Chinese patients with rheumatic diseases. Mod. Rheumatol. 16 (4), 206–213.

Ciancio, G., Colina, M., La Corte, R., et al., 2010. Nicotine-patch therapy on mucocutaneous lesions of Behçet's disease: a case series. Rheumatology (Oxford) 49 (3), 501–504.

Davatchi, F., Sadeghi Abdollahi, B., Tehrani Banihashemi, A., et al., 2009. Colchicine versus placebo in Behçet's disease: randomized, double-blind, controlled crossover trial. Mod. Rheumatol. 19 (5), 542–549.

de Menthon, M., Lavalley, M.P., Maldini, C., et al., 2009. HLA-B51/B5 and the risk of Behçet's disease: a systematic review and meta-analysis of case-control genetic association studies. Arthritis Rheum. 61 (10), 1287–1296.

Demetriades, N., Hanford, H., Laskarides, C., 2009. General manifestations of Behçet's syndrome and the success of CO$_2$-laser as treatment for oral lesions: a review of the literature and case presentation. J. Mass. Dent. Soc. 58 (3), 24–27.

Deniz, E., Guc, U., Buyukbabani, N., Gul, A., 2010. HSP 60 expression in recurrent oral ulcerations of Behçet's disease. Oral Surg. Oral Med. Oral Pathol. Oral Radiol. Endod. 110 (2), 196–200.

Direskeneli, H., Mumcu, G., 2010. A possible decline in the incidence and severity of Behçet's disease: implications for an infectious etiology and oral health. Clin. Exp. Rheumatol. 28 (Suppl. 4), S86–S90.

Escudier, M., Bagan, J., Scully, C., 2006. Behçets syndrome (Adamantiades syndrome). Oral Dis. 12, 78–84.

Evereklioglu, C., 2006. Adamantiades–Behçet disease: an enigmatic process with oral manifestations. Med. Oral Patol. Oral Cir. Bucal 11 (5), E393–E394.

Freysdottir, J., Hussain, L., Farmer, I., et al., 2006. Diversity of gammadelta T cells in patients with Behçet's disease is indicative of polyclonal activation. Oral Dis. 12 (3), 271–277.

Geri, G., Terrier, B., Rosenzwajg, M., et al., 2011. Critical role of IL-21 in modulating T(H)17 and regulatory T cells in Behçet disease. J. Allergy Clin. Immunol. 128 (3), 655–664.

Green, J., Upjohn, E., McCormack, C., et al., 2008. Successful treatment of Behçet's disease with lenalidomide. Br. J. Dermatol. 158 (1), 197–198.

Hamuryudan, V., Hatemi, G., Tascilar, K., et al., 2010. Prognosis of Behçet's syndrome among men with mucocutaneous involvement at disease onset: long-term outcome of patients enrolled in a controlled trial. Rheumatology (Oxford) 49 (1), 173–177.

Hamzaoui, K., Bouali, E., Ghorbel, I., et al., 2011. Expression of Th-17 and RORγt mRNA in Behçet's Disease. Med. Sci. Monit. 17 (4) CR227–CR234.

Hayran, O., Mumcu, G., Inanc, N., 2009. Assessment of minimal clinically important improvement by using Oral Health Impact Profile-14 in Behçet's disease. Clin. Exp. Rheumatol. 27 (2 Suppl 53), S79–S84.

Hirohata, S., 2006. Is the long-term use of systemic corticosteroids beneficial in the management of Behçet's syndrome? Nat. Clin. Pract. Rheumatol. 2 (7), 358–359.

Ideguchi, H., Suda, A., Takeno, M., et al., Behçet disease:evolution of clinical manifestations. Medicine (Baltimore) 90 (2), 125–132.

Jiang, Z., Yang, P., Hou, S., et al., 2010. IL-23R gene confers susceptibility to Behçet's disease in a Chinese Han population. Ann. Rheum. Dis. 69 (7), 1325–1328.

Kaneko, F., Oyama, N., Yanagihori, H., et al., 2008. The role of streptococcal Hypersensitivity in the pathogenesis of Behçet's Disease. Eur. J. Dermatol. 18 (5), 489–498.

Karacayli, U., Mumcu, G., Simsek, I., et al., 2009. The close association between dental and periodontal treatments and oral ulcer course in Behçet's disease: a prospective clinical study. J. Oral Pathol. Med. 38 (5), 410–415.

Keogan, M.T., 2009. Clinical Immunology Review Series: an approach to the patient with recurrent orogenital ulceration, including Behçet's syndrome. Clin. Exp. Immunol. 156 (1), 1–11.

Kernich, C.A., 2006. Patient and family fact sheet. Behçet disease. Neurologist 12 (2), 115–116.

Kiliç, H., Zeytin, H.E., Korkmaz, C., et al., 2009. Low-dose natural human interferon-alpha lozenges in the treatment of Behçet's syndrome. Rheumatology (Oxford) 48 (11), 1388–1391.

Kim, J., Park, J.A., Lee, E.Y., et al., 2010. Imbalance of Th17 to Th1 cells in Behçet's disease. Clin. Exp. Rheumatol. 28 (4 Suppl. 60), S16–S19.

Krause, I., Weinberger, A., 2008. Behçet's disease. Curr. Opin. Rheumatol. 20 (1), 82–87.

Kurata, R., Nakaoka, H., Tajima, A., et al., 2010. TRIM39 and RNF39 are associated with Behçet's disease independently of HLA-B*51 and -A*26. Biochem. Biophys. Res. Commun. 401 (4), 533–537.

Lee, L.A., 2001. Behçet disease. Semin. Cutan. Med. Surg. 20, 53–57.

Matsuda, T., Ohno, S., Hirohata, S., et al., 2003. Efficacy of rebamipide as adjunctive therapy in the treatment of recurrent oral aphthous ulcers in patients with Behçet's disease; a randomised double-blinded, placebo-controlled study. Drugs R D 4, 19–28.

Mizuki, N., Meguro, A., Ota, M., et al., 2010. Genome-wide association studies identify IL23R-IL12RB2 and IL10 as Behçet's disease susceptibility loci. Nat. Genet. 42 (8), 703–706.

Mumcu, G., Inanc, N., Aydin, S.Z., et al., 2009. Association of salivary S. mutans colonisation and mannose-binding lectin deficiency with gender in Behçet's disease. Clin. Exp. Rheumatol. 27 (2 Suppl. 53), S32–S36.

Nanke, Y., Kamatani, N., Okamoto, T., et al., 2008. Irsogladine is effective for recurrent oral ulcers in patients with Behçet's disease: an open-label, single-centre study. Drugs R D 9 (6), 455–459.

Onal, S., Kazokoglu, H., Koc, A., et al., 2011. Long-term efficacy and safety of low-dose and dose-escalating interferon alfa-2a therapy in refractory Behçet uveitis. Arch. Ophthalmol. 129 (3), 288–294.

Sakane, T., Takeno, M., 2000. Current therapy in Behçet's disease. Skin Ther. 5, 3–5.

Seyahi, E., Fresko, I., Melikoglu, M., Yazici, H., 2006. The management of Behçet's syndrome. Acta Reumatol. Port. 31 (2), 125–131.

Stuebiger, N., Hazirolan, D., Pleyer, U., et al., 2011. Anti-TNF agents for Behçet´s disease: analysis of published data on 369 patients. Semin. Arthritis Rheum. 41 (1), 61–70.

Yanagihori, H., Oyama, N., Nakamura, K., et al., 2006. Role of IL-12B promoter polymorphism in Adamantiades–Behçet's disease susceptibility: An involvement of Th1 immunoreactivity against Streptococcus sanguinis antigen. J. Invest. Dermatol. 126 (7), 1534–1540.

Yates, P.A., Michelson, J.B., 2006. Behçet disease. Int. Ophthalmol. Clin. 46 (2), 209–233.

Yazici, Y., Yurdakul, S., Yazici, H., 2010. Behçet's syndrome. Curr. Rheumatol. Rep. 12 (6), 429–435.

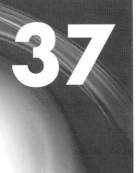

37 Bell palsy

Key Points

- Bell palsy is an acute lower motor neurone face palsy where there is inflammation with demyelination, in the stylomastoid canal
- Most cases are related to viral infections – mainly herpes simplex virus
- Management is with antivirals and corticosteroids

INTRODUCTION

Bell palsy is an acute lower motor neurone facial palsy. There is inflammation of the facial nerve with demyelination, usually in the stylomastoid canal, and oedema further hazarding the blood supply to the nerve interrupting neural transmission. No local or systemic cause can be identified except usually herpes simplex virus (HSV) infection.

INCIDENCE

Bell palsy represents about 50% of all facial palsies, but is rare at possibly around 10 cases per 100 000 population.

AGE

Usually seen in a young adult.

GENDER

Both sexes can be affected.

GEOGRAPHIC

No geographic factors are known.

PREDISPOSING FACTORS

Predisposing factors, found in a minority of cases, include:

- pregnancy
- hypertension
- diabetes
- a chronic granulomatous disorder, such as Crohn disease or orofacial granulomatosis, when the association is often termed Melkersson–Rosenthal syndrome (Ch. 56), or sarcoidosis
- lymphoma
- respiratory infections
- immune defects.

AETIOLOGY AND PATHOGENESIS

Bell palsy is most commonly caused by inflammation and oedema in the facial nerve canal, usually in the stylomastoid canal, causing demyelination of the facial nerve (seventh cranial nerve) (**Table 37.1**) usually due to HSV. Facial palsy may be seen in:

- Herpesviruses
  - Usually associated with herpes simplex virus (HSV)
  - Rarely associated with:
    - varicella-zoster virus (VZV) infection
    - Epstein–Barr virus (EBV) infection
    - cytomegalovirus (CMV) infection
    - human herpesvirus-6 infection
- Retroviruses:
  - HIV infection
  - HTLV-1 infection
- Bacteria:
  - otitis media
  - infections around stylomastoid foramen region
  - *Borrelia burgdorferi* infection (Lyme disease; neuroborreliosis)
  - syphilis
- Kawasaki disease (Ch. 56)
- Heerfordt syndrome (sarcoidosis; Ch. 56)
- Melkersson–Rosenthal syndrome (Ch. 56)
- Disseminated sclerosis.

CLINICAL FEATURES

The facial nerve (see Ch. 20) carries:

- motor nerve impulses to the muscles of the face, and facial expression, and to the stapedius muscle of the stirrup bone (the stapes) in the middle ear
- secretomotor fibres to the lacrimal (tear) glands, and to the submandibular and sublingual salivary glands
- taste from the anterior tongue (**Fig. 37.1**) (via the chorda tympani).

Since the function of the facial nerve is so complex, many symptoms may occur if it is disrupted. Bell palsy may result in twitching, weakness or paralysis of the face; in dryness of the eye or the mouth; and/or in disturbance of taste or hearing. There is:

- acute onset of unilateral facial paralysis over a few hours, maximal within 48 h (**Fig. 37.2**)
- diminished blinking and absence of tearing. Together these can reduce or eliminate the flow of tears across the

Table 37.1 Localization of site of lesion in, and causes of, unilateral facial palsy

Muscles paralysed unilaterally	Lacrimation	Hyperacusis	Sense of taste	Other features	Probable site of lesion	Type of lesion
Lower face	N	–	N	Emotional movement retained ± monoparesis or hemiparesis ± aphasia	Upper motor neurone	Stroke, brain tumour, trauma, HIV infection
All facial muscles	↓	+	↓	± VIth nerve damage	Lower motor neurone Facial nucleus	Disseminated sclerosis
All facial muscles	↓	+	↓	± VIIIth nerve damage	Between nucleus and geniculate ganglion	Fractured base of skull, posterior cranial fossa tumours, sarcoidosis
All facial muscles	N	±	N or ↓	–	Between geniculate ganglion and stylomastoid canal	Otitis media, cholesteatoma, mastoiditis
All facial muscles	N	–	N	–	In stylomastoid canal or extracranially	Bell palsy, trauma, local analgesia (e.g. misplaced inferior dental block), Lyme disease, parotid malignant neoplasm, Guillain–Barré syndrome
Isolated facial muscles	N	–	N	–	Branch of facial nerve extracranially	Trauma, local analgesia

N, normal; +, present; ↓, reduced.

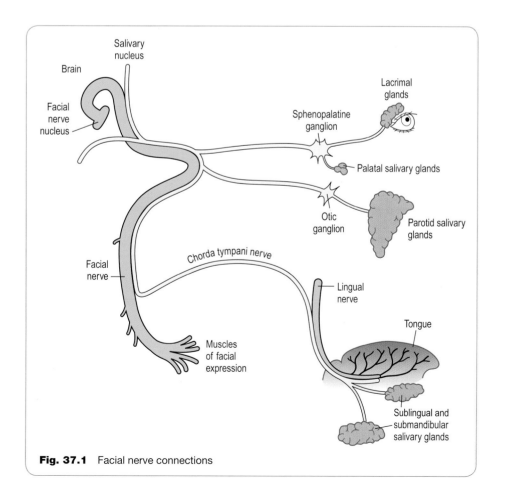

Fig. 37.1 Facial nerve connections

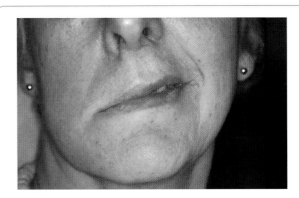

Fig. 37.2 Bell palsy on the right side

eyeball, resulting in drying, erosion, and ulceration of the cornea and the potential loss of the eye.

Occasionally there may be:

- pain in the region of the ear or in the jaw may precede the palsy by a day or two
- complaints of facial numbness, but sensation appears intact on testing
- hyperacusis (heightened sense of hearing due to reduced damping activity of the stapedius because of loss of function of the nerve to the stapedius) or loss of taste (loss of function of the chorda tympani), or loss of lacrimation
- there is a positive family history in up to 10% of patients and recurrent episodes of palsy in up to 10% of patients.

DIAGNOSIS

The history should be directed to exclude facial palsy caused by other factors, such as:

- stroke
- trauma including surgery (parotidectomy) and lacerations physically affecting the facial nerve (e.g. in the parotid region or to the base of the skull), or by underwater diving (barotrauma)
- tumours affecting the facial nerve (e.g. acoustic neuroma or cholesteatoma)
- non-infective inflammatory disorders affecting the facial nerve:
  - disseminated sclerosis
  - connective tissue disease
  - sarcoidosis
  - Melkersson–Rosenthal syndrome
- infections affecting the facial nerve:
  - viral infections (HSV, VZV, EBV, CMV, HIV infection, HTLV-1 infection (Japanese and African-Caribbean patients mainly))
  - bacterial infections (middle ear infections (e.g. otitis media), Lyme disease (camping or walking in areas that may contain deer ticks)).

Bell palsy is less likely to be the diagnosis if:

- the paralysis is slowly progressive or chronic.
- trauma has occurred

- multiple cranial nerves are involved
- there are other neurological features
- there are signs of neoplasia.

The examination should include the following:

- A full neurological examination, especially to exclude a stroke, and to exclude lesions involving other cranial nerves (especially the abducens and vestibulocochlear nerves).
- Examination of the facial nerve; weakness is demonstrated by testing the corneal reflex and asking the patient to close the eyes against resistance, raise the eyebrows, raise the lips to show the teeth, and try to whistle.
- Ear and mouth examination to exclude Ramsay–Hunt syndrome (herpes zoster of the facial nerve ganglion (geniculate ganglion), which causes lesions in the palate and ipsilateral ear, and facial palsy).
- Ear examination, for discharge and other signs of middle ear disease.

Investigations that may be indicated include the following (**Table 37.2**):

- A test for the degree of nerve damage; facial nerve stimulation or needle electromyography may be useful, as may nerve excitability tests, electromyography and electroneuronography.
- A test for loss of hearing; pure tone audiometry is often used.
- A test for taste loss: electrogustometry.
- A test for balance.
- A test for tear production (Schirmer's test), in which a strip of filter paper is placed in the lower conjunctival fornix and the amount of tear production measured.
- MRI or CT imaging of the internal auditory meatus, cerebellopontine angle and mastoid may be needed to exclude an organic lesion such as a tumour – particularly in progressive facial palsy.
- Blood pressure measurement to exclude hypertension.
- Blood tests, which may include:
  - fasting blood sugar levels (to exclude diabetes)
  - serum angiotensin converting enzyme levels to exclude sarcoidosis

Table 37.2 Aids that might be helpful in diagnosis/ prognosis/management in some patients suspected of having Bell palsy*

In most cases	In some cases
Neurological opinion	Audiometry
ENT examination	Facial nerve tests (stimulation,
ESR	needle electromyography,
Blood pressure	electrogustometry, nerve
	excitability tests, electromyography,
	electroneuronography)
	Full blood picture
	Serum ferritin, vitamin B_{12} and
	corrected whole blood folate levels
	Blood glucose
	Serology (HSV, VZV, EBV, CMV, HIV,
	HTLV-1, Lyme disease, syphilis)
	SACE
	ANA
	Lumbar puncture

*See text for details and glossary for abbreviations.

■ serum antinuclear antibodies to exclude connective tissue disease

■ serological tests for HSV or other virus infections, such as HIV, may need to be considered and, in some areas, Lyme disease (tick-borne infection with *Borrelia burgdorferi*) should be excluded by enzyme-linked immunosorbent assay (ELISA) and western blot assay.

■ Occasionally, a lumbar puncture is required.

TREATMENT (see also Chs 4 and 5)

Most patients with Bell palsy (up to 85%) improve spontaneously within a few weeks. However, the after-effects in the remaining 15–40% can be so severe and distressing, that active treatment is warranted (**Table 37.3**). A neurological opinion may be in order.

Patient information is an important aspect in management. The evidence in this controversial area favours use of systemic prednisolone (enteric-coated) within 48–72 h of onset of palsy as this can result in significantly higher complete recovery rates and less synkinesis (see below). The addition of a systemic antiviral (usually valaciclovir) may add marginal benefit.

Complications include the following:

■ The commonest complication of Bell palsy is corneal dryness and scarring due to inadequate eyelid closure. Therefore, during the acute phase, the cornea should be protected with an eye pad. Synthetic tears (hypromellose drops) may help. Protective glasses or clear eye patches are often used to keep the eye moist and to keep foreign materials from entering the eye.

■ Synkinesis: involuntary movements such as eyelid movements accompanying voluntary movements, such as smiling.

■ If paralysis persists and function remains incomplete, the palpebral fissure may narrow, the nasolabial fold deepens and there may be leakage of saliva from the commissure.

FOLLOW-UP OF PATIENTS

The prognosis can be assessed on several factors:

■ Favourable prognostic signs include:
  ■ incomplete paralysis in the first week
  ■ persistence of the stapedial reflex, measured by electroneurography.

■ Bad prognostic signs include:
  ■ an initially complete paralysis (then only 50% recover completely within a week, and few who have not recovered by 2 weeks will do so)
  ■ hyperacusis
  ■ severe taste impairment
  ■ diminished lacrimation or salivation, especially if in older, diabetic or hypertensive patients.

Long-term follow-up is rarely required as most patients recover.

PATIENT INFORMATION SHEET

Bell palsy

▼ Please read this information sheet. If you have any questions, particularly about the treatment or potential side-effects, please ask your doctor.

■ This is fairly common.

■ It affects only the facial nerve; there are no brain or other neurological problems.

■ It may be caused by herpes simplex virus, or other infections.

■ It is not contagious.

■ It disproportionately attacks pregnant women and people who have diabetes, influenza, a cold, or immune problems.

■ There are usually no serious long-term consequences.

■ X-rays, scans and blood tests *may* be required.

■ Treatment takes time and patience; corticosteroids and/or antimicrobials can sometimes help.

■ Most patients begin to get significantly better within 2 weeks, and about 80% recover completely within 3 months.

■ It rarely recurs, but can do so in ~ 5–10%.

Table 37.3 Regimens that might be helpful in management of patient suspected of having Bell palsy

Regimen	Use in primary or secondary care
Likely to be beneficial	Prednisolone (enteric-coated) plus valaciclovir or aciclovir
Unproven effectiveness	Facial nerve decompression Acupuncture
Supportive	Corneal protection Facial exercises

USEFUL WEBSITES

American Academy of Otolaryngology – Head and Neck Surgery, Bell's Palsy. http://www.entnet.org/HealthInformation/bellsPalsy.cfm

Bell's Palsy Information Site: http://www.bellspalsy.ws/

National Institute of Neurological Disorders and Stroke, Bell's Palsy Information. http://www.ninds.nih.gov/disorders/bells/bells.htm

FURTHER READING

Alberton, D.L., Zed, P.J., 2006. Bell's palsy: a review of treatment using antiviral agents. Ann. Pharmacother. 40 (10), 1838–1842.

Axelsson, S., Berg, T., Jonsson, L., et al., 2011. Prednisolone in Bell's palsy related to treatment start and age. Otol. Neurotol. 32 (1), 141–146.

Browning, G.G., 2010. Bell's palsy: a review of three systematic reviews of steroid and anti-viral therapy. Clin. Otolaryngol. 35 (1), 56–58.

Cardoso, J.R., Teixeira, E.C., Moreira, M.D., et al., 2008. Effects of exercises on Bell's palsy: systematic review of randomized controlled trials. Otol. Neurotol. 29 (4), 557–560.

Chen, N., Zhou, M., He, L., et al., 2010. Acupuncture for Bell's palsy. Cochrane Database Syst. Rev (8), CD002914.

Cohen, Y., Lavie, O., Granovsky-Grisaru, S., et al., 2000. Bell's palsy complicating pregnancy: a review. Obstet. Gynecol. Surv. 55, 184–188.

de Almeida, J.R., Al Khabori, M., Guyatt, G.H., et al., 2009. Combined corticosteroid and antiviral treatment for Bell palsy: a systematic review and meta-analysis. JAMA 302 (9), 985–993.

Kennedy, P.G., 2010. Herpes simplex virus type 1 and Bell's palsy–a current assessment of the controversy. J. Neurovirol. 16 (1), 1–5.

Kim, M.S., Yoon, H.J., Kim, H.J., et al., 2006. Bilateral peripheral facial palsy in a patient with human immunodeficiency virus (HIV) infection. Yonsei Med. J. 47 (5), 745–747.

Kim, M.W., Kim, E.H., 2011. Re: Prognostic value of electroneurography in Bell's palsy and Ramsay-Hunt's syndrome. Clin. Otolaryngol. 36 (1), 88–89; author reply 89.

Lackner, A., Kessler, H.H., Walch, C., et al., 2010. Early and reliable detection of herpes simplex virus type 1 and varicella zoster virus DNAs in oral fluid of patients with idiopathic peripheral facial nerve palsy: Decision support regarding antiviral treatment? J. Med. Virol. 82 (9), 1582–1585.

Lampert, L., Wong, Y.J., 2012. Combined antiviral– corticosteroid therapy for Bell palsy yields inconclusive benefit. JADA 143, 57–58.

Lorch, M., Teach, S.J., 2010. Facial nerve palsy: etiology and approach to diagnosis and treatment. Pediatr. Emerg. Care 26 (10), 763–769; quiz 770–773.

McAllister, K., Walker, D., Donnan, P.T., Swan, I., 2011. Surgical interventions for the early management of Bell's palsy. Cochrane Database Syst. Rev (2), CD007468.

McCormick, D.P., 2000. Herpes simplex virus as a cause of Bell's palsy. Rev. Med. Virol. 10, 285–289.

Numthavaj, P., Thakkinstian, A., Dejthevaporn, C., Attia, J., 2011. Corticosteroid and antiviral therapy for Bell's palsy: a network meta-analysis. BMC Neurol. 11, 1.

Quant, E.C., Jeste, S.S., Muni, R.H., et al., 2009. The benefits of steroids versus steroids plus antivirals for treatment of Bell's palsy: a meta-analysis. BMJ 339, b3354.

Quesnel, A.M., Lindsay, R.W., Hadlock, T.A., 2010. When the bell tolls on Bell's palsy: finding occult malignancy in acute-onset facial paralysis. Am. J. Otolaryngol. 31 (5), 339–342.

Ramsey, M.J., DerSimonian, R., Holtel, M.R., et al., 2000. Corticosteroid treatment for idiopathic facial nerve paralysis: a meta-analysis. Laryngoscope 110, 335–341.

Reid, S.R., Hetzel, T., Losek, J., 2006. Temporal bone rhabdomyosarcoma presenting as acute peripheral facial nerve paralysis. Pediatr. Emerg. Care 22 (10), 743–745.

Salinas, R.A., Alvarez, G., Daly, F., Ferreira, J., 2010. Corticosteroids for Bell's palsy (idiopathic facial paralysis). Cochrane Database Syst. Rev. (3), CD001942.

Santos, M.A., Caiaffa Filho, H.H., Vianna, M.F., et al., 2010. Varicella zoster virus in Bell's palsy: a prospective study. Braz. J. Otorhinolaryngol. 76 (3), 370–373.

Shaikh, Z.A., Bakshi, R., Wasay, M., et al., 2000. Magnetic resonance imaging findings in bilateral Bell's palsy. J. Neuroimaging 10, 223–225.

Siddiq, M.A., Hanu-Cernat, L.M., Irving, R.M., 2007. Facial palsy secondary to cholesteatoma: analysis of outcome following surgery. J. Laryngol. Otol. 121, 114–117.

Siol, T., Huber, M., Buchner, H., 2001. Posttraumatic Bell's palsy. Am. J. Psychiatry 158, 322.

Worster, A., Keim, S.M., Sahsi, R., Pancioli, A.M., Best Evidence in Emergency Medicine (BEEM) Group, 2010. Do either corticosteroids or antiviral agents reduce the risk of long-term facial paresis in patients with new-onset Bell's palsy? J. Emerg. Med. 38 (4), 518–523.

Yanagihara, N., Honda, N., Hato, N., et al., 2000. Edematous swelling of the facial nerve in Bell's palsy. Acta Otolaryngol. 120, 667–671.

Burning mouth syndrome (oral dysaesthesia)

38

Key Points

- Burning mouth 'syndrome' (BMS) is a burning sensation, experienced in the absence of identifiable organic aetiological factors
- BMS is seen especially in older women
- BMS may have a psychogenic or neuropathic basis
- BMS most frequently affects the tongue, with persistent discomfort but can affect other sites
- Management is usually with cognitive behavioural therapy or psychoactive medication

INTRODUCTION

A burning sensation in the mouth may be a primary condition, or secondary to identifiable causes (**Fig. 38.1**). Burning mouth 'syndrome' (BMS) – also known as glossopyrosis, glossodynia, oral dysaesthesia or stomatodynia – is the term used when symptoms described usually as a burning sensation, exist in the absence of clinically identifiable oral mucosal disease, when a medical or dental cause has been excluded. BMS is a medically unexplained symptom (MUS). The International Association for the Study of Pain define it as: 'A distinctive nosological entity characterized by unremitting oral burning or similar pain in the absence of detectable mucosal changes'.

INCIDENCE

BMS is a fairly common chronic complaint, affecting up to five persons per 100 000 population.

AGE

BMS is seen especially in middle-aged or older patients.

GENDER

BMS is seen especially in women, in a ratio of about 3:1.

GEOGRAPHIC

BMS is seen worldwide.

PREDISPOSING FACTORS, AETIOLOGY AND PATHOGENESIS

- No precipitating cause for a burning sensation can be identified in over 50% of the patients, but in others, local or systemic factors may be identifiable (**Fig. 38.2**).
- BMS in some appears to follow either:
  - dental intervention
  - an upper respiratory tract infection
  - use of drugs, such as cytotoxics, angiotensin converting enzyme (ACE) inhibitors, clonazepam, antidepressants, hormone replacement therapy, proton pump inhibitors (PPIs) or protease inhibitors (PIs) (**Algorithm 38.1**)
  - exposure to various chemicals or other substances (**Box 38.1**).
- BMS has been associated with immunological changes; it has been hypothesized that the presence of low levels of CD28 cells suggests that BMS might be a pre-autoimmune disease. Cytokines IL-2 and TNF-alpha might play a role in the pathogenesis.

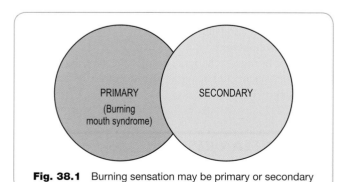

Fig. 38.1 Burning sensation may be primary or secondary

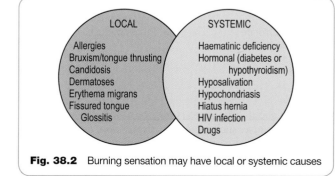

Fig. 38.2 Burning sensation may have local or systemic causes

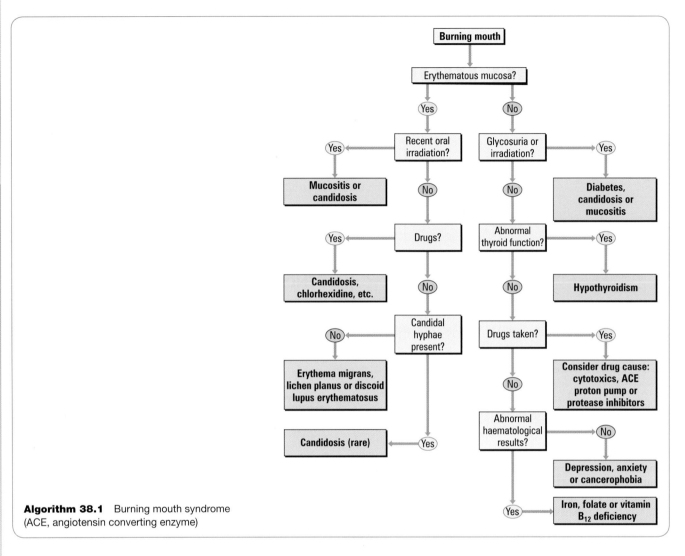

Algorithm 38.1 Burning mouth syndrome (ACE, angiotensin converting enzyme)

BOX 38.1 Substances implicated in causing oral burning sensations

Foods and additives
- Benzoic acid
- Chestnuts
- Cinnamonaldehyde
- Instant coffee
- Nicotinic acid
- Peanuts
- Sodium metabisulphite
- Sorbic acid

Metals
- Cadmium
- Cobalt chloride
- Mercury
- Nickel
- Palladium

Plastics
- Benzoyl peroxide
- Bisphenol A
- Epoxy resins
- Methyl methacrylate
- Octyl gallate
- Propylene glycol

Drugs (Table 54.24)
- Cyctotoxic drugs
- ACE inhibitors
- Protease inhibitors
- Proton pump inhibitors

- BMS in about 20% of cases may be associated with a psychogenic cause, such as anxiety, depression, cancerophobia or concern about a sexually shared infection.
- BMS may be a neuropathic disorder of reduced pain and sensory thresholds. It can follow damage to the cauda

tympani nerve and is increased in frequency in Parkinson's disease. BMS patients are often 'super-tasters' – they have raised sensitivity to taste. Nerve growth factor (NGF) peptide and tryptase activity appear significantly and persistently raised in saliva in BMS. Hypotheses include that BMS is a sympathetic activity-mediated neuropathic disorder induced by traumatic trigeminal nerve injury or varicella-zoster virus infection, or due to:

- changes in the nigrostriatal dopaminergic system, which causes trigeminal excitability, or
- loss of central inhibition from taste damage in the chorda tympani and/or glossopharyngeal nerve (**Fig. 38.3**).
- BMS appears unrelated
  - to contact allergies
  - to sex hormone changes, despite the fact that BMS is often seen in middle-aged or older peri- or postmenopausal females.

CLINICAL FEATURES

BMS most frequently affects the anterior tongue, but it can also affect the palate or, less commonly, the lips or

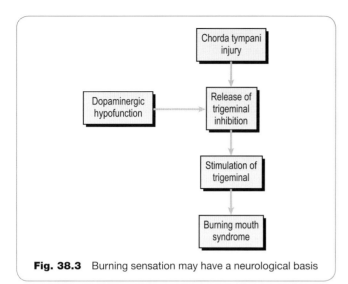

Fig. 38.3 Burning sensation may have a neurological basis

lower alveolus. Three types of BMS have been described on the basis of the pattern of symptoms of burning sensation (**Table 38.1**).

The symptoms are variable and may be:

- of burning, scalding or tingling
- moderately severe (visual analogue scale 5–8)
- bilateral usually
- relieved by eating and drinking, in contrast to pain caused by organic lesions, which is typically aggravated by eating
- relieved by alcohol
- persistent, but does not disturb sleep
- prolonged >4 months.

Patients with BMS often are on medications and have systemic conditions, and there are frequently multiple psychogenic-related complaints, such as:

- dry mouth (>50%)
- bad or altered taste (>10%)
- thirst
- headaches
- chronic back pain
- irritable bowel syndrome
- dysmenorrhoea.

Patients seem only uncommonly to use analgesics to try to control the symptoms. There may be changes in sleep patterns and mood and there have often already been multiple consultations and attempts at treatment.

DIAGNOSIS

Defined clinical conditions that must be excluded, since they can also present with a burning sensation, include (**Fig. 38.2**) (see **Algorithm 38.1**):

- Allergies
- Bruxism/tongue thrusting/restricted tongue space from poor denture construction
- Candidosis
- Dermatoses such as lichen planus, dry mouth and drugs such as ACE inhibitors and protease inhibitors
- Erythema migrans (geographic tongue)
- Fissured tongue
- Glossitis such as caused by haematinic (iron, folic acid or vitamin B) deficiency in about 30%. Magnesium deficiency may underlie some cases
- Hormonal problems, such as diabetes and hypothyroidism, hyposalivation.

Investigations indicated may include psychological screening using, for example, the hospital anxiety and depression (HAD) scale, and laboratory screening (**Table 38.2**) in order to exclude:

- anaemia, a vitamin, iron or trace element deficiency (blood tests)
- diabetes (blood and urine analyses)
- hypothyroidism (blood analyses)
- hyposalivation (salivary flow rates)
- candidosis (oral rinse).

Table 38.2 Aids that might be helpful in diagnosis/prognosis/management in some patients suspected of having burning mouth (oral dysaesthesia)*

In most cases	In some cases
Full blood picture	Allergy testing
Serum ferritin, vitamin B_{12} and corrected whole blood folate levels	Culture and sensitivity
	Psychological assessment
ESR	
Sialometry	
Thyroid function tests	
Blood glucose	

*See text for details and glossary for abbreviations.

Table 38.1 Types of burning mouth syndrome

Type	Symptom pattern	Frequency	Other features
1	No symptoms on waking, but increasing	Unremitting	–
2	Symptoms on waking and through the day	Most common	Unremitting
3	No regular pattern of symptoms	Least common	May remit

BMS is the diagnosis when all organic causes have been excluded, investigations are all negative, and examination shows no:

- clinically detectable signs of mucosal disease
- tenderness or swelling of the tongue or affected area
- neurological or other objective signs.

TREATMENT (see also Chs 4 and 5)

- Few patients have spontaneous remission in the short term, and thus treatment is usually indicated (**Fig. 38.4**); burning mouth syndrome may be controlled by some nerve-calming drugs. About 50% of patients with BMS remit spontaneously within 6 or 7 years.
- Patient information is an important aspect in management.
- Active dental or oral surgical treatment, or attempts at 'hormone replacement', in the absence of any specific indication, should be avoided. Attention to factors such as haematinic deficiencies however, may occasionally be indicated.
- Patients should avoid anything that aggravates symptoms, such as sparkling wines, citrus drinks and spices.
- It is important to clearly acknowledge the reality of the patient's symptoms and distress and never to trivialize or dismiss them.
- Try and explain the psychosomatic background to the problem, ascribing the symptoms to causes for which the patient cannot be blamed.
- Set goals, which include helping the patient cope with the symptoms, rather than attempt any impossible cure.
- Do not repeat examinations or investigations at subsequent appointments, since this only serves to reinforce illness behaviour and health fears.
- Cognitive–behavioural therapy or a specialist referral may be indicated. 'Reattribution' helps manage these patients; it involves demonstrating an understanding of the complaints by taking a history of related physical, mood and social factors, making the patient feel understood and supported, and making the link between symptoms and psychological problems.

- Some patients respond to medication – for example to:
  - topical medication: benzydamine rinse or spray; capsaicin cream 0.025% (Zacin) or 0.075% (Axsain); or a clonazepam tablet sucked locally
  - lysozyme-lactoperoxidase or other mouth wetting agents (for BMS patients with hyposalivation).
  - α-lipoic acid systemically (may have similar effectiveness to capsaicin).
  - Hypericum perforatum, which produces a general reduction in the number of sites with reported burning sensation
  - lafutidine, a histamine H2 receptor antagonist which has a sensitizing effect on capsaicin-sensitive afferent neurons
  - hormone replacement therapy (HRT)
  - antidepressants (**Table 38.3**): shown in controlled trials to be effective for BMS, whether or not the patient is depressed. The pain reduction achieved with antidepressants exceeds that produced by placebos, and most patients with MUS show benefit within 1 week; although antidepressants must be given for at least 2–3 weeks to achieve any antidepressive effect.

Table 38.3 Regimens that might be helpful in management of patient suspected of having burning mouth syndrome

Regimen	Use in primary care
Likely to be beneficial	Cognitive behavioural therapy Topical capsaicin Topical clonazepam Gabapentin Antidepressants (amitriptyline, dosulepin, doxepin, fluoxetine, nortryptiline, trazodone, venlafaxine)
Unproven effectiveness	Alpha lipoic acid Hormone replacement Hypericum perforatum Lafutidine Milnacipran
Supportive	Benzydamine Diet with little acidic, spicy or citrus content Lidocaine Mouth wetting agents

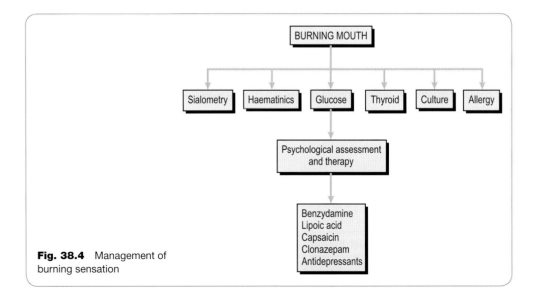

Fig. 38.4 Management of burning sensation

FOLLOW-UP OF PATIENTS

Long-term follow-up in primary care, or as shared care is usually appropriate.

PATIENT INFORMATION SHEET

Burning mouth syndrome

▼ Please read this information sheet. If you have any questions, particularly about the treatment or potential side-effects, please ask your doctor.

- This is a common condition.
- The cause is not usually known, but it may be a nerve hypersensitivity.
- It is not inherited.
- It is not infectious.
- It may occasionally be caused by some mouth conditions, dry mouth, deficiencies, diabetes or drugs.
- It has no long-term consequences.
- Blood tests or biopsy may be required.
- Burning mouth syndrome may be controlled by some nerve-calming drugs.

USEFUL WEBSITES

www.nidcr.nih.gov/oralHealth/Topics/
BurningMouthSyndrome.htm

FURTHER READING

Barker, K.E., Savage, N.W., 2005. Burning mouth syndrome: an update on recent findings. Aust. Dent. J 50 (4), 220–223. quiz 288.

Borelli, V., Marchioli, A., Di Taranto, R., et al., 2010. Neuropeptides in saliva of subjects with burning mouth syndrome: a pilot study. Oral Dis. 16, 365–374.

Borras-Blasco, J., Belda, A., Rosique-Robles, J.D., et al., 2006. Burning mouth syndrome due to efavirenz therapy. Ann. Pharmacother. 40 (7–8), 1471–1472.

Brailo, V., Vueiaeeviae-Boras, V., Alajbeg, I.Z., et al., 2006. Oral burning symptoms and burning mouth syndrome – significance of different variables in 150 patients. Med. Oral Patol. Oral Cir. Bucal 11 (3), E252–E255.

Buchanan, J., Zakrzewska, J., 2002. Burning mouth syndrome. Clin. Evid. 7, 1239–1243.

Carbone, M., Pentenero, M., Carrozzo, M., et al., 2009. Lack of efficacy of alpha-lipoic acid in burning mouth syndrome: a double-blind, randomized, placebo-controlled study. Eur. J. Pain 13 (5), 492.

Cavalcanti, D.R., da Silveira, F.R., 2009. Alpha lipoic acid in burning mouth syndrome – a randomized double-blind placebo-controlled trial. J. Oral Pathol. Med. 38 (3), 254–261.

Cho, G.S., Han, M.W., Lee, B., et al., 2010. Zinc deficiency may be a cause of burning mouth syndrome as zinc replacement therapy has therapeutic effects. J. Oral Pathol. Med. 39 (9), 722–727.

Femiano, F., Gombos, F., Scully, C., et al., 2000. Burning mouth syndrome (BMS): controlled open trial of the efficacy of α-lipoic acid (thioctic acid) on symptomatology. Oral Dis. 6, 274–277.

Gao, J., Chen, L., Zhou, J., Peng, J., 2009. A case-control study on etiological factors involved in patients with burning mouth syndrome. J. Oral Pathol. Med. 38 (1), 24–28.

Grushka, M., Ching, V., Epstein, J., 2006. Burning mouth syndrome. Adv. Otorhinolaryngol. 63, 278–287.

Heckmann, S.M., Heckmann, J.G., Ungethum, A., et al., 2006. Gabapentin has little or no effect in the treatment of burning mouth syndrome – results of an open-label pilot study. Eur. J. Neurol. 13 (7), e6–e7.

Hershkovich, O., Nagler, R.M., 2004. Biochemical analysis of saliva and taste acuity evaluation in patients with burning mouth syndrome, xerostomia and/or gustatory disturbances. Arch. Oral Biol. 49 (7), 515–522.

Ito, M., Kimura, H., Yoshida, K., et al., 2010. Effectiveness of milnacipran for the treatment of chronic pain in the orofacial region. Clin. Neuropharmacol. 33 (2), 79–83.

Just, T., Steiner, S., Pau, H.W., 2010. Oral pain perception and taste in burning mouth syndrome. J. Oral Pathol. Med. 39 (1), 22–27.

López-D'alessandro, E., Escovich, L., 2011. Combination of alpha lipoic acid and gabapentin, its efficacy in the treatment of Burning Mouth Syndrome: A randomized, double-blind, placebo controlled trial. Med. Oral Patol. Oral Cir. Bucal 16 (5), e635–e640.

López-Jornet, P., Camacho-Alonso, F., Andujar-Mateos, P., 2011. A prospective, randomized study on the efficacy of tongue protector in patients with burning mouth syndrome. Oral Dis. 17, 277–282.

López-Jornet, P., Camacho-Alonso, F., Lucero-Berdugo, M., 2008. Quality of life in patients with burning mouth syndrome. J. Oral Pathol. Med. 37 (7), 389–394.

Maina, G., Vitalucci, A., Gandolfo, S., Bogetto, F., 2002. Comparative efficacy of SSRIs and amisulpride in burning mouth syndrome: a single-blind study. J. Clin. Psychiatry 63 (1), 38–43.

Marino, R., Capaccio, P., Pignataro, L., Spadari, F., 2009. Burning mouth syndrome: the role of contact hypersensitivity. Oral Dis. 15, 255–258.

Marino, R., Torretta, S., Capaccio, P., et al., 2010. Different therapeutic strategies for burning mouth syndrome: preliminary data. J. Oral Pathol. Med. 39 (8), 611–616.

Patton, L.L., Siegel, M.A., Benoliel, R., De Laat, A., 2007. Management of burning mouth syndrome: systematic review and management recommendations. Oral Surg. Oral Med. Oral Pathol. Oral Radiol. Endod 103 (Suppl.), S39.e1–S39.e13.

Pekiner, F.N., Demirel, G.Y., Gümrü, B., Ozbayrak, S., 2008. Serum cytokine and T regulatory cell levels in patients with burning mouth syndrome. J. Oral Pathol. Med. 37 (9), 528–534.

Pekiner, F.N., Gümrü, B., Demirel, G.Y., Ozbayrak, S., 2009. Burning mouth syndrome and saliva: detection of salivary trace elements and cytokines. J. Oral Pathol. Med. 38 (3), 269–275.

Purello-D'Ambrosio, F., Gangemi, S., Minciullo, P., et al., 2000. Burning mouth syndrome due to cadmium in a denture wearer. J. Investig. Allergol. Clin. Immunol. 10, 105–106.

Salort-Llorca, C., Mínguez-Serra, M.P., Silvestre, F.J., 2008. Drug-induced burning mouth syndrome: a new etiological diagnosis. Med. Oral Patol. Oral Cir. Bucal 13 (3), E167.

Sardella, A., Lodi, G., Demarosi, F., et al., 2006. Causative or precipitating aspects of burning mouth syndrome: a case-control study. J. Oral Pathol. Med. 35 (8), 466–471.

Sardella, A., Lodi, G., Demarosi, F., et al., 2008. Hypericum perforatum extract in burning mouth syndrome: a randomized placebo-controlled study. J. Oral Pathol. Med. 37 (7), 395–401.

Savage, N.W., Boras, V.V., Barker, K., 2006. Burning mouth syndrome: clinical presentation, diagnosis and treatment. Australas. J. Dermatol. 47 (2), 77–81.

Scala, A., Checchi, L., Montevecchi, M., et al., 2003. Update on burning mouth syndrome: overview and patient management. Crit. Rev. Oral Biol. Med. 14, 275–291.

Steele, J., Bruce, A., Drage, L., Rogers, R., 2008. α-Lipoic acid treatment of 31 patients with sore, burning mouth. Oral Dis. 14, 529–532.

Suarez, P., Clark, G.T., 2006. Burning mouth syndrome: an update on diagnosis and treatment methods. J. Calif. Dent. Assoc. 34 (8), 611–622.

Terai, H., Shimahara, M., 2007. Tongue pain: burning mouth syndrome vs Candida- associated lesion. Oral Dis. 13, 440–442.

Toida, M., Kato, K., Makita, H., et al., 2009. Palliative effect of lafutidine on oral burning sensation. J. Oral Pathol. Med. 38 (3), 262–268.

Zou, Q.H., Li, R.Q., 2011. *Helicobacter pylori* in the oral cavity and gastric mucosa: a meta-analysis. J. Oral Pathol. Med. 40 (4), 317–324.

39 Candidosis (candidiasis)

Key Points

- *Candida* species are common mouth commensals
- *Candida* proliferates if the local ecology changes or if immune defences fall
- Candidosis manifests with red or white lesions and soreness
- Treatment includes correcting the local ecological factors, and/or improving immune defences, together with antifungal medication

INTRODUCTION

Some 50% of the normal population harbour (carry) the fungus *Candida albicans* as a normal oral commensal mainly on the posterior dorsum of tongue (without any disease) and are therefore termed 'Candida carriers'. The opportunistic pathogen grows either as yeasts or hyphae (i.e. it is a *dimorphic* fungus). Actual infection with *Candida* (usually *Candida albicans*) is common mainly in people who are otherwise unwell; candidosis is thus called a 'disease of the diseased'. The importance of *Candida* has increased greatly, particularly as the HIV pandemic extends since, when host defences are compromised, *Candida* typically colonizes mucocutaneous surfaces and causes only superficial infections but in immunocompromised people candidosis is commonly oro-pharyngeal and can be a portal for entry into deeper tissues and invasive candidosis (see Chs 53 and 54).

AETIOLOGY

Host defences against *Candida* species include the following:

- Oral epithelium: a physical barrier.
- Microbial interactions: competition and inhibition by the oral flora.
- Salivary non-immune defences: mechanical cleansing plays a major role but other factors include salivary antimicrobial proteins (AMPs):
  - lysozyme (muramidase): can damage *Candida*, stimulate phagocytosis and agglutinate *Candida*
  - lactoferrin: is antifungal and antibacterial due to binding of iron or altering yeast cell wall permeability
  - lactoperoxidase: is anticandidal via multiple factors (H_2O_2 and halides)
  - glycoproteins antigenically similar to blood group antigens – affect adherence to mucosa
  - histatins
  - antileukoprotease (secretory leukocyte protease; SLIP1)
  - histidine-rich polypeptides
  - calprotectin
  - β-defensin 2.
- Oral immune defences, which include mainly cell-mediated responses:
  - T cells and phagocytes. The full expression of phagocyte effectiveness is dependent on augmentation by cytokines synthesized or induced by T cells, such as lymphokines and IFN-γ. Polymorphonuclear leukocytes (PMNL) and macrophages phagocytose and produce cytokines, such as: myeloperoxidase, tumour necrosis factor (TNF), interferon-γ (IFN-γ), nitric oxide and granulocyte-macrophage colony stimulating factor (GM-CSF).
  - Salivary sIgA antibodies: which aggregate *Candida* organisms and/or prevent adherence.

PATHOGENESIS

- *C. albicans* can switch frequently and reversibly between several variant, heritable, phenotypes associated with changes in micromorphology, physiology and virulence ('colony switching').
- *C. albicans* adhere to the oral epithelial surface via extracellular polymeric materials, including mannoprotein and adhesins.
- Adhesins, such as HWP1 (hyphal wall protein 1), originating from the yeast cell surface, appear important in making hyphal forms adhere more strongly than do yeast forms.
- Hyphae invade the superficial epithelium and penetrate, via enzymes such as the phospholipases, lysophospholipases and aspartyl proteinase (secretory aspartyl proteinases; SAP) (**Fig. 39.1**) as far as the stratum spinosum.
- Epithelial endocytic pathways are key innate immune mechanisms in host defence. Defective endolysosomal maturation may partially explain the inability of oral epithelial cells to kill *C. albicans*.
- *C. albicans* invades oral epithelial cells by inducing its own endocytosis by the adhesin and invasin Als3 and gains access to epithelial vacuolar compartments. *C. albicans* is internalized by oral epithelial cells through actin-dependent clathrin-mediated endocytosis and is taken into vacuolar compartments immediately following its internalization. *Candida*-containing endosomes transiently acquire early

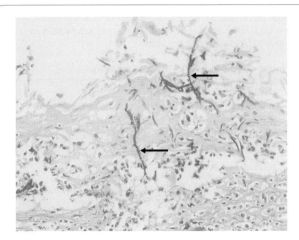

Fig. 39.1 Candidal hyphae stained with periodic acid–Schiff, seen penetrating the epithelium

endosomal marker EEA1, but show marked defects in acquisition of late endosomal marker LAMP1 and lysosomal marker cathepsin D.

- The innate immune system is a first-line defence and involves pattern recognition receptors such as Toll-like receptors and C-type lectin-receptors that not only induce innate immune responses but also modulate cellular and humoral adaptive immunity.
- IL-12: a cytokine family which includes IL-12, IL-23, IL-27, and IL-35 – links to both innate and adaptive immunity systems. An essential component of the response that leads to the generation of Th1-type cytokine responses and protection activity against disseminated candidosis.
- CD4 T-cells are crucial in the regulation of immunity and inflammation; Th1/2, helper cells, together with Th17 and Treg cells are important.
- Th17 and release IL-17 (which recruits neutrophils), IL-21 (which stimulates CD8 or NK cells) and IL-22, the latter stimulating epithelial cells to produce proteins with antimicrobial activity against *Candida*.
- Fungal pattern-recognition receptors such as C-type lectin receptors trigger protective Th17 responses which play the predominant role against mucosal candidiasis. IL-17A and IL-17F are essential for mucocutaneous immunity against *C. albicans*
- Dectin-1, a C-type lectin that recognizes 1,3-beta-glucans from fungi, including *Candida*, is involved in the initiation of the immune response against fungi. Patients bearing the Y238X polymorphism in the DECTIN-1 gene are more likely to be colonized with *Candida* species, compared with patients bearing wild-type DECTIN-1.
- Oral epithelial cells orchestrate an innate response to *C. albicans* via NF-κB and a biphasic MAPK response.
- Activation of NF-κB and the first MAPK response, constituting c-Jun activation, is due to fungal cell wall recognition while the second MAPK phase, constituting MKP1 and c-Fos activation, depends upon hypha formation and fungal burdens – and correlates with the pro-inflammatory responses.
- Activation of the kallikrein–kinin system and other factors result in an inflammatory response in the connective tissue comprising lymphocytes, plasma cells and other leukocytes.

- PMNL migrate into the epithelium in defensive mode, but candidal cell-wall mannans and glycans may impair PMNL chemotaxis, phagocytosis, respiratory burst, T lymphocyte reactivity and the macrophage secretion of tumour necrosis factor (TNF).
- Defective cell-mediated immune responses are commonly associated with mucocutaneous *Candida* infections.

CLINICAL FEATURES

Candidosis (candidiasis; moniliasis) is the state when *Candida species* cause lesions or symptoms:

- The most dominant oral *Candida* species, in decreasing order of frequency, are:
  - *C. albicans*
  - *C. tropicalis*
  - *C. glabrata*
  - *C. parapsilosis*
  - *C. krusei*
  - other *Candida* species
  - other genera which are rare and transient.
- *C. albicans* is the only common cause of oral fungal or yeast infection. *C. albicans* can be differentiated serologically into A and B serotypes, equally distributed in healthy individuals, but there is a significant shift to type B in immunocompromised patients.
- Species other than *C. albicans* (especially *C. krusei*) are increasingly seen, especially in persons with compromised immunity. In HIV disease, for example, *C. dubliniensis* and *C. geotrichium* may appear.
- Antifungal resistance is an increasingly serious clinical reality.

Symptomatic oral candidosis presents as mainly:

- white lesions, in which hyphal forms are common: these include thrush, candidal leukoplakia and chronic mucocutaneous candidosis
- red lesions, in which yeast forms predominate: these include denture-related stomatitis, median rhomboid glossitis, and erythematous candidosis. These may be symptomless, although antibiotic stomatitis and angular cheilitis in particular can cause soreness.

Factors that can increase the liability to oral candidosis are shown in **Box 39.1**. Candidosis may also affect or spread from or to the mouth, from:

- pharynx, oesophagus, and rarely lungs, liver or elsewhere
- anogenital region: candidosis can also be sexually shared (e.g. by vaginal, oral or anal sex)
- skin and nails.

By tradition, the most frequently adopted classification of oral candidosis has been into (**Box 39.2**):

- acute candidosis
- pseudomembranous candidosis (thrush)
- atrophic candidosis
- chronic candidosis
- atrophic candidosis
- hyperplastic candidosis, which was further subdivided into four groups based on localization patterns and endocrine

involvement as follows: chronic oral candidosis (*Candida* leukoplakia); candidosis endocrinopathy syndrome; chronic localized mucocutaneous candidosis; and chronic diffuse candidosis.

A newer classification categorizes candidosis into:

- primary oral candidosis, which is confined to oral and perioral tissues
- secondary oral candidosis, which is distributed in other parts of the body as well as the oral cavity.

DIAGNOSIS OF CANDIDOSIS

Diagnosis can, if necessary, be supported by:

- identification of blastospores and pseudohyphae in stained smears from a lesion
- culture, usually on Sabouraud or dextrose Sabouraud medium
- PCR studies – mainly for detection of invasive candidosis
- occasionally by histology stained by periodic acid–Schiff (PAS).

Table 39.1 Aids that might be helpful in diagnosis/prognosis/management in some patients suspected of having candidosis (candidiasis)*

In most cases	In some cases
Culture and sensitivity Full blood picture	Biopsy Serum ferritin, vitamin B_{12} and corrected whole blood folate levels ESR CD4 counts Serology for antiacetylcholine receptor antibodies Plasma cortisol Plasma calcium and phosphate levels

*See text for details and glossary for abbreviations.

However, the diagnosis of candidosis in most instances is clinical and investigations can be complicated by the facts that:

- up to about 50% of the population are carriers
- any attempt at quantitation of *Candida* is affected by time of sampling and the way in which the specimen is handled.

Since oral candidosis is occasionally associated with nutritional deficiencies or blood dyscrasias, estimates of haemoglobin, white blood cell counts, corrected whole blood folate, vitamin B_{12} and serum ferritin can be important.

Tests of immune function are indicated mainly in HIV disease or chronic mucocutaneous candidosis.

Since some endocrine disorders may be associated with chronic mucocutaneous candidosis, tests of thyroid, parathyroid and adrenocortical function are warranted in selected individuals (**Table 39.1**).

TREATMENT OF CANDIDOSIS
(see also Chs 4 and 5)

Few patients have spontaneous remission unless the condition is solely related to, for example, the use of an antimicrobial, or a topical corticosteroid, and thus, in other cases, treatment is often indicated (**Table 39.2**). Often, in the treatment of fungal infections, attention to the underlying cause will avoid the need for prolonged or repeated courses of treatment. Intermittent or prolonged topical antifungal treatment may be necessary where the underlying cause is unavoidable or incurable. Treatment includes the following measures:

- Avoid or reduce smoking.
- Treat any local predisposing cause, such as hyposalivation.
- Improve oral hygiene; chlorhexidine also has some anticandidal activity.
- Antifungals:
  - topical antifungal agents are useful for most lesions restricted to the oral cavity and are available as suspensions, tablets, gels and creams. Oral suspensions, gels or liquids are useful for patients with dry mouth who may have difficulty in dissolving tablets. Available preparations include: nystatin oral suspension and miconazole

Table 39.2 Regimens that might be helpful in management of patient suspected of having candidosis

Regimen	Use in primary or secondary care
Beneficial	Nystatin Miconazole Fluconazole Itraconazole
Unproven effectiveness	Chlorhexidine Ciclopirox Gentian violet Isotretinoin Probiotics Sodium iodide Yoghurt
Emergent treatments	Caspofungin Posaconazole Voriconazole
Supportive	Smoking cessation ART in HIV infection Benzydamine Diet with little acidic, spicy or citrus content Lidocaine

gel or tablets (intended for topical use), and systemic azoles (used as 'swish and swallow'). Fluconazole, itraconazole and posaconazole are available as suspensions effective against oropharyngeal candidosis, and voriconazole as a liquid. In resource-poor areas, gentian violet is often used; solution at a concentration of 0.00165% does not stain the oral mucosa, is stable and still possesses potent antifungal activity

- systemic antifungals are increasingly used, especially fluconazole (Ch. 5)
- fluconazole-resistant *Candida* may respond to itraconazole, voriconazole or posaconazole.

See also the relevant clinical presentations described below.

PROPHYLAXIS OF CANDIDOSIS

In patients with severe immunosuppression, prevention of colonization and infection is the goal because the oropharyngeal region may be the primary source of initial colonization and allow subsequent spread of the infection.

Those at greatest need for such prophylactic antifungals include patients:

- with HIV disease
- receiving cancer chemotherapy
- on immunosuppressive therapy
- on prolonged antibiotic therapy.

CLINICAL PRESENTATIONS OF CANDIDOSIS

The most common form of oral candidosis is denture-related stomatitis (Ch. 40), and sometimes this is complicated by

angular stomatitis (Ch. 33), again often a *Candida*-related lesion. However, most clinicians are more aware of acute pseudomembranous candidosis ('thrush'), which is not uncommon in neonates, but was rare in older persons before the advent of immunosuppressive therapies and HIV/AIDS. The latter has also highlighted the other red, or erythematous, forms of oral candidosis.

The various types are now discussed in more detail.

WHITE FORMS OF CANDIDOSIS

ACUTE PSEUDOMEMBRANOUS CANDIDOSIS

Thrush is the common title for acute pseudomembranous candidosis, and is so termed because the white flecks resemble the appearance of the breast of the bird of that name.

Incidence

Neonates, who are otherwise healthy but have yet to develop immunity to *Candida* species, may develop thrush, but it is otherwise uncommon in healthy individuals of any age. It is far more common in immunocompromised persons; thrush is a 'disease of the diseased'.

AGE

Can occur at any age.

GENDER

It can occur in either gender.

GEOGRAPHIC

Candidosis is seen worldwide.

Predisposing factors

Predisposing factors include changes in local or systemic immunity in the mouth. Thrush in most patients is related to antibiotic or corticosteroid use, or hyposalivation. However, if these local factors cannot be identified, systemic disease should be suspected – mainly immune defects, such as in terminally ill patients, leukaemia and other malignancies, HIV disease and patients on immunosuppressive treatment.

Aetiology and pathogenesis

Thrush is mainly caused by *C. albicans* but, in infants, *C. parapsilosis* is frequently found. The highest incidence of thrush amongst cancer patients is seen in head neck cancers, where most infections are caused by *C. albicans* but one third of patients harbour non-*C. albicans* strains such as *C. krusei* or *C. glabrata* which are often more resistant to antifungal agents.

The plaques in oral thrush are made up of necrotic material, *Candida* and desquamated parakeratotic epithelia. Oedema and micro-abscesses containing PMNL are found in the outer layers of the epithelium, while the deeper parts show acanthosis and sometimes even dysplasia.

Clinical features

Thrush is classically an acute infection, but it may persist for many months or even years in patients using corticosteroids

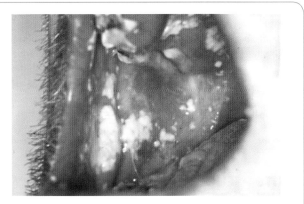

Fig. 39.2 Thrush showing white and red lesions

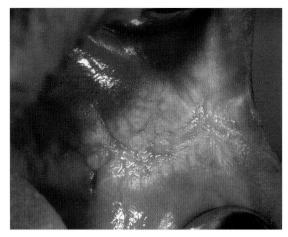

Fig. 39.3 Chronic hyperplastic candidosis, in a typical location

topically or by aerosol, in HIV-infected individuals, and in other immunocompromised patients.

Thrush is characterized by:

- white papules on the surface of the oral mucosa. These may form confluent plaques that resemble milk curds (**Fig. 39.2**). These can be wiped off with gauze to reveal a raw, erythematous and sometimes bleeding base
- complications, which may sometimes be lesions of the mucosa of the upper respiratory tract and the oesophagus, a combination particularly prevalent in HIV-infected patients.

Diagnosis

The diagnosis of thrush is usually clinical and straightforward, but it has been over-diagnosed in the past. In immunosuppressed patients, a Gram-stained smear should be taken to distinguish it from the thrush-like plaques produced by opportunistic bacteria. Hyphae seem to indicate that the *Candida* are acting as pathogens.

Treatment (see also Chs 4 and 5)

Possible predisposing causes should be looked for and dealt with, if possible. Topical polyene antifungals such as nystatin, or imidazoles such as miconazole or fluconazole are often indicated (Ch. 5). With the increasing use of antimycotic therapy, especially in HIV disease, there is a shift towards antifungal-resistant *C. albicans*, as well as the appearance of novel species, such as *C. dubliniensis*, but also towards other species, such as *C. glabrata* and *C. krusei*.

Follow-up of patients

Long-term follow-up as shared care is usually appropriate.

CHRONIC HYPERPLASTIC CANDIDOSIS

Chronic hyperplastic candidosis, or candidal leukoplakia is a persistent white or speckled red/white lesion (**Fig. 39.3**), characterized histologically by parakeratosis and chronic intraepithelial inflammation with fungal hyphae invading the superficial layers of the epithelium. The epithelium of some leukoplakias is invaded by *Candida* hyphae, but it is unclear whether the yeasts are secondary invaders or are causally involved in the development or transformation of leukoplakia.

The cellular changes often include hyperplasia, but cellular atypia, mild or severe dysplasia and ultimately in situ or invasive carcinoma may arise.

Incidence

It is uncommon.

AGE

It is found in adults.

GENDER

It can occur in either gender.

GEOGRAPHIC

It can be found worldwide.

Predisposing factors, aetiology and pathogenesis

C. albicans is the species by far the most commonly isolated from candidal leukoplakia, and it may be predisposed to in a minority of patients by:

- smoking
- iron and folate deficiencies
- defective cell-mediated immunity
- blood group secretor status.

The *Candida* biotypes associated with leukoplakias differ from those isolated from normal oral cavities and those from non-homogeneous leukoplakias such as candidal leukoplakia have higher nitrosation potentials, which might indicate a possible role of specific types in the malignant transformation of these leukoplakias.

Clinical features

Candidal leukoplakias are chronic, discrete raised lesions that vary from small, palpable, translucent, whitish areas to large, dense, opaque plaques, hard and rough to the touch (plaque-like lesions) and are non-homogeneous 'speckled' leukoplakias in up to 50%.

Candidal leukoplakias usually occur on the buccal mucosa on one or both sides, mainly just inside the commissure (**Fig. 39.3**), less often on the tongue dorsum.

Diagnosis

Candidal leukoplakias can be indistinguishable from other leukoplakias except by biopsy when *Candida* hyphae can be seen after staining with periodic acid–Schiff (PAS). Candidal leukoplakia should, therefore, be biopsied both to:

- distinguish it from other non-candidal lesions
- examine for dysplasia.

Treatment (see also Chs 4 and 5)

From 9–40% of candidal leukoplakias may develop into carcinomas. Factors influencing the prognosis may include:

- risk factors, such as tobacco and alcohol use
- whether the lesion is speckled (more dangerous) or homogeneous
- the presence (more dangerous) and degree of epithelial dysplasia
- the management adopted.

In order to improve the prognosis:

- tobacco and alcohol habits should be stopped
- antifungals should be used. The lesions of candidal leukoplakia may prove poorly responsive to polyene antifungal drugs and, in some cases, respond only to systemic fluconazole or itraconazole
- excision is indicated if there is more than mild dysplasia
- the patient should be fully informed about the condition, and reviewed regularly.

Follow-up of patients

Long-term follow-up as shared care is usually appropriate

CHRONIC MUCOCUTANEOUS CANDIDOSIS

In many patients with persistent oral candidosis no local cause or underlying defect can be identified. In general, the more severe the candidosis and the more widespread the sites involved, the greater is the likelihood that an underlying immunological defect (particularly of cell-mediated immunity) can be identified.

Chronic mucocutaneous candidosis (CMC) is not a specific condition, but rather a phenotypic presentation of a spectrum of immunologic, endocrinologic, and autoimmune disorders.

Patients who lack broad T-cell immunity (e.g. those with severe combined immune deficiency syndrome (SCID) or DiGeorge syndrome (CATCH 22)) or patients with severely impaired T-cell function (e.g. patients with HIV/AIDS) are also susceptible to chronic candidal infections but are not usually included in CMC.

CMC is the term given to a heterogeneous group of rare syndromes, sometimes familial in which there is persistent *mucocutaneous* candidosis and, to a lesser extent, *Staphylococcus aureus* infections, and an underlying immune defect is present, that responds poorly to even prolonged topical antifungal treatment.

CMC is associated with a defect in cell-mediated immunity that may either be limited to *Candida* antigens or be part of a more general immune defect. Some forms are due to autosomal recessive deficiency in the cytokine receptor, interleukin-17 receptor A (IL-17RA), others to autosomal dominant deficiency of the cytokine interleukin-17F (IL-17F). Others have a defect of cytokine production (interleukin-2 and IFN-γ) in response to candidal and some bacterial antigens, with reduced Th1 lymphocyte function and enhanced Th2 activity (and increased interleukin-6).

Patients with CMC suffer from chronic candidosis caused mainly by *Candida albicans*, with irremovable whitish patches and deep fissures on the tongue and often the palate as the most common oral manifestations but patients may also have candidal infections of other mucosae, skin and nails. Repeated courses of azole antifungals have led to microevolution and point mutations and the development of azole-resistant isolates. Alternative *Candida* treatment options, other than azoles – such as chlorhexidine, should therefore be considered.

Oral carcinomas have developed in some patients with CMC.

Autoimmune polyendocrinopathy-candidosis (APEC) is a group of rare autosomal recessive diseases, which may involve autoimmune hormonal hypofunction affecting thyroid, parathyroids, gonads and/or pancreas.

Hyper-IgE syndrome (HIES/Job syndrome) is a rare congenital immunodeficiency characterized by mutations in signal transducer and activator of transcription 3, leading to defects in IL-6 and IL-23, and hence Th17 defects. HIES patients develop mucocutaneous candidosis.

Specialist care is indicated (**Table 39.3**).

Table 39.3 Chronic mucocutaneous candidosis (CMC)

Type	Inheritance	Clinical features
Localized CMC	Sporadic	Persistent oral candidosis, oesophagitis, iron deficiency
Diffuse CMC (*Candida* granuloma)	AR or sporadic	Severe chronic oral candidosis, granulomas, susceptibility to bacterial infections
Candidosis–endocrinopathy syndrome (CES)	AR	Mild chronic oral candidosis, pernicious anaemia, hypoparathyroidism, hypoadrenocorticism, diabetes, vitiligo, thyroid disease
Candidosis thymoma syndrome	Sporadic	Chronic oral candidosis, myasthenia gravis, polymyositis, aplastic anaemia

RED (ERYTHEMATOUS) FORMS OF CANDIDOSIS

ATROPHIC CANDIDOSIS (INCLUDING DENTURE-RELATED STOMATITIS (Ch. 40) AND ANGULAR STOMATITIS (Ch. 33))

Erythematous or atrophic candidosis may be seen in denture-related stomatitis, antibiotic- or steroid-induced stomatitis, sometimes in median rhomboid glossitis and, in HIV infection, may develop *de novo*, may precede pseudomembranous candidosis, or may arise as a consequence of persistent acute pseudomembranous candidosis when the pseudomembranes are shed.

ANTIBIOTIC OR STEROID-INDUCED STOMATITIS
Incidence

It is uncommon.

AGE

It can occur at any age.

GENDER

It can occur in either gender.

GEOGRAPHIC

It has no known geographic incidence.

Predisposing factors

Acute oral candidosis may complicate corticosteroid or antibiotic therapy, particularly with long-term, broad-spectrum antimicrobials, such as tetracycline.

Clinical features

There is widespread erythema and soreness of the oral mucosa, sometimes, also with thrush.

Diagnosis

This is a clinical diagnosis, but if the aetiology is not absolutely clear a blood picture and smears for fungal hyphae and culture may be helpful management.

Treatment (see also Chs 4 and 5)
- The causal drug should be stopped if possible.
- Tobacco habits should be stopped.
- Antifungals are indicated. However, the lesions may prove poorly responsive to the polyene antifungal drugs and, therefore, an azole is preferred. Some cases respond only to systemic fluconazole or itraconazole (Ch. 5).

Follow-up of patients

Long-term follow-up is rarely required

MEDIAN RHOMBOID GLOSSITIS

Median rhomboid glossitis (MRG), or glossal central papillary atrophy, is a depapillated rhomboidal area in the centre line of the dorsum of the tongue, just anterior to the sulcus terminalis (**Fig. 39.4**).

Incidence

It is uncommon.

AGE

It can occur at any age.

GENDER

It can occur in either gender.

GEOGRAPHIC

It has no known geographic incidence.

Predisposing factors

Candida species colonize mainly the posterior dorsum of the tongue, even in healthy patients, but MRG is predisposed by:

- smoking
- denture wearing
- corticosteroid sprays/inhalers
- HIV infection.

Aetiology and pathogenesis

Formerly thought to be caused by persistence of the embryonic tuberculum impar, this lesion is now thought to be related to candidosis because:

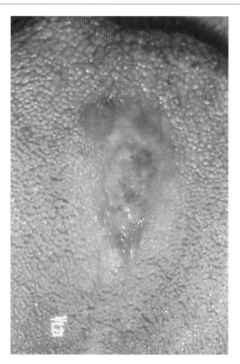

Fig. 39.4 Median rhomboid glossitis

- culture frequently shows *Candida*, although often in a mixed bacterial/fungal microflora
- histopathologically, candidal hyphae infiltrate the superficial layers of the parakeratotic epithelium and a neutrophil infiltrate occupies the epithelium, with elongated hyperplastic rete ridges (pseudoepitheliomatous hyperplasia), and a lymphocyte infiltration in the corium. Thus, there can be a trap for the unwary, since the lesion may be mistaken for a cancer clinically (**Fig. 39.5**) and the histopathology is of pseudo-epitheliomatous hyperplasia – it also mimics cancer.

Clinical features

MRG is only rarely sore, but is more usually detected incidentally by the patient or dentist. It is characterized by:

- an area of papillary atrophy, which is usually flat, reddish or red and white, or occasionally white. It is elliptical or rhomboidal in shape, symmetrically placed centrally at the midline of the tongue, just anterior to the circumvallate papillae (see **Fig. 39.4**)
- occasionally by a hyperplastic, or even lobulated exophytic appearance.

Diagnosis

MRG is usually a clinical diagnosis. Biopsy is indicated if there is any concern it could be a neoplasm; histology shows irregular epithelial hyperplasia, which resembles, but is not, a carcinoma (because of the pseudoepitheliomatous hyperplasia) (**Fig. 39.5**).

Rarely, is there a need for blood picture, smears for fungal hyphae or culture.

Treatment (see also Chs 4 and 5)

- Tobacco habits should be stopped.
- Antifungals are indicated. However, the lesions may prove poorly responsive to the polyene antifungal drugs, and some cases respond only to systemic azoles (Ch. 5).

Follow-up of patients

Long-term follow-up as shared care is usually appropriate.

ERYTHEMATOUS CANDIDOSIS IN HIV DISEASE

Incidence

It is uncommon.

AGE

It can occur at any age.

GENDER

It can occur in either gender.

GEOGRAPHIC

It has no known geographic incidence.

Predisposing factors

- The immunological defect.
- Smoking.
- Corticosteroid therapy.
- Broad-spectrum antibiotic therapy.
- Hyposalivation (from HIV-salivary gland disease, antiretroviral agents or other agents which have this effect) (Ch. 54).

Clinical features

- The clinical presentation is of irregular erythematous macules and/or patches, generally on the dorsum of the tongue, palate or buccal mucosa.
- Lesions are often seen in the central palate and sometimes termed 'thumbprint lesions' (**Fig. 39.6**).
- Lesions on the dorsum of the tongue present as glossitis or depapillated areas.
- There can be an associated angular stomatitis.

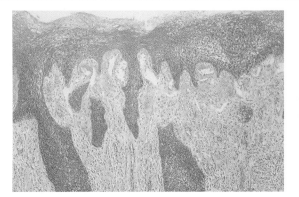

Fig. 39.5 Median rhomboid glossitis, showing histopathological appearance of pseudoepitheliomatous hyperplasia that may lead to confusion with carcinoma

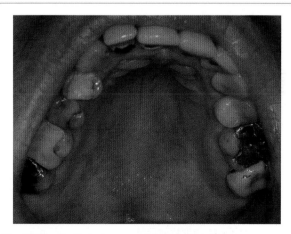

Fig. 39.6 Erythematous candidosis in HIV disease

Diagnosis

This is a clinical diagnosis; biopsy is only rarely indicated. Occasionally there is a need for smears or culture.

Treatment (see also Chs 4 and 5)

- Tobacco habits should be stopped.
- Antiretroviral treatment.
- Candidosis in HIV disease may prove poorly responsive to polyene antifungal drugs, so systemic fluconazole is usually indicated (Ch. 5).

Follow-up of patients

Long-term follow-up by a specialist is usually appropriate.

CHRONIC MULTIFOCAL ORAL CANDIDOSIS

In a minority of apparently healthy individuals, chronic red and/or white candidal infection may be seen in multiple oral sites, without other mucosal or skin candidosis; this is termed 'chronic multifocal oral candidosis' (**Fig. 39.7**). Diagnostic criteria include:

- lesions of >1 month duration
- an absence of predisposing medical conditions. It excludes patients who have received radiotherapy or drugs of the following types: antibiotics, antiinflammatory or immunosuppressive drugs, cytotoxic or psychotropic agents.

Incidence

It is uncommon.

AGE

Adults usually; most of the patients are in their fifth or sixth decade.

GENDER

Most patients are males.

GEOGRAPHIC

No known geographical incidence.

Predisposing factors

Tobacco smoking is a known risk factor.

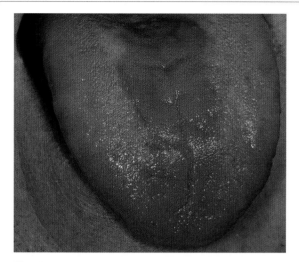

Fig. 39.7 Multifocal candidosis: lingual lesion

Clinical features

Various combinations can be seen, including:

- retrocommissural leukoplakia, which is the most constant component
- angular cheilitis, which is unilateral or bilateral and encountered mainly in denture-wearers
- median rhomboid or erythematous glossitis
- palatal red irregular patches.

Diagnosis

This is a clinical diagnosis. A blood picture, smears for fungal hyphae and culture may help management.

Treatment (see also Chs 4 and 5)

- Tobacco habits should be stopped.
- Antifungals are indicated. However, the lesions may prove poorly responsive to the polyene antifungal drugs and some cases respond only to systemic fluconazole (Ch. 5).

Follow-up of patients

Long-term follow-up by a specialist is usually appropriate.

USEFUL WEBSITES

Medscape, Candidiasis in Emergency Medicine.
  http://www.emedicine.com/emerg/topic76.htm

FURTHER READING

Al-Karawi, Z.M., Manfredi, M., Waugh, A.C.W., et al., 2002. Molecular characterization of *Candida* spp. isolated from the oral cavity of patients from diverse clinical settings. Oral Microbiol. Immunol. 17, 44–49.

Ashman, R.B., Vijayan, D., Wells, C.A., 2011. IL-12 and related cytokines: function and regulatory implications in *Candida albicans* infection. Clin. Dev. Immunol. 2011, 686597.

Böckle, B.C., Wilhelm, M., Müller, H., et al., 2010. Oral mucous squamous cell carcinoma–an anticipated consequence of autoimmune polyendocrinopathy-candidiasis-ectodermal dystrophy (APECED). J. Am. Acad. Dermatol. 62 (5), 864–868.

Casaroto, A.R., Lara, V.S., 2010. Phytomedicines for Candida-associated denture stomatitis. Fitoterapia 81 (5), 323–328.

Collins, C.D., Cookinham, S., Smith, J., 2011. Management of oropharyngeal candidiasis oral miconazole therapy: efficacy, safety, and patient acceptability. Patient Prefer Adherence 5, 369–374.

Conti, H.R., Baker, O., Freeman, A.F., et al., 2011. New mechanism of oral immunity to mucosal candidiasis in hyper-IgE syndrome. Mucosal Immunol 4 (4), 448–455.

Conti, H.R., Gaffen, S.L., 2010. Host responses to *Candida albicans*: Th17 cells and mucosal candidiasis. Microbes Infect. 12 (7), 518–527.

de Resende, M.A., de Sousa, L.V., de Oliveira, R.C., et al., 2006. Prevalence and antifungal susceptibility of yeasts obtained from the oral cavity of older individuals. Mycopathologia 162 (1), 39–44.

Farah, C.S., Lynch, N., McCullough, M.J., 2010. Oral fungal infections: an update for the general practitioner. Aust. Dent. J. 55 (Suppl. 1), 48–54.

Firinu, D., Massidda, O., Lorrai, M.M., et al., 2011. Successful treatment of chronic mucocutaneous candidiasis caused by azole-resistant *Candida albicans* with posaconazole. Clin. Dev. Immunol. 2011, 283239.

Giannini, P.J., Shetty, K.V., 2011. Diagnosis and management of oral candidiasis. Otolaryngol. Clin. North Am. 44 (1), 231–240.

Ianas, V., Matthias, K.R., Klotz, S.A., 2010. Role of posaconazole in the treatment of oropharyngeal candidiasis. Infect Drug Resist 3, 45–51.

Jham, B.C., Chen, H., Carvalho, A.L., Freire, A.R., 2009. A randomized phase III prospective trial of bethanechol to prevent mucositis, candidiasis, and taste loss in patients with head and neck cancer undergoing radiotherapy: a secondary analysis. J. Oral Sci. 51 (4), 565–572.

Lafleur, M.D., Qi, Q., Lewis, K., 2010. Patients with long-term oral carriage harbour high-persister mutants of *Candida albicans*. Antimicrob. Agents Chemother. 54 (1), 39–44.

Lalla, R.V., Bensadoun, R.J., 2011. Miconazole mucoadhesive tablet for oropharyngeal candidiasis. Expert Rev. Anti Infect. Ther. 9 (1), 13–17.

Laudenbach, J.M., Epstein, J.B., 2009. Treatment strategies for oropharyngeal candidiasis. Expert Opin. Pharmacother. 10 (9), 1413–1421.

Liu, X., Hua, H., 2007. Oral manifestation of chronic mucocutaneous candidiasis: seven case reports. J. Oral Pathol. Med. 36 (9), 528–532.

Manfredi, M., McCullough, M.J., Al-Karaawi, Z.M., et al., 2006. Analysis of the strain relatedness of oral *Candida albicans* in patients with diabetes mellitus using polymerase chain reaction-fingerprinting. Oral Microbiol. Immunol. 21 (6), 353–359.

Martin, R., Wächtler, B., Schaller, M., et al., 2011. Host-pathogen interactions and virulence-associated genes during *Candida albicans* oral infections. Int. J. Med. Microbiol. 301 (5), 417–422.

McCullough, M., Patton, L.L., Coogan, M., et al., 2011. New approaches to Candida and oral mycotic infections: Workshop 2A. Adv. Dent. Res. 23 (1), 152–158.

McManus, B.A., McGovern, E., Moran, G.P., et al., 2011. Microbiological screening of Irish patients with autoimmune polyendocrinopathy-candidiasis-ectodermal dystrophy reveals persistence of *Candida albicans* strains, gradual reduction in susceptibility to azoles, and incidences of clinical signs of oral candidiasis without culture evidence. J. Clin. Microbiol. 49 (5), 1879–1889.

Moyes, D.L., Runglall, M., Murciano, C., et al., 2010. A biphasic innate immune MAPK response discriminates between the yeast and hyphal forms of *Candida albicans* in epithelial cells. Cell Host Microbe 16; 8 (3), 225–235.

Naglik, J.R., Fostira, F., Ruprai, J., et al., 2006. *Candida albicans* HWP1 gene expression and host antibody responses in colonization and disease. J. Med. Microbiol. 55 (Pt 10), 1323–1327.

Pankhurst, C., 2011. Oropharyngeal candidiasis. Clin. Evid. 7, 1248–1262.

Pereira, C.A., da Costa, A.C., Machado, A.K., et al., 2010. Enzymatic activity, sensitivity to antifungal drugs and Baccharis dracunculifolia essential oil by Candida strains isolated from the oral cavities of breastfeeding infants and in their mothers' mouths and nipples. Mycopathologia 171 (2), 103–109.

Petruzzi, M., Grassi, F.R., Nardi, G.M., et al., 2010. Sodium iodide associated to salicylic acid in the topical management of chronic oral candidiasis: a randomized trial. J. Biol. Regul. Homeost. Agents 24 (3), 381–384.

Puel, A., Cypowyj, S., Bustamante, J., et al., 2011. Chronic mucocutaneous candidiasis in humans with inborn errors of interleukin-17 immunity. Science 332 (6025), 65–68.

Richardson, R., 2011. Oral candidosis– Clinical challenges of a biofilm disease. CRC Crit. Rev. Microbiol. 37 (4), 328–336.

Scardina, G.A., Ruggieri, A., Messina, P., 2009. Chronic hyperplastic candidosis: a pilot study of the efficacy of 0.18% isotretinoin. J. Oral Sci 51 (3), 407–410.

Sharon, V., Fazel, N., 2010. Oral candidiasis and angular cheilitis. Dermatol. Ther. 23 (3), 230–242.

Siikala, E., Bowyer, P., Richardson, M., 2011. ADH1 expression inversely correlates with CDR1 and CDR2 in *Candida albicans* from chronic oral candidosis in APECED (APS-I) patients. FEMS Yeast Res. 11 (6), 494–498.

Siikala, E., Rautemaa, R., Richardson, M., et al., 2010. Persistent *Candida albicans* colonization and molecular mechanisms of azole resistance in autoimmune polyendocrinopathy-candidiasis-ectodermal dystrophy (APECED) patients. J. Antimicrob. Chemother. 65 (12), 2505–2513.

Soysa, N., Samaranayake, L., Ellepola, A., 2008. Antimicrobials as a contributory factor in oral candidosis – a brief overview. Oral Dis. 14, 138–143.

Soysa, N.S., Samaranayake, L.P., Ellepola, A.N., 2006. Diabetes mellitus as a contributory factor in oral candidosis. Diabet. Med. 23 (5), 455–459.

Subissi, A., Monti, D., Togni, G., Mailland, F., 2010. Ciclopirox: recent nonclinical and clinical data relevant to its use as a topical antimycotic agent. Drugs 70 (16), 2133–2152.

Sullivan, D.J., Moran, G.P., 2011. Differential virulence of *Candida albicans* and *C. dubliniensis*: A role for Tor1 kinase? Virulence 2 (1), 77–81.

Taillandier, J., Esnault, Y., Alemanni, M., 2000. A comparison of fluconazole oral suspension and amphotericin B oral suspension in older patients with oropharyngeal candidiasis. Multicentre Study Group. Age Ageing 29, 117–123.

Vazquez, J.A., Patton, L.L., Epstein, J.B., et al., 2010. Randomized, comparative, double-blind, double-dummy, multicenter trial of miconazole buccal tablet and clotrimazole troches for the treatment of oropharyngeal candidiasis: study of miconazole Lauriad® efficacy and safety (SMiLES). HIV Clin. Trials 11 (4), 186–196.

Webb, A.K., Woolnough, E., 2006. *Candida albicans* infection in adults with cystic fibrosis. J. R. Soc. Med. 99 (Suppl. 46), 13–16.

Wei, X.Q., Rogers, H., Lewis, M.A., Williams, D.W., 2011. The role of the IL-12 cytokine family in directing T-cell responses in oral candidosis. Clin. Dev. Immunol. 2011, 697340.

Weindl, G., Wagener, J., Schaller, M., 2010. Epithelial cells and innate antifungal defense. J. Dent. Res. 89 (7), 666–675.

Williams, D., Lewis, M., 2011. Pathogenesis and treatment of oral candidosis. J. Oral Microbiol. 28, 3.

Williams, D.W., Kuriyama, T., Silva, S., 2011. Candida biofilms and oral candidosis: treatment and prevention. Periodontol 2000 55 (1), 250–265.

Worthington, H.V., Clarkson, J.E., Khalid, T., et al., 2010. Interventions for treating oral candidiasis for patients with cancer receiving treatment. Cochrane Database Syst. Rev. (7), CD001972.

Yan, Z., Young, A.L., Hua, H., Xu, Y., 2011. Multiple oral Candida infections in patients with Sjögren's syndrome – prevalence and clinical and drug susceptibility profiles. J. Rheumatol. 38 (11), 2428–2431.

Zhao, X.R., Villar, C.C., 2011. Trafficking of *Candida albicans* through oral epithelial endocytic compartments. Med. Mycol. 49 (2), 212–217.

Denture-related stomatitis

INTRODUCTION

Denture-related stomatitis (denture sore mouth; chronic atrophic candidosis) consists of mild inflammation and erythema of the mucosa beneath a dental appliance, usually a complete upper denture.

INCIDENCE

Common; in some studies of institutionalized older denture-wearing patients, figures as high as 70% have been found, but it is overall considerably less common in other people, particularly in normal healthy subjects.

AGE

This is a disease mainly of the middle-aged or older.

GENDER

It is slightly more prevalent in women than men.

GEOGRAPHIC

This is seen worldwide.

PREDISPOSING FACTORS

- Dental appliance wearing (mainly maxillary dentures), especially when worn throughout the night, or with a dry mouth, is the major predisposing factor.
- Smoking occasionally predisposes.
- Diabetes or a high carbohydrate diet occasionally predispose.
- Hyposalivation is a occasionally an underlying factor.
- Haematinic deficiencies are a rare underlying factor.
- HIV is a rare underlying factor.
- Factors that are usually *not* significant include:
  - allergy to the dental material (if it were, denture-related stomatitis would affect mucosae other than just that beneath the appliance)
  - trauma; the condition is more common beneath maxillary dentures than mandibular dentures, yet trauma is more common under the latter
  - pharmacological agents.

AETIOLOGY AND PATHOGENESIS

Dentures and other appliances can produce a number of ecological changes, including accumulation of microbial plaque (bacteria and/or yeasts) on and in the fitting surface of the denture and the underlying mucosa. Histological examination of the soft tissue beneath dentures has shown proliferative or degenerative responses with reduced keratinization and thinner epithelium.

Fungi, such as *Candida*, are isolated in up to 90% of persons with denture-related stomatitis, and when *Candida* species are involved in denture-related stomatitis, the more common terms 'Candida-associated denture stomatitis', 'denture-induced candidosis' or 'chronic atrophic candidosis' are used. The most frequently isolated organism is *Candida albicans*. In some persons, the cause appears to be related to a non-specific plaque, which undergoes sequential development, and is finally colonized by *Candida* organisms. Although there is no increased aspartyl proteinase production from the *Candida* involved, the decreased salivary flow and a low pH under the denture probably result in a high *Candida* enzymatic activity, which can cause mucosal inflammation.

Candida, however, are not the only microorganisms associated with denture-related stomatitis; occasionally bacterial infection is responsible, or mechanical irritation has a role.

It not yet clear why only some denture-wearers develop denture stomatitis, since most patients with denture-related stomatitis appear otherwise healthy and they have no serious cell-mediated immune defects, but they may sometimes be deficient in migration-inhibition factor (MIF) and may have overactive suppressor T cells or other T lymphocyte or phagocyte defects.

CLINICAL FEATURES

The characteristic presenting features of denture-related stomatitis are:

- An absence of symptoms. The former term 'denture sore mouth' was a misnomer.
- Chronic erythema and oedema of the mucosa that contacts the fitting surface of the denture, usually a complete upper denture (the denture-bearing area); the mucosa below lower dentures is rarely involved (**Figs 40.1 and 40.2**).
- Uncommon complications, which include:
  - angular stomatitis, and rarely
  - papillary hyperplasia in the vault of the palate (idiopathic papillary epithelial hyperplasia (IPEH), which usually needs to be surgically removed before the appliance is replaced or relined).

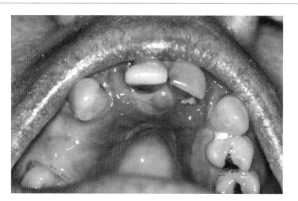

Fig. 40.1 Denture-related stomatitis

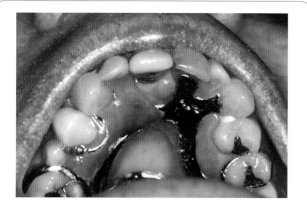

Fig. 40.2 Denture-related stomatitis (denture in situ; same patient as in **Fig. 40.1**)

CLASSIFICATION

Denture-related stomatitis has been classified into three clinical types (Newton types), increasing in severity (**Table 40.1**).

DIAGNOSIS

This is a clinical diagnosis.

A full blood picture, haematinic assays and smears for fungal hyphae and culture may be warranted (**Table 40.2**). If there is angular stomatitis, or other oral or systemic lesions, or a suspicion of an immunocompromising condition, then diabetes and HIV in particular should be excluded.

TREATMENT (see also Chs 4 and 5)

Patient information is probably the most important aspect in management.

Any underlying systemic disease should be treated where possible. Smoking cessation is important.

The denture or other appliance fitting surface and plaque is infested, usually with *Candida albicans*. Scrupulous appliance hygiene is mandatory, with daily thorough brushing.

Table 40.1 Newton classification of denture-related stomatitis

Type	Definition	Comment
1	Localized simple inflammation or a pinpoint hyperaemia	Early lesion usually
2	Erythematous or generalized simple type presenting as more diffuse erythema involving a part of, or the entire, denture-covered mucosa	Common type
3	Granular type (inflammatory papillary hyperplasia) commonly involving the central part of the hard palate and the alveolar ridge	Uncommon

Table 40.2 Aids that might be helpful in diagnosis/prognosis/management in some patients suspected of having denture-related stomatitis*

In most cases	In rare cases
Full blood picture	ESR
Serum ferritin, vitamin B$_{12}$ and corrected whole blood folate levels	HIV test
Blood glucose	
Culture and sensitivity	

*See text for details and glossary for abbreviations.

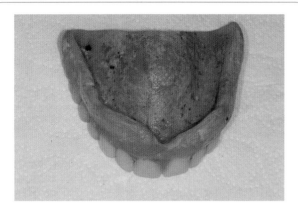

Fig. 40.3 Denture plaque needs removing

The appliance should be removed from the mouth over-night and as much as possible at other times (**Fig. 40.3**), while the denture is cleaned and disinfected. This can be achieved by microwave irradiation for 3 min at 650 W with the appliance immersed in 200 mL of water. Disinfection can also be achieved using an inexpensive option of 10% acetic acid (vinegar) or an antiseptic denture cleanser, and storing the appliance in it overnight. Suitable antiseptic solutions include chlorhexidine or dilute sodium hypochlorite (10 drops of household bleach in a 500 mL container filled with tap water). Hypochlorite however, can turn chrome cobalt dentures black. Many other cleansers are available (alkaline peroxides, alkaline hypochlorites, acids, yeast lytic enzymes), proteolytic enzymes, tea tree oil (*Melaleuca alternifolia*) and *Punica granatum* (dwarf pomegranate).

The mucosal infection is eradicated by brushing the palate and using antifungals for 4 weeks (**Table 40.3**), with the denture removed from the mouth and being disinfected as frequently as possible. Antifungal agents (e.g. miconazole gel) should also be applied to the tissue-contacting surface of the appliance before every re-insertion. Effective topical antifungals include nystatin suspension, miconazole gel or mucoadhesive tablets, or fluconazole suspension, or topical ketoconazole if available, which can be administered concurrently with an oral antiseptic with antifungal activity – such as chlorhexidine. Lacquer or tissue conditioners containing antifungals are also effective

Studies of sensitivity to antifungal agents have shown that isolates from different strains are sensitive to nystatin, but less sensitive to miconazole and fluconazole.

FOLLOW-UP OF PATIENTS

Long-term follow-up in primary care is usually appropriate.

PATIENT INFORMATION SHEET

Denture sore mouth

▼ Please read this information sheet. If you have any questions, particularly about the treatment or potential side-effects, please ask your doctor.
- Denture sore mouth is common but not sore.
- It is caused by a fungus (*Candida*) that usually lives harmlessly in the mouth and elsewhere.
- It is caused mainly by wearing a dental appliance, which allows the fungus to grow.
- It may be precipitated by prolonged appliance-wearing, especially at night.
- It predisposes to sores at the corners of the mouth.
- It has no serious long-term consequences.
- Blood tests, microbiological studies or biopsy may be required.
- It may be controlled by:
  - leaving out the denture, to allow the mouth to heal
  - disinfecting the denture
  - using antifungal creams or gels (e.g. Daktarin) or tablets (e.g. Nystan, Fungilin, Diflucan) regularly for up to 4 weeks
  - the dentures may require adjustment.

PATIENT INFORMATION SHEET

Denture care

▼ Please read this information sheet. If you have any questions, particularly about the treatment or potential side-effects, please ask your doctor.
- If you still have some natural teeth, these will need regular attention, because wearing a denture can encourage food accumulation.
- Keep your dentures as clean as natural teeth. Clean both surfaces of your dentures (inside and outside) after meals and at night. Use washing-up liquid and a toothbrush and lukewarm water and hold it over a basin containing water, in case you drop the denture, which could cause it to break. Never use hot water, as it may alter the denture colour. A disclosing agent, e.g. Rayner's Blue or red food colouring (available at most supermarkets), can be applied with cotton buds, to help you see whether you are cleaning the denture thoroughly enough. If stains or calculus deposits are difficult to remove, try an overnight immersion (e.g. Dentural, Milton or Steradent) or an application of Denclen.
- Your dentures should be left out overnight, so that your mouth has a rest. It is not natural for your palate to be covered all the time, and the chances of getting an infection are increased if the dentures are worn 24 h a day. Ensure you leave the dentures out for at least some time and keep them in water, Dentural or Steradent, or in a damp tissue, as they may distort if allowed to dry out.
- Special precautions for dentures with metal parts: Denclen, Dentural and Milton may discolour metal, so use with care. Brush briefly to remove stains and deposits, rinse well with lukewarm water and do not soak overnight in these solutions.
- Before re-use, brush the dentures to remove loosened deposits.

Table 40.3 Regimens that might be helpful in management of patient suspected of having denture-related stomatitis

Regimen	Use in primary or secondary care
Beneficial	Nystatin Miconazole Fluconazole Itraconazole
Unproven effectiveness	Chlorhexidine Gentian violet Probiotics Punica granatum Yoghurt
Supportive	Chlorhexidine Dental appliance hygiene Smoking cessation

USEFUL WEBSITES

Medscape, Denture Stomatitis. http://emedicine.
    medscape.com/article/1075994

FURTHER READING

Abu-Elteen, K.H., 2000. *Candida albicans* strain
    differentiation in complete denture wearers. New
    Microbiol. 23, 329–337.

Amanlou, M., Beitollahi, J.M., Abdollahzadeh, S.,
    Tohidast-Ekrad, Z., 2006. Miconazole gel compared
    with *Zataria multiflora* Boiss. gel in the treatment of
    denture stomatitis. Phytother. Res. 20, 966–969.

Barnabe, W., de Mendonca Neto, T., Pimenta, F.C., et al.,
    2004. Efficacy of sodium hypochlorite and coconut
    soap used as disinfecting agents in the reduction of
    denture stomatitis, *Streptococcus mutans* and *Candida
    albicans*. J. Oral Rehabil. 31, 453–459.

Casaroto, A.R., Lara, V.S., 2010. Phytomedicines for
    Candida-associated denture stomatitis. Fitoterapia 81,
    323–328.

Catalan, A., Pacheco, J.G., Martinez, A., Mondaca,
    M.A., 2008. In vitro and in vivo activity of *Melaleuca
    alternifolia* mixed with tissue conditioner on *Candida
    albicans*. Oral Surg. Oral Med. Oral Pathol. Oral
    Radiol. Endod. 105, 327–332.

Chandra, J., Mukherjee, P.K., Leidich, S.D., et al., 2001.
    Antifungal resistance of candidal biofilms formed on
    denture acrylic in vitro. J. Dent. Res. 80, 903–908.

Cross, L.J., Bagg, J., Aitchison, T.C., 2000. Efficacy of
    the cyclodextrin liquid preparation of itraconazole
    in treatment of denture stomatitis: comparison
    with itraconazole capsules. Antimicrob. Agents
    Chemother. 44, 425–427.

de Freitas Fernandes, F.S., Pereira-Cenci, T., da Silva,
    W.J., et al., 2011. Efficacy of denture cleansers on
    Candida spp. biofilm formed on polyamide and
    polymethyl methacrylate resins. J. Prosthet. Dent.
    105, 51–58.

de Oliveira, C.E., Gasparoto, T.H., Dionísio, T.J., et al.,
    2010. *Candida albicans* and denture stomatitis:
    evaluation of its presence in the lesion, prosthesis, and
    blood. Int. J. Prosthodont. 23 (2), 158–159.

Dorocka-Bobkowska, B., Zozulinska-Ziolkiewicz,
    D., Wierusz-Wysocka, B., et al., 2010. Candida-
    associated denture stomatitis in type 2 diabetes
    mellitus. Diabetes Res. Clin. Pract. 90 (1), 81–86.

Felton, D., Cooper, L., Duqum, I., et al., 2011. Evidence-
    based guidelines for the care and maintenance of
    complete dentures: a publication of the American
    College of Prosthodontists. J. Prosthodont. 20 (Suppl.
    1), S1–S12.

Golecka-Bakowska, M., Mierzwinska-Nastalska,
    E., Bychawska, M., 2010. Influence of hormone
    supplementation therapy on the incidence of
    denture stomatitis and on chemiluminescent activity
    of polymorphonuclear granulocytes in blood
    of menopausal-aged women. Eur. J. Med. Res.
    15 (Suppl. 2), 46–49.

Hoshi, N., Mori, H., Taguchi, H., et al., 2011.
    Management of oral candidiasis in denture wearers.
    J. Prosthodont. Res. 55 (1), 48–52.

Jainkittivong, A., Aneksuk, V., Langlais, R.P., 2010. Oral
    mucosal lesions in denture wearers. Gerodontology
    27 (1), 26–32.

Jose, A., Coco, B.J., Milligan, S., et al., 2010. Reducing
    the incidence of denture stomatitis: are denture
    cleansers sufficient? J. Prosthodont. 19 (4), 252–257.

Kakol, A., Budtz-Jorgensen, E., 2010. Candida-
    associated denture stomatitis in type 2 diabetes
    mellitus. Diabetes Res. Clin. Pract. 90, 81–86.

Khozeimeh, F., Shahtalebi, M.A., Noori, M., Savabi, O.,
    2010. Comparative evaluation of ketoconazole tablet
    and topical ketoconazole 2% in orabase in treatment
    of Candida-infected denture stomatitis. J. Contemp.
    Dent. Pract. 11, 17–24.

Lyon, J.P., de Resende, M.A., 2006. Correlation between
    adhesion, enzyme production, and susceptibility
    to fluconazole in *Candida albicans* obtained from
    denture wearers. Oral Surg. Oral Med. Oral Pathol.
    Oral Radiol. Endod. 102 (5), 632–638.

Milillo, L., Lo Muzio, L., Carlino, P., et al., 2005.
    Candida-related denture stomatitis: a pilot study of
    the efficacy of an amorolfine antifungal varnish. Int.
    J. Prosthodont. 18, 55–59.

Monsenego, P., 2000. Presence of microorganisms on
    the fitting denture complete surface: study 'in vivo'.
    J. Oral Rehabil. 27, 708–713.

Motta-Silva, A.C., Aleva, N.A., Chavasco, J.K., et al.,
    2010. Erythematous oral candidiasis in patients with
    controlled type II diabetes mellitus and complete
    dentures. Mycopathologia 169 (3), 215–223.

Neppelenbroek, K.H., Pavarina, A.C., Palomari
    Spolidorio, D.M., et al., 2008. Effectiveness of
    microwave disinfection of complete dentures on
    the treatment of Candida-related denture stomatitis.
    J. Oral Rehabil. 35, 836–846.

Pinto, E., Ribeiro, I.C., Ferreira, N.J., et al., 2008.
    Correlation between enzyme production, germ tube
    formation and susceptibility to fluconazole in Candida
    species isolated from patients with denture-related
    stomatitis and control individuals. J. Oral Pathol.
    Med. 37 (10), 587–592.

Pinto, T.M., Neves, A.C., Leao, M.V., Jorge, A.O.,
    2008. Vinegar as an antimicrobial agent for control of
    Candida spp. in complete denture wearers. J. Appl.
    Oral Sci. 16, 385–390.

Salerno, C., Pascale, M., Contaldo, M., et al., 2011.
    Candida-associated denture stomatitis. Med. Oral
    Patol. Oral Cir. Bucal 16 (2), e139–e143.

Song, X., Sun, J., Store, G., et al., 2006. Genotypic
    relatedness of yeasts in thrush and denture
    stomatitis. Oral Microbiol. Immunol.
    21 (5), 301–308.

Vasconcelos, L.C., Sampaio, M.C., Sampaio, F.C.,
    Higino, J.S., 2003. Use of *Punica granatum* as an
    antifungal agent against candidosis associated with
    denture stomatitis. Mycoses 46, 192–196.

Webb, B.C., Thomas, C.J., Whittle, T., 2005. A 2-year
    study of Candida-associated denture stomatitis
    treatment in aged care subjects. Gerodontology
    22, 168–176.

Williams, D.W., Kuriyama, T., Silva, S., 2011.
    Candida biofilms and oral candidosis: treatment and
    prevention. Periodontol 2000 (55), 250–265.

Zomorodian, K., Haghighi, N.N., Rajaee, N., et al.,
    2011. Assessment of Candida species colonization
    and denture-related stomatitis in complete denture
    wearers. Med. Mycol. 49 (2), 208–211.

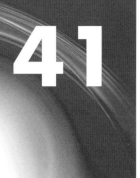
Erythema migrans

INTRODUCTION

Erythema migrans (geographic tongue, benign migratory glossitis) is a common cause of a sore tongue, where the tongue has red patches that resemble a map ('geographic' tongue) (**Fig. 41.1**). It is totally unrelated to erythema migrans of the skin (Lyme disease).

INCIDENCE

It occurs in 1–2% of adults.

AGE

It may be seen at any age.

GENDER

It can occur in either gender.

GEOGRAPHIC

It has no known geographic incidence.

AETIOLOGY AND PATHOGENESIS

- There is a genetic background; there is:
  - often a family history
  - sometimes an HLA association (an increased incidence of HLA-Cw6, DR5 and DRW6 antigens and a decrease in B51 antigen), and an increased incidence of HLA-B15 in atopic patients with erythema migrans
  - an association with IL-1B polymorphism +3954.
- Patients with fissured tongue often have erythema migrans.
- Patients with erythema migrans are typically non-smokers.
- Some patients with erythema migrans have:
  - psoriasis, probably about 4% of cases. Some have a family history of psoriasis. Histologically there is epithelial thinning at the centre of the lesion with an inflammatory infiltrate mainly of polymorphonuclear leukocytes (PMNL), reminiscent of psoriasis – even in patients without psoriasis (**Fig. 41.2**)
  - atopic allergies, such as hay fever, and a few relate the discomfort or oral lesions to various foods (e.g. cheese)
  - diabetes mellitus.
- People with Down syndrome have a higher prevalence of erythema migrans.

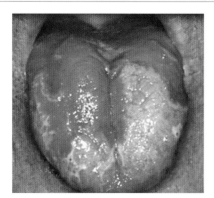

Fig. 41.1 Erythema migrans (geographic tongue), showing typical red lesions with irregular creamy borders

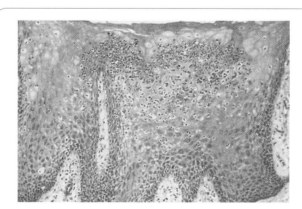

Fig. 41.2 Erythema migrans (geographic tongue), showing typical histopathological features of intra-epithelial foci of leukocytes, resembling psoriasis

CLINICAL FEATURES

- Erythema migrans typically involves the dorsum of the tongue, sometimes the ventrum, and rarely other areas on the oral mucosa.
- There are irregular, pink or red depapillated map-like areas, which change in shape, increase in size, and spread or move to other areas, sometimes within hours (**Figs 41.3 to 41.7**).
- The red areas are often surrounded by distinct yellowish, slightly raised margins.
- There is increased thickness of the intervening filiform papillae.
- It is often asymptomatic.
- A small minority complain of soreness and these patients are virtually invariably middle-aged. If sore, this may be noted especially with acidic foods (e.g. tomatoes, strawberries, pineapple, eggplants or others), walnuts or some cheese. Why the condition should give rise to symptoms after it has presumably been present for decades is unclear.
- Many patients with a fissured tongue (scrotal tongue) also have erythema migrans.

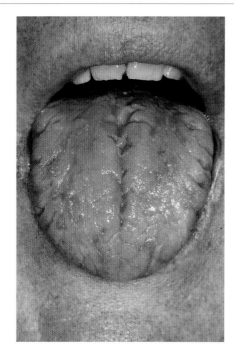

Fig. 41.5 Erythema migrans

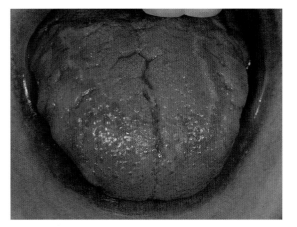

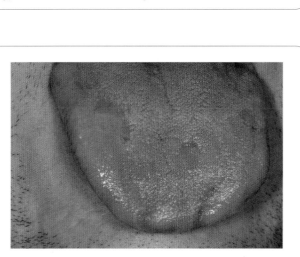

Fig. 41.3 Erythema migrans (geographic tongue), showing typical lesions in a fissured tongue – a common association

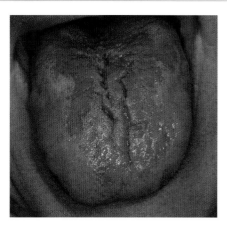

Fig. 41.6 Erythema migrans

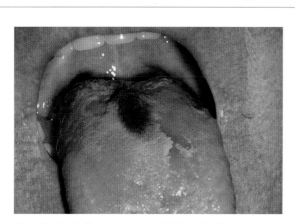

Fig. 41.4 Erythema migrans

Fig. 41.7 Erythema migrans with black hairy tongue

DIAGNOSIS

- The diagnosis is clinical mainly from the history of a migrating pattern and the clinical appearance.
- Very similar lesions may be seen in psoriasis and Reiter syndrome (transiently).
- There also may be confusion with glossitis, lichen planus and lupus erythematosus.
- Blood examination may rarely be necessary to exclude anaemia if there is confusion with a depapillated tongue of glossitis (**Table 41.1**).

TREATMENT (see also Chs 4 and 5)

- Patient information is an important aspect in management.
- There are isolated reports of management with vitamin B, zinc, tetracyclines, corticosteroids, or ciclosporin but

Table 41.1 Aids that might be helpful in diagnosis/prognosis/management in some patients suspected of having erythema migrans*

In some cases
Full blood picture
Serum ferritin, vitamin B_{12} and corrected whole blood folate levels
ESR
Blood glucose

*See text for details and glossary for abbreviations.

reassurance remains the best advice that can be given (**Table 41.2**). Chewing gum or using benzydamine topically can afford symptomatic relief if essential, without adverse effects.

FOLLOW-UP OF PATIENTS

Long-term follow-up is rarely appropriate.

Table 41.2 Regimens that have been trialled in management of patients suspected of having oral erythema migrans

Regimen	Use in primary care
Unproven effectiveness	Ciclosporin Corticosteroids Tetracyclines Vitamins Zinc
Supportive	Benzydamine rinse Chewing gum Diet with little acidic, spicy or citrus content Lidocaine Reassurance

USEFUL WEBSITES

www.ncbi.nlm.nih.gov/pubmedhealth/PMH0002044

FURTHER READING

Abe, M., Sogabe, Y., Syuto, T., et al., 2007. Successful treatment with cyclosporin administration for persistent benign migratory glossitis. J. Dermatol. 34 (5), 340–343.

Assimakopoulos, D., Patrikakos, G., Fotika, C., Elisaf, M., 2002. Benign migratory glossitis or geographic tongue: an enigmatic oral lesion. Am. J. Med 113 (9), 751–755.

Costa, S.C., Hirota, S.K., Takahashi, M.D., et al., 2009. Oral lesions in 166 patients with cutaneous psoriasis: a controlled study. Med. Oral Patol. Oral Cir. Bucal 14 (8), e371–e375.

Daneshpazhooh, M., Moslehi, H., Akhyani, M., Etesami, M., 2004. Tongue lesions in psoriasis: a controlled study. BMC Dermatol. 4 (1), 16.

Daneshpazhooh, M., Nazemi, T.M., Bigdeloo, L., Yoosefi, M., 2007. Mucocutaneous findings in 100 children with Down syndrome. Pediatr. Dermatol. 24 (3), 317–320.

De Biase, A., Guerra, F., Polimeni, A., et al., 2005. Psoriasis of the dorsal surface of the tongue. Minerva Stomatol. 54 (9), 525–529.

Goregen, M., Melikoglu, M., Miloglu, O., Erdem, T., 2010. Predisposition of allergy in patients with benign migratory glossitis. Oral Surg. Oral Med. Oral Pathol. Oral Radiol. Endod. 110 (4), 470–474.

Guimarães, A.L., Correia-Silva, J.de.F, Diniz, M.G., et al., 2007. Investigation of functional gene polymorphisms: IL-1B, IL-6 and TNFA in benign migratory glossitis in Brazilian individuals. J. Oral Pathol. Med. 36 (9), 533–537.

Hernández-Pérez, F., Jaimes-Aveldañez, A., Urquizo-Ruvalcaba, M.de.L., et al., 2008. Prevalence of oral lesions in patients with psoriasis. Med. Oral Patol. Oral Cir. Bucal 13 (11), E703–E708.

Jainkittivong, A., Langlais, R.P., 2005. Geographic tongue: clinical characteristics of 188 cases. J. Contemp. Dent. Pract. 6 (1), 123–135.

Marks, R., Scarff, C.E., Yap, L.M., et al., 2005. Fungiform papillary glossitis: atopic disease in the mouth? Br. J. Dermatol. 153 (4), 740–745.

Miloğlu, O., Göregen, M., Akgül, H.M., Acemoğlu, H., 2009. The prevalence and risk factors associated with benign migratory glossitis lesions in 7619 Turkish dental outpatients. Oral Surg. Oral Med. Oral Pathol. Oral Radiol. Endod. 107 (2), e29–e33.

Pass, B., Brown, R.S., Childers, E.L., 2005. Geographic tongue: literature review and case reports. Dent. Today 24 (8), 54. 56–57; quiz 57.

Saini, R., Al-Maweri, S.A., Saini, D., et al., 2010. Oral mucosal lesions in non oral habit diabetic patients and association of diabetes mellitus with oral precancerous lesions. Diabetes Res. Clin. Pract. 89 (3), 320–326.

Scully, C., Felix, D.H., 2005. Oral medicine – update for the dental practitioner: red and pigmented lesions. Br. Dent. J. 199 (10), 639–645.

Shulman, J.D., Carpenter, W.M., 2006. Prevalence and risk factors associated with geographic tongue among US adults. Oral Dis. 12 (4), 381–386.

Yarom, N., Cantony, U., Gorsky, M., 2004. Prevalence of fissured tongue, geographic tongue and median rhomboid glossitis among Israeli adults of different ethnic origins. Dermatology 209 (2), 88–94.

Zargari, O., 2006. The prevalence and significance of fissured tongue and geographical tongue in psoriatic patients. Clin. Exp. Dermatol. 31 (2), 192–195.

Erythema multiforme

42

Key Points

- Erythema multiforme (EM) is an acute, often recurrent, hypersensitivity reaction
- The cause of EM may remain elusive, but herpes simplex virus and drugs are commonly implicated
- EM affects the mouth with serosanguinous exudates on the lips, and widespread ulceration
- Some patients develop lesions on other mucosae, or skin
- Treatment usually involves corticosteroids

INTRODUCTION

Erythema multiforme (EM) is an acute, often recurrent, non-immediate allergic hypersensitivity reaction affecting muco-cutaneous tissues, seen especially in males, and characterized by serosanguinous exudates on the lips, mouth ulceration and sometimes lesions on other mucosae, or target-like lesions on the skin. Most cases involve oral mucosa only but some more widespread cases (Stevens–Johnson syndrome (SJS) and toxic epidermal necrolysis (TEN); Ch. 56) are severe cutaneous adverse reactions (SCARs) and, though rare (affecting approximately 1 or 2:1 000 000 annually) are medical emergencies as they are potentially fatal.

INCIDENCE

Erythema multiforme is uncommon.

AGE

Younger adults (peaks between 20 and 40 years of age) are affected; 20% of cases occur in children.

GENDER

It is more common in males.

GEOGRAPHIC

It is seen worldwide.

PREDISPOSING FACTORS

There may be a genetic predisposition to EM, with HLA associations including:

- HLA–B12: individuals are 3 times more likely to develop EM
- HLA DQ3: in patients with herpes-simplex-associated EM (HAEM)
- HLA DQB1*0402: in patients with extensive mucosal EM
- HLA-B15 (B62), HLA-B35, HLA-A33, HLA-DR53 and HLA-DQB1*0301: in patients with recurrent EM.

AETIOLOGY AND PATHOGENESIS

The trigger for EM is unclear in most patients but, where a trigger can be identified, it is mainly (**Boxes 42.1** and **42.2**):

- infective agents: herpes simplex virus is implicated in 70% of recurrent EM (herpes-associated EM; HAEM). Numerous other organisms, particularly mycoplasmas, have also been implicated
- drugs: especially NSAIDs, anticonvulsants, allopurinol and antimicrobials
- immune conditions: such as BCG or hepatitis B immunization
- food additives or chemicals: such as benzoates, nitrobenzene, perfumes, terpenes.

SJS/TEN, the far more serious disorders, are assumed or identified to be caused by drugs in most cases. NSAIDs, antibiotics, and anticonvulsants are the most common triggers but several drugs are at 'high risk' of inducing TEN/SJS including: allopurinol, trimethoprim-sulfamethoxazole and other

---

BOX 42.1 Main aetiological factors in erythema multiforme

- Chemicals
- Drugs
- Immunization
- Infections
- Radiation therapy

BOX 42.2 Advanced list of aetiological factors in erythema multiforme

Infections
- Viruses:
    - cytomegalovirus
    - Epstein-Barr virus
    - hepatitis C
    - herpes simplex virus 1 and 2
    - human immunodeficiency virus
    - orf
    - varicella zoster virus
- Bacterial:
    - *Mycoplasma pneumoniae*
- Fungal:
    - histoplasmosis

Drugs (see Table 54.15)
- Allopurinol
- Aminopenicillins
- Anticonvulsants
- Antimicrobials
- Carbamazepine
- Cephalosporins

Vaccines
- BCG
- Diphtheria-tetanus
- Hepatitis B
- Smallpox

Immune disorders
- Graft-versus-host disease
- Inflammatory bowel disease
- Polyarteritis nodosa
- Sarcoidosis
- Systemic lupus erythematosus

Food additives or chemicals
- Benzoates
- Nitrobenzene
- Perfumes
- Terpenes

Radiation therapy

---

sulphonamide antibiotics, aminopenicillins, cephalosporins, quinolones, carbamazepine, phenytoin, phenobarbital and NSAIDs of the oxicam-type. Genetic susceptibility to SJS and TEN is likely as exemplified by the strong association observed in Han Chinese between a genetic marker, the human leukocyte antigen HLA-B*1502, and SJS induced by carbamazepine.

Human leukocyte antigen (HLA)-restricted presentation of antigens (drugs or their metabolites) to T lymphocytes initiates the immune reactions of SJS/TEN. The manifestation of a disregulated immune reaction against epithelial cells (**Fig. 42.1**) with the appearance in the epithelium of cytotoxic effector cells, mainly activated CD8$^+$ T lymphocytes and macrophages, and neutrophils, causing keratinocyte apoptosis leading to satellite cell necrosis and thus sub- and intra-epithelial vesiculation (**Fig. 42.2**). The Fas/FasL system is not significantly expressed in typical EM but in extensive mucocutaneous disease such as SJS and TEN, this apoptosis has a pivotal role. Humoral and cellular components of the innate immune response have been identified in association with SJS/TEN. Activated monocytes and macrophages may produce several 'alarmins' or endogenous damage-associated molecular patterns. Natural killer (NK) cells contribute through secretion of effector molecules such as granulysin. The innate immunity receptor CD94/NKG2C is expressed by NK cells and cytotoxic T lymphocytes in SJS/TEN and triggers degranulation in response to human leukocyte antigen-E-expressing keratinocytes. During the early stages, apoptosis mediates keratinocyte death – in which Fas-FasL pathway activation is involved. CD8$^+$ T cell cytotoxicity is mediated by the perforin-granzyme pathway. Cytokines from T lymphocytes, macrophages or keratinocytes may participate by activating keratinocytes and enhancing their expression of Fas and FasL, or by promoting the skin recruitment of lymphocytes by upregulating adhesion molecules. CD4$^+$ and particularly CD8$^+$ T cells producing type 1 and type 2 cytotoxic cytokines. Cytotoxic T cells or natural killer (NK) cells release a cytotoxic protein granulysin. Subsequently, there may be an expansion of apoptosis involving the interaction of Fas ligand (sFasL) with its receptor Fas.

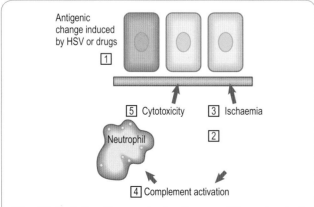

Fig. 42.1 Aetiopathogenesis of erythema multiforme (see text)

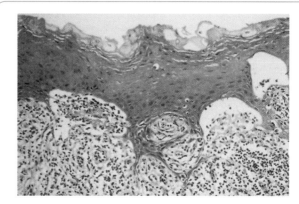

Fig. 42.2 Histopathology of erythema multiforme showing mainly sub-epithelial vesiculation

CLINICAL FEATURES

EM may present a wide spectrum of severity, from the much more common mild limited disease (minor EM) often involving only the mouth, to a severe, widespread and life-threatening illness (TEN), with ill-defined clinical distinctions between the intermediate forms (EM major and SJS) (**Table 42.1**).

ORAL LESIONS

Most patients with EM (70%), of either minor or major forms, have oral lesions, which typically:

- Precede lesions on other stratified squamous epithelia, or may arise in isolation.
- Present with:
- lips that become swollen and cracked, bleeding, and crusted (**Fig. 42.3**)
  - diffuse and widespread macules that progress through to blisters and ulceration
  - lesions on the non-keratinized mucosae and most pronounced in the anterior mouth (**Fig. 42.4**).
  - recur in about 25%; the periodicity can vary from weeks to years, attacks usually lasting 10–20 days occurring once or twice a year.
- Resolve after about 6 episodes.

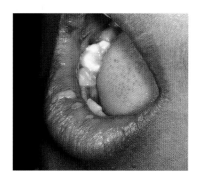

Fig. 42.4 Erythema multiforme

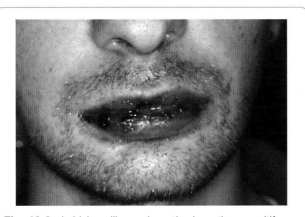

Fig. 42.3 Labial swelling and crusting in erythema multiforme

SKIN LESIONS

Skin lesions seen in major EM:

- commonly affect the distal extremities, especially the extensor surfaces of the arms, legs, elbows, knees, dorsum of hands and feet
- vary in type (hence the term erythema *multiforme*) but are usually macules that are symmetric, round, erythematous and slightly pruritic or non-itchy and may evolve into papules or plaques that frequently display a circumferential pallor and evolve into target or iris lesions. The well-demarcated centre of the papule forms a necrotic ulcer, which results in a depressed white, yellow or grey area surrounded by a red edge and then a pale oedematous ring; a bright red margin may surround this pale ring.

There may also be blistering.

OTHER MUCOSAL LESIONS

Other mucosal lesions, seen in major EM may include:

- eye involvement: may cause lacrimation and photophobia
- genital lesions: painful and may result in urinary retention.

Table 42.1 Differentiation of erythema multiforme, SJS, and TEN

	Oral erosions	Erosions of other mucosae	Skin target lesions	Other skin lesions	Body surface area epidermal detachment (%)
Erythema multiforme minor	+	−	± Typical targets	Raised atypical targets	<10
Erythema multiforme major/SJS	+	+	−	Flat atypical targets, confluent purpuric macules on the face and trunk	<10
SJS and TEN overlap	+	+	−	Flat atypical targets	10–30
TEN	+	+	−	Flat atypical targets	>30

FORMS OF EM

The extent of involvement of different mucosae is the distinguishing feature between minor and major forms:

- Minor erythema multiforme:
  - affects only one site (mouth alone, or skin or other mucosae)
  - rashes are various, but are typically 'iris' or 'target' lesions or bullae on the extremities.
- Major erythema multiforme:
  - in about 30% of cases begins with a prodrome, from within 1–3 weeks of starting a new drug, lasting 1–2 weeks before the onset of the mucocutaneous manifestations, and often also with flu-like symptoms, sore throat, headache, arthralgias, myalgias or fever
  - widespread lesions appear and affect the mouth, but also other sites such as skin, eyes, genitals, pharynx, larynx and/or oesophagus. Skin involvement may present with bullous and other rashes with epidermal detachment involving <10% of the body surface. Ocular changes that resemble those of mucous membrane pemphigoid (dry eyes and symblepharon) may result. Genital changes may include balanitis, urethritis and vulval ulcers. *HSV-induced EM major* is characterized by mucosal erosions plus typical or raised atypical targets usually on the extremities and/or the face; *drug-induced EM major* is characterized by mucosal erosions plus widespread distribution of flat atypical targets or purpuric macules on the trunk, face and extremities.
- Stevens–Johnson syndrome (SJS) and toxic epidermal necrolysis (TEN) are extreme forms of major EM, with widespread blistering, and potentially other complications such as pneumonia, arthritis, nephritis or myocarditis. There are no factors reliably predictive for the progression of EM to these extreme forms. Initially, SJS/TEN present with non-specific symptoms, followed by an acute macular erythematous rash with bullae, a positive Nikolsky sign and a separation of large sheets of epidermis from the dermis and extensive blistering and shedding of the skin similar to that seen in large burns. Besides the skin, mucous membranes such as oral, genital, anal, nasal, and conjunctival mucosa are frequently involved. SJS and TEN are considered to be two ends of a spectrum, differing only by their extent of skin detachment. SJS affects <10% of the skin surface, and has an average mortality rate of 1–5%, whereas involvement of 10–30% of body surface area is called SJS/TEN overlap. TEN is the most severe form and includes denudation of >30% of surface area and is associated with a significant mortality of 25–30%. Mortality rates can be even higher in older patients and those with a large surface area of epidermal detachment.

DIAGNOSIS

A diagnosis of erythema multiforme can be difficult to readily establish, as there can be a need to differentiate from viral stomatitides, pemphigus, and the subepithelial immune blistering disorders (pemphigoid and others):

- The diagnosis of EM is mainly clinical; the Nikolsky sign is negative.
- It may be helpful to undertake serological testing for HSV or *Mycoplasma pneumoniae*, or for other micro-organisms (**Table 42.2**).

Table 42.2 Aids that might be helpful in diagnosis/prognosis/management in some patients suspected of having erythema multiforme*

In most cases	In some cases
Dermatological/gynaecological opinion Nikolsky sign Biopsy	Full blood picture Serum ferritin, vitamin B$_{12}$ and corrected whole blood folate levels ESR Serology (HSV, mycoplasma) G6PD and TPMT levels Blood pressure Blood glucose

*See text for details and glossary for abbreviations.

- Biopsy of perilesional tissue, with histological and immunostaining examination, are essential if a specific diagnosis is required. The histopathology can be variable and immunostaining is not specific – but typically shows:
  - intraepithelial oedema and spongiosis early on
  - satellite cell necrosis (individual eosinophilic necrotic keratinocytes surrounded by lymphocytes)
  - Keratinocyte necrosis and dermal inflammation containing eosinophils may occur in drug-related cases
  - immune deposits: fibrin and C3 at the epithelial basement membrane zone
  - vacuolar degeneration of the junctional zone and severe papillary oedema
  - sub- or intraepithelial vesiculation
  - increased vascularity
  - perivascular lymphocytic infiltrate (CD4$^+$ more than CD8$^+$ T lymphocytes) with a few neutrophils and occasional eosinophils
  - perivascular IgM, C3 and fibrin deposits.

Diagnosis of SJS/TEN relies mainly on clinical signs (the Nikolsky sign is often positive), together with a skin biopsy – histopathology showing typical full-thickness epidermal necrolysis.

TREATMENT (see also Chs 4 and 5)

Spontaneous healing can be slow; up to 3 weeks in minor EM and up to 6 weeks in EM major:

- No specific treatment is available, but specialist care is indicated.
- Patient information is an important aspect in management.
- Early ophthalmologic and dermatological consultations are needed.
- Precipitating factors, when identified, should be treated.
- Oral hygiene should be improved with 0.2% aqueous chlorhexidine mouthbaths.
- Antimicrobials may be indicated (**Table 42.3**):
  - aciclovir or valaciclovir in EM related to herpes simplex virus
  - tetracycline in EM related to *Mycoplasma pneumoniae*.
- *Patients with minor EM* often respond to topical corticosteroids (Ch. 5), though systemic corticosteroids may also be required.

Table 42.3 Regimens that might be helpful in management of patient suspected of having erythema multiforme

Regimen	Use in primary care (minor erythema multiforme)	Use in secondary care (severe oral involvement and/or extraoral involvement/major erythema multiforme)*
Likely to be beneficial	Topical corticosteroids	Systemic corticosteroids (controversial)
Unproven effectiveness	Antivirals Antibacterials	Azathioprine Intravenous immunoglobulins Ciclosporin Cyclophosphamide Dapsone Levamisole Mycophenolate mofetil Pentoxifylline Plasmapheresis Thalidomide Ulinastatin
Supportive	Chlorhexidine Benzydamine Diet with little acidic, spicy or citrus content Lidocaine	In-patient care

*See text for SJS/TEN care.

- Topical corticosteroids are the primary therapeutic agents used to treat ulcerative mucosal lesions, which have an immunologically-based aetiology such as erythema multiforme. Typically a medium potency corticosteroid such as betamethasone or a higher potency one such as fluocinonide or beclomethasone are required, moving to a super-potent topical corticosteroid, e.g. clobetasol, if the benefit is inadequate (Tables 5.5 and 42.3). Patients should be instructed to apply a small quantity of the agent three times daily, refraining from speaking, eating and drinking for the subsequent 0.5 h. A theoretical concern is that long-term immunosuppression might predispose to neoplastic change. In long-term use, candidosis can arise and thus topical antifungal medication such as miconazole may be prudent. The more major concern – of adrenal suppression with long-term and/or repeated application – has rarely been addressed, although the topical preparations noted in Ch. 5 (apart from super potent halogenated corticosteroids when used several times a day) appear not to cause a significant problem. Specific treatment with immunosuppressive drugs or immunoglobulins has not shown an improved outcome in most studies and remains controversial.
- *Patients with major EM* may need admission for hospital care. Supportive care is important. A complete blood count, urea and electrolytes, ESR, CRP or PV, liver function tests, and cultures from blood, sputum and erosive areas should be taken. A liquid diet and intravenous fluid therapy may be necessary, and electrolytes and nutritional support should be started early on. Specific treatment with immunosuppressive drugs or immunoglobulins has not shown an improved outcome in most studies and remains controversial, but major EM is still often treated with topical and systemic corticosteroids (prednisolone (enteric-coated)) and/or steroid-sparing immunosuppressive agents (**Table 42.3**) (Ch. 5).
- *Patients with SJS or TEN* require urgent admission in a burn or intensive care unit, the prompt withdrawal of the suspected drug, fluid and electrolyte replacement

and topical wound care. No systemic treatment has been established as standard and therefore treatment is primarily symptomatic and supportive and involves a multidisciplinary approach. In the early exudating phase, the use of an airfluidized bed combined with gentle debridement are recommended. Next, an alternating pressure mattress and silver impregnated absorbent dressings should be used. During the re-epithelialization phase, antiseptic or antibiotic creams overlaid with nonadherent dressings favour an optimized moist and bacteria-controlled environment. The use of corticosteroids has largely been abandoned and the role of immunosuppressants, despite some success, is not considered as a standard. Plasmapheresis is reported to lead to some success, with improvement of clinical conditions and survival. The use of human intravenous immunoglobulins (IVIGs) is controversial but they may have a place in the management of severe disease. Oral lesions are managed additionally, as above.

PROPHYLACTIC CARE
Avoid triggers.

Pharmacogenomic studies may be used to predict the risk of adverse reactions from drugs such as carbamazepine and other aromatic antiepileptic drugs, allopurinol and abacavir. Different ethnic populations show variations in genetic associations. For example, there is a strong association between carbamazepine-induced SJS/TEN and HLA-B*1502 in Southeast Asian patients but not in Caucasian and Japanese. HLA-B*5801 is associated with allopurinol-induced SJS/TEN in Caucasian and Asian patients, including Japanese.

FOLLOW-UP OF PATIENTS

Long-term follow-up as shared care is usually appropriate for minor erythema multiforme.

USEFUL WEBSITES

www.ncbi.nlm.nih.gov/pubmedhealth/PMH0001854/

FURTHER READING

Abe, R., 2008. Toxic epidermal necrolysis and Stevens-Johnson syndrome: soluble Fas ligand involvement in the pathomechanisms of these diseases. J. Dermatol. Sci. 52 (3), 151–159.

Aihara, M., 2011. Pharmacogenetics of cutaneous adverse drug reactions. J. Dermatol. 38 (3), 246–254.

Ayangco, L., Rogers III, R.S., 2003. Oral manifestations of erythema multiforme. Dermatol. Clin. 21, 198.

Bellón, T., Blanca, M., 2011. The innate immune system in delayed cutaneous allergic reactions to medications. Curr. Opin. Allergy Clin. Immunol. 11 (4), 292–298.

Borchers, A.T., Lee, J.L., Naguwa, S.M., et al., 2008. Stevens-Johnson syndrome and toxic epidermal necrolysis. Autoimmun. Rev. 7 (8), 598–605.

Caproni, M., Antiga, E., Parodi, A., et al., 2006. Elevated circulating CD40 ligand in patients with erythema multiforme and Stevens–Johnson syndrome/toxic epidermal necrolysis spectrum. Br. J. Dermatol. 154 (5), 1006–1007.

Caproni, M., Torchia, D., Schincaglia, E., et al., 2006. Expression of cytokines and chemokine receptors in the cutaneous lesions of erythema multiforme and Stevens–Johnson syndrome/toxic epidermal necrolysis. Br. J. Dermatol. 155 (4), 722–728.

Caproni, M., Torchia, D., Schincaglia, E., et al., 2006. The CD40/CD40 ligand system is expressed in the cutaneous lesions of erythema multiforme and Stevens–Johnson syndrome/toxic epidermal necrolysis spectrum. Br. J. Dermatol. 154 (2), 319–324.

Chung, W.H., Hung, S.I., 2010. Genetic markers and danger signals in Stevens-Johnson syndrome and toxic epidermal necrolysis. Allergol. Int. 59 (4), 325–332.

Del Pozzo-Magana, B.R., Lazo-Langner, A., Carleton, B., et al., 2011. A systematic review of treatment of drug-induced Stevens-Johnson syndrome and toxic epidermal necrolysis in children. J. Popul. Ther. Clin. Pharmacol. 18, e121–e133.

Farthing, P., Bagan, J.V., Scully, C., 2005. Mucosal disease series. Number IV. Erythema multiforme. Oral Dis. 11 (5), 261–267.

Gerull, R., Nelle, M., Schaible, T., 2011. Toxic epidermal necrolysis and Stevens-Johnson syndrome: a review. Crit. Care Med. 39 (6), 1521–1532.

Greenberger, P.A., 2006. 8. Drug allergy. J. Allergy Clin. Immunol. 117 (2 Suppl. Mini-Primer), S464–S470 8.

Halevy, S., 2010. Stevens-Johnson syndrome and toxic epidermal necrolysis—updates and innovations. Harefuah 149 (3), 186–190, 193.

Harr, T., French, L.E., 2010a. Severe cutaneous adverse reactions: acute generalized exanthematous pustulosis, toxic epidermal necrolysis and Stevens-Johnson syndrome. Med. Clin. North Am. 94 (4), 727–742.

Harr, T., French, L.E., 2010. Toxic epidermal necrolysis and Stevens-Johnson syndrome. Orphanet J. Rare Dis. 5, 39.

Hoffman, L.D., Hoffman, M.D., 2006. Dapsone in the treatment of persistent erythema multiforme. J. Drugs Dermatol. 5 (4), 375–376.

Hussain, W., Craven, N.M., 2005. Toxic epidermal necrolysis and Stevens-Johnson syndrome. Clin. Med. 5 (6), 555–558.

Khalili, B., Bahna, S.L., 2006. Pathogenesis and recent therapeutic trends in Stevens–Johnson syndrome and toxic epidermal necrolysis. Ann. Allergy Asthma Immunol. 97 (3), 272–280, quiz 281–3, 320.

Knowles, S., Shear, N.H., 2009. Clinical risk management of Stevens-Johnson syndrome/toxic epidermal necrolysis spectrum. Dermatol. Ther. 22 (5), 441–451.

Lee, M.T., Hung, S.I., Wei, C.Y., Chen, Y.T., 2010. Pharmacogenetics of toxic epidermal necrolysis. Expert Opin. Pharmacother. 11 (13), 2153–2162.

Lissia, M., Mulas, P., Bulla, A., Rubino, C., 2010. Toxic epidermal necrolysis (Lyell's disease). Burns 36 (2), 152–163.

Nagy, N., McGrath, J.A., 2010. Blistering skin diseases: a bridge between dermatopathology and molecular biology. Histopathology 56 (1), 91–99.

Paquet, P., Piérard, G.E., 2010. Topical treatment options for drug-induced toxic epidermal necrolysis (TEN). Expert Opin. Pharmacother. 11 (15), 2447–2458.

Reese, D., Henning, J.S., Rockers, K., et al., 2011. Cyclosporine for SJS/TEN: a case series and review of the literature. Cutis 87 (1), 24–29.

Rozieres, A., Vocanson, M., Saïd, B.B., et al., 2009. Role of T cells in nonimmediate allergic drug reactions. Curr. Opin. Allergy Clin. Immunol. 9 (4), 305–310.

Sanchis, J.M., Bagán, J.V., Gavaldá, C., et al., 2010. Erythema multiforme: diagnosis, clinical manifestations and treatment in a retrospective study of 22 patients. J. Oral Pathol. Med. 39 (10), 747–752.

Struck, M.F., Hilbert, P., Mockenhaupt, M., et al., 2010. Severe cutaneous adverse reactions: emergency approach to non-burn epidermolytic syndromes. Intensive Care Med. 36 (1), 22–32.

Tartarone, A., Lerose, R., 2010. Stevens-Johnson syndrome and toxic epidermal necrolysis: what do we know? Ther. Drug. Monit. 32 (6), 669–672.

Tripathi, A., Ditto, A.M., Grammer, L.C., et al., 2000. Corticosteroid therapy in an additional 13 cases of Stevens–Johnson syndrome: a total series of 67 cases. Allergy Asthma Proc. 21, 101–105.

Wohrl, S., Loewe, R., Pickl, W.F., et al., 2005. EMPACT syndrome. J. Dtsch Dermatol. Ges. 3 (1), 39–43.

Worswick, S., Cotliar, J., 2011. Stevens-Johnson syndrome and toxic epidermal necrolysis: a review of treatment options. Dermatol. Ther. 24 (2), 207–218.

Herpesvirus infections

43

Key Points

- Herpesviruses are DNA viruses that can be transmitted in body fluids such as saliva, contracted in early life, characterized by latency and reactivated during immunosuppression
- Herpes simplex virus (HSV) causes primary herpetic stomatitis and recurrent herpes labialis or intraoral recurrences
- Herpes zoster varicella virus causes chickenpox and shingles
- Epstein–Barr virus causes infectious mononucleosis, and also nasopharyngeal carcinoma, lymphomas and hairy leukoplakia
- Cytomegalovirus causes some salivary infections
- Human herpesviruses 6 and 7 cause rashes and possibly drug hypersensitivity syndrome
- Human herpesvirus 8 causes Kaposi sarcoma
- Some herpesviruses are linked to oncogenicity
- A range of antiherpesvirus drugs is now available

INTRODUCTION

Herpesviruses (from Greek *herpein* = to creep) are DNA viruses that are mostly:

- contracted in early life
- transmitted in saliva and other secretions
- characterized by latency
- reactivated during immunosuppression - when they are associated with more severe and protracted disorders, particularly in HIV infection, in cancer patients and in those immunosuppressed after organ grafts.

Herpesviruses and the orofacial disorders with which they may be associated are shown in **Table 43.1**. Some herpesviruses can cause malignant tumours (i.e. are *oncogenic*).

HERPES SIMPLEX VIRUS INFECTIONS

The term 'herpes' is often used loosely to refer to infections with herpes simplex virus (HSV), a ubiquitous virus that commonly produces lesions in the mouth, oropharynx and anogenital region. Generally speaking, herpetic infections are caused above the belt (oral or oropharyngeal) mainly by HSV-1, but caused below the belt (genital or anal) by HSV-2.

PRIMARY HSV INFECTIONS

Primary oral infection is often subclinical between the ages of 2 and 4 years and is a common cause of 'teething'. Herpetic stomatitis (gingivostomatitis) is:

- the primary clinical infection with HSV
- usually caused by HSV-1
- seen mainly in children
- increasingly seen in older patients, when it is sometimes due to HSV-2 transmitted sexually.

INCIDENCE

Common, especially in resource-poor persons.

Age

Primary stomatitis is seen mainly in children and adolescents. Oropharyngeal herpes is seen mainly in adolescents and recurrences are seen mainly in adults.

Gender

Both sexes are affected.

Geographic

Common in children in resource - poor areas. Also seen in adults, especially in resource - rich areas.

PREDISPOSING FACTORS

- Close contact with infected individuals, such as in play groups or sexually, predisposes to infection.
- HSV is contracted from infected saliva or other body fluids after an incubation period of approximately 4–7 days.
- HSV-1 can cause oral or oropharyngeal infection, usually via infection from saliva, and is most frequent and at a younger age in resource-poor groups.
- HSV-2 can cause severe oropharyngeal infection, usually via orogenital or oro–anal sexual contact, via infected semen, saliva or other body fluids. It is more common in the sexually active and is most frequent amongst female prostitutes (75%) and men who have sex with men (80%). HSV-1 genital infection is less common and usually less severe than HSV-2 infection.
- Neonatal HSV infections are potentially dangerous as they may lead to disseminated involvement and encephalitis, and often leave neurological sequelae.
- Patients with immune defects are liable to severe and/or protracted and/or disseminated HSV infections.

AETIOLOGY AND PATHOGENESIS

- HSV must contact mucosae or abraded skin to initiate infection.

277

Table 43.1   Herpesvirus infections and their known possible oral sequelae

Herpesvirus	Abbreviation	Typical primary infection	Common clinical oral sequelae	Other known possible sequelae, particularly in immunocompromised patients
Herpes simplex	HSV-1	Stomatitis	Herpes labialis	Ulcers Erythema multiforme Bell palsy
Herpes simplex	HSV-2	Anogenital herpes	Recurrent herpes	Ulcers
Herpes varicella-zoster	VZV	Chickenpox	Zoster	Jaw necrosis
Epstein–Barr virus	EBV	Glandular fever	Fatigue	Hairy leukoplakia Lymphomas Nasopharyngeal carcinoma
Cytomegalovirus	CMV	Glandular fever	?	Ulcers
Human herpesvirus-6	HHV-6	Rash	?	Drug hypersensitivity syndrome
Human herpesvirus-7	HHV-7	Rash	?	–
Human herpesvirus-8	HHV-8 or KSHV (Kaposi sarcoma herpesvirus)	Rash	Kaposi sarcoma	Castleman disease Primary effusion lymphoma

- HSV surface glycoproteins mediate cell attachment and penetration.
- HSV is neuroinvasive and neurotoxic and infects neurones of dorsal root and autonomic ganglia.
- HSV remains latent thereafter in the ganglion, usually the trigeminal ganglion, but can be reactivated and result in clinical recrudescence (see below).
- *Primary* infection is when a susceptible (non-immune) individual develops infection.
- *Initial* infection occurs when an individual who has antibodies to either HSV-1 or HSV-2 is infected with the other virus type for the first time.
- *Recurrent* infection occurs when an individual who has contracted either HSV-1 or HSV-2 reactivates the latent virus.
- HSV is also implicated in Bell palsy (see Ch. 37), erythema multiforme (see Ch. 42), herpetic encephalitis and Alzheimer disease.

CLINICAL FEATURES

Some 50% of primary HSV infections are subclinical but the main features of clinical disease are that:

- often there is fever and/or malaise
- the mouth or oropharynx is sore (herpetic stomatitis); this probably explains many instances of 'teething'.

Other features include:

- a single episode of oral vesicles, which may be widespread, and break down to leave oral ulcers. These are initially pin-point, but fuse to produce irregular painful ulcers (**Fig. 43.1**)
- gingival oedema, erythema and ulceration
- the cervical lymph nodes may be enlarged and tender. Usually, several nodes in the anterior triangle of the neck (especially the jugulodigastric nodes) are enlarged but posterior triangle

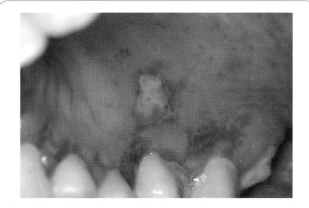

Fig. 43.1   Herpetic stomatitis; ulcers in the palate

and nodes elsewhere are not enlarged, unless there are systemic complications or lesions in other sites
- there is no hepatosplenomegaly, unless there are systemic complications or lesions elsewhere.

DIAGNOSIS

- Diagnosis is largely clinical.
- Herpetic stomatitis should be differentiated from other causes of mouth ulcers (see Ch. 21), especially herpangina, hand, foot and mouth disease, chickenpox and shingles, erythema multiforme and leukaemia. Full blood picture is warranted.
- Viral studies which are occasionally used for diagnosis include (**Table 43.2**):
  - polymerase chain reaction detection of HSV-DNA: sensitive and rapid, but expensive
  - antibody detection of HSV antigens (direct fluorescent antibody; DFA): sensitive and rapid serology for detection of a rising titre of serum antibodies; confirmatory, but only gives the diagnosis retrospectively; conventional

Table 43.2 Aids that might be helpful in diagnosis/prognosis/management in some patients suspected of having herpesvirus infections*

In most cases	In some cases
Full blood picture	Serum ferritin, vitamin B$_{12}$ and corrected whole blood folate levels
	ESR
	HSV, VZV, HIV, EBV, CMV, KSHV serology, direct fluorescent immunostaining or PCR

*See text for details and glossary for abbreviations.

enzyme-linked immunosorbent assays (ELISA) for serum antibodies have poor sensitivity and specificity, while newer assays based on gG-1 HSV glycoproteins are comparable with Western blot assays

- culture: takes days to give a result
- electron microscopy: not always available
- smears for viral damaged cells: now rarely used.

TREATMENT (see also Chs 4 and 5)

Although patients eventually have spontaneous remission, treatment is indicated particularly to reduce fever and control pain (**Table 43.3**). Patient information is an important aspect in management:

- Pregnant women and neonates must receive urgent specialist care. HSV infection in pregnancy can cause foetal disorders ranging from minor issues to death, herpes being one of the peri-natal infections causing the so-called TORCH syndrome or complex (toxoplasmosis; rubella; cytomegalovirus; herpes) (Ch. 57).
- Adequate fluid intake is important, especially in children.
- Antipyretics/analgesics, such as paracetamol help relieve pain and fever.
- A soft bland diet may be needed, as the mouth can be very sore.
- Local antiseptics (0.2% aqueous chlorhexidine mouthwashes) may aid resolution of the lesions.
- Antivirals may be effective if used systemically within 5 days of symptoms, though they do not reduce the frequency of subsequent recurrences; 100–200 mg aciclovir tablets 5 times daily, or sugar-free oral suspension (200 mg/5 mL) 5 times daily or valaciclovir or famciclovir.

Table 43.3 Regimens that might be helpful in management of patient suspected of having herpetic stomatitis

Regimen	Use in primary or secondary care*
Beneficial	Aciclovir, valciclovir or famciclovir
Supportive	Adequate hydration
	Benzydamine
	Chlorhexidine
	Diet with little acidic, spicy or citrus content
	Lidocaine
	Paracetamol

*Specialist care for neonates, pregnant or immunocompromised people.

- Aciclovir must be used systemically with care in pregnancy, older patients, renal disease, or when infused (Ch. 5). Systemic antivirals are useful especially in neonates, pregnancy and in immunocompromised patients; but all such patients should be seen by a specialist.

FOLLOW-UP OF PATIENTS

Long-term follow-up is rarely required.

RECURRENT HSV INFECTIONS

INCIDENCE

Up to 15% of the population have recurrent HSV-1 infections. – usually lip lesions (herpes labialis).

Age

They occur mainly in adults.

Gender

Both genders are affected.

Geographic

Herpes labialis is the most common form of recurrence and is seen mainly in sunny climes.

PREDISPOSING FACTORS

Reactivating factors include:

- sunlight
- fever, such as caused by upper respiratory tract infection (hence herpes labialis is often termed 'cold' sores)
- trauma
- immunosuppression.

AETIOLOGY AND PATHOGENESIS

HSV-1 is latent in the trigeminal ganglion after primary infection. The virus can be reactivated, is shed into saliva, and there may be clinical recrudescence, recurrently, to produce herpes labialis or, occasionally, intraoral ulceration.

CLINICAL FEATURES

Features of recurrent herpes labialis are:

- lip lesions at the mucocutaneous junction (**Fig. 43.2**)
- lesions may be preceded by pain, burning, tingling or itching, and begin as macules that rapidly become papular, then vesicular for about 48 h, then become pustular, and scab within 72–96 h and heal without scarring
- widespread recalcitrant lesions may appear in immunocompromised patients.

Features of recurrent intraoral herpes include:

- in apparently healthy patients: a small crop of ulcers over the greater palatine foramen, following a palatal local anaesthetic injection, presumably because of the trauma (**Fig. 43.3**). This can mimic zoster
- in immunocompromised patients: chronic, often dendritic, ulcers, frequently on the tongue dorsum.

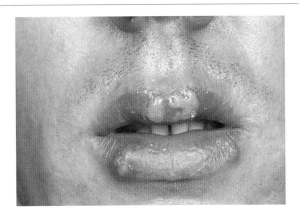

Fig. 43.2 Herpes labialis

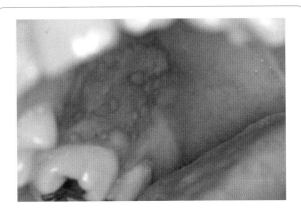

Fig. 43.3 Recurrent intraoral herpes

DIAGNOSIS

- Differential diagnosis of herpes labialis is mainly from zoster, impetigo, or carcinoma (rarely). Diagnosis is largely clinical, although viral studies are used very occasionally.
- Diagnosis of recurrent intraoral herpes in healthy patients is mainly from zoster. Diagnosis is largely clinical and viral studies are used very occasionally.
- Diagnosis of recurrent intraoral herpes in immunocompromised patients can be difficult since the lesions can mimic many other causes of oral ulceration. Clinical diagnosis tends to underestimate the frequency of these lesions and viral studies may be needed, particularly as there may be co-infection with other agents such as CMV.

TREATMENT (see also Chs 4 and 5)

- Patient information is an important aspect in management.
- Patients should avoid any triggers they have identified. For example, if sunlight is a trigger, they should use a good quality sun block. Getting enough sleep and taking a good diet may be helpful.
- Once a lesion appears, most patients will have spontaneous remission within 1 week to 10 days, but the condition is both uncomfortable and unsightly, and, thus, early treatment is indicated.
- Antivirals will achieve maximum benefit only if given in the prodrome or early in the disease (Ch. 5), and may be indicated in herpes labialis especially in:
  - patients who have severe, widespread or persistent lesions
  - immunocompromised persons.
- Lip lesions in healthy patients may be minimized with topical penciclovir 1% cream or aciclovir 5% cream applied from the prodrome, every 2h whilst awake (Ch. 5; **Table 43.4**). Penciclovir may be marginally the more effective.

Table 43.4 Regimens that might be helpful in management of patient suspected of having recurrent herpes simplex lesions

Regimen	Use in primary care (herpes labialis)	Use in secondary care (severe oral involvement and/or extraoral involvement), or immunocompromised
Beneficial	Topical penciclovir or aciclovir	Systemic aciclovir, valciclovir or famciclovir
Likely to be beneficial	Protective hydrocolloid patches	
Unproven effectiveness	Soft lasers Cetrimide Chlorocresol Dimeticone Docosanol Geranium oil Idoxuridine Inosine Lemon balm mint extract Lysine Melatonin Monocaprin Silica gel Tea tree oil Tromantidine Urea	
Supportive	Lip balm	

- Lip lesions in immunocompromised patients may require systemic aciclovir or other antivirals, such as valaciclovir or famciclovir (the precursor of penciclovir).
- Recurrent intraoral herpes in healthy patients can be managed with symptomatic treatment with a soft diet and adequate fluid intake, antipyretics/analgesics (paracetamol), and local antiseptics (0.2% aqueous chlorhexidine mouthwashes). Systemic aciclovir or other antivirals, such as valciclovir or famciclovir may be indicated for persistent lesions.
- Recurrent intraoral herpes in immunocompromised patients is difficult to manage and systemic aciclovir or other antivirals may well be needed. A soft diet and adequate fluid intake, antipyretics/analgesics (paracetamol elixir) and local antiseptics (0.2% aqueous chlorhexidine mouthwashes) may help. Antiviral resistance is becoming a significant problem to immunocompromised persons, especially those with a severe immune defect.
- Other therapies tried for recurrent herpes are shown in **Table 43.4**.
- There is insufficient evidence to support use of many other preparations including echinacea, eleuthero, zinc or aloe vera.
- Reliably effective anti-herpes vaccines are not currently available.

FOLLOW-UP OF PATIENTS

Long-term follow-up in primary care is usually appropriate.

HERPES VARICELLA-ZOSTER VIRUS INFECTIONS

PRIMARY VZV INFECTIONS

Chickenpox (varicella) is the primary infection with the virus.

Incidence

Chickenpox is common.

Age

It mainly occurs in children.

Gender

Both sexes are affected.

Geographic

No known geographic incidence, it occurs worldwide.

Predisposing factors

Chickenpox is highly contagious and VZV is readily spread by droplets.

Aetiology

After this primary infection, the virus remains latent in dorsal root ganglia.

Clinical features

- The incubation period is 14–21 days.
- Some 50% of VZV infections are subclinical.

- Clinical features include:
  - rash: often very prominent and seen mainly on the face and trunk; consists of itchy papules then vesicles, pustules and scabs, in crops
  - fever
  - malaise
  - irritability
  - anorexia
  - mouth ulcers: indistinguishable from HSV, but no associated gingivitis
  - cervical lymphadenitis.

Diagnosis

The diagnosis is on clinical grounds. A rising antibody titre is confirmatory. Differentiation is from other mouth ulcers, especially herpes simplex and other viral infections.

Treatment (see also Chs 4 and 5)

- Patient information is an important aspect in management.
- Most patients will have spontaneous remission within 1 week to 10 days.
- Symptomatic care is important (see Ch. 4).
- Antivirals can be beneficial if given early in the disease (**Table 43.5**). 100–200 mg aciclovir tablets 5 times daily, or sugar-free oral suspension (200 mg/5 mL) 5 times daily, or valaciclovir or famciclovir are useful prophylaxis (especially in neonates, pregnancy and in immunocompromised patients).
- Neonates and pregnant women should receive specialist care and are usually treated with antivirals. Immunocompromised patients should receive specialist care and are usually treated with antivirals and immune globulin.

Prevention of VZV infections

A VZV vaccine is available.

Follow-up of patients

Long-term follow-up is rarely required.

RECURRENT VZV INFECTIONS

Recurrence of VZV, which has been latent in dorsal root ganglia, causes zoster, or shingles. The word 'zoster' comes from the Greek for 'belt', since the lesion occurs in a belt-like distribution.

Table 43.5 Regimens that might be helpful in management of patient suspected of having chickenpox

Regimen	Use in primary or secondary care*
Likely to be beneficial	Aciclovir or valaciclovir or famciclovir orally or parenterally
Supportive	Adequate hydration Benzydamine Diet with little acidic, spicy or citrus content Lidocaine Paracetamol

*Specialist care for neonates, pregnant or immunocompromised people.

Incidence

Zoster is uncommon.

Age

It occurs mainly in adults, especially the older.

Gender

Both sexes are affected.

Geographic

Seen worldwide.

Predisposing and protective factors

Zoster mainly affects the older, or immunocompromised patients, such as in HIV infection, leukaemia or cancer. Zoster has become a fairly common feature in HIV-infected patients treated with HAART (see Ch. 5).

Fresh fruit appears to be associated with a reduced risk of developing zoster.

Aetiology and pathogenesis

Reactivation of VZV latent in sensory ganglia.

Clinical features

▪ The main features are pain and a rash in one dermatome (the area of skin and mucosa supplied by a sensory nerve). However, herpes zoster in children is often painless, but older people are more likely to get zoster as they get older, and the disease tends to be more severe. Early or late in the disease a rash is absent (and in zoster sine herpete).
▪ Most zoster is seen in the thoracic region; 30% is in the trigeminal region.
▪ Pain occurs before, with and after the rash.
▪ Rash is unilateral vesiculating then scabbing in dermatome (**Fig. 43.4**).

▪ Mouth ulcers are seen in maxillary or mandibular zoster only:
  ▪ mandibular zoster: ipsilateral on buccal and lingual mucosa
  ▪ maxillary: ipsilateral on palate and vestibule.
▪ Post-herpetic neuralgia (see Ch. 52) is the condition when the pain persists long after the rash has healed.

Diagnosis

Diagnosis is clinical; differentiation from toothache and other causes of ulcers, especially HSV, is important.

Treatment (see also Chs 4 and 5)

▪ Antivirals given within 72 h of the onset of zoster inhibit VZV replication, may help pain and healing and can reduce the severity and duration of zoster – and minimize post-herpetic neuralgia (PHN: **Table 43.6**) with minimal side effects, but antivirals do not reliably prevent PHN (Ch. 52). Antiviral treatment is recommended for all immunocompetent patients over 50 years of age. 400–800 mg aciclovir tablets 5 times daily, or sugar-free oral suspension, for 7 days, or valaciclovir 1000 mg 3 times daily for 7 days, or famciclovir 500 mg 3 times daily for 7 days are useful. Addition of systemic corticosteroids may be beneficial in reducing PHN in patients over 50. In ophthalmic zoster, valaciclovir 1000 mg 3 times daily is indicated, and an ophthalmological opinion, since there can be corneal ulceration.
▪ Immunocompromised patients should receive specialist care and are usually treated with antivirals and immune globulin.
▪ Analgesics are also needed. The evidence base supports the oral use of tricyclic antidepressants, certain opioids, and gabapentinoids in PHN. Topical therapy with lidocaine patches and capsaicin is similarly supported. Intrathecal administration of methylprednisolone appears to be highly effective, but its safety requires further evaluation.

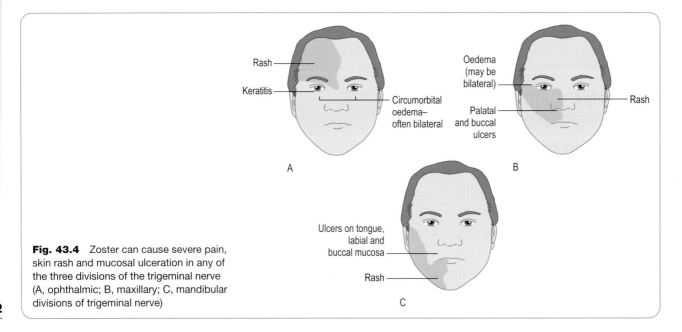

Fig. 43.4 Zoster can cause severe pain, skin rash and mucosal ulceration in any of the three divisions of the trigeminal nerve (A, ophthalmic; B, maxillary; C, mandibular divisions of trigeminal nerve)

Table 43.6 Regimens that might be helpful in management of patient suspected of having zoster

Regimen	Use in primary care	Use in secondary care (severe oral involvement and/or extraoral involvement) or immunocompromised
Likely to be beneficial	Aciclovir, valaciclovir or famciclovir orally or parenterally Systemic-gabapentinoids Opioids Tricyclic antidepressants	Aciclovir, valaciclovir or famciclovir orally or parenterally Systemic-gabapentinoids Opioids Tricyclic antidepressants Intrathecal methylprednisolone
Supportive	Topical-lidocaine patches or capsaicin	

Follow-up of patients

Long-term follow-up as shared care is usually appropriate

EPSTEIN–BARR VIRUS INFECTION

EBV is a ubiquitous virus that commonly produces 'glandular fever', 'infectious mononucleosis' or 'mono', often with lesions in the mouth and oropharynx.

INCIDENCE

It is common, especially in resource-poor conditions.

Age

Infection is common among young adults (especially students) and is often subclinical. By adulthood, 90–95% of people have been infected with EBV.

Gender

Both sexes are affected.

Geographic

Common in resource - poor areas. Also seen in adolescents and adults in resource - rich areas.

PREDISPOSING FACTORS

- Close contact with infected individuals, such as sexually, predisposes to EBV infection, which appears to be spread by close oral contact, such as kissing ("the kissing disease").
- EBV is found in pharyngeal epithelium and appears in the saliva from patients with infectious mononucleosis and for several months after apparent recovery.
- EBV is contracted from infected saliva or other body fluids after an incubation period of approximately 20–40 days.
- EBV is contracted earlier in resource-poor persons than in resource-rich persons
- Patients with immune defects are liable to severe and/or protracted infections or EBV may be reactivated, leading to viral shedding, recurrence of infectious mononucleosis or, rarely, producing lymphoproliferative disease.

CLINICAL FEATURES

The clinical features of EBV infection are as follows:

- A glandular fever syndrome termed 'infectious mononucleosis' which includes mainly:
  - lymphadenopathy
  - sore throat
  - fever
  - malaise
  - rashes.

Symptoms of mononucleosis are non-specific and may include: fever, malaise, headache, myalgia, rashes, hepatomegaly, splenomegaly and others. Recovery can take weeks or months and the virus thereafter remains latent in pharyngeal and/or salivary epithelial cells. Particular features predominate in some patients:

- The anginose type of infectious mononucleosis (sore-throat type) is characterized by a sore oedematous throat with soft palate petechiae and a whitish exudate on the tonsils. Pharyngeal oedema may threaten the airway.
- The glandular type of infectious mononucleosis is characterized mainly by general lymph node enlargement and splenomegaly.
- The febrile type of infectious mononucleosis is characterized mainly by fever.

COMPLICATIONS

Complications are rare but may include:

- autoimmune haemolysis (and cold agglutinins)
- CNS involvement (meningitis, encephalitis, etc.)
- erythema multiforme
- hepatomegaly or hepatitis
- jaundice (from hepatic involvement or haemolysis)
- pericarditis or myocarditis
- pneumonitis
- splenic rupture
- thrombocytopenia.

EBV is also implicated in:

- rashes of a non-allergic nature affecting the extensor surfaces of the limbs in patients taking ampicillin or amoxicillin with infectious mononucleosis or lymphatic leukaemia
- hairy leukoplakia (Ch. 53)
- chronic infection, which may cause persistent malaise
- Burkitt and some other lymphomas
- post-transplantation lymphoproliferative disorder (PTLD; Ch. 54)
- nasopharyngeal carcinoma (NPC: see Ch. 57).

Table 43.7 Regimens that might be helpful in management of patient suspected of having infectious mononucleosis (i.m.)

Regimen	Use in primary care	Use in secondary care (severe oral involvement and/or extraoral involvement)
Likely to be beneficial		Systemic corticosteroids if airway threatened, or there is haemolysis or thrombocytopenia Valaciclovir in complicated i.m.
Supportive	Adequate hydration Benzydamine Diet with little acidic, spicy or citrus content Lidocaine Paracetamol	

DIAGNOSIS

- Differentiation from other glandular fever syndromes caused by CMV, HHV-6, HIV or *Toxoplasma* infection is important.
- Investigations are indicated: characteristic of infectious mononucleosis are:
  - mononucleosis: large numbers of atypical mononuclear cells in the blood
  - serological changes such as heterophil antibodies (human antibodies which agglutinate animal (sheep and horse) erythrocytes and are detectable by the Paul–Bunell (Paul–Bunell–Davidson) or Monospot tests) and antibody to EBV viral capsid antigen (VCA). IgM anti-EBV reflects a current infection
  - abnormal liver function tests.

TREATMENT (see also Chs 4 and 5)

- Treatment is aimed at easing the symptoms, and can usually be done at home with rest, fluids, and over-the-counter medications and analgesia/antipyretic such as paracetamol or NSAIDs. Serious complications are rare but contact sports and heavy physical activity should be banned, to avoid splenic rupture.
- No specific reliably effective antiviral treatment is available (**Table 43.7**). Valaciclovir may be helpful in complicated mononucleosis.
- Systemic corticosteroids are required if there is pharyngeal oedema severe enough to hazard the airway.

FOLLOW-UP OF PATIENTS

Long-term follow-up as shared care is usually appropriate.

CYTOMEGALOVIRUS INFECTION

Cytomegalovirus (CMV) is a ubiquitous herpesvirus that infects most persons at some time during their lives and thereafter remains latent. It has been termed the 'salivary gland inclusion virus' since there are inclusion bodies seen histopathologically in salivary glands of infected people. These strikingly enlarged cells (the property of 'cytomegaly', from which CMV acquires its name) contain intranuclear inclusions that have the histopathological appearance of owl's eyes. CMV affects especially the CNS and arguably causes the most morbidity and mortality of all herpesviruses.

INCIDENCE

It is common, especially in resource-poor conditions.

Age

Infection is common among young children and is often subclinical.

Gender

Both sexes are affected.

Geographic

Common in children in resource-poor conditions. Also seen in adolescents and adults in resource-rich conditions.

PREDISPOSING FACTORS

- Close contact with infected individuals predisposes to infection.
- CMV can also be transmitted via saliva, blood, sexually and transplacentally, and in transplantation.
- CMV is contracted from infected saliva, urine, semen or other body fluids after an incubation period of approximately 20–40 days.
- Patients with immune defects are liable to severe and/or protracted infections, or CMV may be reactivated.

CLINICAL FEATURES

- Transplacental CMV infection may cause abortion, learning disability or other defects (see TORCH syndrome; Ch. 57), and the affected child excretes CMV in urine for months or years after birth and is a major reservoir of the virus.
- CMV infection in normal children or adults is usually asymptomatic.
- CMV infection in some otherwise apparently healthy children and adults causes the CMV mononucleosis syndrome ('infectious lymphocytosis') of headache, back and abdominal pain, sore throat, fever and atypical lymphocytosis, but with a negative Paul–Bunell test.
- Immunocompromised patients may be infected with CMV, or latent CMV may be reactivated. In these patients, CMV acts as an opportunistic infection and may cause various clinical syndromes with viral dissemination leading to multiple organ system involvement, the most important clinical manifestations consisting of CMV pneumonitis, GI disease, and retinitis. They also excrete the virus in body fluids.
- The long-term health consequences of CMV infection may include atherosclerosis, immunosenescence, and an increased risk of malignancy.

DIAGNOSIS

- Differentiation from other glandular fever syndromes caused by EBV, HHV-6, HIV or *Toxoplasma* infection is important.
- Virus isolation and serology may be of value in the diagnosis.

TREATMENT (see also Chs 4 and 5)

Treatment is usually symptomatic, although the immunocompromised host needs specialist care, when antivirals such as ganciclovir are used. Valaciclovir may prevent CMV infections and valganciclovir may treat them in immunocompromised patients.

FOLLOW-UP OF PATIENTS

Long-term follow-up in secondary care in usually appropriate.

OTHER HUMAN HERPESVIRUSES

- HHV-6 is usually associated with a rash in children, but has also been implicated in some cases of:
  - glandular-fever-type syndromes (see Ch. 3)
  - facial palsy
  - drug-induced hypersensitivity syndromes, manifesting with lymphadenopathy (Ch. 6).

- HHV-7 is not of any known relevance to oral health.
- HHV-8 (now termed Kaposi sarcoma herpesvirus (KSHV)) is transmitted mainly sexually and strongly associated mainly with Kaposi sarcoma (Ch. 53).

PATIENT INFORMATION SHEET
Cold sores

▼ Please read this information sheet. If you have any questions, particularly about the treatment or potential side-effects, please ask your doctor.
- These are common.
- They are not inherited.
- They are caused by a virus (herpes simplex), which lives in nerves.
- They are infectious and the virus can be transmitted by kissing.
- They may be precipitated by sun exposure, stress, injury or immune problems.
- They have no long-term consequences.
- Blood tests or biopsy may be required.
- Cold sores may be controlled by some antiviral creams or tablets, best used early on.

USEFUL WEBSITES

Herpes Viruses Association, About cold sores. http://www.herpes.org.uk/coldsores.html

Herpes.com, Overview. http://www.herpes.com/overview.shtml

Herpes.com, Reference Information. http://www.herpes.com/references.shtml

MedlinePlus, Herpes Simplex. http://www.nlm.nih.gov/medlineplus/herpessimplex.html

Wikipedia, Herpesviridae. http://en.wikipedia.org/wiki/Herpesviridae

FURTHER READING

Agren, S.H., 2006. Therapeutic options for herpes labialis: Experimental and natural therapies. Cutis 78 (3), 182.

Ammatuna, P., Campisi, G., Giovannelli, L., et al., 2001. Presence of Epstein–Barr virus, cytomegalovirus and human papilloma virus in normal oral mucosa of HIV-infected and renal transplant patients. Oral Dis. 7, 34–40.

Arduino, P.G., Porter, S.R., 2008. Herpes Simplex Virus Type 1 infection: overview on relevant clinico-pathological features. J. Oral Pathol. Med. 37 (2), 107–121.

Birek, C., 2000. Herpesvirus-induced diseases: oral manifestations and current treatment options. J. Calif. Dent. Assoc. 28, 911–921.

Cernik, C., Gallina, K., Brodell, R.T., 2008. The treatment of herpes simplex infections: an evidence-based review. Arch. Intern. Med. 168 (11), 1137–1144.

Elad, S., Zadik, Y., Hewson, I., et al., 2010. A systematic review of viral infections associated with oral involvement in cancer patients: a spotlight on Herpesviridea. Support Care Cancer 18 (8), 993–1006.

Femiano, F., Gombos, S., Scully, C., 2001. Recurrent herpes labialis; efficacy of topical therapy with penciclovir compared with acyclovir (aciclovir). Oral Dis. 7, 31–32.

Femiano, F., Gombos, S., Scully, C., 2005. Recurrent herpes labialis; pilot study of the efficacy of zinc therapy. J. Oral Pathol. Oral Med. 34, 423–425.

Gilbert, S.C., 2006. Oral shedding of herpes simplex virus type 1 in immunocompetent persons. J. Oral Pathol. Med. 35 (9), 548–553.

Goldenberg, D., Golz, A., Netzer, A., et al., 2001. Epstein–Barr virus and cancers of the head and neck. Am. J. Otolaryngol. 22, 197–205.

Goldman, B.D., 2000. Herpes serology for dermatologists. Arch. Dermatol. 136, 1158–1161.

Gómez-Moreno, G., Guardia, J., Ferrera, M.J., et al., 2010. Melatonin in diseases of the oral cavity. Oral Dis. 16 (3), 242–247.

Hargate, G., 2006. A randomised double-blind study comparing the effect of 1072-nm light against placebo for the treatment of herpes labialis. Clin. Exp. Dermatol. 31 (5), 638–641.

Hempenstall, K., Nurmikko, T.J., Johnson, R.W., et al., 2005. Analgesic therapy in postherpetic neuralgia: a quantitative systematic review. PLoS Med. 2 (7), e164.

Karlsmark, T., Goodman, J.J., Drouault, Y., et al., 2008. Randomized clinical study comparing COMPEED® cold sore patch to acyclovir cream 5% in the treatment of herpes simplex labialis. J. Eur. Acad. Dermatol. Venereol. 22 (10), 1184–1193.

Kimberlin, D.W., Lin, C.Y., Jacobs, R.F., et al., 2001. Natural history of neonatal herpes simplex virus infections in the acyclovir era. Pediatrics 108, 223–229.

Knaup, B., Schunemann, S., Wolff, M.H., 2000. Subclinical reactivation of herpes simplex virus type 1 in the oral cavity. Oral Microbiol. Immunol. 15, 281–283.

Kolokotronis, A., Louloudiadis, K., Fotiou, G., et al., 2001. Oral manifestations of infections of infections due to varicella zoster virus in otherwise healthy children. J. Clin. Pediatr. Dent. 25, 107–112.

Leao, J.C., Porter, S.R., Scully, C., 2000. Human herpesvirus 8 and oral health care: an update. Oral Surg. Oral Med. Oral Pathol. Oral Radiol. Endod. 90, 694–704.

Mustafa, M.B., Arduino, P.G., Porter, S.R., 2009. Varicella zoster virus: review of its management. J. Oral Pathol. Med. 38 (9), 673–688.

Nasser, M., Fedorowicz, Z., Khoshnevisan, M.H., Shahiri Tabarestani, M., 2008. Acyclovir for treating primary herpetic gingivostomatitis. Cochrane Database Syst. Rev (4) CD006700.

Nunes Oda, S., Pereira Rde, S., 2008. Regression of herpes viral infection symptoms using melatonin and

SB-73: comparison with Acyclovir. J. Pineal. Res. 44 (4), 373–378.

Perfect, M.M., Bourne, N., Ebel, C., Rosenthal, S.L., 2005. Use of complementary and alternative medicine for the treatment of genital herpes. Herpes 12 (2), 38–41.

Rice, A.S., Maton, S., 2001. Postherpetic Neuralgia Study Group. Gabapentin in postherpetic neuralgia: a randomised, double blind, placebo controlled study. Pain 94 (2), 215–224.

Samonis, G., Mantadakis, E., Maraki, S., 2000. Orofacial viral infections in the immunocompromised host. Oncol. Rep. 7, 1389–1394.

Skulason, S., Holbrook, W.P., Thormar, H., et al., 2012. A study of the clinical activity of a gel combining monocaprin and doxycycline: a novel treatment for herpes labialis. J. Oral Pathol. Med. 41 (1), 61–67.

Spruance, S.L., Bodsworth, N., Resnick, H., et al., 2006. Single-dose, patient-initiated famciclovir: a randomized, double-blind, placebo-controlled trial for episodic treatment of herpes labialis. J. Am. Acad. Dermatol. 55, 47–53.

Treister, N.S., Woo, S.B., 2010. Topical n-docosanol for management of recurrent herpes labialis. Expert Opin. Pharmacother. 11 (5), 853–860.

Walsh, D.E., Griffith, R.S., Behforooz, A., 1983. Subjective response to lysine in the therapy of herpes simplex. J. Antimicrob. Chemother. 12 (5), 489–496.

Whitley, R.J., Roizman, B., 2001. Herpes simplex virus infections. Lancet 357, 1513–1518.

Woo, S.B., Challacombe, S.J., 2007. Management of recurrent oral herpes simplex infections Oral Surgery. Oral Med. Oral Path Oral Radiol. Endod. 103, S12. e1–S12.e18.

Zschocke, I., Reich, C., Zielke, A., et al., 2008. Silica gel is as effective as aciclovir cream in patients with recurrent herpes labialis: results of a randomized, open-label trial. J. Dermatolog. Treat. 19 (3), 176–181.

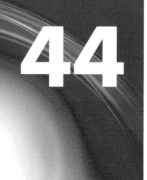

44 Keratoses

INTRODUCTION

Increased keratin (hyperkeratosis or keratosis) can produce a clinical white lesion in the mouth which, on histopathology shows only benign hyperplasia (benign keratosis).

AETIOLOGY AND PATHOGENESIS

Keratosis can arise from a number of aetiological factors, such as:

- friction
- tobacco or betel habits.

Microscopically, there is usually benign hyperplasia with:

- simple orthokeratosis
- parakeratosis with epithelial hyperplasia and minimal inflammation
- hyperkeratosis with minimal if any dysplasia.

FRICTIONAL KERATOSIS

White lesions caused by repeated trauma, such as from food, the teeth, toothbrushing or dental appliances.

INCIDENCE

Frictional keratosis is common.

Age

It occurs in the middle-aged and older patient.

Gender

It occurs in more men than women.

Geographic

It is seen worldwide.

PREDISPOSING FACTORS

Repeated trauma such as from the teeth, food or dental appliances.

AETIOLOGY, PATHOGENESIS AND CLINICAL FEATURES

- Frictional keratosis is not uncommonly seen on edentulous ridges, especially in the partially dentate, and then presumably caused by the friction from mastication (**Fig. 44.1**). It may be bilateral (bilateral alveolar ridge keratosis; BARK).
- Horizontal white lines in the buccal mucosa (see Fig. 24.3) and sometimes on the margins of the tongue at the occlusal lines (linea alba), are common, often bilateral, and are most prevalent in anxious women, especially those with other psychologically related disorders. Masseteric hypertrophy and/or tooth attrition may be associated.
- Cheek biting (morsicatio buccarum) may also fairly commonly be seen in anxious individuals. Habitual cheek biting causes red and white lesions with a rough surface, invariably restricted to the lower labial and/or buccal mucosa near the occlusal line, often bilateral, but sometimes just in one area around a commissure. In the early stages, the patches are pale and translucent, but later become dense and white, sometimes with a rough surface.
- Rarely, more severe self-mutilation is seen in psychiatric disorders, learning disability or some rare syndromes, e.g. Lesch–Nyhan syndrome and familial dysautonomia (Riley–Day syndrome).

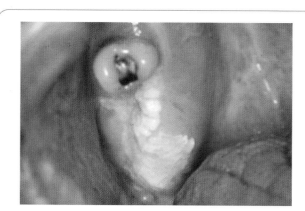

Fig. 44.1 Frictional keratosis on the alveolar ridge

DIAGNOSIS

The diagnosis is clinical and differentiation is mainly from white sponge naevus (Ch. 57), leukoplakia and lichen planus. If the patient or clinician have concerns, biopsy is warranted.

TREATMENT (see also Chs 4 and 5)

Patient information is an important aspect in management. Frictional keratosis is completely benign, and does not require treatment. There is no evidence that continued minor trauma alone has any carcinogenic potential, but, if the patient is causing the lesion from some habit, that should be stopped. Apart from removing irritants and ceasing habits, no active treatment is required.

TOBACCO-INDUCED KERATOSES

Tobacco is a common cause of mild keratosis seen especially on the palate, lip (occasionally nicotine stained) and at the commissures, along with nicotine-stained teeth. Men especially are affected. Malignant change is rare.

However, tobacco use is one of the major risk factors for oral carcinoma and, if smoked, also predisposes to cancers elsewhere in the upper aerodigestive tract, bladder and other sites. Tobacco use should thus be discouraged; nicotine patches or the drug Zyban (bupropion) or Champix (varenicline) may help users break the habit.

STOMATITIS NICOTINA
Definition

Stomatitis nicotina (known as smoker's palate, smoker's keratosis, nicotinic stomatitis, stomatitis palatini, leukokeratosis nicotina palate) is a diffuse white lesion covering most of the hard palate, typically related to pipe or cigar smoking.

Incidence

It is uncommon.

AGE

It occurs in middle-aged or older adults.

GENDER

It occurs in more men than women.

GEOGRAPHIC

It is seen worldwide.

Predisposing factors

Smoker's keratosis is seen usually among heavy, long-term pipe smokers and some cigar smokers or reverse cigarette smoking, less commonly in cigarette smokers.

Aetiology and pathogenesis

Presumably the hyperkeratosis is related to tobacco products and/or heat.

Clinical features

The appearances of smoker's keratosis are distinctive in that the palate is affected, but any part protected by a denture is

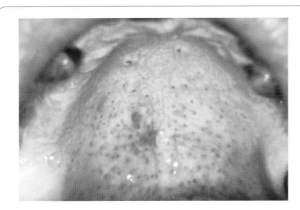

Fig. 44.2 Stomatitis nicotina

spared. The teeth are often stained from the tobacco exposure. The lesion has two components, namely:

- white thickening of the palatal mucosa due to hyperkeratosis (**Fig. 44.2**)
- inflammatory swelling of minor mucous glands, which show as red spots against the white hyperkeratosis, as small umbilicated swellings with red centres.

Diagnosis

The diagnosis is clinical but, if the patient or clinician have concerns, biopsy is warranted. Darier disease (Ch. 56) has a similar clinical appearance. Apart from removing irritants and ceasing habits, no active treatment is required.

The condition is not known to be potentially malignant, but the patient may develop premalignant changes at other sites in the upper aerodigestive tract.

Treatment (see also Chs 4 and 5)

Patient information is an important aspect in management. Few patients have spontaneous remission and the patient should be encouraged to stop the causative habit.

SNUFF-DIPPERS' KERATOSIS AND OTHER SMOKELESS TOBACCO OR BETEL LESIONS

Snuff or betel may produce white hyperkeratotic lesions caused by snuff-dipping (holding flavoured tobacco powder in the oral sulcus or vestibule), together with gingival recession at the site of use, often the buccal sulcus. Malignant change is rare.

Incidence

It is uncommon.

AGE

It occurs in adults.

GENDER

It occurs equally in men and women.

GEOGRAPHIC

Snuff-dipping may be more common in North America and Scandinavia; betel use is mainly in Asians (**Figs 44.3** and **44.4**).

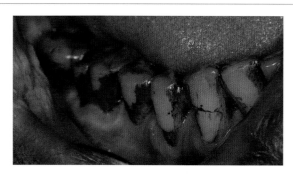

Fig. 44.3 Betel chewing in a Bangladeshi person who developed keratosis in the adjacent buccal mucosa

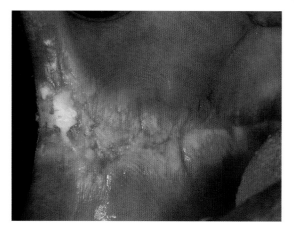

Fig. 44.4 Betel-induced keratosis (same patient as Fig. 44.3)

Predisposing factors

The risk factors are tobacco- or betel-chewing or snuff-dipping.

Aetiology and pathogenesis

Oral snuff appears to cause more severe clinical changes than does tobacco-chewing, but dysplasia is more likely in tobacco chewers. Snuff-dipping is associated predominantly with verrucous keratoses, which can progress to verrucous carcinoma, occasionally, but only after several decades of use.

Clinical features

There is typically a white lesion in the buccal sulcus.

Diagnosis

The diagnosis is clinical but, if the patient or clinician have concerns, biopsy is warranted.

Treatment (see also Chs 4 and 5)

Patient information is an important aspect in management. Few patients have spontaneous remission and, thus, habit cessation is indicated (**Table 44.1**). Apart from removing irritants and ceasing habits, no active treatment is required. Snuff dippers' lesions will resolve on stopping the habit even after 25 years of use.

Follow-up of patients with keratosis

Long-term follow-up as shared care is usually appropriate.

Table 44.1 Aids that might be helpful in diagnosis/prognosis/management in some patients suspected of having keratosis

In many cases	In some cases
Biopsy Stop self-mutilation, tobacco, betel or alcohol use	Excise if dysplastic

FURTHER READING

Alexander, R.E., Wright, J.M., Thiebaud, S., 2001. Evaluating, documenting and following up oral pathological conditions. A suggested protocol. J. Am. Dent. Assoc. 132, 329–335.

Awan, K.H., Morgan, P.R., Warnakulasuriya, S., 2011. Utility of chemiluminescence (ViziLite™) in the detection of oral potentially malignant disorders and benign keratoses. J. Oral Pathol. Med. 40 (7), 541–544.

Natarajan, E., Woo, S.B., 2008. Benign alveolar ridge keratosis (oral lichen simplex chronicus): A distinct clinicopathologic entity. J. Am. Acad. Dermatol. 58 (1), 151–157.

Woo, S.B., Lin, D., 2009. Morsicatio mucosae oris – a chronic oral frictional keratosis, not a leukoplakia. J. Oral Maxillofac. Surg. 67 (1), 140–146.

Odontogenic cysts and tumours

INTRODUCTION

Odontogenic cysts and tumours are defined as lesions of the jaws and gingiva derived from odontogenic epithelium. The aetiology of these lesions however, is quite unclear.

ODONTOGENIC CYSTS

A cyst is a pathological cavity having liquid, semi-liquid or gaseous contents. It is frequently, but not always, lined with epithelium.

Most cysts of the jaws arise from odontogenic epithelium. These are relatively common lesions – most are inflammatory cysts (about 55% of all jaw cysts), dentigerous cysts (22%) or odontogenic keratocysts (keratocystic odontogenic tumours; 19%).

There is an overall male predominance and the mandible is affected three times as commonly as the maxilla.

Most odontogenic cysts are benign, but occasionally tumours or squamous cell carcinomas may arise within.

AETIOLOGY AND PATHOGENESIS

The main pathogenic factors include the following:

- Epithelial proliferation – either stimulated by inflammation in the case of radicular cysts, or occurring with genetic stimulation in the case of keratocystic odontogenic tumours and probably the glandular odontogenic cysts.
- Hydrostatic or osmotic factors: may play a part in cyst growth since the cyst wall acts as a semipermeable membrane.
- Keratin formation: may be prominent in keratocystic odontogenic tumours.
- Bone resorbing factors: such as prostaglandins and collagenase.
- Cytokines: IL-1-alpha, TNF-alpha, MCP-1 (*Monocyte chemotactic protein-1*), and RANTES (regulated upon activation, normal T-cell expressed, and secreted (also known as CCL5)), levels are significantly higher in radicular cyst fluids than those in the residual cysts.

CLINICAL FEATURES

Odontogenic cysts are often discovered as an incidental finding on imaging (**Fig. 45.1**). They are generally symptomless, slow-growing and may reach a large size before they give rise to symptoms, such as:

- swelling: cysts in bone initially produce a smooth bony hard lump with normal overlying mucosa but, as the bone thins, it may crackle on palpation rather like an egg shell (termed 'egg shell cracking'). When the overlying bone is resorbed, the cyst may show through as a bluish fluctuant swelling (**Fig. 45.2**)
- discharge: usually into the mouth
- pain: due to secondary infection.

DIAGNOSIS

The diagnosis of an odontogenic cyst is based on an adequate history, clinical examination and appropriate investigations,

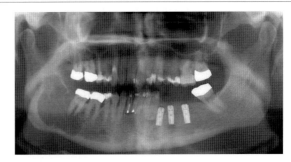

Fig. 45.1 Mandibular odontogenic tumour revealed on dental pantomograph

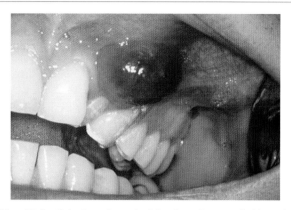

Fig. 45.2 Odontogenic cyst arising from the non-vital lateral incisor

Table 45.1 Aids that might be helpful in diagnosis/prognosis/management in some patients suspected of having odontogenic cyst or tumour*

In most cases	In some cases
Radiography	MRI
Biopsy	Aspiration

*See text for details and glossary for abbreviations.

such as pulp vitality testing and radiographs (both intraoral and extraoral) of associated teeth, together with aspiration and analysis of cyst fluids, and histopathology (**Table 45.1**).

TREATMENT (see also Chs 4 and 5)

Odontogenic cysts are managed either by enucleation or by marsupialization (**Table 45.2**):

■ Enucleation is the complete removal of the cyst: the benefit is that all the cyst tissue is available for histological examination and the cyst cavity will usually heal uneventfully with minimal aftercare. Enucleation is potentially problematic however, if the cyst involves the apices of adjacent vital teeth, as the surgery may deprive the teeth of their blood supply and render them non-vital.

■ Marsupialization is the partial removal of the cyst: the benefit is that it is somewhat less invasive than enucleation and tooth vitality is retained but it requires considerable aftercare and good patient cooperation in keeping the cavity clean whilst it resolves. In order to keep the cavity open, a 'bung' or acrylic plug is usually inserted in the opening, often attached to a denture or acrylic splint. The bung stops most food collecting

Table 45.2 Regimens that might be helpful in management of patient suspected of having odontogenic cyst or tumour

Regimen	Use in secondary care (severe oral involvement and/or extraoral involvement)
Likely to be beneficial	Enucleation Marsupialization

in the cavity, but the cavity must still be syringed by the patient after each meal. Healing is slower than after enucleation: marsupialized cyst cavities may take up to 6 months to close down to the extent of becoming 'self-cleansing'. The other disadvantage of marsupialization is that not all the cyst lining is available to histopathological examination, and this could lead to misdiagnosis.

INFLAMMATORY CYSTS

Inflammatory cysts are by far the most common of all jaw cysts and arise in association with a non-vital tooth.

Aetiology and pathogenesis

The epithelial lining of inflammatory cysts is derived from the rests of Malassez, which proliferate to produce thick, irregular, often incomplete squamous epithelium, with granulation tissue forming the cyst wall in the denuded areas (**Fig. 45.3**). Depending on the nature of the inflammatory response, there may be areas of chronic inflammation, or acute inflammation with abscess formation. Cholesterol crystal clefts are often present and mucous cells may be found. The cyst fluid is usually watery, but may be thick and viscid with cholesterol crystal clefts giving it a shimmering appearance. The cysts have capsules of collagenous fibrous connective tissue and cause bone resorption and may become quite large.

Bacterial endotoxins may initiate epithelial proliferation together with complement activation and T lymphocyte infiltration, T cells releasing contributory inflammatory cytokines-interleukins, IL-1 and IL-6, in particular. Osmosis plays a role in cyst expansion. Prostaglandins, collagenases and matrix metalloproteinases plus gene products NF-κB ligand (RANKL) and osteoprotegerin (OPG) appear to be associated with the bone destruction both in periapical cysts and periapical granulomas. The Runx2 (core-binding protein (cbfa)1/polyoma enhancer-binding protein (pebp)2alphaA) a DNA-binding transcriptional molecule expressed in osteoprogenitor cells, and transforming growth factor (TGF-β2) are involved in the new bone formation.

Clinical features

They include the following:

■ Radicular cyst (dental or periapical cyst): where the cyst is associated with the apex of a non-vital tooth. Occasionally,

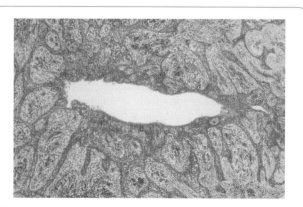

Fig. 45.3 Developing radicular cyst

a radicular cyst may develop on the lateral aspect of a root, where the stimulus has been an inflammatory reaction arising from necrotic pulp in a lateral root canal. Radicular cysts are seen especially where:

- a non-vital pulp is infected
- endodontic treatment has failed
- a root has fractured and there is a perforation
- a root is retained.
- Residual cysts: these arise where an inflammatory cyst (usually a radicular cyst) remains after the removal of the non-vital tooth or root from which it arose.

Diagnosis

The diagnosis is based on history, clinical examination and appropriate investigations, such as pulp vitality testing and radiographs (both intraoral and extraoral) of associated teeth, aspiration and analysis of cyst fluids, and histopathology. Protein p63 expression may be useful to identify cyst types with a more aggressive and invasive phenotype.

Treatment (see also Chs 4 and 5)

The treatment of inflammatory cysts depends on whether or not the involved non-vital tooth is to be retained. Conventional intra-canal endodontic treatment will often lead to the resolution of very small radicular cysts, but regular radiographic review is necessary until there has been complete resolution of the cyst. If, when the tooth has been root-filled, the cyst does not resolve, or if the cyst is of such a size that it is unlikely to resolve with endodontic treatment alone, surgery is indicated – either enucleation or marsupialization.

Follow-up

This is mainly in primary care.

DEVELOPMENTAL CYSTS
Dentigerous (follicular) cyst

Dentigerous cyst is the second most common odontogenic cyst. This develops within the normal dental follicle that surrounds an unerupted tooth, or from degeneration of the stellate reticulum, or an accumulation of fluid between the layers of the reduced enamel epithelium. The lining typically consists of flattened stratified epithelium.

CLINICAL FEATURES

The dentigerous cyst is most frequently found in areas where unerupted teeth are found – mandibular third molars, maxillary third molars and maxillary canines, in decreasing order of frequency. These cysts may grow to a large size, displace the tooth with which they are associated, or rarely cause resorption of adjacent tooth roots

DIAGNOSIS

Diagnosis is usually made by clinical and radiographic assessment – when the follicular space exceeds 5 mm from the crown it is likely that a cyst is present. However, odontogenic keratocysts and ameloblastomas may occasionally mimic the radiological appearances of follicular cysts. Aspiration may be helpful in differentiating the lesions

TREATMENT (see also Chs 4 and 5)

Treatment may be either marsupialization, allowing the tooth to erupt, or enucleation, with removal of the associated tooth. Rarely squamous cell carcinoma or ameloblastomas arise within a dentigerous cyst.

Eruption cysts

Eruption cysts are considered as minor soft tissue forms of dentigerous cysts. In these cases, the involved teeth are usually prevented from eruption by dense fibrous tissue overlying them. They often burst spontaneously before eruption of the associated tooth, and only require excision if impeding normal eruption. Then, a narrow window can be excised over the erupting tooth.

FOLLOW-UP

This is mainly in secondary care.

KERATOCYSTIC ODONTOGENIC TUMOUR (KCOT: ODONTOGENIC KERATOCYST; OKC; PRIMORDIAL CYST)

The KCOT is the least common, but most dangerous odontogenic cyst. KCOT can be associated with the naevoid basal cell carcinoma syndrome (NBCCS: Gorlin syndrome) (see Ch. 56). By definition, most KCOTs develop instead of a tooth, arising from the dental lamina or remnants, while some, particularly in the posterior mandible, may develop from basal cell off-shoots or hamartomas from the overlying gingival epithelium. They may be associated with the PTCH gene on chromosome 9 and the epithelium may harbour *patched* (PTCH) mutations, leading to constitutive activity of the embryonic *Hedgehog* (Hh) signalling pathway.

KCOT growth has been attributed to osmolality of the cyst fluid, and to various bone-resorbing factors, including collagenases, IL-1, matrix metalloproteinases and parathyroid-hormone-related protein.

Clinical features

The KCOT is a great mimic; it may have many clinical appearances, and may be seen over a wide age range. Most involve the mandibular angle and may expand to occupy the major part of the ramus as a radiolucent lesion. They may sometimes be multilocular. They may resorb the cortical plates and expand into the soft tissues, envelop unerupted teeth giving a dentigerous appearance or displace teeth but not resorb them. KCOTs are generally painless, and often grow to a large size before giving rise to symptoms, unless they become secondarily infected.

Diagnosis

Diagnosis may be suggested by clinical features supported by imaging, and aspiration and estimation of soluble protein level in aspirated cyst fluid may be an aid to the diagnosis, since a protein level of <4 g/100 mL suggests KCOT, whereas a value >5 g/100 mL suggests a radicular or dentigerous cyst, or rarely a cystic ameloblastoma. The demonstration of keratin squames in an aspirate is virtually diagnostic of a KCOT. The diagnosis of KCOT is confirmed on histological grounds.

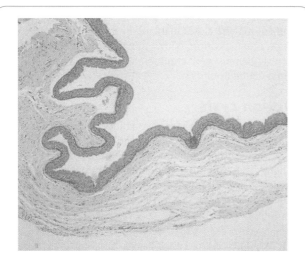

Fig. 45.4 Keratocystic odontogenic tumour (low power view)

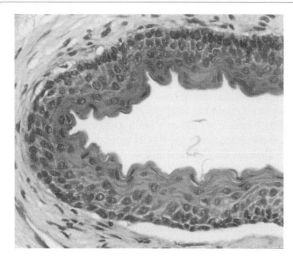

Fig. 45.5 Keratocystic odontogenic tumour (high power)

The cyst lining usually has a characteristic appearance of a regular keratinized stratified squamous epithelium, commonly five to eight cell layers thick and without rete pegs (**Figs 45.4 and 45.5**). There is a well-defined basal layer predominantly of columnar, but occasionally cuboidal, cells. Desquamated keratin is often present within the cyst lumen and the fibrous wall is usually thin.

Treatment (see also Chs 4 and 5)

Gorlin syndrome should be excluded – especially if the lesions are bilateral and/or in young people. Although there is some dispute over the most appropriate treatment for keratocysts, all authors agree that the cyst lining should be meticulously removed. Small unilocular lesions should be thoroughly enucleated. Large or multiloculated cysts should be excised with a margin of surrounding bone. KCOTs tend to recur following removal; recurrence rates can be as high as 60%.

Follow-up

This is mainly in secondary care. Long-term clinical and radiographic follow-up is mandatory as recurrences may occur many years after initial treatment.

One KCOT variant (orthokeratinized odontogenic cyst) is almost always found in a dentigerous association, usually around the mandibular third molar. It does not have a hyperchromatic basal layer and produces only orthokeratin, is not associated with basal cell naevus syndrome and acts much less aggressively.

OTHER ODONTOGENIC CYSTS

Other odontogenic cysts are uncommon and their pathogenesis is far from clear. They include:

- Glandular odontogenic cyst (GOC; sialo-odontogenic cyst): usually presents in the anterior mandible as a painless, slow-growing swelling and a large, multiloculated, well-defined radiolucency. It contains mucous cells and duct-like structures that may mimic central mucoepidermoid carcinoma. Characteristic histopathological features include epithelial spherules/'knobs'/whorls, cuboidal eosinophilic cells, goblet cells, intraepithelial glandular/microcystic ducts, variations in lining width, ciliated cells and mucous pools/mucous-lined crypts, which, with expression of p53 and Ki67, may aid the diagnosis. GOC tends to be aggressive and may recur following curettage.
- Gingival cysts of adults: which arise from epithelial rests in the gingivae and are found only in soft tissue in the lower premolar areas.
- Gingival cysts of infants: which arise from remnants of the dental lamina and are located in the corium below the surface epithelium. They are generally asymptomatic. Bohn nodules and Epstein pearls are similar lesions with which gingival cysts sometimes are confused (see Ch. 56).
- Developmental lateral periodontal cysts: which are most commonly associated with the mandibular premolar area and occasionally the maxillary anterior region and arise from the postfunctional dental lamina. As described earlier, cysts of inflammatory origin are found to lie on the lateral aspect of a non-vital tooth, and must be distinguished from a developmental lateral periodontal cyst.
- Paradental cysts: also of inflammatory origin and most frequently found on the lateral aspect of the roots of partially erupted mandibular third molars where there is an associated history of pericoronitis.

Treatment

Treatment of all these cysts is generally by enucleation.

FOLLOW-UP

Follow-up is mainly in secondary care.

ODONTOGENIC TUMOURS

Odontogenic tumours may consist predominantly of odontogenic epithelium, ectomesenchyme, or both (see Box 31.1). Enamel, dentine and their precursors are also present in a number of other lesions and then their presence is usually indicated by inclusion of the prefix 'odonto' (e.g. ameloblastic fibro-odontoma, odontoameloblastoma, ameloblastic odontosarcoma):

- Odontogenic tumours consisting predominantly of epithelium arise from odontogenic epithelium, but it is uncertain whether this epithelium is derived from the enamel organ itself, the remnants of the dental lamina (cell rests of Serre) or Hertwig root sheath (cell rests of Malassez), the epithelium of odontogenic cysts (particularly the dentigerous cyst), or from the oral mucosa.
- Odontogenic tumours composed of odontogenic connective tissue originate from the ectomesenchymal portion of the tooth germ, either from the dental papilla or the dental follicle.
- Odontogenic tumours of mixed origin consist both of odontogenic epithelium and ectomesenchyme and, during the period of active growth contain both ameloblastic epithelium and odontoblastic tissue, but, when completely developed, consist principally of enamel, dentine, cementum or combinations thereof.

Most odontogenic tumours (75%) are odontomas and benign. The second most common is ameloblastoma (12%), which is locally aggressive – followed by odontogenic myxoma, adenomatoid odontogenic tumour (AOT), ameloblastic fibro-odontoma, ameloblastic fibroma, calcifying odontogenic cyst and odontogenic fibroma.

Altered expression of platelet-derived endothelial cell growth factor/thymidine phosphorylase (PD-ECGF/TP) and of angiopoietins in ameloblastic tumours may be responsible for aggressive behaviour.

Classification

The World Health Organization (1992), related to the tissues of origin and histopathological features. The following main changes were proposed in 2005:

- Odontogenic tumours are not only 'related to' odontogenic tissues but are derived from them.
- The stroma of the epithelial tumour group is of a fibrous nature and does not contain any ectomesenchymal component.
- Subtypes of ameloblastomas are differentiated (intra-, extraosseous, desmoplastic, unicystic).
- Eponyms are no longer used in the revised classification.
- The AOT is reclassified as an epithelial odontogenic tumour.
- A neoplastic and non-neoplastic line of the ameloblastic fibroma and ameloblastic fibrodentinoma is proposed.
- The calcifying ghost cell odontogenic tumour is included in the classification.
- The simple and the WHO type of odontogenic fibroma are included in the classification.
- Ameloblastic carcinoma is differentiated from malignant (metastasizing) ameloblastoma.
- The term carcinoma in intraosseous (peripheral) ameloblastoma is introduced. Also, the malignant epithelial odontogenic ghost cell tumour is termed calcifying ghost cell odontogenic carcinoma.
- The clear cell odontogenic tumour is termed clear cell odontogenic carcinoma.
- The so-called pseudocysts are termed 'cavities' (aneurysmal bone cavity, simple bone cavity, lingual and buccal mandibular bone cavity, focal marrow-containing jaw cavity).

Treatment and follow-up of patients with odontogenic tumours

Secondary care is usually appropriate.

AMELOBLASTOMA (ADAMANTINOMA)

The ameloblastoma is the most common odontogenic neoplasm – a locally invasive lesion arising from the dental lamina, Hertwig sheath, the enamel organ, or the lining of dental follicles/dentigerous cysts. Fos (a transcription factor) and TNFRSF (tumour necrosis factor receptor super family) genes are overexpressed.

Clinical features and diagnosis

Ameloblastomas are more frequent in males, and usually appear after the age of 40 years, although unicystic variants occur in adolescence. The tumour is not uncommon in people of African heritage compared to the lower incidence in white people.

The initial detection of an ameloblastoma is likely to be a 'chance finding', but, when the tumour is evident clinically, there is a slow-growing, painless, expansile swelling of bone. Some 80% are found in the mandible, most in the posterior mandible. The lesion expands to produce progressive facial deformity and intraorally there may be evidence of malocclusion and mobile teeth. Eventually the bone is perforated and soft tissues involved.

Diagnosis

A monocystic (unicystic) or polycystic ('soap bubble') radiolucency is evident. Diagnosis is confirmed by histological examination of a biopsy specimen. Ameloblastomas are composed of epithelial cells arranged as a peripheral layer of ameloblast-like cells around a central area of cells resembling stellate reticulum (**Fig. 45.6**). Two main histological types are seen: follicular and plexiform types. In the follicular type, discrete islands (follicles) of epithelial cells are evident, whereas in the plexiform type the epithelium forms continuous anastomosing strands. Enamel formation is not evident, presumably because no odontogenic mesenchyme is present to give the critical inductive forces. Histological variations occasionally seen include granular cells, squamous metaplasia and keratinization, areas of calcification and variable degrees of vascularity. There appears to be little correlation between these histological patterns and the clinical course of the tumour but features such as increased cellular

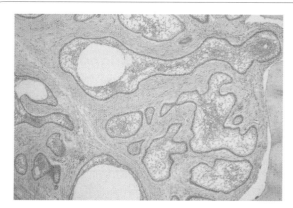

Fig. 45.6 Ameloblastoma

pleomorphism and mitotic activity suggest that the lesions will behave more aggressively.

Treatment (see also Chs 4 and 5)

Ameloblastomas expand rather than destroy bone, but there is also some local invasion. The treatment of choice, therefore, is surgical excision of the tumour together with removal of a margin of normal bone but retention of the lower border of the mandible.

Metastatic dissemination is rare and usually occurs by aspiration to the lungs following longstanding local disease or previous surgical intervention.

ODONTOGENIC MYXOMA (MYXOMA OF THE JAWS)
Clinical features and diagnosis

Odontogenic myxoma is derived from odontogenic mesenchyme and usually occurs in adolescents and young adults (10–40 years), more frequently in females than males, and usually in the posterior region of the mandible. Maxillary lesions are characterized by extensive involvement of the alveolar bone, antrum and zygomatic process. Clinically, the myxoma is an intrabony lesion that slowly expands the bony cortex and only perforates later. The lesion is rarely painful, but there may be loosening and displacement of the teeth.

Radiographic examination shows a well-defined unilocular or multilocular ('soap bubble') radiolucency, which may extend between the roots of the teeth and, thus, a scalloped margin is seen. On microscopic examination of biopsy specimens, spindle/stellate shaped cells are present in an intercellular mucoid stroma, sometimes containing nests of epithelial cells. Fibrous tissue and collagen are frequently evident throughout the lesion ('fibromyxoma'). There is widespread infiltration of the surrounding bone.

Treatment (see also Chs 4 and 5)

Myxomas infiltrate and, therefore, should be treated with surgical excision of the tumour and removal of a margin of normal bone.

ADENOMATOID ODONTOGENIC TUMOUR (AOT: ADENOAMELOBLASTOMA)

AOT is an uncommon and benign odontogenic tumour.

Clinical features and diagnosis

The AOT may be remembered as the 'two-thirds tumour' since:

- it most commonly occurs in the second and third decades of life
- two-thirds of cases are seen in females
- two-thirds of cases occur in the anterior maxilla
- two-thirds of cases are associated with an impacted tooth (usually the canine).

Clinically, the lesion presents as a gradually increasing intrabony swelling, which is occasionally painful.

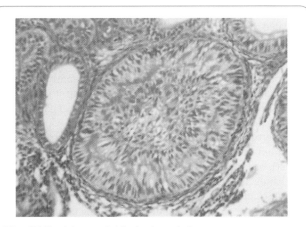

Fig. 45.7 Adenomatoid odontogenic tumour

On radiographs, the tumour appears as a unilocular radiolucency sometimes with radio-opaque foci. A clinical provisional diagnosis should include either a lateral periodontal cyst or a dentigerous cyst, particularly as, in the latter case, the tumour is sometimes associated with an unerupted tooth.

On histological examination, the tumour is encapsulated and consists of sheets and strands of epithelial cells arranged as convoluted bands and tubular structures (**Fig. 45.7**). In the tubular structures, ameloblast-like cells are arranged radially around spaces containing a homogeneous eosinophilic material. The nature of this material is unknown, although suggestions have included pre-enamel, pre-dentine, amyloid and basement membrane material. Separate from the homogeneous material, foci of calcification frequently are evident throughout the lesion. The tumour contains little intervening mesenchymal stroma, although cystic degeneration of this tissue is common.

Treatment (see also Chs 4 and 5)

Conservative surgical excision is indicated since the AOT is not locally invasive and does not recur.

CALCIFYING EPITHELIAL ODONTOGENIC TUMOUR (CEOT; PINDBORG TUMOUR)
Clinical features and diagnosis

CEOT is rare, benign, but aggressive, and has been reported in all age groups (10–90 years), but manifests most commonly as a progressive painless swelling of the jaws at approximately 40 years of age. It has no gender predilection and is most frequent in the mandibular premolar-molar region. It is associated with an unerupted or impacted tooth in 50% of cases. Rarely, it is extraosseous in more anterior parts of the mouth.

Radiographically, the tumour usually appears as a radiolucency containing focal opacities. Histological examination shows three distinct features:

- Sheets of epithelial cells (containing tonofilaments, desmosomes and hemi-desmosomes), which are pleomorphic and contain abnormal nuclei. In places, these cells are characterized by a clear cytoplasm, and hence have been termed 'clear cells'. Mitoses are rare.

- Amyloid, with characteristic green birefringence with Congo red stain; positive fluorescence with thioflavine T.
- Concentric masses of calcified tissues: often closely associated with the epithelial cells.

Treatment (see also Chs 4 and 5)

The CEOT is locally invasive and, therefore, treated with surgical excision plus a margin of normal bone.

CALCIFYING EPITHELIAL ODONTOGENIC CYST
Clinical features and diagnosis

Calcifying epithelial odontogenic cyst (CEOC) is extremely rare, and most commonly presents in adults younger than 40 years. Either jaw of either sex may be affected, but most are anterior to the first molar.

Clinically, there is a slowly enlarging, painless swelling of the jaws, which, on radiographic examination, appears as a well-defined unilocular or multilocular radiolucency containing flecks of opacity. Embedded teeth and/or denticle-like structures are not infrequent findings.

Microscopically, the tumour may be solid or cystic. In cystic lesions, the cyst wall is lined by odontogenic epithelium resembling that in an ameloblastoma, with peripheral ameloblast-like cells in close association with more central cells comparable to the stratum intermedium and the stellate reticulum. In places, the epithelial cells undergo aberrant keratinization to form large eosinophilic cells without a nucleus, termed 'ghost cells'. With further development, large masses of keratin accumulate and a foreign body giant cell reaction may be evoked if there is breakdown of the epithelial cyst lining. Foci of calcification and dentine-like material frequently are present throughout the specimen.

Treatment (see also Chs 4 and 5)

Conservative enucleation is usually adequate.

KERATINIZING AND CALCIFYING ODONTOGENIC CYST (KCOC OR GORLIN CYST)
Clinical features and diagnosis

KCOC is a neoplasm with cystic tendencies arising from a more mature enamel epithelium than does the ameloblastoma and, accordingly, has less growth potential. KCOC has no age, sex, or location predilections and may be found anywhere in the jaws. Up to one-fourth of lesions are found in peripheral soft tissues (e.g. gingiva). They appear as nondescript radiolucencies that may contain flecks of opacity. The lesions are lined by an epithelium that is similar in appearance to ameloblastoma, but the cells have no nuclei and are called ghost cells (ghost epithelium) – which eventually herniate into the connective tissue, causing a connective tissue foreign body response that results in dentinoid dystrophic calcification and the formation of granulation tissue.

Treatment (see also Chs 4 and 5)

These lesions are surgically removed and rarely recur.

ODONTOGENIC FIBROMA
Clinical features and diagnosis

Odontogenic fibroma is a rare tumour that may be peripheral or central. The tumour generally presents in close relation to the root of a tooth, the crown of an unerupted tooth, or in the site of a tooth that is congenitally missing. Histologically, the lesion consists of fibrous tissue which has a similar appearance to the dental pulp, but contains small nests of odontogenic epithelium.

Treatment (see also Chs 4 and 5)

Conservative enucleation is the treatment of choice.

AMELOBLASTIC FIBROMA
Clinical features and diagnosis

Ameloblastic fibroma is a tumour that occurs in young adults (15–25 years) presenting as a slow, painless jaw expansion and appears as a unilocular radiolucency. Infrequently, the tumour may be associated with an unerupted tooth.

Histologically, odontogenic epithelium is present as small islands, elongated strands, or terminal buds of peripheral ameloblast-like cells and central stellate reticulum cells. The odontogenic mesenchyme resembles the dental papilla. Surrounding the epithelial component there is frequently a cellular hyaline material. Uncommonly, dentine or dentinoid may be present, and this has led to the term 'ameloblastic fibro-dentinoma' being used. In some instances young enamel may also be found in close relationship with the dentinoid, and these tumours are known as ameloblastic fibro-odontomas.

Treatment (see also Chs 4 and 5)

Management is by conservative enucleation.

AMELOBLASTIC FIBRO-SARCOMA
Clinical features and diagnosis

Malignant counterparts of the ameloblastic fibroma are very rare. The lesions are preceded by pain and are characterized by a rapid enlargement of the jaw. Biopsy shows an odontogenic epithelial component similar to that found in an ameloblastic fibroma, whereas the mesenchymal tissues resemble a fibrosarcoma with cellular pleomorphism, tumour giant cells and numerous, atypical mitotic figures. Variations in which dentinoid are found are known as ameloblastic fibro-dentinosarcomas and if there is also rudimentary enameloid present, these have been called ameloblastic fibro-odontosarcomas.

Treatment (see also Chs 4 and 5)

Treatment involves radical surgery.

TUMOUR-LIKE LESIONS

ODONTOMES

Odontomes are calcified hamartomatous malformations of dental hard tissues and consist of dental tissues in normal relationship one to another (**Fig. 45.8**). Odontomes have been

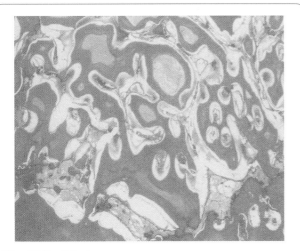

Fig. 45.8 Odontome

classified according to the type and spatial arrangement of the dental tissues as follows:

- compound type (compound composite odontomes): consist of multiple small simple denticles embedded in fibrous connective tissue within a fibrous capsule. Multiple lesions may be seen in Gardner syndrome (Ch. 56)
- complex type (complex composite odontomes): consist of an irregular mass of all the dental tissues.

Clinical features

Odontomes typically present in children and adolescents, more commonly in females than males, and show a distinct predilection for the premolar-molar region of the mandible. Typically, they behave like teeth: they grow to a certain size and then tend to erupt with ulceration of the overlying mucosa. Alternatively, they may go unnoticed or, if located over the crown of an unerupted tooth, may prevent its eruption. They may displace adjacent teeth or impede eruption.

Diagnosis

Radiographically, the lesions appear as small well-defined radio-opacities.

Treatment (see also Chs 4 and 5)

The lesions should be excised, but considerable mechanical difficulty may be encountered.

ENAMEL PEARLS

Rarely, disturbances in odontogenesis cause small deposits of enamel, termed enamel pearls (enamelomas), usually between the roots of the first permanent molars. No treatment is required.

DENTINOMA

Focal deposits of dentine or osteodentine have been found overlying the crown of unerupted mandibular molar teeth in young adults and have been termed 'dentinomas'. The lesions are usually asymptomatic and appear as chance findings, as opacities on radiographic examination. No treatment is required.

CEMENTOMA

Cementum is normally deposited on tooth roots throughout life to compensate for occlusal wear; an excess of such physiological deposition is termed 'hypercementosis'. The common causes of hypercementosis are chronic periapical infection, a functionless tooth, a reaction to increased stress on the tooth, and Paget disease. Hypercementosis is often symptomless and causes complications only during exodontia. No other treatment is required.

Alternatively, cementum may be deposited neoplastically, when the lesion is termed a 'cementoma'– uncommon lesions, which include:

- benign cementoblastoma
- gigantiform cementoma
- periapical cemental dysplasia
- cementifying fibroma.

DENS INVAGINATUS

Dens invaginatus arises because, during odontogenesis, a portion of the enamel organ protrudes, or invaginates, into the dental papilla. Thus, when development has been completed, the affected and distorted tooth (dilated odontome) contains a cavity that is completely or partially lined by enamel, radiographically resembling a tooth within a tooth (dens in dente). Dens invaginatus occurs in children and adolescents, shows no sex predilection, commonly affects the permanent dentition, usually the upper lateral incisor or an upper anterior tooth, and not infrequently is bilateral. The degree of invagination may be mild to severe, presents as a small pit on the palatal surface of the affected tooth, and the defect collects plaque and food debris, as a result of which there is often caries and consequently pulpitis and periapical infection.

Routine conservation is adequate for mild defects but, in more severe cases, particularly where there is pulpitis or periapical infection, extraction is needed.

DENS EVAGINATUS (TALON CUSP)

In this instance, an evagination causes a nodule usually on the occlusal surface of mandibular premolars, but may be seen buccally or lingually on other teeth. It is most common in Mongoloid races.

GEMINATED ODONTOME

A geminated odontome is a large abnormal tooth that is actually composed of two joined teeth, resulting either from partial division of a tooth germ, or from the fusion of adjacent tooth germs. Gemination is seen mainly anteriorly; the crowns may be separate or divided by a groove. Similarly, the roots may be fused or separate.

USEFUL WEBSITES

Modern Pathology (Nature Publishing Group), Odontogenic Cysts, Odontogenic Tumors, Fibroosseous, and Giant Cell Lesions of the Jaws. http://www.nature.com/modpathol/journal/v15/n3/full/3880527a.html

The University of Texas Medical Branch, Odontogenic Cysts and Tumors. http://www.utmb.edu/otoref/grnds/Odontogenic-tumor_2002-02/Odontogenic-Tumors-2002-02.htm

FURTHER READING

Bernaerts, A., Vanhoenacker, F.M., Hintjens, J., et al., 2006. Imaging approach for differential diagnosis of jaw lesions: a quick reference guide. JBR-BTR 89 (1), 43–46.

Bernaerts, A., Vanhoenacker, F.M., Hintjens, J., et al., 2006. Tumors and tumor-like lesions of the jaw mixed and radiopaque lesions. JBR-BTR 89 (2), 91–99.

Bernaerts, A., Vanhoenacker, F.M., Hintjens, J., et al., 2006. Tumors and tumor-like lesions of the jaw: radiolucent lesions. JBR-BTR 89 (2), 81–90.

Blanas, N., Freund, B., Schwartz, M., et al., 2000. Systematic review of the treatment and prognosis of the odontogenic keratocyst. Oral Surg. Oral Med. Oral Pathol. Oral Radiol. Endod. 90, 553–558.

Buchner, A., Merrell, P.W., Carpenter, W.M., 2006. Relative frequency of central odontogenic tumors: a study of 1,088 cases from Northern California and comparison to studies from other parts of the world. J. Oral Maxillofac. Surg. 64 (9), 1343–1352.

Buchner, A., Merrell, P.W., Carpenter, W.M., 2006. Relative frequency of peripheral odontogenic tumors: a study of 45 new cases and comparison with studies from the literature. J. Oral Pathol. Med. 35 (7), 385–391.

Chirapathomsakul, D., Sastravaha, P., Jansisyanont, P., 2006. A review of odontogenic keratocysts and the behavior of recurrences. Oral Surg. Oral Med. Oral Pathol. Oral Radiol. Endod. 101 (1), 5–9.

Darling, M.R., Daley, T.D., 2006. Peripheral ameloblastic fibroma. J. Oral Pathol. Med. 35 (3), 190–192.

Ezsias, A., 2001. Longitudinal in vivo observations on odontogenic keratocyst over a period of 4 years. Int. J. Oral Maxillofac. Surg. 30, 80–82.

Ghandhi, D., Ayoub, A.F., Pogrel, M.A., et al., 2006. Ameloblastoma: a surgeon's dilemma. J. Oral Maxillofac. Surg. 64 (7), 1010–1014.

Gomes, C.C., Duarte, A.P., Diniz, M.G., Gomez, R.S., 2010. Review article: Current concepts of ameloblastoma pathogenesis. J. Oral Pathol. Med. 39 (8), 585–591.

Gomes, C.C., Oliveira Cda, S., Castro, W.H., et al., 2009. Clonal nature of odontogenic tumours. J. Oral Pathol. Med. 38 (4), 397–400.

Grachtchouk, M., Liu, J., Wang, A., et al., 2006. Odontogenic keratocysts arise from quiescent epithelial rests and are associated with deregulated hedgehog signaling in mice and humans. Am. J. Pathol. 169 (3), 806–814.

Haring, P., Filippi, A., Bornstein, M.M., et al., 2006. The 'globulomaxillary cyst' a specific entity or a myth? Schweiz. Monatsschr. Zahnmed. 116 (4), 380–397.

Hisatomi, M., Asaumi, J., Konouchi, H., et al., 2003. MR imaging of epithelial cysts of the oral and maxillofacial region. Eur. J. Radiol. 48 (2), 178–182.

Iida, S., Fukuda, Y., Ueda, T., et al., 2006. Calcifying odontogenic cyst: radiologic findings in 11 cases. Oral Surg. Oral Med. Oral Pathol. Oral Radiol. Endod. 101 (3), 356–362.

Jones, A.C., Prihoda, T.J., Kacher, J.E., et al., 2006. Osteoblastoma of the maxilla and mandible: a report of 24 cases, review of the literature, and discussion of its relationship to osteoid osteoma of the jaws. Oral Surg. Oral Med. Oral Pathol. Oral Radiol. Endod. 102 (5), 639–650.

Jones, A.V., Craig, G.T., Franklin, C.D., 2006. Range and demographics of odontogenic cysts diagnosed in a UK population over a 30-year period. J. Oral Pathol. Med. 35 (8), 500–507.

Jones, A.V., Franklin, C.D., 2006. An analysis of oral and maxillofacial pathology found in adults over a 30-year period. J. Oral Pathol. Med. 35 (7), 392–401.

Kanno, C.M., Gulinelli, J.L., Nagata, M.J., et al., 2006. Paradental cyst: report of two cases. J. Periodontol. 77 (9), 1602–1606.

Kaplan, I., Anavi, Y., Hirshberg, A., 2008. Glandular odontogenic cyst: a challenge in diagnosis and treatment. Oral Dis. 14, 575–581.

Kumamoto, H., 2006. Molecular pathology of odontogenic tumors. J. Oral Pathol. Med. 35 (2), 65–74.

Kuroyanagi, N., Sakuma, H., Miyabe, S., et al., 2008. Ameloblastoma, calcifying epithelial odontogenic tumor, and glandular odontogenic cyst show a distinctive immunophenotype with some myoepithelial antigen expression. J. Oral Pathol. Med. 37 (3), 177–184.

Lau, S.L., Samman, N., 2006. Recurrence related to treatment modalities of unicystic ameloblastoma: a systematic review. Int. J. Oral Maxillofac. Surg. 35 (8), 681–690.

Meningaud, J.P., Oprean, N., Pitak-Arnnop, P., Bertrand, J.C., 2006. Odontogenic cysts: a clinical study of 695 cases. J. Oral Sci. 48 (2), 59–62.

Muglali, M., Komerik, N., Bulut, E., et al., 2008. Cytokine and chemokine levels in radicular and residual cyst fluids. J. Oral Pathol. Med. 37 (3), 185–189.

Myoung, H., Hong, S.P., Hong, S.D., et al., 2001. Odontogenic keratocyst: review of 256 cases for recurrence and clinicopathologic parameters. Oral Surg. Oral Med. Oral Pathol. Oral Radiol. Endod. 91, 328–333.

Noffke, C., Raubenheimer, E.J., 2002. The glandular odontogenic cyst: clinical and radiological features; review of the literature and report of nine cases. Dentomaxillofac. Radiol. 31 (6), 333–338.

Philipsen, H.P., Reichart, P.A., 2002. Revision of the 1992-edition of the WHO histological typing of odontogenic tumours. A suggestion. J. Oral Pathol. Med. 31 (5), 253–258.

Philipsen, H.P., Reichart, P.A., 2006. Classification of odontogenic tumours. A historical review. J. Oral Pathol. Med. 35 (9), 525–529.

Philipsen, H.P., Reichart, P.A., Siar, C.H., et al., 2007. An updated clinical and epidemiological profile of the adenomatoid odontogenic tumour: a collaborative retrospective study. J. Oral Pathol. Med. 36 (7), 383–393.

Regezi, J.A., 2002. Odontogenic cysts, odontogenic tumors, fibro-osseous, and giant cell lesions of the jaws. Mod. Pathol. 15 (3), 331–341.

Shear, M., 2002. The aggressive nature of the odontogenic keratocyst: is it a benign cystic neoplasm? Part 1. Clinical and early experimental evidence of aggressive behaviour. Oral Oncol. 38 (3), 219–226.

Shear, M., 2002. The aggressive nature of the odontogenic keratocyst: is it a benign cystic neoplasm? Part 2. Proliferation and genetic studies. Oral Oncol. 38 (4), 323–331.

Shear, M., 2002. The aggressive nature of the odontogenic keratocyst: is it a benign cystic neoplasm? Part 3. Immunocytochemistry of cytokeratin and other epithelial cell markers. Oral Oncol. 38 (5), 407–415.

Shear, M., Speight, P.M. (Ed.), 2007. Cysts of the oral and maxillofacial regions. fourth ed. Blackwell, Oxford.

Sklavounou, A., Iakovou, M., Kontos-Toutouzas, J., et al., 2005. Intra-osseous lesions in Greek children and adolescents. A study based on biopsy material over a 26-year period. J. Clin. Pediatr. Dent 30 (2), 153–156.

Slater, L.J., 2006. Botryoid odontogenic cyst versus glandular odontogenic cyst. Int. J. Oral Maxillofac. Surg. 35 (8), 775.

Suyama, Y., Kubota, Y., Ninomiya, T., Shirasuna, K., 2008. Immunohistochemical analysis of interleukin-1 alpha, its type I receptor and antagonist in keratocystic odontogenic tumors. J. Oral Pathol. Med. 37 (9), 560–564.

Vargas, P.A., Carlos-Bregni, R., Mosqueda-Taylor, A., et al., 2006. Adenomatoid dentinoma or adenomatoid odontogenic hamartoma: what is the better term to denominate this uncommon odontogenic lesion? Oral Dis. 12 (2), 200–203.

Warnakulasuriya, S., Nagao, T., Shimozato, K., 2009. Prognostic factors for keratocystic odontogenic tumor (odontogenic keratocyst): analysis of clinico-pathologic and immunohistochemical findings in cysts treated by enucleation. J. Oral Pathol. Med. 38 (4), 386–392.

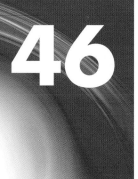

Orofacial granulomatosis

INTRODUCTION

Orofacial granulomatosis (OFG) is an uncommon condition very similar to Crohn disease, due to granulomatous inflammation (**Fig. 46.1**) and often presents with granulomatous cheilitis, a rare, chronic swelling of the lip. OFG can also manifest with angular stomatitis and/or cracked lips (**Fig. 46.2**), ulcers, mucosal tags, cobble-stoning or gingival hyperplasia.

INCIDENCE

It is uncommon.

AGE

The onset is usually in adolescents and young adult life and has no known racial predilection.

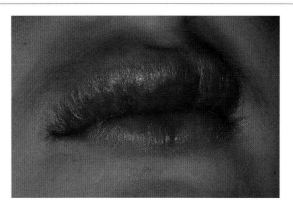

Fig. 46.1 Granulomatous cheilitis – persistent painless diffuse swelling

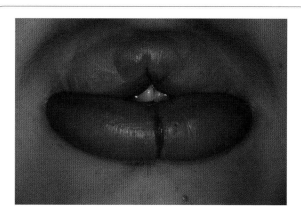

Fig. 46.2 Granulomatous cheilitis (same patient as **Fig. 46.1**)

GENDER

Either gender but males may predominate.

GEOGRAPHIC

No known geographic incidence.

PREDISPOSING FACTORS

OFG sometimes arises from an adverse reaction to various foods or additives which include cinnamic aldehyde, benzoates, butylated hydroxyinosole or dodecyl gallate (in margarine), or menthol (in peppermint oil). Others have or develop, gastrointestinal Crohn disease or sarcoidosis; others have a postulated reaction to other antigens (e.g. metals, such as cobalt), or paratuberculosis or mycobacterial stress protein mSP65.

AETIOLOGY AND PATHOGENESIS

The cause of OFG is unknown, but it may be related to, or may be, Crohn disease and there may be a genetic predisposition. A delayed type of hypersensitivity reaction appears to be involved, although the exact antigen inducing the immunological reaction appears to vary in individual patients. The inflammatory response is:

- probably mediated by cytokines such as tumour necrosis factor (TNF) alpha, and by protease-activated receptors

(PARs), matrix metalloproteinases (MMPs) and cyclo-oxygenases (COXs)

- submucosal and chronic with many Th1 and mononuclear, IL-1 producing cells and large, active, dendritic B cells
- associated with non-caseating granulomas in the lamina propria, which appear to cause lymphatic obstruction and lymphoedema, resulting in the clinical swellings (**Fig. 46.3**).

CLINICAL FEATURES

OFG presents with:

- Non-tender swelling and enlargement of one or both lips (**Figs 46.1** and **46.2**). At the first episode the swelling typically subsides completely in hours or days, but after recurrent attacks the swelling may persist, slowly increases in degree and eventually becomes permanent. The lip involved may feel soft, firm or nodular on palpation. Swellings involve, in decreasing order of frequency, the lip and one or both cheeks. Less commonly, lingual, palatal, gingival and buccal swellings also may occur. The forehead, the eyelids or one side of the scalp may be involved as well or in isolation. The normal lip architecture is eventually chronically altered by the persistence of lymphoedema and non-caseating granulomas in the lamina propria. Once chronicity is established, the enlarged lip appears cracked and fissured, with reddish brown discolouration and scaling becomes painful and eventually acquires the consistency of firm rubber.
- Thickening and folding of the oral mucosa produces a 'cobblestone' type of appearance and mucosal tags (**Figs 46.4 – 46.6**). Purple granulomatous enlargements may appear on the gingiva.
- Ulcers appear: classically involving the buccal sulcus where they appear as linear ulcers, often with granulomatous masses flanking them.
- The attacks of OFG are sometimes accompanied by:
  - fever and mild constitutional symptoms, including headache and even visual disturbance
  - loss of sense of taste and decreased salivary gland secretion
  - cervical lymph node enlargement
  - central nervous system defects are sometimes reported, but the significance of the resulting symptoms is easily

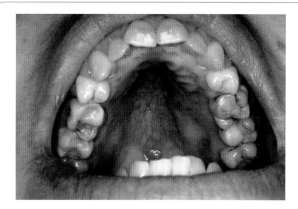

Fig. 46.4 Granulomatous cobblestoning in palate

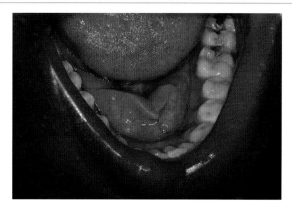

Fig. 46.5 Granulomatous swelling in floor of mouth ("staghorn sign")

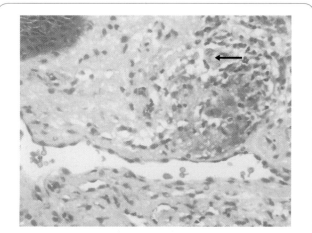

Fig. 46.3 OFG; granuloma arrowed

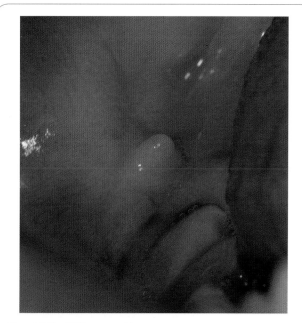

Fig. 46.6 OFG mucosal tag

overlooked as they are very variable, sometimes simulating disseminated sclerosis, but often with a poorly defined association of psychotic and neurological features. Autonomic disturbances may occur

◼ occasionally, deficits of cranial nerves (olfactory, facial, auditory, glossopharyngeal, vagus and hypoglossal) may arise. Facial palsy occurs in up to 30% of cases, more commonly develops late, but may precede the attacks of swelling by months or years. Though intermittent at first, the palsy is lower motor neurone type and may become permanent. It may be unilateral or bilateral, and partial or complete and is part of the Melkersson–Rosenthal syndrome (see Ch. 56).

◼ A fissured or plicated tongue (seen in 20–40% of cases), which is part of the Melkersson–Rosenthal syndrome, present from birth.

DIAGNOSIS

The early attacks of OFG may be impossible to clinically differentiate from angioedema, but persistence of the swelling between attacks should suggest the diagnosis. Similar swelling may also be seen in a range of conditions including:

◼ Melkersson–Rosenthal syndrome (Ch. 56), Miescher cheilitis (Ch. 56), Crohn disease or sarcoidosis.
◼ Lymphomas.
◼ Infections: rare cases of lip or oral swelling related to tuberculosis or leprosy have been reported. Agents such as *Borrelia burgdorferi* have been discounted as causes of OFG.
◼ Liver transplantation – mucosal lesions similar to OFG have been reported.
◼ Foreign body reactions.
◼ Rarely, Ascher syndrome, although the swelling of the lip is caused by redundant salivary tissue and is associated with blepharochalasia and present from childhood (see Ch. 56).

The many causes of oedema of the lips make the diagnosis one based on exclusion, on clinical signs and on histological examination. This is supported by blood tests, radiology, endoscopy, and biopsy to differentiate the above (**Table 46.1**). Lesional biopsy is often indicated but, during the early stages, may show

only lymphoedema and perivascular lymphocytic infiltration. However, with time, the infiltrate usually becomes more dense and pleomorphic, and small focal granulomas are formed, which in OFG are indistinguishable from those of Crohn disease or sarcoidosis. Patch tests and RAST may be indicated to exclude reactions to various foodstuffs or additives. Both standard and urticarial patch testing are used to detect such allergies. Elimination diets have also been shown to be diagnostic in some patients.

Investigation of the gastrointestinal tract (endoscopy, radiography and biopsy) is mandatory to exclude Crohn disease; endoscopic and histologic intestinal abnormalities are common in younger patients even when there are no gastrointestinal symptoms. Sarcoidosis may be excluded by chest radiography, serum angiotensin converting enzyme, and a gallium scan, and a tuberculin skin test may also be indicated.

TREATMENT (see also Chs 4 and 5)

Reactions to dietary components should be sought and possible provoking substances avoided (**Table 46.2**). Elimination diets may be warranted and many patients respond. OFG may be an initial manifestation of Crohn disease and so careful surveillance and specialist care are recommended. Management is to treat recalcitrant lesions medically. Conservative management usually includes topical corticosteroids, intralesional corticosteroid injections (such as low-volume, high-concentrate, extended-release triamcinolone) or topical tacrolimus. Oral clofazimine 100–200 mg daily for 3–6 months (hyperpigmentation and raised liver enzymes are adverse effects) may be helpful. Other therapies include NSAIDs, sulfasalazine, antibiotics such as metronidazole, antimalarials such as hydroxychloroquine, mast cell stabilizers, or low-dose methotrexate. Rarely, cheiloplasty is indicated.

EMERGENT TREATMENTS

If OFG fails to respond to diet or topical measures, systemic immunomodulators may be required, under specialist supervision. These include anti-TNF therapies such as thalidomide, adalumimab or infliximab, but should be used only with caution.

Table 46.1 Aids that might be helpful in diagnosis/prognosis/management in some patients suspected of having orofacial granulomatosis*

In most cases	In some cases
Gastroenterological opinion	Patch tests
Biopsy	RAST
Full blood picture	Elimination diet
Serum ferritin, vitamin B$_{12}$	G6PD and TPMT levels
and corrected whole blood	Blood pressure
folate levels	Blood glucose
ESR	DEXA (dual-emission X-ray
SACE	absorptiometry)
Chest radiography	
Gastrointestinal imaging,	
endoscopy, biopsy	
Tuberculin testing	

*See text for details and glossary for abbreviations.

Table 46.2 Regimens that might be helpful in management of patient suspected of having orofacial granulomatosis

Regimen	Use in primary care	Use in secondary care (severe oral involvement and/or extraoral involvement)
Likely to be beneficial	Dietary modification (antigen exclusion) Intralesional corticosteroids Topical corticosteroids Topical tacrolimus	Clofazimine Corticosteroids Thalidomide
Unproven effectiveness	Topical pimecrolimus	Hydroxychloroquine Metronidazole Sulfasalazine
Emergent treatments		Infliximab Adalumimab

FOLLOW-UP OF PATIENTS

Long-term follow-up as shared care is usually appropriate.

PATIENT INFORMATION SHEET
Orofacial granulomatosis (OFG)

▼ Please note this is our provisional diagnosis which must be confirmed by tests. If you have any questions, particularly about the treatment or potential side-effects, please ask.
■ OFG is an uncommon condition.

■ The cause is unknown but it may be immunological.
■ It is not thought to be inherited.
■ It is not thought to be infectious.
■ It usually has no long-term consequences but related conditions such as Crohn disease may affect the gut and other tissues.
■ Some patients have food or food additive intolerance or allergy: most commonly this is to cinnamaldehyde, carnosine, monosodium glutamate, cocoa, carbone, or sunset yellow.
■ Blood tests, X-rays, biopsy, allergy tests and other investigations are often required–mainly to exclude Crohn disease, sarcoidosis and allergies.
■ OFG may be controlled by avoiding allergens, or by using medicines.

USEFUL WEBSITES

Circa, Children with Crohns and Colitis. http://www.cicra.org/

Dermnet, N.Z., Orofacial granulomatosis. http://dermnetnz.org/site-age-specific/orofacial-granulomatosis.html

Emedicine, Cheilitis Granulomatosa (Miescher-Melkersson-Rosenthal Syndrome). http://emedicine.medscape.com/article/1075333-overview

FURTHER READING

Al Johani, K., Moles, D., Hodgson, T., et al., 2009. Onset and progression of clinical manifestations of orofacial granulomatosis. Oral Dis. 15, 214–219.

Alawi, F., 2005. Granulomatous diseases of the oral tissues: differential diagnosis and update. Dent. Clin. North Am. 49 (1), 203–221.

Barry, O., Barry, J., Langan, S., et al., 2005. Treatment of granulomatous cheilitis with infliximab. Arch. Dermatol. 141 (9), 1080–1082.

Bradley, P.J., Ferlito, A., Devaney, K.O., Rinaldo, A., 2004. Crohn's disease manifesting in the head and neck. Acta Otolaryngol. 124 (3), 237–241.

Elliott, E., Campbell, H., Escudier, M., 2011. Experience with anti-TNF-α therapy for orofacial granulomatosis. J. Oral Pathol. Med. 40 (1), 14–19.

Feller, M., Huwiler, K., Schoepfer, A., et al., 2010. Long-term antibiotic treatment for Crohn's disease: systematic review and meta-analysis of placebo-controlled trials. Clin. Infect. Dis. 50, 473–480.

Fitzpatrick, L., Healy, C.M., McCartan, B.E., et al., 2011. Patch testing for food-associated allergies in orofacial granulomatosis. J. Oral Pathol. Med. 40 (1), 10–13.

Gaya, D.R., Aitken, S., Fennell, J., et al., 2006. Anti-TNF-α therapy for orofacial granulomatosis: proceed with caution. Gut 55 (10), 1524–1525.

Grave, B., McCullough, M., Wiesenfeld, D., 2009. Orofacial granulomatosis – a 20-year review. Oral Dis. 15, 46–51.

Hodgson, T.A., Buchanan, J.A., Porter, S.R., 2004. Orofacial granulomatosis. J. Oral Pathol. Med 33 (4), 252.

Kavala, M., Südoan, S., Can, B., Sargül, S., 2004. Granulomatous cheilitis resulting from a tuberculide. Int. J. Dermatol. 43, 524–527.

Khouri, J.M., Bohane, T.D., Day, A.S., 2005. Is orofacial granulomatosis in children a feature of Crohn's disease? Acta Paediatr. 94 (4), 501–504.

Kim, S.K., Lee, E.S., 2010. Orofacial granulomatosis associated with Crohn's disease. Ann. Dermatol. 22, 203–305.

Leao, J.C., Hodgson, T., Scully, C., Porter, S., 2004. Review article: orofacial granulomatosis. Aliment Pharmacol. Ther. 20 (10), 1019–1027.

Mignogna, M.D., Fedele, S., Lo Russo, L., et al., 2004. Effectiveness of small-volume, intralesional, delayed-release triamcinolone injections in orofacial granulomatosis: a pilot study. J. Am. Acad. Dermatol. 51 (2), 265–268.

Mignogna, M.D., Pollio, A., Leuci, S., et al., 2012. Clinical behaviour and long-term therapeutic response in orofacial granulomatosis patients treated with intralesional triamcinolone acetonide injections alone or in combination with topical pimecrolimus 1%. J. Oral Pathol. Med. Jun 15. [Epub ahead of print].

O'Neill, I., Scully, C., 2012. Biologics in oral medicine: oral Crohns disease and orofacial granulomatosis. Oral Disease Mar 15 Epub.

Patel, P., Barone, F., Nunes, C., et al., 2010. Subepithelial dendritic B cells in orofacial granulomatosis. Inflamm. Bowel Dis. 16 (6), 1051–1060.

Saalman, R., Sundell, S., Kullberg-Lindh, C., et al., 2010. Long-standing oral mucosal lesions in solid organ-transplanted children–a novel clinical entity. Transplantation 89 (5), 606–611.

Sanderson, J., Nunes, C., Escudier, M., et al., 2005. Oro-facial granulomatosis: Crohn's disease or a new inflammatory bowel disease? Inflamm. Bowel Dis. 11 (9), 840–846.

Scully, C., Felix, D.H., 2005. Oral medicine – update for the dental practitioner lumps and swellings. Br. Dent. J. 199 (12), 763–770.

Singh, G., Haneef, N.S., 2005. Leprosy masquerading as Melkersson–Rosenthal syndrome. Indian J. Lepr. 77 (3), 273–276.

Staines, K.S., Green, R., Felix, D.H., 2007. The management of fistulizing oral Crohn's disease with infliximab. J. Oral Pathol. Med 36 (7), 444–446.

Tan, O., Atik, B., Calka, O., 2006. Plastic surgical solutions for Melkersson–Rosenthal syndrome: facial liposuction and cheiloplasty procedures. Ann. Plast. Surg. 56 (3), 268–273.

Tilakaratne, W.M., Freysdottir, J., Fortune, F., 2008. Orofacial granulomatosis: review on aetiology and pathogenesis. J. Oral Pathol. Med. 37 (4), 191–195.

Tonkovic-Capin, V., Galbraith, S.S., Rogers 3rd, R.S., et al., 2006. Cutaneous Crohn's disease mimicking Melkersson–Rosenthal syndrome: treatment with methotrexate. J. Eur. Acad. Dermatol. Venereol. 20 (4), 449–452.

Tuxen, A.J., Orchard, D., 2010. Childhood and adolescent orofacial granulomatosis is strongly associated with Crohn's disease and responds to intralesional corticosteroids. Australas. J. Dermatol. 5, 124–126.

van der Waal, R.I., Schulten, E.A., van der Meij, E.H., et al., 2002. Cheilitis granulomatosa: overview of 13 patients with long-term follow-up–results of management. Int. J. Dermatol. 41, 225–229.

White, A., Nunes, C., Escudier, M., et al., 2006. Improvement in orofacial granulomatosis on a cinnamon- and benzoate-free diet. Inflamm. Bowel Dis. 12, 508–514.

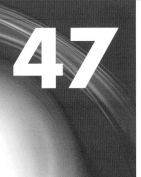

47 Pemphigoid

Key Points

- Mucous membrane pemphigoid (MMP) is a group of chronic autoimmune diseases affecting mucous membranes and/or skin
- The autoantibodies are directed against epithelial basement membrane zone (BMZ) proteins, especially integrin and epiligrin
- Immune deposits result in a subepithelial split and blistering
- Oral lesions in all types include bullae and erosions and desquamative gingivitis
- Other mucosae, e.g. conjunctivitae may be involved
- Diagnosis is achieved by biopsy with immunostaining
- Treatment is usually with corticosteroids, tetracyclines or dapsone

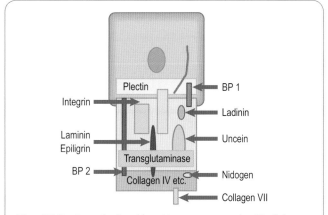

Fig. 47.2 Complexity of hemidesmosome and epithelial basement membrane zone. IMSEBD are caused by autoantibodies to these proteins (BP, bullous pemphigoid)

INTRODUCTION

Pemphigoid and pemphigus along with erythema multiforme produce vesicles and bullae (blisters) and are thus termed vesiculobullous disorders. The vesiculobullous disorders include two groups of autoimmune blistering mucocutaneous diseases:

- The pemphigoid subset: mediated by autoantibodies that target the extracellular components that link the epithelial basement membrane components either to the lowermost layer of epithelial cells or to the lamina propria components (subepithelial blistering, or immune-mediated subepithelial blistering diseases – IMSEBD). This region, the epithelial basement membrane zone (BMZ), has a highly complex structure composed of an array of proteins. Autoantibodies directed against these proteins can produce a range of disorders (**Figs 47.1** and **47.2**), which all show similar clinical features and immune deposits at the BMZ and subepithelial splitting of epithelium from the lamina

propria. Special immune studies are required to separate these similar phenotypes.

- The pemphigus subset: mediated by autoantibodies that target the extracellular components that link one epithelial cell to another (intra-epithelial blistering) (see Ch. 48).

Pemphigoid is the term given to a group of subepithelial immunologically mediated vesiculobullous disorders that affect stratified squamous epithelium and are characterized by damage to one of the protein constituents of the basement membrane zone (BMZ) anchoring filament components. A number of other subepithelial vesiculobullous disorders may produce similar clinical features (**Box 47.1**) of blisters, erosions and desquamative gingivitis.

Pemphigoid is the term given when the IMSEBD is associated with IgG autoantibodies directed against specific hemidesmosomal antigens such as BP antigen, alpha

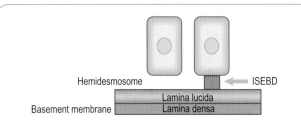

Fig. 47.1 Immune mediated subepithelial blistering diseases – lesion at basement membrane zone (BMZ)

BOX 47.1 Subepithelial vesiculobullous disorders

- Pemphigoid variants
- Dermatitis herpetiformis
- Acquired epidermolysis bullosa
- Toxic epidermal necrolysis
- Erythema multiforme
- Dermatitis herpetiformis
- Linear IgA disease
- Chronic bullous dermatosis of childhood

integrin or epiligrin (laminin 322). Several disorders in the pemphigoid group can cause oral lesions but the main types that involve the mouth are termed 'mucous membrane pemphigoid' (MMP) in which mucosal (oral, ocular, genital, laryngeal) lesions predominate, but skin lesions are rare. Antibodies are to bullous pemphigoid antigen 1 and 2 (BP or BPAG1 and BPAG2), epiligrin (laminin 322), laminin 6, type VII collagen, α6β4 integrin and antigens with unknown identities (a 45-kd protein, uncein, a 168-kd epithelial protein, and a 120-kd epithelial protein. There are two main subsets ocular cicatricial pemphigoid (OCP) and oral pemphigoid (OP):

- OCP: affects mainly the conjunctivae and may cause scarring (anti-epiligrin antibodies)
- OP: oral lesions only with no scarring process (anti-integrin antibodies).

However, most of the literature has failed to distinguish these types, since their distinction has only recently been recognized, and, therefore, the following discussion groups them together as mucous membrane pemphigoid.

MUCOUS MEMBRANE PEMPHIGOID (MMP)

MMP (or sometimes termed 'benign mucous membrane pemphigoid') is a chronic autoimmune disease of the mucous membranes mainly.

INCIDENCE

This lesion is not uncommon.

Age

The onset is usually in the fifth to sixth decades.

Gender

Pemphigoid is twice as common in females.

Geographic

There is no known geographic incidence.

PREDISPOSING FACTORS

- A genetic predisposition is suggested by an HLA-DQB1*0301 allele association (with haplotypes DQB1*0302, 0303 and 06, and especially the DRB1*1101 DQB1*0301).
- The precipitating event is unclear in most cases.
- A few cases are drug-induced (e.g. by furosemide, penicillamine, NSAIDS, captopril, antimicrobials (Table 54.13)) or radiation induced (UV light or X-irradiation).

AETIOLOGY AND PATHOGENESIS

Histologically, MMP is characterized by junctional separation at the level of the epithelial basement membrane zone, giving rise to a sub-basilar split as in other forms of pemphigoid (**Fig. 47.3**). The pathogenesis probably includes complement-mediated sequestration of leukocytes, with resultant cytokine and leukocyte enzyme release and detachment of the basal

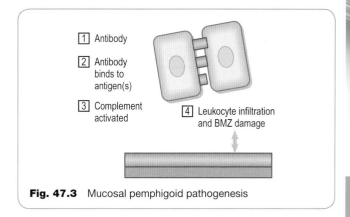

Fig. 47.3 Mucosal pemphigoid pathogenesis

cells from the BMZ (**Fig. 47.4**). MMP is characterized immunologically by:

- circulating autoantibodies to basement membrane zone components, which are classically of IgG class (97%) with C3 (78%), but sometimes IgA (27%) or IgM (12%) (**Table 47.1**)
- deposition of immunoglobulins and complement components at the epithelial basement membrane zone (BMZ), suggesting antibodies are directed against the basement membrane.

CLINICAL FEATURES

The oral lesions in pemphigoid affect especially the gingivae and palate, and may include:

- Bullae or vesicles, but not commonly, due to them breaking from the trauma of eating and speaking (**Fig. 47.5**). Blisters if present are tense, may sometimes be blood-filled and can remain intact for days, similar to those of angina bullosa haemorrhagica (localized oral purpura), often on the soft palate. Pressure on the blister may cause it to spread (Nikolsky sign).
- Persistent irregular erosions or ulcers which result from the blisters bursting and typically are covered with a yellowish fibrinous slough and have surrounding inflammatory erythema, thus somewhat resembling erosive lichen planus, except that no white lesions are present (**Fig 47.6**). They may also resemble erythema multiforme, or late lesions of pemphigus.
- Desquamative gingivitis; this is the most common oral finding and is characterized by erythematous, tender gingiva, usually in a patchy, rather than continuous distribution (**Fig. 47.7**). Sole involvement of the gingiva is not uncommon and is frequently misdiagnosed as inflammatory periodontal disease. There may be erosions and ulcers.
- Scarring, but only rarely in the mouth.

The majority of affected individuals with MMP have oral involvement only, but in some:

- untreated ocular involvement can lead to blindness mainly due to conjunctival scarring (leading to entropion, symblepharon or ankyloblepharon) (**Fig. 47.8**)
- laryngeal scarring may lead to stenosis
- nasal lesions may bleed and crust
- genital involvement can be a source of great morbidity
- skin blisters may rarely be seen

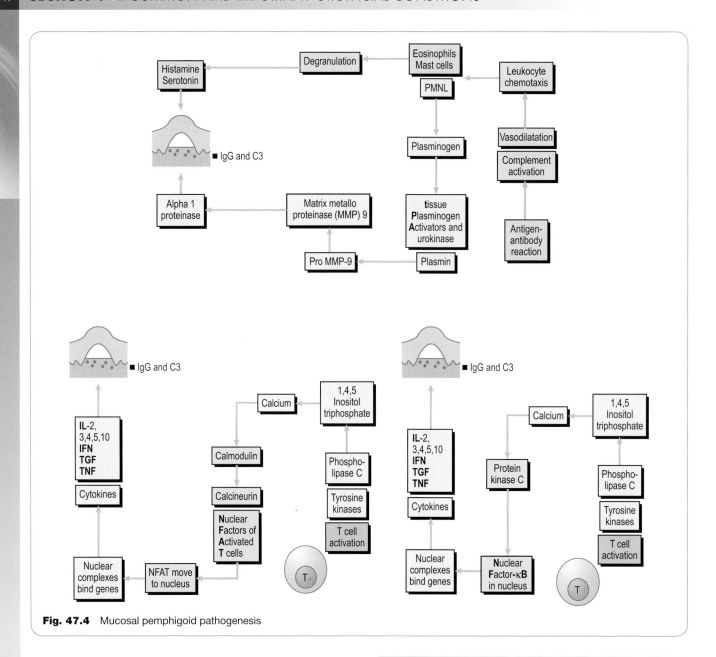

Fig. 47.4 Mucosal pemphigoid pathogenesis

Table 47.1 Main antigens implicated in subepithelial disorders

Disease	Main antigens
Bullous pemphigoid	BP1, BP2*
Mucous membrane pemphigoid	BP1, BP2 (BP180), Laminin 5[†], β4 integrin, α6 integrin or type VII collagen
Linear IgA disease	97 kDa, 45 kDa
Epidermolysis bullosa acquisita	Type VII collagen
Toxic epidermal necrolysis	105 kDa

*BP, bullous pemphigoid.
[†]Also known as laminin 322, epiligrin, nicein, kalinin and BM600.

Fig. 47.5 Mucosal pemphigoid may present with blisters, which break to leave erosions

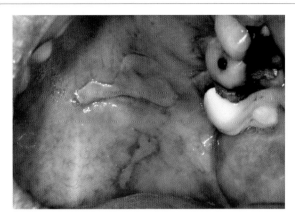

Fig.47.6 Pemphigoid erosions in palate

Table 47.2 Aids that might be helpful in diagnosis/prognosis/ management in some patients suspected of having pemphigoid*

In most cases	In some cases
Nikolsky sign	Dermatological/gynaecological
Biopsy and	opinion
Immunofluorescence	Serum BP-180 antibodies
Ophthalmic opinion	Full blood picture
	Reticulocyte count
	Haptoglobin level
	Liver function
	Renal function
	Serum ferritin, vitamin B_{12}
	and corrected whole blood folate
	levels
	ESR
	G6PD and TPMT levels
	Blood pressure
	Blood glucose
	DEXA (dual-emission X-ray
	absorptiometry)

*See text for details and glossary for abbreviations.

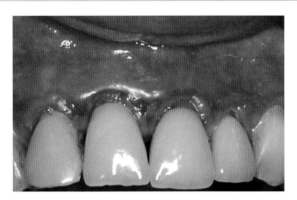

Fig. 47.7 Mucosal pemphigoid commonly presents with desquamative gingivitis

- associated autoimmune disorders
- associations with parkinsonism, cerebrovascular events and disseminated sclerosis have been suggested
- internal malignancy such as lymphoma may be present in some patients with anti-epiligrin (anti-laminin 322) pemphigoid but patients with antibodies to α6 integrin may have a possible reduced relative risk for developing cancer.

DIAGNOSIS

The oral lesions of pemphigoid should be differentiated mainly from lichen planus, pemphigus, angina bullosa haemorrhagica, dermatitis herpetiformis and linear IgA disease or, occasionally, acquired epidermolysis bullosa or erythema multiforme.

The pemphigoid variants are indistinguishable one from another clinically, and by light microscopy and therefore, biopsy of perilesional tissue, with histological and immunostaining examination is essential to the diagnosis (**Table 47.9**). The incisional biopsy specimen exhibits subepithelial clefting following staining with haematoxylin and eosin (**Fig. 47.10**).

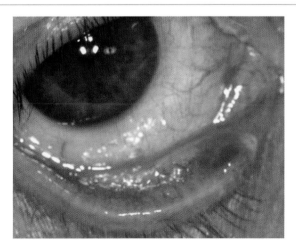

Fig. 47.8 Mucosal pemphigoid may cause ocular disease and scarring

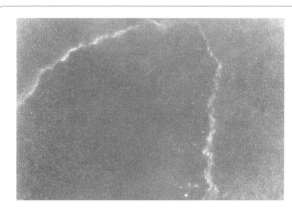

Fig. 47.9 Mucosal pemphigoid linear immune deposits at BMZ

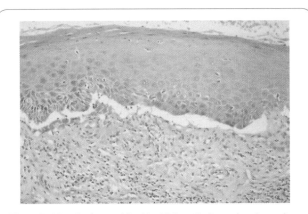

Fig. 47.10 Oral pemphigoid – histopathology showing sub-epithelial split and vesiculation

Direct immunofluorescence microscopy (DIF) detects deposits at the epithelial basement membrane zone (**Fig. 47.10**). Indirect immunofluorescence microscopy (IIF) microscopy detects epithelial basement membrane zone-binding autoantibodies in serum. Indirect immunofluorescence on salt-split substrate (ssIIF) uses epithelial substrates in which the lamina lucida of the basement membrane zone has been split at the middle, leaving the target antigens for the serum

autoantibodies of pemphigoid and epidermolysis bullosa acquisita to the roof and the base of the split substrate, respectively, thus distinguishing these two diseases. In mucous membrane pemphigoid however, serum autoantibodies can bind to the roof, base, or both, corresponding to the heterogeneity of the target antigens recognized by these autoantibodies. ELISA to BP 180 antigen in serum may be positive.

TREATMENT (see also Chs 4 and 5)

Few patients with pemphigoid have spontaneous remission and, thus, treatment is often indicated (**Algorithm 47.1; Table 47.3**). Patient information is an important aspect in management.

- An International Consensus on MMP categorized patients into 'low-risk' and 'high-risk' groups based upon the site(s) of involvement, with 'low-risk' patients defined as having only oral mucosal or oral and skin involvement and 'high-risk' patients as having involvement of the ocular, genital, nasopharyngeal, esophageal, and/or laryngeal mucosae, and requiring more aggressive treatment (see below).
- Systemic manifestations of pemphigoid must be given attention. Ocular manifestations have been reported in up to 20% of patients and, left untreated, can lead to blindness and thus an ophthalmological consultation is essential. Patients with MMP should also be questioned about the

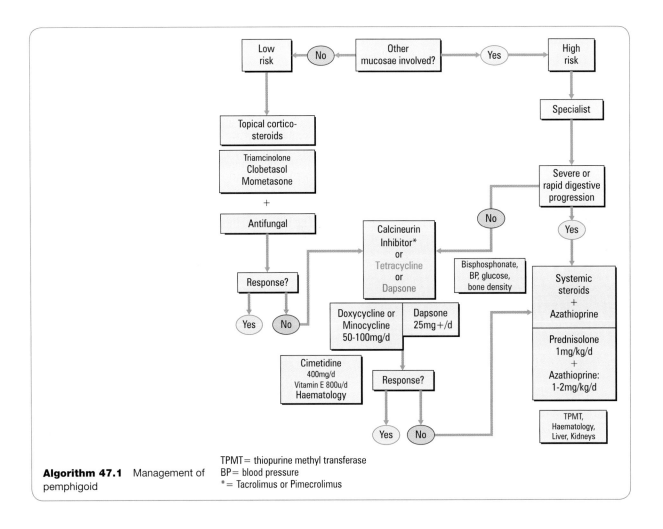

Algorithm 47.1 Management of pemphigoid

TPMT = thiopurine methyl transferase
BP = blood pressure
* = Tacrolimus or Pimecrolimus

Table 47.3 Regimens that might be helpful in management of patient suspected of having pemphigoid

Regimen	Use in primary care	Use in secondary care (severe oral involvement and/or extraoral involvement)
Likely to be beneficial	Topical corticosteroids (e.g. betamethasone, clobetasol propionate) or tacrolimus or pimecrolimus	Systemic dapsone, minocycline, corticosteroids Or other immunosuppressives such as azathioprine, mycophenolate mofetil or intravenous immunoglobulins
Unproven effectiveness	Tetracyclines ± nicotinamide	
Emergent treatments		Etanercept Infliximab
Supportive	Chlorhexidine Benzydamine Diet with little acidic, spicy or citrus content Lidocaine Triclosan	

presence of other mucosal symptoms, which might indicate genital or laryngeal involvement. Multidisciplinary treatment is indicated for 'high-risk' patients.

- Most patients have oral pemphigoid alone and respond well to topical corticosteroids or tacrolimus though some advocate use of tetracyclines (minocycline or doxycycline) alone or plus nicotinamide, or dapsone.
- Topical corticosteroids are the primary therapeutic agents used to treat ulcerative mucosal lesions, which have an immunologically-based aetiology such as pemphigoid. A mild potency agent such as hydrocortisone is rarely effective and more typically a medium potency corticosteroid such as betamethasone or a higher potency one such as fluocinonide or beclomethasone are required, moving to a super-potent topical corticosteroid, e.g. clobetasol, if the benefit is inadequate (Tables 5.5 and 47.3). Patients should be instructed to apply a small quantity of the agent three times daily, refraining from speaking, eating and drinking for the subsequent 0.5 h. A theoretical concern is that long-term immunosuppression might predispose to neoplastic change. In long-term use, candidosis can arise and thus topical antifungal medication such as miconazole may be prudent. The more major concern (of adrenal suppression with long-term and/or repeated application) has rarely been addressed, although the topical preparations noted in Ch. 5 (apart from super potent halogenated corticosteroids when used several times a day) appear not to cause a significant problem.
- Desquamative gingivitis associated with pemphigoid often responds well to topical corticosteroids or tacrolimus, which are most effective if used in a vacuum-formed custom tray or veneer worn during sleep. Oral hygiene improvement is often needed, as secondary infection may inhibit healing.
- Tetracycline (a capsule of 100 mg doxycycline dissolved in 10 mL water) can be as a mouth rinse then swallowed, to provide relief and reduce ulcer duration, but should be restricted to adults.
- Dapsone starting at 25–50 mg per day, increasing monthly by 25–50 mg until clinical remission is achieved or until the maximum tolerated dose (usually 200 mg per day). Patients should first be screened including a glucose-6-phosphate dehydrogenase level due to the risk of haemolysis.

Monitoring during therapy is required to assess for adverse effects including dose-related haemolytic anaemia and methaemoglobinemia, and other idiosyncratic adverse effects such as agranulocytosis and hepatitis (Ch. 5).

- Good oral hygiene should be maintained; chlorhexidine or triclosan mouthwashes may help.
- Antiinflammatory agents: there is a spectrum of topical agents, such as benzydamine, that may help in the management of discomfort in pemphigoid.
- In 'high-risk' patients or if pemphigoid fails to respond to these measures, systemic immunomodulators may be required, under specialist supervision. Severe pemphigoid may need to be treated with systemic corticosteroids or immunosuppression using azathioprine, cyclophosphamide, methotrexate, mycophenolate mofetil or intravenous immunoglobulins but these are of variable benefit and/or can give rise to serious adverse effects.

EMERGENT TREATMENTS

Etanercept or infliximab for high-risk patients.

FOLLOW-UP OF PATIENTS

Long-term follow-up as shared care is usually appropriate but if there are severe oral lesions or other sites involved, specialist follow-up is appropriate.

PATIENT INFORMATION SHEET
Pemphigoid

▼ Please read this information sheet. If you have any questions, particularly about the treatment or potential side-effects, please ask your doctor.

- This is an uncommon condition.
- The cause is unknown, but it may be immunological.
- It is not thought to be inherited.
- It is not thought to be infectious.
- It occasionally affects the skin or other sites.
- It usually has no long-term consequences.
- Blood tests and biopsy are often required.
- Pemphigoid may be controlled, but rarely cured with medicines.
- You should seek advice from an ophthalmologist.

USEFUL WEBSITES

American Autoimmune Related Diseases Association:
http://www.aarda.org/

FURTHER READING

Alexandre, M., Brette, M.D., Pascal, F., et al., 2006. A prospective study of upper aerodigestive tract manifestations of mucous membrane pemphigoid. Medicine (Baltimore) 85, 239–252.

Arash, A., Shirin, L., 2008. The management of oral mucous membrane pemphigoid with dapsone and topical corticosteroid. J. Oral Pathol. Med. 37 (6), 341–344.

Arduino, P., Farci, V., D'Aiuto, F., et al., 2011. Periodontal status in oral mucous membrane pemphigoid: initial results of a case-control study. Oral Dis. 17, 90–94.

Assmann, T., Becker, J., Ruzicka, T., et al., 2004. Topical tacrolimus for oral cicatricial pemphigoid. Clin. Exp. Dermatol. 29, 674–676.

Bagan, J., Lo Muzio, L., Scully, C., 2005. Mucous membrane pemphigoid. Oral Dis. 11, 197–218.

Canizares, M.J., Smith, D.I., Conners, M.S., et al., 2006. Successful treatment of mucous membrane pemphigoid with etanercept in 3 patients. Arch. Dermatol. 142 (11), 1457–1461.

Carrozzo, M., Arduino, P., Bertolusso, G., et al., 2009. Systemic minocycline as a therapeutic option in predominantly oral mucous membrane pemphigoid: a cautionary report. Int. J. Oral Maxillofac. Surg. 38 (10), 1071–1076.

Challacombe, S.J., Setterfield, J., Shirlaw, P., et al., 2001. Immunodiagnosis of pemphigus and mucous membrane pemphigoid. Acta Odontol. Scand. 59, 226–234.

Chan, L.S., Ahmed, A.R., Anhalt, G.J., et al., 2002. The first international consensus on mucous membrane pemphigoid: definition, diagnostic criteria, pathogenic factors, medical treatment, and prognostic indicators. Arch. Dermatol. 138, 370–379.

Daoud, Y., Amin, K.G., Mohan, K., et al., 2005. Cost of intravenous immunoglobulin therapy versus conventional immunosuppressive therapy in patients with mucous membrane pemphigoid: a preliminary study. Ann. Pharmacother. 39, 2003–2008.

Darling, M.R., Daley, T., 2005. Blistering mucocutaneous diseases of the oral mucosa – a review: part 1. Mucous membrane pemphigoid. J. Can. Dent. Assoc. 71 (11), 851–854.

Demitsu, T., Yoneda, K., Iida, E., et al., 2009. A case of mucous membrane pemphigoid with IgG antibodies against all the alpha3, beta3 and gamma2 subunits of laminin-332 and BP180 C-terminal domain, associated with pancreatic cancer. Clin. Exp. Dermatol. 34 (8), e992–e994.

Egan, C.E., Lazarova, Z., Darling, T.N., et al., 2001. Anti-epiligrin cicatricial pemphigoid and relative risk for cancer. Lancet 357, 1850–1851.

Endo, Y., Tsuji, M., Shirase, T., et al., 2011. Angioimmunoblastic T-cell lymphoma presenting with both IgA-related leukocytoclastic vasculitis and mucous membrane pemphigoid. Eur. J. Dermatol. 21 (2), 274–276.

Fukushima, S., Egawa, K., Nishi, H., et al., 2008. Two cases of anti-epiligrin cicatricial pemphigoid with and without associated malignancy. Acta Derm. Venereol. 88 (5), 484–487.

Heffernan, M.P., Bentley, D.D., 2006. Successful treatment of mucous membrane pemphigoid with infliximab. Arch. Dermatol. 142, 1268–1270.

Higgins, G.T., Allan, R.B., Hall, R., et al., 2006. Development of ocular disease in patients with mucous membrane pemphigoid involving the oral mucosa. Br. J. Ophthalmol. 90 (8), 964–967.

Ingen-Housz-Oro, S., Prost-Squarcioni, C., Pascal, F., et al., 2005. Cicatricial pemphigoid: treatment with mycophenolate mofetil. Ann. Dermatol. Venereol. 132, 13–16.

Lazarova, Z., Salato, V.K., Lanschuetzer, C.M., et al., 2008. IgG anti-laminin-332 autoantibodies are present in a subset of patients with mucous membrane, but not bullous, pemphigoid. J. Am. Acad. Dermatol. 58 (6), 951–958.

Leao, J., Ingafou, M., Khan, A., et al., 2008. Desquamative gingivitis: retrospective analysis of disease associations of a large cohort. Oral Dis. 14, 556–560.

Letko, E., Gürcan, H.M., Papaliodis, G.N., et al., 2007. Relative risk for cancer in mucous membrane pemphigoid associated with antibodies to the beta4 integrin subunit. Clin. Exp. Dermatol. 32 (6), 637–641.

Mahmood, S., Lim, Z.Y., Benton, E., et al., 2009. Mucous membrane pemphigoid following reduced intensity conditioning allogeneic haematopoietic SCT for biphenotypic leukaemia. Bone Marrow Transplant. 45 (1), 195–196.

Malik, M., Gürcan, H.M., Christen, W., Ahmed, A.R., 2007. Relationship between cancer and oral pemphigoid patients with antibodies to alpha6-integrin. J. Oral Pathol. Med. 36 (1), 1–5.

Mitsuya, J., Hara, H., Ito, K., et al., 2008. Metastatic ovarian carcinoma-associated subepidermal blistering disease with autoantibodies to both the p200 dermal antigen and the gamma 2 subunit of laminin 5

showing unusual clinical features. Br. J. Dermatol. 158 (6), 1354–1357.

Popovsky, J.L., Camisa, C., 2000. New and emerging therapies for diseases of the oral cavity. Dermatol. Clin. 18, 113–125.

Rashid, K.A., Gurcan, H.M., Ahmed, A.R., 2006. Antigen specificity in subsets of mucous membrane pemphigoid. J. Invest. Dermatol. 126 (12), 2631–2636.

Rashid, K.A., Stern, J.N., Ahmed, A.R., 2006. Identification of an epitope within human integrin alpha 6 subunit for the binding of autoantibody and its role in basement membrane separation in oral pemphigoid. J. Immunol. 176 (3), 1968–1977.

Sacher, C., Rubbert, A., Konig, C., et al., 2002. Treatment of recalcitrant cicatricial pemphigoid with the tumor necrosis factor alpha antagonist etanercept. J. Am. Acad. Dermatol. 46, 113–115.

Sadler, E., Lazarova, Z., Sarasombath, P., Yancey, K.B., 2007. A widening perspective regarding the relationship between anti-epiligrin cicatricial pemphigoid and cancer. J. Dermatol. Sci. 47 (1), 1–7.

Salzano, S., Arduino, P., Zambruno, G., et al., 2006. OC9 Successful use of mycophenolate mofetil in combination with minocycline in a woman with severe predominantly oral mucous membrane pemphigoid: a case report. Oral Dis. 12, 11.

Suresh, L., Martinez Calixto, L.E., Radfar, L., 2006. Successful treatment of mucous membrane pemphigoid with tacrolimus. Spec. Care Dentist. 26, 66–70.

Takahara, M., Tsuji, G., Ishii, N., et al., 2009. Mucous membrane pemphigoid with antibodies to the beta(3) subunit of Laminin 332 in a patient with acute myeloblastic leukemia and graft-versus-host disease. Dermatology 219 (4), 361–364.

Tricamo, M.B., Rees, T.D., Hallmon, W.W., et al., 2006. Periodontal status in patients with gingival mucous membrane pemphigoid. J. Periodontol. 77 (3), 398–405.

Yancey, K.B., Egan, C.A., 2000. Pemphigoid: clinical, histologic, immunopathologic and therapeutic considerations. JAMA 284, 350–356.

Young, A.L., Bailey, E.E., Colaço, S.M., 2011. Anti-laminin-332 mucous membrane pemphigoid associated with recurrent metastatic prostate carcinoma: hypothesis for a paraneoplastic phenomenon. Eur. J. Dermatol. 21 (3), 401–404.

Pemphigus 48

Key Points

- Pemphigus is a group of potentially life-threatening chronic autoimmune diseases characterized by epithelial blistering affecting mucocutaneous surfaces
- Autoantibodies in the most common variant, pemphigus vulgaris, are directed against desmoglein in epithelial desmosomes
- Immune deposits result in intra-epithelial splitting (acantholysis)
- Epithelial blistering and erosions often manifest first in the mouth
- Diagnosis is confirmed by biopsy and immunostaining
- Treatment needs specialist advice and systemic immunomodulation

INTRODUCTION

This is a potentially lethal condition. Pemphigus is the term for a group of chronic autoimmune diseases characterized by epithelial blistering affecting mucocutaneous surfaces, the term being derived from the Greek (*pemphix* = bubble or blister). Autoantibodies are directed against desmosomes (epithelial adhesion proteins) that bind stratified squamous epithelial cells together and that have a complex protein structure (**Fig. 48.1**). There are several variants of pemphigus due to autoantibodies directed against the different desmosome constituents (especially desmogleins) and, since the resultant damage is at different levels within the epithelium, clinical manifestations may vary somewhat (**Fig. 48.2**). The main types are:

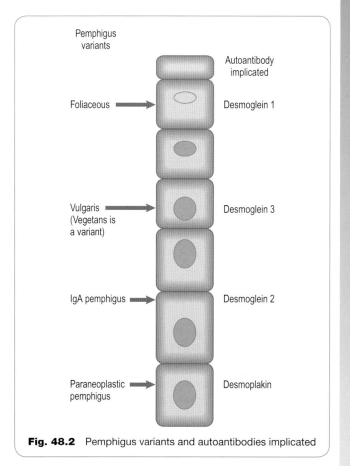

Fig. 48.2 Pemphigus variants and autoantibodies implicated

- Pemphigus vulgaris: the most common pemphigus variant, and the form responsible for most oral lesions seen – is associated with antibodies against desmoglein (Dsg) 3, a constituent of oral epithelial intercellular cement and, when there is skin involvement, also with anti-Dsg 1. Oral and skin lesions are inevitable. This type of pemphigus includes the uncommon variant pemphigus vegetans.
- Pemphigus foliaceus: skin lesions are invariable but oral lesions are rare, and the main antigen is Dsg 1. This type of pemphigus includes the uncommon variant pemphigus erythematosus (Senear–Usher syndrome).
- Paraneoplastic pemphigus: oral lesions are invariable but skin lesions are rare and the main antigen is distinct from Dsg. This type of pemphigus is seen in association with neoplasms such as lymphoproliferative disorders – lymphomas and Castleman disease (Ch. 56).

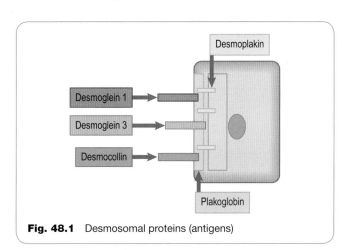

Fig. 48.1 Desmosomal proteins (antigens)

Pemphigus is one of the vesiculobullous disorders, along with for example, pemphigoid and erythema multiforme.

PEMPHIGUS VULGARIS

INCIDENCE

Pemphigus vulgaris is a rare disease.

Age

Pemphigus vulgaris is found mainly in middle-aged and older patients.

Gender

There is a female predisposition.

Geographic

Pemphigus vulgaris predominately occurs in middle-aged patients of Ashkenazi Jewish, Asian or Mediterranean descent.

PREDISPOSING FACTORS

- There is a fairly strong genetic background to pemphigus vulgaris, seen in people from the groups above, and an HLA association with HLA DRB1*04 and DRB1*14 alleles (and haplotypes DRB1*0402, 1401 and DQB1*0302, 1503).
- Some cases have been triggered by:
  - medications (captopril and penicillamine, which contain sulphydryl groups, and rifampicin and diclofenac (Table 54.14))
  - radiation
  - surgery
  - certain foods, such as garlic
  - emotional stress.

AETIOLOGY AND PATHOGENESIS

- Serum antibodies, mainly IgG (particularly IgG4 class) are directed predominantly against desmosomes in stratified squamous epithelia. Intercellular immune deposits (mainly IgG and C3), are detectable intraepithelially (**Fig. 48.3**).
- The antigen–antibody response on epithelial surfaces activates plasminogen to plasmin, leading to damage to desmosomal

cadherin-type epithelial cell adhesion molecules, particularly Dsg 3 and plakoglobin. This causes loss of cell–cell contact (acantholysis), and thus intraepithelial vesiculation (**Figs 48.4** and **48.5**).

- Since oral epithelium expresses largely Dsg 3, but skin expresses Dsg 1 as well as Dsg 3, damage by antibodies against Dsg 3 results in oral lesions at an early stage, whereas skin integrity is maintained by Dsg 1. However, if Dsg 1 antibodies appear, cutaneous lesions result and the disease tends to be more severe (**Table 48.1**).
- Other autoimmune diseases, such as myasthenia gravis and systemic lupus erythematosus, are occasionally associated.

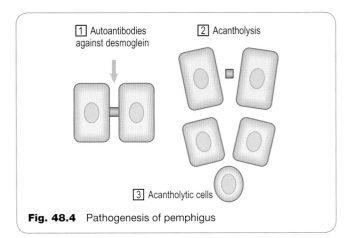

Fig. 48.4 Pathogenesis of pemphigus

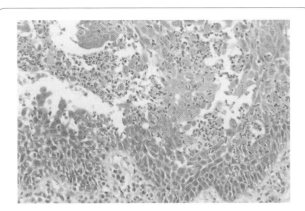

Fig. 48.5 Histopathology showing acantholysis in pemphigus with intra-epithelial vesiculation

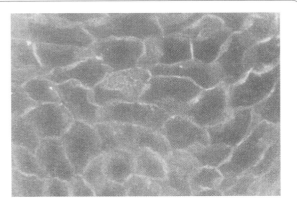

Fig. 48.3 Immunofluorescence in pemphigus showing intercellular antibodies directed against desmoglein

Table 48.1 Antibodies to desmogleins in pemphigus vulgaris

Pemphigus vulgaris lesions	Dsg 3	Dsg 1
Mucosal mainly	+	–
Mucocutaneous	+	+

CLINICAL FEATURES

Pemphigus vulgaris is the most severe form of pemphigus, and typically runs a chronic course, causing blisters and scabs on the skin and also blisters, erosions and ulcers on the mucosae of the:

- mouth
- pharynx
- larynx
- oesophagus
- nose
- conjunctiva
- anogenital region.

Pemphigus vulgaris often begins with blister formations (bullae) occurring in the mouth and on the scalp. The blisters are soft and are easily broken. The Nikolsky sign (the spreading of a blister by pressure) is positive.

Oral lesions in pemphigus vulgaris:

- are common
- may be an early manifestation
- may be the sole manifestation for a considerable time
- are vesiculobullous, but readily rupture, new bullae developing as the older ones rupture and ulcerate
- form erosions, which are irregular and initially red with a whitish surround (**Fig. 48.6**), but later are yellowish as a slough forms (**Fig. 48.7**)
- are seen mainly on the:
  - soft palate and posterior hard palate
  - buccal mucosa
  - lips
  - gingiva, where lesions usually comprise severe desquamative or erosive gingivitis; flaps of peeling tissue with red erosions or deep ulcerative craters are seen, mainly on the attached gingivae.

In the absence of systemic treatment, oral lesions are almost invariably followed by involvement of the skin (**Fig. 48.8**) or, occasionally, other epithelia, such as the oesophagus.

DIAGNOSIS

- The differential diagnosis for pemphigus often includes other pemphigus variants and:
  - pemphigoid
  - erythema multiforme and toxic epidermal necrolysis
  - pyostomatitis vegetans.

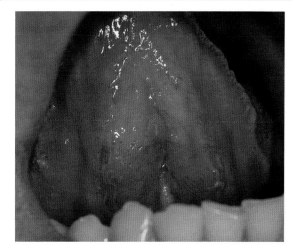

Fig. 48.7 Pemphigus; lesions become erosions with a yellowish slough

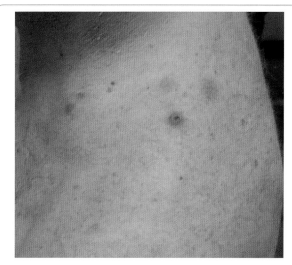

Fig. 48.8 Pemphigus skin lesions

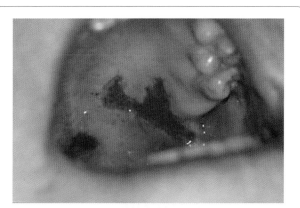

Fig. 48.6 Pemphigus; early red oral lesions

- A careful history and physical examination are important, but biopsy of perilesional tissue, with histological and immunostaining examination are essential (**Table 48.2**). Direct immunofluorescence microscopy (DIF) detects deposits at the epithelial cell surfaces. In paraneoplastic pemphigus, DIF usually reveals deposits at both the epithelial cell surfaces and the epithelial basement membrane zone. Serum should be collected for titres of antibody to epithelial intercellular cement, which may help guide treatment. Serum autoantibodies to Dsg are best detected using both normal human skin and monkey oesophagus by enzyme-linked immunosorbent assay (ELISA). The most specific serodiagnosis is using ELISA anti-dsg3. Indirect immunofluorescence microscopy (IIF) detects epithelial cell surface-binding autoantibodies. The titre of circulating autoantibodies corresponds to the severity of disease in pemphigus.

Table 48.2 Aids that might be helpful in diagnosis/prognosis/management in some patients suspected of having pemphigus*

In most cases	In some cases
Nikolsky sign Biopsy and immunofluorescence Dermatological/gynaecological opinion ELISA to desmogleins Full blood picture G6PD and TPMT levels Blood pressure Blood glucose DEXA (dual-emission X-ray absorptiometry)	Serum ferritin, vitamin B_{12} and corrected whole blood folate levels ESR

*See text for details and glossary for abbreviations.

- In addition to binding to squamous epithelial cell surfaces (e.g. skin, oesophagus substrates), circulating autoantibodies from patients with paraneoplastic pemphigus also label transitional epithelium (e.g. rat bladder).

TREATMENT (see also Chs 4 and 5)

Before the introduction of corticosteroids, pemphigus vulgaris typically was fatal – mainly from dehydration or secondary systemic infections. Pemphigus vulgaris remains a life-threatening disorder, though current treatment, largely based on systemic immunosuppression, has reduced the mortality significantly – to about 10% (**Table 48.3**). Specialist involvement and patient information are, thus, important. Patients with severe oral lesions should also be seen by a dermatologist and possibly:

Table 48.3 Regimens that might be helpful in management of patient suspected of having pemphigus

Regimen	Use in secondary care (severe oral involvement and/or extraoral involvement)
Likely to be beneficial	Corticosteroids Azathioprine Ciclosporin mofetil Mycophenolate Gold Dapsone Chlorambucil Cyclophosphamide Levamisole Intravenous immunoglobulins Immmunoadsorption
Unproven effectiveness	Anti-TNF drugs (sulfasalazine, pentoxifylline or thalidomide)
Emergent treatments	Rituximab
Supportive	Benzydamine Chlorhexidine Diet with little acidic, spicy or citrus content Lidocaine

Table 48.4 Monitoring protocol for patients with pemphigus on systemic corticosteroid therapy during the first 3 months of therapy

Daily	Weekly	Monthly
Diet low in sodium and carbohydrate	Clinical oral examination	Titre of serum antiepithelial antibodies
Blood pressure estimation	Body weight estimation	Blood glucose assay
Recording of symptomatology	Recording of symptomatology	DEXA (dual-emission X-ray absorptiometry)

- pulmonary specialist, for patients with paraneoplastic pemphigus, and particularly if the patients have symptoms or signs suggestive of respiratory difficulty
- gastroenterologist: to detect possible oesophageal involvement.

Systemic therapy, often with corticosteroids (e.g. prednisolone (enteric-coated) at least 60 mg/day) is usually essential, unless there are only localized oral lesions, when topical corticosteroids or intralesional corticosteroids may suffice for a time (**Table 48.4**). Once under control, the dosage of prednisolone can be tapered or adjuncts added, or immunoadsorption considered. Adjuncts or alternatives include are shown in **Table 48.3**. For recalcitrant pemphigus, peptide-based immunoadsorption (Globaffin adsorber system) can remove considerable amounts of the autoantibodies from the patient with significant and prolonged clinical benefit and minimal adverse effects.

It is thus usually possible to eventually induce complete and durable remissions, permitting systemic therapy to be safely discontinued without a flare in disease activity. The proportion of patients in whom this can be achieved increases steadily with time, and therapy can be discontinued in approximately 75% of patients after 10 years.

- Systemic manifestations of pemphigus must be given priority but dental professionals can help achieve and maintain oral health. Oral lesions are persistent, and are often recalcitrant even when cutaneous lesions are controlled by treatment. In these cases, oral care should include:
  - Good oral hygiene should be maintained; chlorhexidine or triclosan mouthwashes may help.
  - Antiinflammatory agents may help; there is a spectrum of topical agents, such as benzydamine, that may help.
- Topical corticosteroids typically a higher potency one such as fluocinonide or beclomethasone are required, moving to a super-potent topical corticosteroid, e.g. clobetasol, or oral use of prednisolone enema 20 mg in 100 mL if the benefit is inadequate (Tables 5.5 and 48.3).

EMERGENT TREATMENTS

Severe pemphigus may respond to rituximab.

FOLLOW-UP OF PATIENTS

Long-term follow-up in secondary care is appropriate.

PATIENT INFORMATION SHEET

Pemphigus

▼ Please read this information sheet. If you have any questions, particularly about the treatment or potential side-effects, please ask your doctor.
- This is a rare condition.
- It is an immunological disease, the immune reaction damaging the skin.
- It is most commonly seen in persons from around the Mediterranean.
- It is not usually inherited.
- Pemphigus is not known to be infectious.
- It affects the mouth, skin and other sites.
- Uncontrolled it is a very dangerous condition.
- Blood tests and biopsy are usually required.
- Strong drugs such as corticosteroids are normally needed to control pemphigus.
- Advice is available from:
  - Pemphigus Vulgaris Network, Flat C, 26 St. German's Road, London SE23 1RJ
  - National Pemphigus Vulgaris Foundation, PO Box 9606, Berkeley, CA 94709-0606, USA. Tel. (+ 1) 510 527 4970.

USEFUL WEBSITES

American Autoimmune Related Diseases Association:
http://www.aarda.org/
National Pemphigus Foundation: http://www.pemphigus.org/

FURTHER READING

Akman, A., Kacaroglu, H., Yilmaz, E., Alpsoy, E., 2008. Periodontal status in patients with pemphigus vulgaris. Oral Dis. 14, 640–643.

Amagai, M., 2000. Towards a better understanding of pemphigus autoimmunity. Br. J. Dermatol. 143, 237–238.

Beissert, S., Werfel, T., Frieling, U., et al., 2006. A comparison of oral methylprednisolone plus azathioprine or mycophenolate mofetil for the treatment of pemphigus. Arch. Dermatol. 142 (11), 1447–1454.

Black, M., Mignogna, M., Scully, C., 2005. Pemphigus. Oral Dis. 11, 119–130.

Bystryn, J.C., Jiao, D., 2006. IVIg selectively and rapidly decreases circulating pathogenic autoantibodies in pemphigus vulgaris. Autoimmunity 39 (7), 601–607.

Challacombe, S.J., Setterfield, J., Shirlaw, P., et al., 2001. Immunodiagnosis of pemphigus and mucous membrane pemphigoid. Acta Odontol. Scand. 59, 226–234.

Chams-Davatchi, C., Daneshpazhooh, M., 2005. Prednisolone dosage in pemphigus vulgaris. J. Am. Acad. Dermatol. 53 (3), 547.

Cozzani, E., Cacciapuoti, M., Parodi, A., et al., 2000. Desmosomes and their autoimmune pathologies. Eur. J. Dermatol. 10, 255–261.

Craythorne, E., du Viver, A., Mufti, G.J., Warnakulasuriya, S., 2011. Rituximab for the treatment of corticosteroid refractory pemphigus vulgaris with oral and skin manifestations. J. Oral Pathol. Med. 40 (8), 616–620.

Darling, M.R., Daley, T., 2006. Blistering mucocutaneous diseases of the oral mucosa – a review: part 2. Pemphigus vulgaris. J. Can. Dent. Assoc. 72 (1), 63–66.

Edelson, R.L., 2000. Pemphigus – decoding the cellular language of cutaneous autoimmunity. N. Engl. J. Med. 343, 60–61.

El Tal, A.K., Posner, M.R., Spigelman, Z., Ahmed, A.R., 2006. Rituximab: a monoclonal antibody to CD20 used in the treatment of pemphigus vulgaris. J. Am. Acad. Dermatol. 55 (3), 449–459.

el-Darouti, M., Marzouk, S., Abdel Hay, R., et al., 2009. The use of sulfasalazine and pentoxifylline (low-cost antitumour necrosis factor drugs) as adjuvant therapy for the treatment of pemphigus vulgaris: a comparative study. Br. J. Dermatol 161 (2), 313–319.

Eming, R., Rech, J., Barth, S., et al., 2006. Prolonged clinical remission of patients with severe pemphigus upon rapid removal of desmoglein-reactive autoantibodies by immunoadsorption. Dermatology 212 (2), 177–187.

Fatourechi, M.M., el-Azhary, R.A., Gibson, L.E., 2006. Rituximab: applications in dermatology. Int. J. Dermatol 45 (10), 1143–1155.

Femiano, F., Gombos, F., Nunziata, M., et al., 2005. Pemphigus mimicking aphthous stomatitis. J. Oral Pathol. Med. 34 (8), 508–510.

Femiano, F., Gombos, F., Scully, C., 2002. Pemphigus vulgaris with oral involvement; evaluation of two different systemic corticosteroid therapeutic protocols. J. Eur. Acad. Dermatol. Venereol. 16, 353–356.

Fortuna, G., Mignogna, M.D., 2011. Clinical guidelines for the use of adjuvant triamcinolone acetonide injections in oropharyngeal pemphigus vulgaris: the oral medicine point of view. J. Oral Pathol. Med. 40 (4), 359–360.

Harman, K.E., Gratian, M.J., Shirlaw, P.J., et al., 2002. The transition of pemphigus vulgaris into pemphigus foliaceus: a reflection of dermoglein 1 and 3 autoantibody levels in pemphigus vulgaris. Br. J. Dermatol. 146, 684–687.

Hertl, M., 2000. Humoral and cellular autoimmunity in autoimmune bullous skin disorders. Int. Arch. Allergy Immunol. 122, 91–100.

Iamaroon, A., Boonyawong, P., Klanrit, P., et al., 2006. Characterization of oral pemphigus vulgaris in Thai patients. J. Oral Sci. 48 (1), 43–46.

Kricheli, D., David, M., Frusic-Zlotkin, M., et al., 2000. The distribution of pemphigus vulgaris IgG subclasses and their reactivity with desmoglein 3 and 1 in pemphigus patients and their first-degree relatives. Br. J. Dermatol. 143, 337–342.

Kumaran, M.S., Kanwar, A.J., 2006. Efficacy of topical PGE2 in recalcitrant oral lesions of pemphigus vulgaris: a clinical trial. J. Eur. Acad. Dermatol. Venereol. 20 (7), 898–899.

Mignogna, M.D., Lo Muzio, L., Mignogna, R.E., et al., 2000. Oral pemphigus: long term behaviour and clinical response to treatment with deflazacort in sixteen cases. J. Oral Pathol. Med. 29, 145–152.

Niedermeier, A., Worl, P., Barth, S., et al., 2006. Delayed response of oral pemphigus vulgaris to rituximab treatment. Eur. J. Dermatol. 16 (3), 266–270.

Popovsky, J.L., Camisa, C., 2000. New and emerging therapies for diseases of the oral cavity. Dermatol. Clin. 18, 113–125.

Schmidt, E., Hunzelmann, N., Zillikens, D., et al., 2006. Rituximab in refractory autoimmune bullous diseases. Clin. Exp. Dermatol. 31 (4), 503–508.

Schmidt, E., Seitz, C.S., Benoit, S., et al., 2007. Rituximab in autoimmune bullous diseases: mixed responses and adverse effects. Br. J. Dermatol. 156 (2), 352–356.

Scully, C., Challacombe, S.J., 2002. Pemphigus vulgaris: update on etiopathogenesis, oral manifestations and management. Crit. Rev. Oral Biol. Med. 13, 397–408.

Sirois, D.A., Fatahzadeh, M., Roth, R., et al., 2000. Diagnostic patterns and delays in pemphigus vulgaris: experience with 99 patients. Arch. Dermatol. 136, 1569–1570.

Tabrizi, M.N., Chams-Davatchi, C., Esmaeeli, N., et al., 2007. Accelerating effects of epidermal growth factor on skin lesions of pemphigus vulgaris: a double-blind, randomized, controlled trial. J. Eur. Acad. Dermatol. Venereol. 21 (1), 79–84.

Vaillant, L., Huttenberger, B., 2005. Acquired bullous diseases of the oral mucosa. Rev. Stomatol. Chir. Maxillofac. 106 (5), 287–297.

Werth, V.P., Fivenson, D., Pandya, A.G., et al., 2008. Multicenter randomized, double-blind, placebo-controlled, clinical trial of dapsone as a glucocorticoid-sparing agent in maintenance-phase pemphigus vulgaris. Arch. Dermatol. 144 (1), 25–32.

Yeh, S.W., Sami, N., Ahmed, R.A., 2005. Treatment of pemphigus vulgaris: current and emerging options. Am. J. Clin. Dermatol. 6 (5), 327–342.

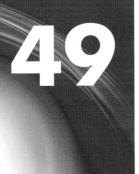

49 Salivary neoplasms

Key Points

- A wide range of different uncommon neoplasms can affect the salivary glands, but most are epithelial neoplasms, present as unilateral swelling of the parotid and are benign. The 'rule of nines' is an approximation that states that 9 out of 10 salivary gland tumours:
  - affect the parotid
  - are benign
  - are pleomorphic salivary adenomas (PSAs)
- Intra-oral salivary gland neoplasms are more likely to be malignant compared with those in major glands
- Treatment of all neoplasms is largely surgical

INTRODUCTION

The wide range of different neoplasms that can affect the salivary glands has been classified by the World Health Organization (**Box 49.1**). The epithelial neoplasms, which are the most important, can be memorized by the mnemonic 'A Most Acceptable Classification' – most are benign but some are malignant (**Tables 49.1** and **49.2**):

- **A**denomas: benign
- **M**ucoepidermoid tumour: intermediate level of malignancy (see below)
- **A**cinic cell tumour: intermediate malignancy (see below)
- **C**arcinomas such as adenoid cystic carcinoma, polymorphous low grade adenocarcinoma, and others.

Most salivary gland neoplasms are epithelial, presenting as a unilateral swelling of the parotid and most are benign (**Fig. 49.1**). This can be remembered by the 'rule of nines' (an approximation) that states that 9 out of 10 salivary gland neoplasms:

- affect the parotid
- are benign
- are pleomorphic salivary adenomas (PSAs).

The next most common neoplasm is carcinoma. Other neoplasms of major salivary glands are usually monomorphic adenomas (such as adenolymphomas), mucoepidermoid tumours or acinic cell tumours. Minor gland neoplasms are more often malignant (**Fig. 49.1**).

INCIDENCE

Salivary gland neoplasms are uncommon.

AGE

Most salivary gland neoplasms are seen in older people. In adults, 10–25% are malignant but in children, 50% are malignant.

GENDER

There is overall a female predisposition to salivary gland neoplasms.

GEOGRAPHIC

Salivary gland neoplasms are more common in certain geographical locations. Inuits, for example, have an increased prevalence.

PREDISPOSING FACTORS

There is a correlation between salivary gland and breast cancer.

AETIOLOGY AND PATHOGENESIS

The aetiology is largely unknown, but associations have included:

- Tobacco smoking: at least in Warthin tumour.
- Infections such as:
  - KSHV (Kaposi syndrome herpesvirus) infection or Epstein–Barr virus (EBV) infection in Warthin tumour
  - EBV infection, at least in salivary lymphoepithelial carcinomas in Asian patients and Inuits
  - SV40 (simian virus 40) infection, at least in pleomorphic salivary adenoma.
- Occupation: rubber manufacturing, plumbing industry, woodworking, hairdressing, mineral exposure (nickel, chromium, cement, asbestos, silica)
- Ionizing radiation exposure, as in:
  - survivors of the atomic explosions in Japan in 1945 (mucoepidermoid carcinomas, pelomorphic adenomas and Warthin tumours)
  - the use of iodine-131 in the treatment of thyroid disease
  - radiotherapy to the head and neck, including cranial irradiation
  - radiographs to the head and neck
  - exposure to ultraviolet radiation.

BOX 49.1 WHO classification of salivary gland tumours

Malignant epithelial tumours
- Acinic cell carcinoma   8550/3
- Mucoepidermoid carcinoma   8430/3
- Adenoid cystic carcinoma   8200/3
- Polymorphous low-grade adenocarcinoma   8525/3
- Epithelial-myoepithelial carcinoma   8562/3
- Clear cell carcinoma, not otherwise specified   8310/3
- Basal cell adenocarcinoma   8147/3
- Sebaceous carcinoma   8410/3
- Sebaceous lymphadenocarcinoma   8410/3
- Cystadenocarcinoma   8440/3
- Low-grade cribriform cystadenocarcinoma
- Mucinous adenocarcinoma   8480/3
- Oncocytic carcinoma   8290/3
- Salivary duct carcinoma   8500/3
- Adenocarcinoma, not otherwise specified   8140/3
- Myoepithelial carcinoma   8982/3
- Carcinoma ex pleomorphic adenoma   8941/3
- Carcinosarcoma   8980/3
- Metastasizing pleomorphic adenoma   8940/1
- Squamous cell carcinoma   8070/3
- Small cell carcinoma   8041/3
- Large cell carcinoma   8012/3
- Lymphoepithelial carcinoma   8082/3
- Sialoblastoma   8974/1

Benign epithelial tumours
- Pleomorphic adenoma   8940/0
- Myoepithelioma   8982/0
- Basal cell adenoma   8147/0
- Warthin tumour   8561/0
- Oncocytoma   8290/0
- Canalicular adenoma   8149/0
- Sebaceous adenoma   8410/0
- Lymphadenoma:
  - sebaceous   8410/0
  - non-sebaceous   8410/0
- Ductal papillomas:
  - inverted ductal papilloma   8503/0
  - intraductal papilloma   8503/0
  - sialadenoma papilliferum   8406/0
- Cystadenoma   8440/0

Soft tissue tumours
- Haemangioma   9120/0

Haematolymphoid tumours
- Hodgkin lymphoma
- Diffuse large B-cell lymphoma   9680/3
- Extranodal marginal zone B-cell lymphoma   9699/3

Secondary tumours
Morphology code of the International Classification of Diseases for Oncology (ICD-O) (821) and the Systematized Nomenclature of Medicine (http://snomed.org). Behaviour is coded /0 for benign tumours, /3 for malignant tumours and /1 for borderline or uncertain behaviour.

- Other radiation: concern about mobile telephones predisposing to epithelial parotid gland malignancy and mucoepidermoid carcinoma has not been resolved though they may almost double the risk of head tumours according to some studies.

Table 49.1 The more common benign salivary gland epithelial neoplasms

Neoplasm	Comment
Pleomorphic salivary adenoma (PSA)	Most common
Warthin tumour	Second most common benign neoplasm; associated with tobacco smoking; often multiple, sometimes bilateral; frequency increasing
Myoepithelioma	Rare
Basal cell adenoma	Older patients affected
Oncocytoma	Older patients affected May follow irradiation May be bilateral
Canalicular adenoma	Most common in upper lip, and in older patients

Table 49.2 The more common malignant salivary gland epithelial neoplasms

Neoplasm	Comment
Carcinoma ex-PSA	Variable prognosis
Acinic cell carcinoma	Mainly in parotid Poor prognosis
Mucoepidermoid carcinoma	Most common malignancy
Adenoid cystic carcinoma	Poor prognosis
Polymorphous low grade adenocarcinoma	Most are seen in palate; good prognosis
Epithelial-myoepithelial carcinoma	Most in major glands; variable prognosis

- Genetics:
  - genes expressed or altered in salivary neoplasms (**Table 49.3**) include particularly the PLAG1 (pleomorphic adenoma gene 1) on chromosome 8 and changes in 19p, particularly at 19p13 in PSAs
  - p53 and Mcm-2 in areas of malignant transformation in PSAs and recurrences
  - C-kit expression is common in salivary gland cancers
  - MECT1-MAML2 gene rearrangement is seen in most mucoepidermoid carcinomas with cyclic AMP response element-binding protein (CREB)-regulated transcription coactivator (CRTC1-MAML2) rearrangement in high-grade neoplasms
  - MYB-NFIB translocations have been identified in adenoid cystic carcinomas
  - ETV6-NTRK3 translocation is seen in mammary analogue secretory carcinoma, a newly described salivary gland neoplasm.

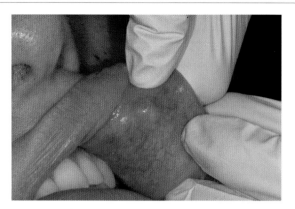

Fig. 49.1 Salivary neoplasm in lip

Table 49.3 Molecular changes in salivary gland neoplasms

	VEGFR	EGFR	HER-2	c-kit
Mucoepidermoid tumour	50%	40%	25%	rare
Adenocarcinoma	65	40	20	rare
Adenoid cystic carcinoma	85	20	rare	80

CLINICAL FEATURES

The main clinical feature of a neoplasm is salivary gland swelling (**Fig. 49.2**; see also Fig. 10.4). A swelling, especially if persistent, may be a neoplasm in the gland or in an intrasalivary lymph node. A history of gradual painless gland enlargement suggests a benign process. A malignant neoplasm may also be symptomless but is suggested by:

- facial palsy
- sensory loss
- pain
- difficulty swallowing
- trismus
- rapid growth.

Clinical examination may reveal an obvious swelling in the case of the parotid outlining the gland anteriorly to the ear, and causing eversion of the ear lobe. However, some neoplasms are small and the presentation may be of pain only.

The gland affected may be relevant:

- parotid neoplasms are largely PSAs
- submandibular gland neoplasms are also usually PSAs but malignant neoplasms contribute up to one-third of all submandibular neoplasms
- sublingual gland neoplasms are exceedingly rare, but virtually all are malignant
- minor salivary glands neoplasms are PSAs in around 50%, and most of the remainder are malignant, such as carcinomas and adenoid cystic carcinomas. Minor salivary gland neoplasms most commonly arise in the palate, but may be seen in the buccal mucosa or upper lip, rarely in the tongue or lower lip.

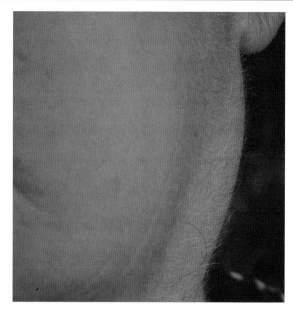

Fig. 49.2 Salivary gland (parotid) neoplasm

DIAGNOSIS

- A detailed history and examination are essential (**Table 49.4**).
- Ultrasonography (US) is diagnostically useful and readily available. Due to their relatively superficial anatomic location, distinct borders and homogenous echotexture, the major salivary glands are ideally positioned for ultrasonographic assessment, the advantages which include high diagnostic accuracy, non-invasiveness, lack of radiation exposure, as well as high reproducibility and low costs. Benign neoplasms are typically hypoechoic but with defined margins. Irregular shape, irregular borders, blurred margins and a hypoechoic inhomogeneous structure are suggestive of malignancy.
- Ultrasound-guided fine needle aspiration (US-FNA) cytology is almost invariably indicated since US alone cannot give equivocal results. However, negative or non-diagnostic cytologic results cannot always guarantee the lesion is benign; careful consideration of US features and cytological results is necessary to avoid false reassurance. Preoperative needle biopsy has a high neoplasm detection rate in experienced hands, more if ultrasound- or CT-guided, although some advocate leaving this until perioperatively if malignancy is likely, because neoplasm cells can be seeded in the needle track.

Table 49.4 Aids that might be helpful in diagnosis/prognosis/management in some patients suspected of having salivary neoplasm*

In most cases	In some cases
Ultrasound	Sialography
Biopsy	Full blood picture
MRI	Serum ferritin, vitamin B_{12} and corrected whole blood folate levels
	ESR

*See text for details and glossary for abbreviations.

- MRI particularly (or CT) is a sensitive means of neoplasm detection when US suggests a neoplasm or the result is equivocal. Reports are now emerging of the successful use of PET or PET/CT.
- Sialography may reveal a filling defect or gland displacement, but is a relatively imprecise and non-specific.

TREATMENT (see also Chs 4 and 5)

- Early detection carries the best prognosis.
- Surgical excision is the treatment of choice both for benign and malignant neoplasms; the main hazard is facial nerve damage and palsy. Even PSAs require early removal since, in a minority of cases, carcinoma arises (carcinoma ex-PSA).
- Some malignant salivary neoplasms, such as adenoid cystic carcinoma, invade bone and neural tissues preferentially and therefore wide excision is required.
- Radiotherapy is sometimes used as an adjunct postoperatively in treatment of malignant neoplasms where prognosis is poor, or for palliation. Adverse effects may cause hyposalivation, hearing loss, optic nerve damage and mastoiditis (Ch. 54).
- Chemotherapy has had some beneficial but transient effects, has not significantly increased survival, is usually palliative alone and has adverse effects (Ch. 54). Agents trialed have included cisplatin, carpboplatin, cyclophosphamide, epirubicin, gemcitabine, vinorelbine, mitoxantrone, doxorubicin, paclitaxel, and 5-fluorouracil as single agents or in various combinations.

EMERGENT THERAPIES

- Targetted therapies are emerging but thus far have failed to improve local control, or survival. Since C-kit is overexpressed in many salivary gland carcinomas, clinical trials with single-agent imatinib have been tried but proved negative. Bortezomib has been trialed but has not been reliably beneficial. Expression of epidermal growth factor receptor EGFR (ErbB1 and ErbB2) has provided a rationale for trials with trastuzumab, cetuximab, gefitinib, and lapatinib. Vascular endothelial growth factor (VEGF), might also be a sensible target (**Table 49.5**).

Table 49.5 Regimens that might be helpful in management of patient suspected of having salivary neoplasm

Regimen	Use in secondary care
Likely to be beneficial	Excision
Unproven effectiveness	Radiotherapy Chemotherapy
Emergent treatments	Bortezomib Cetuximab Dasatinib Gefitinib Lapatinib Trastuzumab

FOLLOW-UP OF PATIENTS

Long-term follow-up in secondary care is usually appropriate.

SPECIFIC SALIVARY GLAND NEOPLASMS

The more important neoplasms only are discussed here.

PLEOMORPHIC SALIVARY ADENOMA (PSA: MIXED SALIVARY GLAND TUMOUR)

PSA appears to originate from ductal epithelium, which proliferates to contribute to duct-like spaces, sheets of epithelial cells and sometimes areas of squamous metaplasia (**Fig. 49.3**). There are also areas reminiscent of connective tissue, such as cartilage. The admixture of epithelial elements with what resembles fibrous, myxoid or cartilage tissue, leads to the name 'mixed tumour'. These lesions usually have a thin fibrous capsule, but this is not complete and neoplastic cells may be seen in or outside the capsule. Various genetic abnormalities can be seen – especially involving chromosomes 8 and/or 12, and PLAG-1 and HMG1-C genes.

PSA is the most common salivary gland neoplasm, and:

- usually a slow-growing, lobulated, rubbery swelling with normal overlying skin, but a bluish appearance if intraoral
- usually benign. However, it recurs if excision is inadequate (around 3% recur in 5 years). The neoplasm is poorly encapsulated and parotid adenomas are in intimate relationship with the facial nerve, both of which make complete excision difficult to guarantee.

Malignant change in PSA (carcinoma ex-pleomorphic adenoma) is uncommon, and is actually a category of tumours rather than a single type – and there are both aggressive and indolent versions. These neoplasms should be:

- Further qualified as to type/grade of carcinoma and extent, since both intracapsular and minimally invasive neoplasms have a fair prognosis. Malignant change though uncommon, is suggested clinically by:
  - rapid growth
  - pain

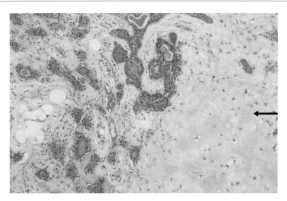

Fig. 49.3 Pleomorphic salivary adenoma with characteristic epithelial islets and chondroid matrix (arrowed)

■ fixation to deep tissues
■ facial palsy.

■ Malignant change is confirmed histopathologically by obvious malignant features within the benign cellular picture.

WARTHIN TUMOUR (PAPILLARY CYSTADENOMA LYMPHOMATOSUM OR ADENOLYMPHOMA)

Warthin tumour is found virtually only in the parotid, and:

■ is found mainly in smokers, in people with autoimmune disease, or those exposed to radiation
■ accounts for about 1:10 parotid neoplasms
■ is benign
■ is multiple in about 20% and bilateral in 5%
■ may rarely be associated with other salivary neoplasms such as PSA, or other malignant disease.

Columnar cells surround lymphocytes in a folded (papillary) lining to cystic spaces (**Fig. 49.4**). Chromosome 11q and 19p translocations may be present.

ONCOCYTOMA (ONCOCYTIC OR OXYPHIL ADENOMA)

Oncocytoma is exceedingly rare, and:

■ is found virtually only in the parotid
■ in 20% of cases is in people exposed to radiation
■ is extremely rare
■ affects mainly the older patient
■ is benign.

The characteristic of this neoplasm is that it consists of cords of large eosinophilic cells with small nuclei (oncocytes).

ADENOID CYSTIC CARCINOMA

Adenoid cystic carcinoma is rare and:

■ slow growing
■ malignant, with a tendency to infiltrate, spread perineurally and metastasize.

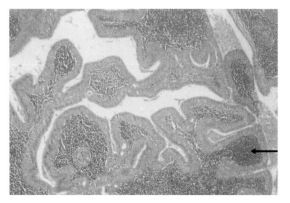

Fig. 49.4 Warthin tumour; papillary cystadenoma lymphomatosum (lymphocytes arrowed)

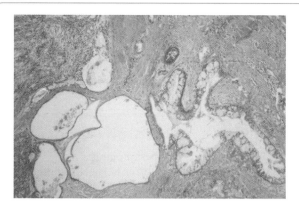

Fig. 49.5 Adenoid cystic carcinoma showing typical 'Swiss-cheese' appearance

Rounded islands of small darkly staining cells surrounding multiple clear areas of varying size (Swiss-cheese appearance) are characteristic (**Fig. 49.5**). Adenoid cystic carcinomas are graded based on pattern, with solid areas correlating with a worse prognosis. They occasionally transform to highly aggressive pleomorphic high-grade carcinomas with frequent nodal metastases. Chromosome 6q, 8q and 12q abnormalities may be present and several chromosome regions (e.g. 1p32-p36, 6q23-q27) are of prognostic interest.

ACINIC CELL TUMOUR

Acinic cell tumour is very rare, and:

■ is found virtually only in the parotid
■ is usually malignant, although all grades of malignancy have been reported and, although generally considered of low grade malignancy, they can recur, metastasize, or even prove lethal. Acinic cell tumours comprise large cells with a granular basophilic cytoplasm with spaces between some cells. The cells resemble serous cells of normal salivary glands. Aggressive histopathological parameters (anaplasia, necrosis, and mitoses) are predictive of poor outcome.

MUCOEPIDERMOID TUMOUR

Mucoepidermoid tumour accounts for up to 10% of salivary gland neoplasms, but is the most common childhood salivary neoplasm, and:

■ is slow-growing
■ is benign or of low-grade malignancy.

The mucoepidermoid tumour consists of large pale mucus-secreting cells (hence 'muco') surrounded by squamous epithelial cells (hence 'epidermoid') (**Fig. 49.6**). Chromosome 11q and 19p translocations may be present, with HER-2 gene overexpression. This neoplasms is graded using standard schemes in a 3-tier manner with the intermediate-grade category shows the most variability between grading systems and thus the most controversy in management. The

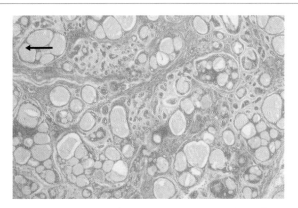

Fig. 49.6 Mucoepidermoid tumour; mucus-secreting cells arrowed

MECT1-MAML2 translocation t(11;19)(q21;p13) may prove to be an objective marker that can help to further stratify difficult cases.

NON-EPITHELIAL SALIVARY NEOPLASMS

- Malignant lymphomas are the next most common neoplasms found in salivary glands. Sjögren syndrome is recognized as predisposing to lymphomas. An intermediate stage between the salivary gland swelling in Sjögren syndrome and lymphomas is termed the 'benign lymphoepithelial lesion', a histological rather than a clinical condition. It has recently been suggested that the lymphoepithelial lesion represents a localized lymphomatous process.

  HIV disease also predisposes to lymphomas, mainly non-Hodgkin's lymphomas, which are Epstein–Barr virus-related (Ch. 53).

- Others (e.g. juvenile haemangioma).
- Secondary neoplasms.
- Unclassified neoplasms.
- Tumour-like lesions (benign lymphoepithelial lesion, sialosis, oncocytosis).

USEFUL WEBSITES

Medscape, Salivary Gland Neoplasms. http://emedicine.medscape.com/article/852373

FURTHER READING

Adelstein, D.J., Rodriguez, C.P., 2011. What is new in the management of salivary gland cancers? Curr. Opin. Oncol. 23 (3), 249–253.

Alterio, D., Jereczek-Fossa, B.A., Griseri, M., et al., 2011. Three-dimensional conformal postoperative radiotherapy in patients with parotid tumors: 10 years' experience at the European Institute of Oncology. Tumori 97 (3), 328–334.

Berrington de Gonzalez, A., Curtis, R.E., Kry, S.F., et al., 2011. Proportion of second cancers attributable to radiotherapy treatment in adults: a cohort study in the US SEER cancer registries. Lancet Oncol. 12 (4), 353–360.

Bradley, P., Huntinas-Lichius, O., 2011. Salivary Gland Disorders and Diseases: Diagnosis and Management. Thieme, Stuttgart.

Bradley, P., McClelland, L., Mehta, D., 2007. Paediatric salivary gland epithelial neoplasms. ORL J. Otorhinolaryngol. Relat. Spec. 69 (3), 137–145.

Brennan, P.A., Herd, M.K., Howlett, D.C., et al., 2012. Is ultrasound alone sufficient for imaging superficial lobe benign parotid tumours before surgery? Br. J. Oral Maxillofac. Surg. 50 (4), 333–337.

Burke, C.J., Thomas, R.H., Howlett, D., 2011. Imaging the major salivary glands. Br. J. Oral Maxillofac. Surg. 49 (4), 261–269.

Cavalcanti de Araújo, V., Orsini, Machado de Sousa, S., Carvalho, Y.R., Soares de Araújo, N., 2000. Application of immunohistochemistry to the diagnosis of salivary gland tumors. Appl. Immunohistochem. Mol. Morphol. 8 (3), 195–202.

Chen, C.H., Liu, B.Y., Wan, J.T., et al., 2001. Expression of epidermal growth factor in salivary gland adenoid cystic carcinoma. Proc. Natl. Sci. Counc. 25 (2), 90–96.

Chenevert, J., Barnes, L.E., Chiosea, S.I., 2011. Mucoepidermoid carcinoma: a five-decade journey. Virchows Arch. 458 (2), 133–140.

Cho, H.W., Kim, J., Choi, J., et al., 2011. Sonographically guided fine-needle aspiration biopsy of major salivary gland masses: a review of 245 cases. AJR Am. J. Roentgenol. 196 (5), 1160–1163.

Clauditz, T.S., Reiff, M., Gravert, L., et al., 2011. Human epidermal growth factor receptor 2 (HER2) in salivary gland carcinomas. Pathology 43 (5), 459–464.

Debaere, D., Vander Poorten, V., Nuyts, S., et al., 2011. Cyclophosphamide, doxorubicin, and cisplatin in advanced salivary gland cancer. B-ENT 7 (1), 1–6.

Duan, Y., Zhang, H.Z., Bu, R.F., 2011. Correlation between cellular phone use and epithelial parotid gland malignancies. Int. J. Oral Maxillofac. Surg. 40 (9), 966–972.

Elledge, R., 2009. Current concepts in research related to oncogenes implicated in salivary gland tumourigenesis: a review of the literature. Oral Dis. 15, 249–254.

Feinstein, T.M., Lai, S.Y., Lenzner, D., et al., 2011. Prognostic factors in patients with high-risk locally advanced salivary gland cancers treated with surgery and postoperative radiotherapy. Head Neck 33 (3), 318–323.

Geyer, J.T., Deshpande, V., 2011. IgG4-associated sialadenitis. Curr. Opin. Rheumatol. 23 (1), 95–101.

Gouveris, H., Lehmann, C.G., Heinrich, U.R., et al., 2011. Genomic changes in salivary gland pleomorphic adenomas detected by comparative genomic hybridization. Neoplasma 58 (2), 97–103.

Grimminger, C., Schmidt, M., Ahlbrecht, A., et al., 2011. Limitations of modern imaging techniques in detection of parotid carcinoma. J. Oral Maxillofac. Surg. 69 (6), 1826–1830.

Haddad, R.I., Colevas, A.D., Krane, J.F., et al., 2003. Herceptin in patients with advanced or metastatic salivary gland carcinomas. A phase II study. Oral Oncol. 39 (7), 724–727.

Hippocrate, A., Oussaief, L., Joab, I., 2011. Possible role of EBV in breast cancer and other unusually EBV-associated cancers. Cancer Lett. 305 (2), 144–149.

Hoffmann, M., Troch, M., Eidherr, H., et al., 2011. 90Y-ibritumomab tiuxetan (Zevalin) in heavily pretreated patients with mucosa associated lymphoid tissue lymphoma. Leuk. Lymphoma 52 (1), 42–45.

Hunt, J.L., 2011. An update on molecular diagnostics of squamous and salivary gland tumors of the head and neck. Arch. Pathol. Lab. Med. 135 (5), 602–609.

Iyer, N.G., Kim, L., Nixon, I.J., et al., 2010. Factors predicting outcome in malignant minor salivary gland tumors of the oropharynx. Arch. Otolaryngol. Head Neck Surg. 136 (12), 1240–1247.

Jeffers, L., Webster-Cyriaque, J.Y., 2011. Viruses and salivary gland disease (SGD): lessons from HIV SGD. Adv. Dent. Res. 23 (1), 79–83.

Laurie, S.A., Licitra, L., 2006. Systemic therapy in the palliative management of advanced salivary gland cancers. J. Clin. Oncol. 24 (17), 2673–2678.

Le Tourneau, C., 2010. Molecularly targeted therapy in head and neck cancer. Bull. Cancer 97 (12), 1453–1466.

Levis, A.G., Minicuci, N., Ricci, P., et al., 2011. Mobile phones and head tumours. The discrepancies in cause-effect relationships in the epidemiological studies – how do they arise? Environ. Health 10 (59).

Lim, J.J., Kang, S., Lee, M.R., et al., 2003. Expression of vascular endothelial growth factor in salivary gland carcinomas and its relation to p53, Ki-67 and prognosis. J. Oral Pathol. Med. 32 (9), 552–561.

Madani, G., Beale, T., 2006. Tumors of the salivary glands. Semin. Ultrasound CT MR 27 (6), 452–464.

Matthiesen, C., Thompson, S., Steele, A., et al., 2010. Radiotherapy in treatment of carcinoma of the parotid gland, an approach for the medically or technically inoperable patient. J. Med. Imaging Radiat. Oncol. 54 (5), 490–496.

Michelow, P., Dezube, B.J., Pantanowitz, L., 2012. Fine needle aspiration of salivary gland masses in HIV-infected patients. Diagn. Cytopathol 40 (8), 684–690.

Milano, A., Longo, F., Basile, M., et al., 2007. Recent advances in the treatment of salivary gland cancers: Emphasis on molecular targeted therapy. Oral Oncol. 43, 729–734.

Nutting, C.M., Morden, J.P., Harrington, K.J., et al., 2011. Parotid-sparing intensity modulated versus conventional radiotherapy in head and neck cancer (PARSPORT): a phase 3 multicentre randomised controlled trial. Lancet Oncol. 12 (2), 127–136.

O'Neill, I.D., 2008. New insights into the nature of Warthin's tumour. J. Oral Pathol. Med. 38 (1), 145–149.

O'Sullivan, E.M., Higginson, I.J., 2010. Clinical effectiveness and safety of acupuncture in the treatment of irradiation-induced xerostomia in patients with head and neck cancer: a systematic review. Acupunct. Med. 28 (4), 191–199.

Pederson, A.W., Salama, J.K., Haraf, D.J., et al., 2011. Adjuvant chemoradiotherapy for locoregionally advanced and high-risk salivary gland malignancies. Head Neck Oncol. 3 (1), 31.

Penner, C.R., Folpe, A.L., Budnick, S.D., 2002. C-kit Expression Distinguishes Salivary Gland Adenoid Cystic Carcinoma from Polymorphous Low-Grade Adenocarcinoma. Mod. Pathol. 15 (7), 687–691.

Raguse, J.D., Gath, H.J., Bier, J., et al., 2004. Docetaxel (Taxotere) in recurrent high grade mucoepidermoid carcinoma of the major salivary glands. Oral Oncol. 40 (2), 5–7.

Rutt, A.L., Hawkshaw, M.J., Lurie, D., Sataloff, R.T., 2011. Salivary gland cancer in patients younger than 30 years. Ear Nose Throat J. 90 (4), 174–184.

Scianna, J.M., Petruzzelli, G.J., 2007. Contemporary management of tumors of the salivary glands. Curr. Oncol. Rep. 9 (2), 134–138.

Seethala, R.R., 2011. Histologic grading and prognostic biomarkers in salivary gland carcinomas. Adv. Anat. Pathol. 18 (1), 29–45.

Soares, A.B., Altemani, A., de Araújo, V.C., 2011. Study of histopathological, morphological and immunohistochemical features of recurrent pleomorphic adenoma: an attempt to predict recurrence of pleomorphic adenoma. J. Oral. Pathol. Med. 40 (4), 352–358.

Stachiw, N., Hornig, J., Gillespie, M.B., 2010. Minimally-invasive submandibular transfer (MIST) for prevention of radiation-induced xerostomia. Laryngoscope 120 (Suppl. 4), S184.

Taylor, M.J., Serpell, J.W., Thomson, P., 2011. Preoperative fine needle cytology and imaging facilitates the management of submandibular salivary gland lesions. ANZ J. Surg. 81 (1–2), 70–74.

Thariat, J., Vedrine, P.O., Orbach, D., 2011. Salivary gland tumors in children. Bull. Cancer 98 (7), 847–855.

Vered, M., Dayan, D., 2007. Histochemical, immunohisto-chemical and cytogenetic markers in salivary gland tumor pathology. Future Oncol. 3 (1), 49–53.

Vissink, A., Mitchell, J.B., Baum, B.J., et al., 2010. Clinical management of salivary gland hypofunction and xerostomia in head-and-neck cancer patients: successes and barriers. Int. J. Radiat. Oncol. Biol. Phys. 78 (4), 983–991.

Sjögren syndrome

50

Key Points

- Sjögren syndrome (SS) is the association of dry mouth and dry eyes
- SS is an autoimmune disorder
- 90% of SS patients are older females
- Dry eyes and mouth alone are termed sicca syndrome or primary SS (SS-1)
- Dry eyes and mouth with a connective tissue disease are termed secondary SS (SS-2)
- Dry mouth predisposes to difficulties speaking and swallowing
- Complications may include caries, candidiosis and sialadenitis – and lymphoma
- Diagnosis is confirmed by detection of serum autoantibodies SS-A and SS-B, and other investigations. Diagnosis can be aided by ultrasound and a labial salivary gland biopsy
- Management is with sialogogues and salivary substitutes (mouth wetting agents) and preventive dentistry

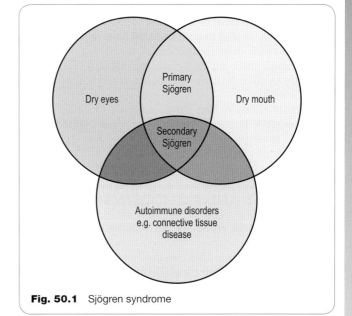

Fig. 50.1 Sjögren syndrome

INTRODUCTION

Sjögren syndrome (SS; Gougerot–Sjögren syndrome) is an autoimmune disorder in which immunocytes damage the salivary, lacrimal and other exocrine glands and is thus termed an autoimmune exocrinopathy. Dry mouth and dry eyes are seen with lymphoid infiltrates in these and other exocrine glands, and serum autoantibodies as discussed below (**Fig. 50.1**). SS has two major forms (**Table 50.1**):

- Primary Sjögren syndrome (SS-1): in which dry eyes and dry mouth are seen in the absence of a connective tissue disease. Uncommon and sometimes termed 'sicca syndrome', but the latter term is also used non-specifically for dry mouth and eyes.
- Secondary Sjögren syndrome (SS-2) is more common: dry eyes and dry mouth are seen together with other autoimmune diseases, usually primary biliary cirrhosis (PBC) or a connective tissue – most usually (in descending order of frequency):
  - rheumatoid arthritis (RA)
  - systemic lupus erythematosus
  - polymyositis
  - scleroderma
  - mixed connective tissue disease.

Table 50.1 Sjögren syndrome: comparison of subtypes

Feature	SS-1	SS-2
Connective tissue disease	–	+
Oral involvement	More severe	Less common
Ocular involvement	More common	Less common
Recurrent sialadenitis	More common	Less common
Lymphoma	More common	Less common
Main serum autoantibody	SS-B	SS-A

INCIDENCE

SS is uncommon, although the very rarity may lead to underdiagnosis.

AGE

SS can affect any age, but the onset is most common in middle-age or older.

321

GENDER

The majority of patients affected by SS are women.

GEOGRAPHIC

There is no known geographic incidence to SS.

PREDISPOSING FACTORS

See **Fig. 50.2**.

- Several genetic risk factors such as STAT-4 (signal transducer and activator of transcription 4), IRF (interferon responsive factor), ILT6 (immunoglobulin-like transcript 6) and the haplotype HLA-B8/DR3, especially with HLADRB1*15-DRB1*0301 have been identified in SS. People with SS also more commonly have family members with other autoimmune disorders.
- In addition, there are environmental risk factors, including possibly viral infections. A Sjögren-like syndrome can be produced by:
  - viruses (Epstein–Barr virus, hepatitis C virus, retroviruses (HIV, human T lymphotropic virus 1 (HTLV-1))).
  - IgG4 syndrome (see below)
  - graft-versus-host-disease (see Ch. 54)

AETIOLOGY AND PATHOGENESIS

Sjögren syndrome (SS) is an autoimmune epithelitis (exocrinopathy).

In animal models of SS, environmental triggers such as infection by Epstein–Barr virus (EBV) and/or oestrogen deficiency can lead to innate immune reactions followed by autoimmune epithelitis.

In humans, syndromes similar to SS can be produced by viruses as above – particularly in HTLV-I-associated myelopathy (HAM)). Viruses can induce expression of B cell activating factor (BAFF) by salivary gland epithelial cells via TLR (toll like receptor)- and IFN (interferon)-dependent and -independent pathways (see below).

In mice at least, IRF5 and STAT4 gene polymorphisms are involved in the activation of type I IFN pathways, the isolated stimulation of innate immunity resulting in dryness, which precedes lymphocytic infiltrates in salivary glands.

Immunologically-activated or apoptotic glandular epithelial cells might drive autoimmune-mediated tissue injury with upregulation of type I IFN-regulated genes, abnormal expression of B-cell-activating factor (BAFF) and activation of the interleukin IL-23-type 17 helper T cell pathway.

Endogenous LINE-1 (L1) retroelements may be potential triggers of type I IFN activation in SS, possibly through TLR dependent or independent pathways. Endogenous retroelements include human endogenous retroviruses (HERVs) which exist in an endogenous form, viral sequences being integrated into the human germ line and vertically transmitted, which probably represent footprints merged in the genome over 25 million years ago. It has been speculated that transcription of some HERV genes may lead to the expression of HERV proteins that may regulate the immune response, act as superantigens, or induce development of antibodies against them that might cross-react with self-proteins.

In SS, IFN-gamma is upregulated, and CD40 can be further induced by IFN-gamma and IL-1beta cytokines, but not by tumour necrosis factor-alpha (TNF-alpha), IL-4, IL-6, granulocyte-macrophage colony-stimulating factor (GM-CSF) or IFN-alpha.

The antigen CD40 is constitutively expressed by salivary ductal epithelial cells and endothelial cells and on infiltrating lymphocytes but not by acinar cells, myoepithelial cells or fibroblasts. CD40 enhances expression of adhesion molecule intercellular adhesion molecule-1 (ICAM-1)/CD54, but not MHC class I or class II (HLA-DR) molecules.

In SS, salivary glands express functional TLRs including TLR2, -3 and -4. TLR-induced signalling typically culminates in activation of NF-κB, mitogen-activated protein kinase (MAPK) pathways, IRF, as well as production of inflammatory and immune cytokines.

In SS, there may be intrinsic activation of epithelial cells through the MAP kinase pathway. Epidermal growth factor receptor (EGF-R) and Akt phosphorylation, and nuclear expression of NF-κB p65 are increased in salivary epithelial cells.

SS progresses through a number of stages:

- SS pathogenesis is related mainly to B cell dysregulation, in part, from the survival and activation of self-reactive B cells, which produce tissue-damaging pathogenic autoantibodies. Early hypergammaglobulinaemia and autoantibody production: serum autoantibodies (especially antinuclear antibodies SS-A (Ro) and SS-B (La)) are common in SS-1. In SS-2 antibodies are mainly against SS-B (La), ds DNA and other extractable nuclear antigens.
- Decreased salivary gland function with early periductal lymphocytic infiltration of the submandibular glands only, but antibody deposition in the submandibular and parotid glands.
- Lymphocytic infiltration of the submandibular, parotid and lacrimal glands with B and T (mainly CD4) lymphocytes and plasma cells causes progressive exocrine glandular acinar destruction along with interstitial lung disease and mild renal disease. CD166 (a ligand for CD6) is highly expressed on salivary epithelial cells, encouraging migration of CD27 memory B cells (Bm) into the glands. B cell-activating factor BAFF causes patients with primary SS to show an increase in Bm2 cells and a decrease in memory Bm5 cells in the salivary glands. The IFN-BAFF-B lymphocyte pathogenic axis is possibly pivotal: BAFF, a member of the TNF family, is a survival factor for peripheral B cells.
- Large B-cell lymphoma.

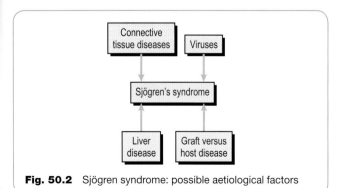

Fig. 50.2 Sjögren syndrome: possible aetiological factors

The autoimmune response in SS usually mainly affects exocrine glands, particularly the salivary, lacrimal, and vaginal. The epithelial cells in salivary glands of patients with SS are activated, bearing characteristics of antigen-presenting cells – inappropriate expression of class II HLA and co-stimulatory molecules. Salivary gland epithelial cells may participate in the development of the glandular inflammatory reactions via the expression and function of several TLR molecules. TLR-3 signalling pathway in the salivary epithelium appears to extend beyond the induction of innate immune responses and to involve the activation of programmed-cell death via anoikis. TLR signalling and antigen presentation may drive the autoimmune response and local autoantibody production in SS. Fragmentation of autoantigens such as La (SS-B) or alpha-fodrin during programmed cell death causes the redistribution of these autoantigens, leading to the production of the autoantibodies (**Fig. 50.3**).

The autoantibodies found in SS are commonly against ribonucleoproteins, especially Sjögren syndrome-A (termed SS-A or Ro), and SS-B (or La autoantibodies). There may also be other autoantibodies (e.g. alpha-fodrin, alpha-amylase, muscarinic M3 receptor, carbonic anhydrase, actin, salivary duct).

There is periductal infiltration initially mainly by B but later mainly by T lymphocytes (**Fig. 50.4**). One theory is that SS is caused by a deficiency of suppressor T lymphocytes and subsequent overactivity of B-lymphocytes, with release of interleukin-10 (IL-10), production of type I IFN and inflammatory cytokines and the production of autoantibodies. The interferon-inducible Ifi-200/HIN-200 gene family proteins are regulators of cell proliferation and differentiation involved in both the apoptotic and inflammatory processes.

Activated CD4+ T helper type 1 (Th1) lymphocytes, B-cells, macrophages and dendritic cells, as well as a network of cytokines including interferon-γ (IFNγ), TNF-α and interleukin (IL)1β, cause tissue destruction and dysfunction and IL-6 often acts as the end stage effector cytokine in this cascade. Interleukin-6 is upregulated in serum, peripheral circulating lymphocytes and saliva of SS patients, and significantly correlates with the degree of infiltration in the gland and the number of extra-glandular features.

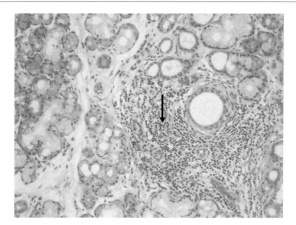

Fig. 50.4 Sjögren syndrome: histopathology showing dense lymphocytic periductal infiltrate (focal sialadenitis) (arrowed)

The distribution of the membrane pore channel (water channel) protein aquaporin-5 is abnormal in SS, perhaps as a result of paracrine effect of TNF-alpha, and the neurogenic regulation of the salivary gland also becomes impaired (**Fig. 50.5**). Anti-muscarinic 3 receptor antibody plays an important role in cholinergic hyper-responsiveness in SS.

There is lymphocyte-mediated destruction of exocrine glandular acini but, although the gland acini atrophy, the duct epithelium tends to persist and proliferates – sometimes to the extent that the duct lumens may become obliterated, producing islets of epithelium known as 'epimyoepithelial islands'.

The fully developed lesion of SS in major glands thus appears as a dense mass of lymphocytes interspersed by islands of epithelium, a pattern termed the 'benign lymphoepithelial lesion' (BLL). Occasionally, BLL exists in the absence of serological and other features of SS.

B-cell lymphoproliferation may eventually lead to pseudolymphoma or even true lymphoma (**Fig. 50.6**).

CLINICAL FEATURES

The early manifestations may be non-specific, such as fatigue, arthralgia, and Raynaud phenomenon, and it can be 8–10 years from the initial symptoms to full-blown disease. SS ultimately presents with a clinical spectrum that ranges from an organ-specific autoimmune process to a systemic disorder (**Box 50.1**). Other autoimmune disorders associated with SS may include systemic lupus erythematosus, scleroderma, mixed connective tissue disease, primary biliary cirrhosis, hyperthyroidism (Graves disease) or hypothyroidism (Hashimoto thyroiditis). Mothers with SS can pass autoantibodies across the placenta into the foetal circulation – leading to foetal heart block.

Features of SS may include:

■ Eye complaints, including sensations of grittiness, soreness, itching, dryness, blurred vision or light intolerance. The eyes may be red with infection of the conjunctivae and soft crusts at the angles (keratoconjunctivitis sicca). The lacrimal glands may swell.

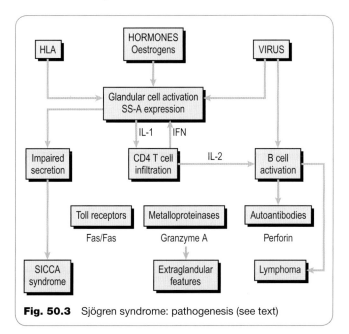

Fig. 50.3 Sjögren syndrome: pathogenesis (see text)

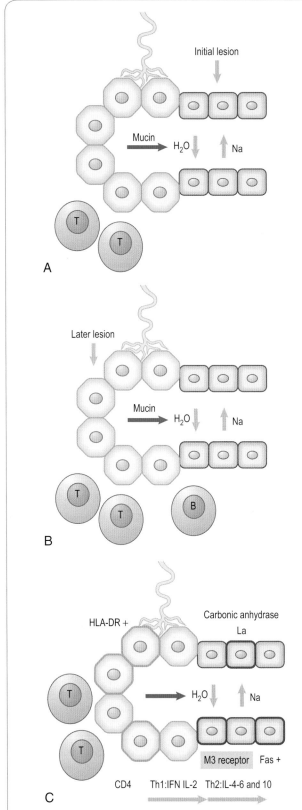

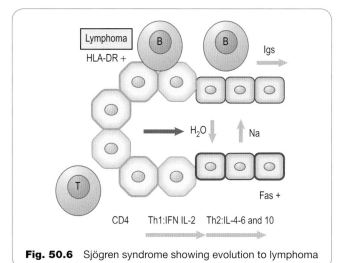

Fig. 50.6 Sjögren syndrome showing evolution to lymphoma

BOX 50.1   Sjögren syndrome main features

Oral signs and symptoms
- Dry mouth
- Cracker sign
- Burning
- Salivary swelling and sialadenitis
- Caries
- Candidosis
- Abnormal taste
- Malodour

Ocular signs and symptoms
- Foreign body sensation
- Inability to tear
- Light intolerance

Others
- Fatigue
- Fever
- Kidney, muscle, nerve, liver, joint, thyroid involvement
- Connective tissue disease

Fig. 50.5 Sjögren syndrome showing evolution of salivary lesion

- Oral complaints (often the presenting feature), include:
  - xerostomia: often the most frequent and obvious clinical component, although not all patients complain of dry mouth (**Fig. 50.7**) – and some may have obvious hyposalivation
  - soreness or burning sensation
  - difficulty eating dry foods, such as biscuits (the cracker sign)
  - difficulties in controlling dentures
  - difficulties in speech: there may be a clicking quality of the speech as the tongue tends to stick to the palate
  - difficulties in swallowing
  - complications such as unpleasant taste or loss of sense of taste; oral malodour; caries; candidosis; sialadenitis.

Oral and salivary gland examinations are important. The mouth may appear dry, and on examination there may be objective:

- hyposalivation
- tendency of the mucosa to stick to a dental mirror

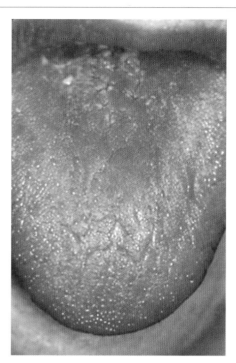

Fig. 50.7 Sjögren syndrome showing dry mouth

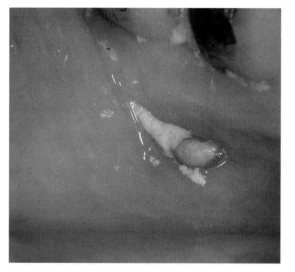

Fig. 50.8 Sjögren syndrome showing food residues in vestibule

- food residues (**Fig. 50.8**)
- lack of salivary pooling
- frothiness of saliva and absence of frank salivation from major gland duct orifices
- a characteristic tongue appearance; lobulated, usually red, surface with partial or complete depapillation
- in advanced cases – obviously dry and glazed oral mucosae.

ORAL COMPLICATIONS

- Unpleasant taste, or loss of sense of taste.
- Malodour.

- Candidosis: common and may cause soreness and redness of the oral mucosa or angular cheilitis.
- Dental caries: tends to be severe, affect smooth surfaces and is difficult to control.
- Ascending (suppurative) sialadenitis is a hazard.
- Salivary gland enlargement:
  - usually caused by the SS inflammatory process
  - if intermittent may be caused by bacterial ascending infection (acute sialadenitis; **Fig. 50.9**)
  - occasionally is massive and associated with enlargement of the regional lymph nodes, a condition called 'pseudolymphoma'
  - rarely is due to true lymphoma (see below).
- Extraoral (extra-glandular) complications of SS (**Fig. 50.10**):
  - connective tissue disease in SS usually precedes the onset of dry eyes and dry mouth, and, therefore, patients presenting with dry eyes and dry mouth alone probably have primary SS, unless a connective tissue disease manifests within about 1 year
  - Raynaud phenomenon (Ch. 57)
  - arthralgia
  - myalgia
  - fatigue
  - skin ulceration or rash
  - dyspnoea
  - dry vagina
  - bruising, bleeding and purpura
  - numbness and other neurological features, including orofacial sensory loss, orofacial pain or facial palsy, and other cranial neuropathies.
- Associations of SS can include:
  - other autoimmune diseases (see above)
  - gastro-oesophageal reflux disease (GORD)
  - sarcoidosis occasionally.

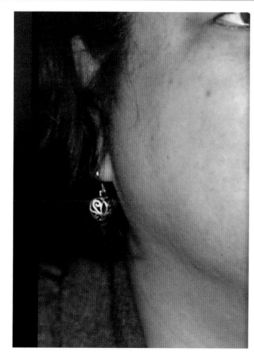

Fig. 50.9 Sjögren syndrome showing salivary swelling

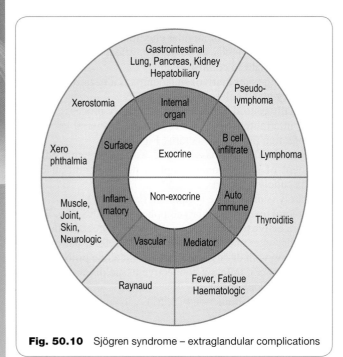

Fig. 50.10 Sjögren syndrome – extraglandular complications

Lymphoproliferative diseases in SS are mostly seen in primary SS, as B-cell lymphoproliferation in mucosal-associated lymphoid tissue (MALT) and may manifest as a pseudolymphoma, or can develop into monoclonal gammopathies (such as Waldenstrom's macroglobulinaemia); free light chains; mixed monoclonal cryoglobulins; non-Hodgkin lymphoma of the diffuse large B-cell type, or extranodal marginal zone B-cell lymphomas of the mucosa-associated lymphoid tissue type.

- Patients with SS have a 15–40-fold increased risk of the development of B-cell non-Hodgkin lymphoma. This is <1 case per 100 patients per year; 2% of cases at 5 years and up to 5% of cases with time.

- Genotypic studies of lymphomas have documented immunoglobulin gene rearrangement across the full spectrum of lymphoid infiltrates in the salivary gland including:
  - reactive lymphoepithelial sialadenitis (LESA)
  - borderline cases with halos of monocytoid cells surrounding epimyoepithelial islets
  - cases with fully developed marginal zone lymphoma (MZL).
- Most lymphomas complicating SS arise in mucosal extranodal sites, especially the salivary glands.
- Most lymphomas are low-grade marginal zone B-cell lymphoma with long-term survival.
- MZL is diagnosed from broad strands of monocytoid B-cells surrounding and invading epimyoepithelial islets, and monotypic immunoglobulin expression.
- The treatment and prognosis of SS lymphoma depends on the lymphoma type and stage.
- Lymphomas may be most likely where there is severe clinical disease and if there has been cytotoxic chemotherapy or salivary irradiation. Pseudolymphoma or frank lymphoma should be suspected when there is:
  - persistent salivary gland enlargement
  - lymphadenopathy
  - hepatosplenomegaly (**Table 50.2**).

Lymphomas may be predicted if there are features such as:

- fevers
- palpable purpura
- leg ulcers
- peripheral neuropathy
- lymphopenia with low CD4 counts
- hypocomplementaemia
- cryoglobulinaemia.

Benign lymphoepithelial lesions of the salivary glands do not necessarily require surgical treatment. For lymphomas, an oncological opinion is indicated; chemotherapy or rituximab may be required. Lymphomas have also been treated with radioimmunotherapy using (90)Y-ibritumomab tiuxetan.

Table 50.2 Features of lymphoproliferation in Sjögren syndrome

Features	Pseudolymphoma	Lymphoma
Parotid swelling	+	+
Lymphadenopathy	+	+
Hepatosplenomegaly	+	+
Vasculitis	+	+
Pulmonary infiltrates	+	+
Others	−	Fever Leg ulcers Palpable purpura Peripheral neuropathy
Laboratory findings	Hypergammaglobulinaemia	Hypergammaglobulinaemia Anaemia Hypocomplementaemia (low C3 and low C4) Lymphopenia (low CD4 counts and CD4/CD8 ratio) Mixed cryoglobulinaemia

IgG4 SYNDROME

Mikulicz disease (MD) was the term given to the condition of persistent salivary and lacrimal gland enlargement. Many cases previously classified as Mikulicz disease, Küttner tumour, and orbital pseudotumour (idiopathic orbital inflammation) show increased numbers of IgG4-positive plasma cells, and some also show elevated levels of serum IgG4, supporting the evolving concept of IgG4-associated sialadenitis/dacroadenitis.

IgG4 syndrome presents with enlargement of one of more salivary gland(s) and/or lacrimal gland(s). Histologically it is characterized by a dense polyclonal lymphoplasmacytic infiltrate, often associated with germinal centres, fibrosis and obliterative phlebitis. IgG4-bearing plasma cells are nearly always present, as is an increased ratio of IgG4 to IgG containing plasma cells. Serum immunoglobulin IgG4 is raised. Complications include multifocal fibrosclerosing disease with autoimmune pancreatitis, retroperitoneal fibrosis, tubulointerstitial nephritis, autoimmune hypophysitis and Riedel thyroiditis.

In IgG4 syndrome compared to SS, the incidence of dry eyes, dry mouth and arthralgias is lower, while allergic rhinitis, bronchial asthma, sclerosing pancreatitis, interstitial nephritis and interstitial pneumonitis are more common; IgG4 syndrome is *not* associated with anti-Ro/SS-A and anti-La/SS-B autoantibodies; and only a few patients have RF and ANA (low serum titres). There is good responsiveness to systemic corticosteroids or anti-CD20 (rituximab).

DIAGNOSIS OF SJOGREN SYNDROME

A subjective feeling of dry mouth (xerostomia) is common in the general population, although reduced salivary flow (hyposalivation) is not always confirmed by objective studies (see Ch. 8). Indeed, of older people, some 16–25% complain of xerostomia – usually caused by drugs. SS is one cause of hyposalivation. The diagnosis of SS is confirmed mainly from the history, clinical examination and investigation findings including:

- ocular symptoms
- oral symptoms
- ocular signs
- autoantibodies and other blood tests
- salivary gland studies (**Table 50.3**).

The American–European diagnostic criteria (revised) for Sjögren syndrome are shown in **Box 50.2**. If SS is suspected and there is objective hyposalivation, specialist referral is warranted since a range of investigations may be needed (**Table 50.4**), as the differential diagnosis may include:

- Viral infections:
  - hepatitis C virus
  - HIV
  - HTLV-1
  - EBV
  - sarcoidosis
  - IgG4 syndrome
- Glandular deposits in:
  - haemochromatosis
  - lipoproteinaemias
  - amyloidosis
  - lymphomas.

AUTOANTIBODIES AND OTHER BLOOD TESTS

Blood tests may be indicated to:

- Examine for SS-A and SS-B, which may have diagnostic value in patients with unexplained parotid swelling and may antedate clinical evidence of SS by months or years. SS-A/Ro and La/SS-B are the hallmark antibodies in primary SS, are present in 60–70%, associated with an earlier disease onset, glandular dysfunction and extraglandular manifestations as well as with other B cells activation markers. Autoantibody assays can be extremely helpful in diagnosis, and are readily available, inexpensive and fairly non-invasive.
- Assess ESR, CRP or PV (raised in SS).
- Exclude similar syndromes seen in IgG4 syndrome (raised IgG4 levels), sarcoidosis (raised SACE levels) and infections (e.g. hepatitis C virus, EBV, HTLV-1 or HIV) (serologically tested).
- Exclude anaemia (common in rheumatoid arthritis and SS).
- Examine for CD4 levels, serum complement and immunoglobulin levels, cryoglobulins and monoclonal immunoglobulins (may help lymphoma prediction).

Table 50.3 Main investigations in Sjögren syndrome

Investigation	Typical findings	Comments
Sialometry	Reduced salivary flow rate	Non-specific, but non-invasive, readily available and often used
Lacrimal flow	Reduced on Schirmer test	Non-specific, but non-invasive, readily available and often used
Autoantibodies	ANA SS-A SS-B	Non-invasive, readily available and often used
Ultrasonography	Hypoechogenicity	Non-invasive, readily available and often used
Salivary gland biopsy	Focal lymphocytic infiltrate Acinar atrophy Fibrosis	More specific, invasive, readily available and sometimes used
Sialography	Sialectasis	Non-specific, but often available though uncommonly used

---

BOX 50.2 Sjögren syndrome revised American–European diagnostic criteria*

SS is diagnosed if 4 of these 6 criteria are positive (especially if histopathology and serology are positive) or if there are ocular symptoms or oral symptoms, plus any 2 of the other 4 criteria.

I. Ocular symptoms
At least one of these 3:
- daily persistent troublesome dry eyes for >3 months
- recurrent sensation of sand or gravel
- need to use teardrops >3 times daily

II. Oral symptoms
At least one of these 3:
- daily feeling of dry mouth >3 months
- recurrent or persistently swollen salivary glands as adult
- frequently drink liquids to aid swallowing dry foods

III. Ocular signs
At least one of these 2:
- Schirmer <5mm in 5 min
- Rose–Bengal score >4 on van Bijsterveld scoring

IV. Histopathology
- Focus score >1 on LSG†

V. Salivary gland involvement
At least one of these abnormal:
- unstimulated whole salivary flow <1.5mL in 15 min
- sialography: diffuse sialectasis
- scintigraphy: reduced concentration/uptake/excretion

VI. Serum autoantibodies
At least one of these:
- SS-A (Ro)
- SS-B (La)

Revised rules for classification
For primary SS
In patients without any potentially associated disease, primary SS may be defined as follows:
a. The presence of any 4 of the 6 items is indicative of primary SS, as long as either item IV (histopathology) or VI (serology) is positive
b. The presence of any 3 of the 4 objective criteria items (that is, items III, IV, V, VI)
c. The classification tree procedure represents a valid alternative method for classification, although it should be more properly used in clinical-epidemiological survey

For secondary SS
In patients with a potentially associated disease (for instance, another well defined connective tissue disease), the presence of item I or item II plus any 2 from among items III, IV, and V may be considered as indicative of secondary SS.

Exclusion criteria:
- Past head and neck radiation treatment
- Hepatitis C infection
- Acquired immunodeficiency syndrome (AIDS)
- Pre-existing lymphoma
- Sarcoidosis
- Graft-versus-host disease
- Use of anticholinergic drugs (since a time shorter than 4-fold the half life of the drug)

*Focus = cluster of 50 or more lymphocytes in a labial salivary gland (LSG).
† Focus score = average number of foci in a 4mm² area.

Table 50.4 Aids that might be helpful in diagnosis/prognosis/management in some patients suspected of having Sjögren syndrome*

In most cases	In some cases
Sialometry	Sialography
Ultrasonography or MRI	Salivary scinitiscanning
Antinuclear antibodies (ANA)	Salivary gland biopsy
SS-A and SS-B antibodies	Rheumatological opinion
Rheumatoid factor (RF)	Urinalysis
Serum immunoglobulin levels	Full blood picture
Serum immunoglobulin IgG4 levels	Serum ferritin, vitamin B_{12} and corrected whole blood folate levels
Serum complement	ESR
CD4 counts	Serology, viral (HCV, HIV, HTLV-1, EBV)
Cryoglobulins	Blood glucose
Eye tests, e.g. Schirmer	Chest radiography
Ophthalmological opinion	Serum angiotensin-converting enzyme (SACE)
	Serum calcium and phosphate

*See text for details and glossary for abbreviations.

SALIVARY GLAND STUDIES

Salivary gland functional studies such as sialometry, and ultrasound may be indicated (**Box 50.2**, **Table 50.3**, **Algorithms 50.1** and **50.2**). Biopsy, sialography and scintigraphy are occasionally used

Salivary flow measurements (sialometry)

Objective evidence of diminished salivary flow includes a:

- decreased resting secretion rate of whole saliva <1.5mL in 15min: this is more closely associated with symptoms of xerostomia than are stimulated flow rates
- decreased stimulated flow rate.

Ultrasonography

This is proving to be useful for evaluating salivary gland disease and may replace other diagnostic techniques, such as sialography or salivary scintigraphy as it is inexpensive and non-invasive. The diagnosis is considered positive for SS if the major glands show hypoechoic areas, echogenic streaks and/or irregular gland margins on US. It is also helpful in excluding lymphoma.

Salivary gland biopsy

Biopsy of salivary glands in the diagnosis of SS can show focal sialadenitis – the characteristic histopathological feature. LSG histology, if used with a focus score (FS), provides a reproducible and objective evaluation of severity of inflammation. A focus is defined as an aggregate containing 50 or more mononuclear cells; the FS is the number of such aggregates in each 4mm² area. The mononuclear cells are predominantly T-helper inducer cells. The FS is reliable only where gland lobes with acinar atrophy and interstitial fibrosis are excluded, and where an adequately large specimen is examined. The threshold FS generally used for diagnosis of SS is one focus per 4mm², though others use slightly higher thresholds. Other

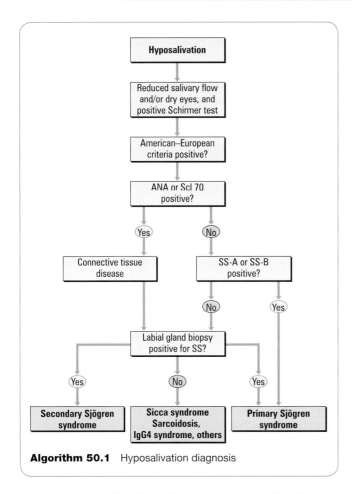

Algorithm 50.1 Hyposalivation diagnosis

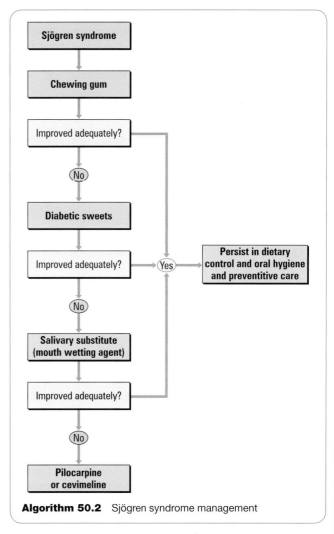

Algorithm 50.2 Sjögren syndrome management

features such as fibrosis or fatty atrophy, duct dilatation and hyperplasia, however, are non-specific.

Focal sialadenitis in an adequate LSG biopsy (at least 4–5 lobules) appears to be sensitive and disease-specific but invasive and controversial: quantitative immunohistochemistry (QIH) may be helpful in lymphoma prediction.

Sialography

Sialography in SS may show peripheral sialectasis; this is the most typical finding, it is most sensitive using oil-based contrast media and is seen particularly in parotid glands, may correlate with histological scores and scintigraphy, but is not universally employed.

Salivary scintiscanning

Salivary scanning (scintigraphy) may in SS show diminished radionuclide uptake and spontaneous secretion, or reduced secretion following citric acid or pilocarpine stimulation. Changes correlate with sialographic, flow rate and LSG histological changes, but are non-specific and so it is uncommonly used. Quantitative registration of uptake and secretion phases with correction for vascular background might improve the diagnostic and monitoring value of salivary scintigraphy.

Magnetic resonance imaging

MRI can be helpful in quantifying glandular parenchyma according to the size of nodules, ducts, and cavities structure and functional glandular changes using diffusion-weighted MR imaging and dynamic MR sialography.

Sialochemistry

Analysis of saliva composition (sialochemistry) for the diagnosis and monitoring of salivary disease has had some enthusiastic proponents, but has been of no real practical value. It could prove to be of value in monitoring the disease process in view of the non-invasive nature. The diagnostically and prognostically most promising recent sialochemical findings in SS have been of raised levels of:

- lactoferrin
- beta$_2$-microglobulin
- interleukin-6
- lysozyme
- sodium, chloride, albumin, IgA and IgG (however, these are non-specific and rarely correlate with salivary flow or histological changes).

TREATMENT (see also Chs 4 and 5)

- Sjögren syndrome remains an incurable condition, since no therapeutic modality has been identified that reliably modifies the course of the disease, but emergent treatments may change this (see below).
- Patient information is an important aspect in management.

- A specialist physician or rheumatologist should be referred to when the patient who suffers any connective tissue or other systemic disorders. Patients with severe extraglandular manifestations are usually treated by a physician with systemic corticosteroids, hydroxychloroquine and other immunosuppressive drugs.
- A specialist ophthalmologist should be referred when the patient who has dry eyes, ocular involvement being assessed by:
  - Schirmer test for lacrimal flow
  - tear break-up time
  - corneal abrasions (stain with rose Bengal)
  - methylcellulose eye drops or, ligation or cautery of the nasolacrimal duct may be appropriate care.
- Other aspects of care include the following, for which the dental professional is the expert (**Table 50.5**):
  - for care of a dry mouth it can be helpful for the patient to: sip water or other fluids throughout the day; protect the lips with lip salve; take small bites of food; eat slowly; eat soft, creamy foods (casseroles, soups) or cool foods with a high liquid content (melon, ice cream); and to moisten foods with water, gravies, sauces, extra oil, dressings, sour cream, mayonnaise or yoghurt
  - it is wise for the patient to avoid: mouth-breathing; any drugs that may produce hyposalivation (e.g. tricyclic antidepressants); alcohol (including in mouthwashes); smoking; caffeine (coffee, some soft drinks); dry foods, such as biscuits (or moisten in liquid first); spicy foods; and oral healthcare products containing sodium lauryl sulphate, which may irritate the mucosa. A humidifier may also help
  - mouth wetting agents (salivary substitutes) may help symptomatically. Various apart from water, those that are available, include: methylcellulose; Saliva Orthana and Oralbalance are particularly useful since they contain fluoride (e.g. Glandosane or Luborant) (see Ch. 5), or

mucin. However, there may be religious or cultural objections to use of mucin by some Muslims, Hindus, Jews and Rastafarians
  - salivation may be stimulated by using: chewing gums (containing xylitol or sorbitol, not sucrose); diabetic sweets; cholinergic drugs, such as pilocarpine or cevimeline that stimulate salivation (sialogogues) – which should be used by the specialist as discussed in Ch. 8; and transglossal electrical stimulation.
- Oral complications should be avoided or managed by:
  - avoiding sugary foods
  - keeping the mouth clean
  - using fluorides and amorphous calcium phosphate (ACP)
  - using mouthwashes of chlorhexidine.
- Dental caries is best controlled by dietary control of sucrose intake, and the daily use of fluorides as toothpastes, mouthwashes and gels (1% sodium fluoride gels or 0.4% stannous fluoride gels).
- Candidosis may cause soreness or burning and, thus, should be treated with antifungals until there is neither erythema nor symptoms. Topical antifungals in liquid form, such as nystatin suspension, are the most effective and acceptable. Other preparations such as miconazole are also effective. Fluconazole, itraconazole and posaconazole are available as suspensions effective against oropharyngeal candidosis, and voriconazole as a liquid – preparations which may find favour for use in patients with SS. Dentures should be left out of the mouth at night and stored in sodium hypochlorite solution, chlorhexidine or benzalkonium chloride to disinfect. An antifungal, such as miconazole gel, or nystatin ointment, should be spread on the denture before reinsertion
- Bacterial sialadenitis needs treating with a penicillinase-resistant antibiotic, such as flucloxacillin.

EMERGENT TREATMENTS

Increasingly, consideration is being given to systemic therapy of SS under specialist supervision. Ciclosporin, azathioprine, methotrexate, leflunomide and mycophenolic acid have produced little if an benefit and/or have had unacceptable adverse effects. Recently there have been attempts to control the underlying autoimmune pathogenic mechanisms with, for example, chimeric humanized anti-CD20 (rituximab) or anti-CD22 (epratuzumab) therapy. A single course of rituximab can be effective in reducing disease activity in primary SS patients for up to six to nine months. In contrast there appears to be little benefit from use of anti-TNF or anti-IFN-alpha therapies. Salivary stimulation by intraoral electrical devices may emerge as a viable treatment.

FOLLOW-UP OF PATIENTS

Sjögren syndrome, particularly the primary type, and especially when clinically severe, carries a small potential for lymphoma development, necessitating regular monitoring, perhaps every six months, which can be carried out by the general medical or dental practitioner. If there is any change causing concern, particularly the development of a salivary swelling or lump, lymphadenopathy or hepatosplenomegaly a specialist opinion should best be obtained. Clinical and investigative predictive features are detailed above but pointers to

Table 50.5 Regimens that might be helpful in management of patient suspected of having Sjögren syndrome

Regimen	Use in primary care	Use in secondary care (severe oral involvement and/or extraoral involvement)
Likely to be beneficial	Sialogogues	Corticosteroids Antimalarials
Unproven effectiveness	Acupuncture Capparis masaikai Intraductal corticosteroid instillations Nizatidine	Anti-IFN agents Anti-TNF agents Sialoendoscopy Non-steroidal immunosuppressive
Emergent treatments	Electrostimulation	Anti-CD20 (rituximab) Anti-CD22 (epratuzumab) Stem cell transplant
Supportive	Antifungals Humidifier Moist diet Mouth wetting agents	

lymphoma development include the presence of fever, purpura, neuropathies, leg ulcers, hypocomplementaemia, cryoglobulinaemia and low CD4 count.

PATIENT INFORMATION SHEET

Sjögren syndrome

▼ Please read this information sheet. If you have any questions, particularly about the treatment or potential side-effects, please ask your doctor.

- This is an uncommon condition.
- The cause is unknown but it is immunological and possibly viral.
- It is not known to be infectious.
- It is not usually inherited.
- Dry mouth is common.
- Other mouth problems may include soreness, tooth decay and salivary swelling.
- Dry eyes are commonly found.
- Joint and other problems may be associated.
- Rarely, a very few patients may, after years, develop a tumour. You should get yourself checked regularly.
- X-rays, blood tests and biopsy may well be required.
- Symptoms can usually be controlled but not cured with simple drugs.
- Advice is available from: British Sjögren Syndrome Association, PO Box 10867, Birmingham, B16 0ZW.

USEFUL WEBSITES

Arthritis Link: http://www.arthritislink.com/
British Sjögren's Syndrome Association: http://www.bssa.uk.net/
Sjögren's Syndrome Foundation: http://www.sjogrens.org/

FURTHER READING

Aframian, D., Helcer, M., Livni, D., et al., 2007. Pilocarpine treatment in a mixed cohort of xerostomic patients. Oral Dis. 13, 88–92.

Amado, F., Lobo, M.J., Domingues, P., et al., 2010. Salivary peptidomics. Expert Rev. Proteomics 7 (5), 709–721.

Balada, E., Ordi-Ros, J., Vilardell-Tarrés, M., 2009. Molecular mechanisms mediated by human endogenous retroviruses (HERVs) in autoimmunity. Rev. Med. Virol. 19 (5), 273–286.

Balada, E., Vilardell-Tarrés, M., Ordi-Ros, J., 2010. Implication of human endogenous retroviruses in the development of autoimmune diseases. Int. Rev. Immunol. 29 (4), 351–370.

Bayetto, K., Logan, R.M., 2010. Sjögren's syndrome: a review of aetiology, pathogenesis, diagnosis and management. Aust. Dent. J. 55 (Suppl. 1), 39–47.

Becker, H., Pavenstaedt, H., Willeke, P., 2010. Emerging treatment strategies and potential therapeutic targets in primary Sjögren's syndrome. Inflamm. Allergy Drug Targets 9 (1), 10–19.

Bialek, E.J., Jakubowski, W., Zajkowski, P., et al., 2006. US of the major salivary glands: anatomy and spatial relationships, pathologic conditions, and pitfalls. Radiographics 26 (3), 745–763.

Bikker, A., van Woerkom, J.M., Kruize, A.A., et al., 2010. Increased expression of interleukin-7 in labial salivary glands of patients with primary Sjögren's syndrome correlates with increased inflammation. Arthritis Rheum. 62 (4), 969.

Chikui, T., Okamura, K., Tokumori, K., et al., 2006. Quantitative analyses of sonographic images of the parotid gland in patients with Sjögren's syndrome. Ultrasound Med. Biol. 32 (5), 617–622.

Colella, G., Cannavale, R., Vicidomini, A., Itro, A., 2010. Salivary gland biopsy: a comprehensive review of techniques and related complications. Rheumatology (Oxford) 49 (11), 2117–2121.

da Silva Marques, D.N., da Mata, A.D., Patto, J.M., et al., 2011. Effects of gustatory stimulants of salivary secretion on salivary pH and flow in patients with Sjögren's syndrome: a randomized controlled trial. J. Oral Pathol. Med. 40 (10), 785–792.

Deshmukh, U.S., Nandula, S.R., Thimmalapura, P.R., et al., 2009. Activation of innate immune responses through Toll-like receptor 3 causes a rapid loss of salivary gland function. J. Oral Pathol. Med. 38 (1), 42–47.

Fox, P.C., Bowman, S.J., Segal, B., et al., 2008. Oral involvement in primary Sjögren syndrome. J. Am. Dent. Assoc. 139 (12), 1592–1601.

Fragoulis, G.E., Moutsopoulos, H.M., 2011. IgG4 Syndrome: Old Disease, New Perspective. J. Rheumatol. 37, 1369.

Gutta, R., McLain, L., McGuff, S.H., 2008. Sjögren syndrome: a review for the maxillofacial surgeon. Oral Maxillofac. Surg. Clin. North Am. 20 (4), 567–575.

Hernández-Molina, G., Leal-Alegre, G., Michel-Peregrina, M., 2011. The meaning of anti-Ro and anti-La antibodies in primary Sjögren's syndrome. Autoimmun. Rev. 10 (3), 123–125.

Jonsson, R., Haga, H.J., Gordon, T.P., 2000. Current concepts on diagnosis, autoantibodies and therapy in Sjögren's syndrome. Scand. J. Rheumatol. 29, 341–348.

Leung, K., McMillan, A., Cheung, B., Leung, W., 2008. Sjögren's syndrome sufferers have increased oral yeast levels despite regular dental care. Oral Dis. 14, 163–173.

Lu, Q., Renaudineau, Y., Cha, S., et al., 2010. Epigenetics in autoimmune disorders: highlights of the 10th Sjögren's syndrome symposium. Autoimmun. Rev. 9 (9), 627–630.

Mahoney, E.J., Spiegel, J.H., 2003. Sjögren's disease. Otolaryngol. Clin. North Am. 36 (4), 733–745.

Manoussakis, M.N., Kapsogeorgou, E.K., 2010. The role of intrinsic epithelial activation in the pathogenesis of Sjögren's syndrome. J. Autoimmun. 35 (3), 219–224.

Manoussakis, M.N., Moutsopoulos, H.M., 2000. Sjögren's syndrome: autoimmune epithelitis. Baillière's Best Pract. Res. Clin. Rheumatol. 14, 73–95.

Manoussakis, M.N., Spachidou, M.P., Maratheftis, C.I., 2010. Salivary epithelial cells from Sjögren's syndrome patients are highly sensitive to anoikis induced by TLR-3 ligation. J. Autoimmun. 35 (3), 212–218.

Mansour, M.J., Al-Hashimi, I., Wright, J.M., 2007. Coexistence of Sjögren's syndrome and sarcoidosis: a report of five cases. J. Oral Pathol. Med. 36 (6), 337–341.

Mariette, X., Gottenberg, J.E., 2010. Pathogenesis of Sjögren's syndrome and therapeutic consequences. Curr. Opin. Rheumatol. 22 (5), 471–477.

Mavragani, C.P., Crow, M.K., 2010. Activation of the type I interferon pathway in primary Sjögren's syndrome. J. Autoimmun. 35 (3), 225–231.

Mavragani, C.P., Moutsopoulos, N.M., Moutsopoulos, H.M., 2006. The management of Sjögren's syndrome. Nat. Clin. Pract. Rheumatol. 2 (5), 252–261.

Meiners, P.M., Vissink, A., Kallenberg, C.G., et al., 2011. Treatment of primary Sjögren's syndrome with anti-CD20 therapy (rituximab). A feasible approach or just a starting point? Expert Opin. Biol. Ther 11 (10), 1381–1394.

Minozzi, F., Galli, M., Gallottini, L., et al., 2009. Stomatological approach to Sjögren's syndrome: diagnosis, management and therapeutical timing. Eur. Rev. Med. Pharmacol. Sci. 13 (3), 201–216.

Mondini, M., Costa, S., Sponza, S., et al., 2010. The interferon-inducible HIN-200 gene family in apoptosis and inflammation:implication for autoimmunity. Autoimmunity 43 (3), 226–231.

Moutsopoulos, N.M., Moutsopoulos, H.M., 2001. Therapy of Sjögren's syndrome. Springer Semin. Immunopathol. 23, 131–145.

Nakamura, H., Kawakami, A., Eguchi, K., 2006. Mechanisms of autoantibody production and the relationship between autoantibodies and the clinical manifestations in Sjögren's syndrome. Transl. Res. 148 (6), 281–288.

Ohara, T., Itoh, Y., Itoh, K., 2000. Reevaluation of laboratory parameters in relation to histological findings in primary and secondary Sjögren's syndrome. Intern. Med. 39, 457–463.

O'Neill I, Scully C. 2012. Biologics in oral medicine: Sjogren syndrome: Oral Diseases Mar 13 Epub.

Perosa, F., Prete, M., Racanelli, V., Dammacco, F., 2010. CD20-depleting therapy in autoimmune diseases: from basic research to the clinic. J. Intern. Med. 267 (3), 260–277.

Prochorec-Sobieszek, M., Wagner, T., 2005. Lympho-proliferative disorders in Sjögren's syndrome. Otolaryngol. Pol. 59 (4), 559.

Ramos-Casals, M., Loustaud-Ratti, V., De Vita, S., et al., 2005. Sjögren syndrome associated with hepatitis C virus: a multicenter analysis of 137 cases. Medicine (Balt) 84 (2), 81–89.

Ramos-Casals M, Brito-Zeron P, Siso-Almirall A., et al., 2012. Topical and systemic medications for the treatment of primary Sjrogen syndrome Nat. Rev. Rheumatol May 1 Epub.

Ramos-Casals, M., Tzioufas, A.G., Stone, J.H., et al., 2010. Treatment of primary Sjögren syndrome: a systematic review. JAMA 304 (4), 452–460.

Rehman, H.U., 2003. Sjögren's syndrome. Yonsei Med. J. 44 (6), 947–954.

Reyes, S.L.I., Leon, B.F., Rozas, V.M.F., et al., 2006. BAFF: A regulatory cytokine of B lymphocytes involved in autoimmunity and lymphoid cancer. Rev. Med. Chil. 134 (9), 1175–1184.

Roescher, N., Tak, P., Illei, G., 2009. Cytokines in Sjögren's syndrome. Oral Dis. 15, 519–526.

Rotter, N., Schwarz, S., Jakob, M., et al., 2010. Salivary gland stem cells: Can they restore radiation-induced salivary gland dysfunction?. HNO 58 (6), 556–563.

Routsias, J.G., Tzioufas, A.G., 2010. Autoimmune response and target autoantigens in Sjögren's syndrome. Eur. J. Clin. Invest. 40 (11), 1026–1036.

Routsias, J.G., Tzioufas, A.G., 2010. B-cell epitopes of the intracellular autoantigens Ro/SSA and La/SSB: tools to study the regulation of the autoimmune response. J. Autoimmun. 35 (3), 256–264.

Salaffi, F., Argalia, G., Carotti, M., et al., 2000. Salivary gland ultrasonography in the evaluation of primary Sjögren's syndrome. Comparison with minor salivary gland biopsy. J. Rheumatol. 27, 1229–1236.

Salomonsson, S., Rozell, B.L., Heimburger, M., et al., 2009. Minor salivary gland immunohistology in the diagnosis of primary Sjögren's syndrome. J. Oral Pathol. Med. 38 (3), 282–288.

Scully C, Georgakopoulos E. 2012. Oral Involvement In Ramos-Casals M, Stone JH, Moutsopoulos HM, "sjrogen syndrome: diagnosis and therapeutics" Springer, Berlin. pp 85-106.

Shacham, R., Puterman, M.B., Ohana, N., Nahlieli, O., 2011. Endoscopic treatment of salivary glands affected by autoimmune diseases. J. Oral Maxillofac. Surg. 69 (2), 476–481.

Shihoskisc, Shiboski C.H., Criswell, L.A., et al., 2012. American College or Rheumatology Classification Criteria for Sjogrens syndrome. Arthritis Care and Research 64, 475–487.

Shimizu, M., Okamura, K., Yoshiura, K., et al., 2006. Sonographic diagnostic criteria for screening Sjögren's syndrome. Oral Surg. Oral Med. Oral Pathol. Oral Radiol. Endod. 102 (1), 85–93.

Skopouli, F.N., Dafni, U., Loannidis, J.P., et al., 2000. Clinical evolution, and morbidity and mortality of primary Sjögren's syndrome. Semin. Arthritis Rheum. 29, 296–304.

Solans-Laqué, R., López-Hernandez, A., Angel Bosch-Gil, J., et al., 2011. Risk, Predictors, and Clinical Characteristics of Lymphoma Development in Primary Sjögren's Syndrome. Semin. Arthritis Rheum. 41 (3), 415–423.

Spachidou, M.P., Bourazopoulou, E., Maratheftis, C.I., et al., 2007. Expression of functional Toll-like receptors by salivary gland epithelial cells: increased mRNA expression in cells derived from patients with primary Sjögren's syndrome. Clin. Exp. Immunol. 147 (3), 497–503.

Stea, E.A., Routsias, J.G., Samiotaki, M., et al., 2007. Analysis of parotid glands of primary Sjögren's syndrome patients using proteomic technology reveals altered autoantigen composition and novel antigenic targets. Clin. Exp. Immunol. 147 (1), 81–89.

Strietzel, F., Martín-Granizo, R., Fedele, S., 2007. Electrostimulating device in the management of xerostomia. Oral Dis. 13, 206–213.

Takagi, Y., Kimura, Y., Nakamura, H., et al., 2010. Salivary gland ultrasonography: can it be an alternative to sialography as an imaging modality for Sjögren's syndrome? Ann. Rheum. Dis. 69 (7), 1321.

Theander, E., Henriksson, G., Ljungberg, O., et al., 2006. Lymphoma and other malignancies in primary Sjögren's syndrome: a cohort study on cancer incidence and lymphoma predictors. Ann. Rheum. Dis. 65 (6), 796–803.

Thomas, B.L., Brown, J.E., McGurk, M., 2010. Salivary gland disease. Front. Oral Biol. 14, 129–146.

Tobón, G.J., Saraux, A., Pers, J.O., Youinou, P., 2010. Emerging biotherapies for Sjögren's syndrome. Expert Opin. Emerg. Drugs 15 (2), 269–282.

Townsend, M.J., Monroe, J.G., Chan, A.C., 2010. B-cell targeted therapies in human autoimmune diseases: an updated perspective. Immunol. Rev. 237 (1), 264–283.

Tran, S.D., Sumita, Y., Khalili, S., 2011. Bone marrow-derived cells: A potential approach for the treatment of xerostomia. Int. J. Biochem. Cell Biol. 43 (1), 5–9.

Vakaloglou, K.M., Mavragani, C.P., 2011. Activation of the type I interferon pathway in primary Sjögren's syndrome: an update. Curr. Opin. Rheumatol. 23 (5), 459–464.

van Woerkom, J.M., Kruize, A.A., Barendregt, P.J., et al., 2006. Clinical significance of quantitative immunohistology in labial salivary glands for diagnosing Sjögren's syndrome. Rheumatology (Oxford) 45 (4), 470.

Vitali, C., Bombardieri, S., Jonsson, R., et al., 2002. Classification criteria for Sjögren's syndrome: a revised version of the European criteria proposed by the American–European Consensus Group. Ann. Rheum. Dis. 61, 554–558.

von Bültzingslöwen, I., Sollecito, T.P., Fox, P.C., Daniels, T., 2007. Salivary dysfunction associated with systemic diseases: systematic review and clinical management recommendations. Oral Surg. Oral Med. Oral Pathol. Oral Radiol. Endod 103, S57. e1–S57.e15.

Voulgarelis, M., Moutsopoulos, H.M., 2008. Mucosa-associated lymphoid tissue lymphoma in Sjögren's syndrome: risks, management, and prognosis. Rheum. Dis. Clin. North Am. 34 (4), 921.

Voulgarelis, M., Tzioufas, A.G., 2010. Pathogenetic mechanisms in the initiation and perpetuation of Sjögren's syndrome. Nat. Rev. Rheumatol. 6 (9), 529–537.

Yamamoto, M., Takahashi, H., Ohara, M., et al., 2006. A new conceptualization for Mikulicz's disease as an IgG4-related plasmacytic disease. Mod. Rheumatol. 16 (6), 335–340.

Temporomandibular joint pain–dysfunction syndrome

51

Key Points

- Temporomandibular joint (TMJ) pain–dysfunction syndrome refers to a common triad of jaw clicking, jaw locking (or limitation of opening) and/or pain
- This afflicts young people mainly, typically teenagers or young adults, especially females
- Trauma and stress appear to predispose
- Diagnosis is essentially clinical
- Management is variously by rest, exercise or other therapies

INTRODUCTION

The temporomandibular joints (TMJ) are complex joints that need to work in concert, are essential to mastication, and are probably the most used joints in the body. Temporomandibular joint pain–dysfunction syndrome (TMPD; myofascial pain dysfunction (MFD), facial arthromyalgia (FAM), mandibular dysfunction, or mandibular stress syndrome) refers to a common triad of joint symptoms:

- jaw clicking
- jaw locking (or limitation of movements)
- orofacial pain.

TMPD is not only one of the most common orofacial complaints but also one of the controversial areas in dentistry in terms of suggested aetiopathogenesis, diagnosis and management.

INCIDENCE

The prevalence is at least 12% of the general population, but these symptoms have been reported at some time by up to 88% – with as many as 25% reporting severe symptoms.

AGE

This disorder afflicts young adults mainly, typically teenagers and up to 20–30 years of age.

GENDER

More patients are females than males.

GEOGRAPHIC

No known geographic incidence.

PREDISPOSING FACTORS

Trauma and stress appear to predispose, especially anything that causes excessive mouth opening.

AETIOLOGY AND PATHOGENESIS

TMJ dysfunction is a symptom complex of multifactorial aetiology, which almost certainly represents a psychological response to stress that becomes chronic through increasing muscle tension affecting the muscles of mastication (mainly the temporalis, masseter and pterygoid muscles). Muscle hyperactivity can release lactic acid and other components that can cause pain.

The two heads of the lateral pterygoid muscle have separate actions, the lower contracting during mouth opening, the superior head contracting during closing, to steady the meniscus as it moves back with the condyle into the glenoid fossa. During mouth closing the lower head is electromyographically silent. In TMJ dysfunction patients, the lower head of the lateral pterygoid muscle contracts during the closing phase (when it should be relaxed). It has been suggested that anterior displacement of the TMJ meniscus, perhaps from a tear of the posterior capsule, prevents the superior head from acting effectively. The lower head perhaps attempts to help stabilize the meniscus. This might explain why this muscle is tender on palpation in TMJ dysfunction patients. Anterior displacement of the meniscus has been demonstrated by TMJ arthrography and found at operation in some TMJ dysfunction patients. Patients may be classified as having: no meniscus displacement; anterior displacement with reduction (excessive forward movement during opening which relocates on closing); and anterior displacement without reduction, when the meniscus remains anterior to the condyle in a buckled-up fashion, such that there is a reduced joint space and the articular surface of the condyle is close to the articular surface of the glenoid fossa. This latter situation predisposes to subsequent osteoarthritis.

Hypotheses as to TMPD however, are many, and facts are few.

TRAUMA

- Trauma which is obvious, including from road accidents, sports injuries, fights and dental treatment or extractions is common and can occasionally be followed by TMJ dysfunction.
- TMJ dysfunction can also be secondary to microtrauma and subsequent muscle hyperactivity. Microtrauma can

result from prolonged mouth opening, as in dental treatment sessions, general anaesthesia, choir singing, wind instrument playing, or parafunctions, such as day-time jaw clenching or night-time tooth grinding (bruxism), and habits, such as chewing a pen or pencil.

- Trauma can result in muscle spasm or hyperactivity.

MUSCLE HYPERACTIVITY

- Psychological stress can also cause muscle hyperactivity. Muscle hyperactivity has been demonstrated in TMJ patients during activities, such as school examinations and watching horror films.
- 50–70% of patients (twice as common as controls) have experienced stressful life events in the 6 months before onset. These problems concerning work, money, health, loss and interpersonal relationships probably have a causative role by inducing anxiety, which then produces increased jaw muscle activity.
- Depression and shortage of sleep are considered important risk indicators.

CONTROVERSIAL SUGGESTED CAUSES

Abnormalities in the dental occlusion are controversial as causes of TMJ dysfunction. There is no neurophysiological evidence to support a primary aetiological role for the occlusion in TMJ dysfunction and many people with gross malocclusions have no TMJ dysfunction. There is no significant difference in the incidence of occlusal abnormalities between TMJ dysfunction patients and control subjects, nor is there any evidence for a relationship between orthodontic treatment (or the wearing of orthodontic headgear) and TMJ dysfunction.

CLINICAL FEATURES

Symptoms are highly variable, but dysfunction is usually unilateral and characterized by one or more of the following features:

- Recurrent clicking in the TMJ: clicking occurs either on attempted mouth opening or closing. Often the click allows the completion of that phase of mandibular movement. Sometimes clicking ceases and the jaw locks either open or closed. Clicks are not diagnostic, since they are common in normal TM joints. A grating noise (crepitus) may signify intra-articular arthritic change, and there may be crepitus at any point of jaw movement, especially with lateral movements.
- Jaw locking or limitation of movement: limitation of opening may be intermittent, with jaw 'locking'. There may be deviation of the jaw to the affected side on attempted opening with variable jaw deviation or locking, but rarely severe trismus. If there is reduced mouth opening this often suggests bilateral disease. Limitation may be more obvious on awakening, especially after nocturnal grinding. In some others, the limitation increases throughout the day.
- Pain in the joint and/or surrounding muscles and elsewhere ipsilaterally: the main site is usually preauricular, but can radiate to the back of the mouth, down the neck, up to the temple or behind the ear. Pain may occur at an early

stage or sometimes after the onset of clicking or stiffness of the jaw. It may range from a vague dull ache to an acute pain. Patients with a night-time clenching or grinding habit (bruxism) may awake with joint pain which abates during the day. The symptoms of individuals who clench or grind during working hours tend to worsen towards evening, and sometimes have a psychogenic basis. The pain may be aggravated by chewing or other jaw movements. The masseters, temporalis and pterygoid muscles may be tender to palpation, but there is no detectable swelling. Sometimes pain is more clearly sited in a single jaw muscle, and sometimes trigger points can be located. Some patients may also complain of headaches, neck aches, and lower back pain. Female cases have significantly fewer children and are more likely to have never been pregnant, possibly due to fibromyalgia.

DIAGNOSIS

Diagnosis of TMPD is mainly on clinical grounds but it is crucial to exclude organic disease in the TMJ or elsewhere and referred to the area, since even lung cancers have caused pain which simulates TMPD (**Table 51.1**). Self-rating assessments for psychological factors may be helpful. The occlusion and any dental appliances should also be assessed. Some clinicians use local anaesthetic injected in or around the joint to exclude TMJ arthritis as a cause. Symptoms can be quantified by the Helkimo indices based on both patient information (anamnestic dysfunction index, Ai) and clinical findings (clinical dysfunction index, Di) (**Table 51.2**). These indices include a numerical scoring system. Many patients presenting for treatment can be graded as AiII DiII/DiIII.

IMAGING

Any osseous changes in organic TMJ disease, such as osteoarthrosis or rheumatoid arthritis are unlikely, in the absence of long-standing disease, to be revealed by imaging. Indeed, radiographic changes are uncommon and the condylar position as seen on radiography is unreliable for diagnosis and does not indicate meniscus displacement. Imaging is rarely indicated but MRI, CT, CBCT, OPT or transpharyngeal,

Table 51.1 Aids that might be helpful in diagnosis/ prognosis/management in some patients suspected of having temporomandibular joint pain–dysfunction syndrome*

In most cases	In some cases
–	Radiography of jaw, TMJ
	CT/MRI
	Full blood picture
	ESR
	Serum uric acid
	ANA
	RF
	Arthrography
	Chest imaging

*See text for details and glossary for abbreviations.

Table 51.2 Helkimo indices

Anamnestic index (Ai)	Symptoms	Clinical dysfunction index (Di)	Dysfunction
0	None	0	None
I	Mild; TMJ sounds; feelings of stiffness of the jaws	I	Mild
II	More severe: difficulty in opening the mouth wide; locking; fixation; pain on movement; facial and jaw pain	II	Moderate
		III	Severe

transcranial oblique lateral or transorbital condylar radiographic views can be helpful if there is:

- a history of trauma
- significant limitation of movement, change in occlusion or a mandibular shift
- sensory or motor alteration
- a real possibility of organic joint or other disease.

Arthrography is rarely indicated.

CONTROVERSIAL 'DIAGNOSTIC' PROCEDURES

There is no reliable scientific evidence to support the regular use of other suggested aids such as:

- jaw tracking (mandibular kinesiology)
- electromyography
- electrovibratography
- sonography
- thermography.

TREATMENT (see also Chs 4 and 5)

Patient information is an important aspect in management. TMJ dysfunction appears not to lead to long-term joint damage and some patients have spontaneous remission: thus, treatment is not always indicated. There is no indication, for example, for attempting treatment for TMJ clicks that are otherwise symptomless. However, in persons who complain of pain, treatment may be worthwhile (**Table 51.3**). The aims of treatment are to:

- control immediate pain
- lower psychological stress (reassure)
- eliminate TMJ damage.

POSSIBLE TREATMENTS

There is a wide range of treatments offered for TMJ dysfunction, including physical, medical, psychological and surgical approaches but conservative approaches are typically successful. The level of placebo response and the response from reassurance is impressive, and conservative measures are at least partially successful in up to 90% – usually within 6 months. Of the other 10%, half may be functional and respond to psychotropic medication and the rest are chronic pain sufferers.

Table 51.3 Regimens that might be helpful in management of patient suspected of having temporomandibular pain–dysfunction

Regimen	Use in primary or secondary care
Likely to be beneficial	Anxiolytics or muscle relaxants (e.g. benzodiazepines such as diazepam or temazepam) Occlusal splint (overlay appliance) Reassurance
Unproven effectiveness	Immobilization of jaw Mandibular orthopaedic repositioning appliance Occlusal reconstruction
Supportive	Reassurance Rest

Medical treatments include:

- rest
- heat
- cold
- analgesics (NSAIDs); topical NSAIDs may help: ibuprofen gel (5% or 10%), ketoprofen 2.5%, or diclofenac 4% gel and patch are available
- muscle relaxants (e.g. benzodiazepines)
- antidepressants (e.g. tricyclics)
- injections
- trigger-point (peri-articular) local analgesics
- intra-articular corticosteroids.
- transcutaneous electrical nerve stimulation.

Psychological treatments include:

- behaviour modification/biofeedback
- hypnosis.
- psychiatric treatment
- group therapy.

A typical treatment regimen includes:

- rest
- avoidance of trauma, wide opening and abnormal habits
- warmth, massage and remedial jaw exercises to control discomfort
- analgesics: nonsteroidal antiinflammatory agents such as aspirin can be helpful. Ibuprofen-containing gel applied to

the area may help. Injection of local analgesics into painful sites, or the spraying of coolants, such as trichlorofluoromethane onto the areas, can ease pain and break the cycle

- muscle relaxants such as oral clonazepam 0.25 mg/day, temazepam 10 mg, or baclofen 10 mg three times daily can help provide relief.

Use biobehavioural modalities (psychotherapy, biofeedback, relaxation), or anxiolytic agents such as:

- diazepam 2 mg three times daily
- lorazepam 1 mg/day
- alprazolam 0.25 mg three times daily.

If these conservative modalities prove insufficient, it may be helpful to:

- use plastic splints on the occlusal surfaces (occlusal splints). It is unclear how these function, but they increase the vertical dimension, may reduce joint loading, eliminate faulty occlusal interferences, and probably most importantly provide cognitive awareness of damaging oral habits and engender a placebo effect. In any event, at least 40% benefit symptomatically, especially from hard splints (**Fig. 51.1**)
- relieve obvious occlusal interferences and to correct prosthetic discrepancies, such as an incorrect vertical dimension; however, any possible benefits from major occlusal alterations must be set against a high placebo response and the important role of reassurance.

The remaining subgroup of 5–10% of patients may need treatment for prominent psychological problems by either medication or psychiatric therapy. The very small minority of patients who fail to respond to the above measures may require local corticosteroid (triamcinolone or depomedrone) or hyaluronate or a sclerosant therapy. Surgery may be required for the very small number of remaining non-responders, especially those with obvious intra-articular pathology (osteoarthritis).

Surgical treatments include:

- condylotomy (rarely, high condylar shave; high partial condylectomy indicated)
- capsular rearrangement
- silicone or Teflon implants
- auriculotemporal nerve section.

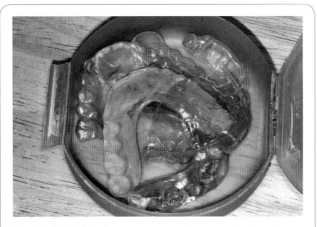

Fig. 51.1 Splints for temporomandibular pain-dysfunction syndrome

FOLLOW-UP OF PATIENTS

Long-term follow-up in primary care is usually appropriate.

PATIENT INFORMATION SHEET

Temporomandibular pain–dysfunction

▼ Please read this information sheet. If you have any questions, particularly about the treatment or potential side-effects, please ask your doctor.

- This is a common condition.
- It appears to be related to stress, damage or habits involving the teeth and joints.
- It is not inherited.
- There are no serious long-term consequences; arthritis does not result.
- The symptoms usually clear spontaneously after some months.
- Various treatments, such as rest, exercises, drugs, ointments, splints or adjustments to the teeth may help.

PATIENT INFORMATION SHEET

Temporomandibular pain–dysfunction:Four steps to manage jaw pain

▼ Please read this information sheet. If you have any questions, particularly about the treatment or potential side-effects, please ask your doctor.

- Rest yourself and your jaw:
  - relax and practice stress reduction
  - exercise regularly
  - eat soft foods and avoid hard, crusty foods like nuts or hard bread or those that need chewing a great deal
  - chew on your back teeth, not the front ones
  - eat small bites
  - sleep on your side.
- Avoid joint or muscle damage by avoiding:
  - contact sports (wear a mouthguard if you must play contact sports)
  - excessive jaw use in yawning, grinding and clenching
  - chewing gum
  - habits, such as biting finger nails, pens and pencils or lip
  - long dental appointments or general anaesthesia
  - cradling the telephone between head and shoulder
  - wind instrument playing.
- Reduce muscle pain with analgesics and by applying:
  - cold packs for 10 min every 3 h for 72 h after injury
  - hot packs for 20 min every 3 h to uninjured joints/muscles.
- Re-educate the jaw opening:
  - open your mouth with a hinge movement
  - exercise your jaw twice daily, opening 5 times in front of a mirror, ensuring the jaw opens vertically downwards without deviating sideways.
- Exercise your jaw three times daily for 5 min:
  - close your mouth on the back teeth
  - put the tip of your tongue on the palate behind your front teeth
  - move the tongue back across the palate as far as it will go
  - keep the tongue in this position with the teeth closed for 10 s
  - open your mouth slowly until the tongue starts to leave the palate
  - keep that position for 10 s
  - close your mouth
  - repeat over 5 min.

USEFUL WEBSITES

American Academy of Orofacial Pain: http://www.aaop.org/

National Institute of Dental and Craniofacial Research, Temporomandibular Joint and Muscle Disorders. http://www.nidcr.nih.gov/OralHealth/Topics/TMJ/

FURTHER READING

Benoliel, R., Svensson, P., Heir, G., et al., 2011. Persistent orofacial muscle pain. Oral Dis. 17, 23–41.

Epstein, J.B., Caldwell, J., Black, G., 2001. The utility of panoramic imaging of the temporomandibular joint in patients with tempomandibular disorders. Oral Surg. Oral Med. Oral Pathol. Radiol. Endod. 92, 236–239.

Haketa, T., Kino, K., Sugisaki, M., et al., 2006. Difficulty of food intake in patients with temporomandibular disorders. Int. J. Prosthodont. 19 (3), 266–270.

Kim, H.I., Lee, J.Y., Kim, Y.K., Kho, H.S., 2010. Clinical and psychological characteristics of TMD patients with trauma history. Oral Dis. 16, 188–192.

Lele, S., Hooper, L., 2004. Pharmacological interventions for pain in patients with temporomandibular disorders (TMD). Cochrane Database Syst. Rev. CD004715.

MacFarlane, T.V., Gray, R.J.M., Kincey, J., et al., 2001. Factors associated with the temporomandibular disorder pain–dysfunction syndrome (PDS): Manchester case–control study. Oral Dis. 7, 321–330.

Nilsson, I.M., List, T., Drangsholt, M., 2006. The reliability and validity of self-reported temporomandibular disorder pain in adolescents. J. Orofac. Pain 20 (2), 138–144.

Otuyemi, O.D., Owotade, F.J., Ugboko, V.I., et al., 2000. Prevalence of signs and symptoms of temporomandibular disorders in young Nigerian adults. J. Orthod. 27, 61–66.

Raphael, K.G., Marbach, J.J., 2000. Comorbid fibromyalgia accounts for reduced fecundity in women with myofascial face pain. Clin. J. Pain 16, 29–36.

Sato, F., Kino, K., Sugisaki, M., et al., 2006. Teeth contacting habit as a contributing factor to chronic pain in patients with temporomandibular disorders. J. Med. Dent. Sci. 53 (2), 103–109.

Selaimen, C.M., Jeronymo, J.C., Brilhante, D.P., Grossi, M.L., 2006. Sleep and depression as risk indicators for temporomandibular disorders in a cross-cultural perspective: a case-control study. Int. J. Prosthodont. 19 (2), 154–161.

Takemura, T., Takahashi, T., Fukuda, M., et al., 2006. A psychological study on patients with masticatory muscle disorder and sleep bruxism. Cranio 24 (3), 191–196.

Trigeminal and other neuralgias

Key Points

- Trigeminal neuralgia (TN) consists of severe paroxysmal orofacial pain which last a few seconds
- TN is one of the most severe pains known
- Pain is in one or more divisions of the trigeminal nerve
- Pain is sometimes triggered by touching areas or by certain daily activities, such as eating, talking, washing the face, shaving or cleaning the teeth
- There is no neurological deficit
- Organic causes of neuralgia must be excluded by history, physical examination and special investigations
- Treatment is primarily and essentially medical, with an anticonvulsant, such as carbamazepine
- Surgery is reserved for recalcitrant TN

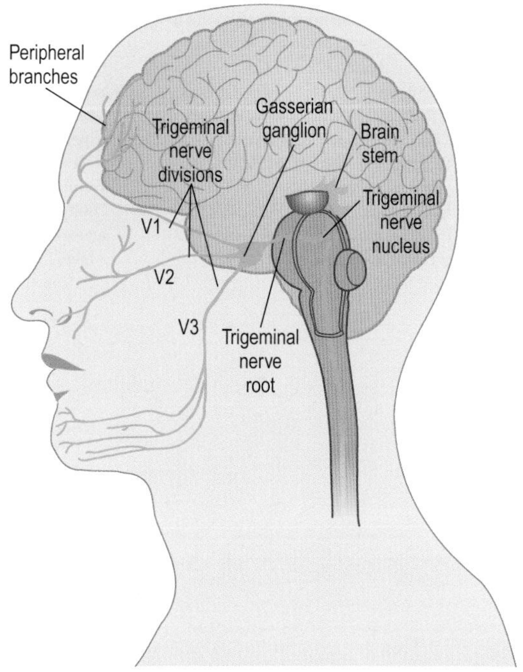

Fig. 52.1 Trigeminal nerve anatomy

INTRODUCTION

'Neuralgia' means pain in a nerve. Trigeminal neuralgia (TN) is a disorder of the trigeminal nerve that consists of episodes of unilateral intense, stabbing, electric shock-like pain in the areas of the face where the branches of the nerve are distributed – lips, eyes, nose, scalp, forehead, upper jaw or lower jaw. TN is not fatal, but it is universally considered to be one of the most painful afflictions known.

Sensory innervation of the mouth, face and scalp depends on the trigeminal (fifth cranial) nerve (**Figs 52.1** and **52.2**), so that disease affecting this nerve can cause not only orofacial pain but also sensory loss, or, indeed, both, sometimes with serious implications; it is important to exclude malignant disease as a cause (Ch. 17).

Trigeminal neuralgia may occur in tumours of the trigeminal nerve (e.g. neuroma), with lesions affecting the trigeminal nerve at the cerebellopontine angle and in disseminated sclerosis or cerebral neoplasms, and these cases are termed secondary or symptomatic TN (STN), when there may be detectable physical signs – initially a reduced corneal reflex, progressing to trigeminal sensory loss. Trigeminal neuralgia however, much more frequently has no *clinically obvious* neurological cause (termed idiopathic TN, or ITN) and is then usually ascribed to pressure on the trigeminal nerve from an adjacent but atherosclerotic artery (see below).

TRIGEMINAL NEURALGIA WITH NO CLINICALLY OBVIOUS NEUROLOGICAL CAUSE

This is also known as idiopathic trigeminal neuralgia (ITN), benign paroxysmal trigeminal neuralgia, trigeminal neuralgia and tic doloureux.

INCIDENCE

Uncommon, probably about 4 cases per 100 000 population, although TN is the most common neurological cause of facial pain.

Age

ITN onset is mainly in the 50–70 year age group (STN tends to arise in younger patients).

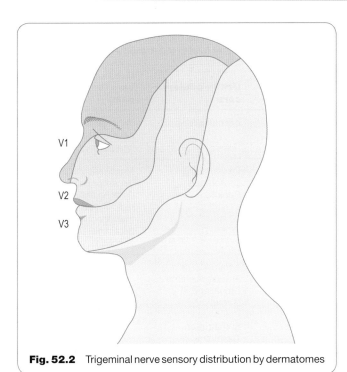

Fig. 52.2 Trigeminal nerve sensory distribution by dermatomes

Gender

ITN is slightly more common in women.

Geographic

There is no known geographic incidence.

PREDISPOSING FACTORS

No predisposing factors have been identified for *idiopathic* trigeminal neuralgia, but emotional or physical stress can increase the frequency and severity of attacks.

AETIOLOGY AND PATHOGENESIS

ITN has an unclear aetiology, but one hypothesis is that there may be compression around the trigeminal nerve root in the posterior cranial fossa, close to the pons, possibly due to the superior cerebellar artery becoming atherosclerotic and, therefore, less flexible, and then pressing on the trigeminal nerve roots, causing demyelination and neuronal discharge.

STN (symptomatic or secondary TN) is severe orofacial pain suggestive of TN, but an organic cause is detectable. STN is usually seen in younger people and/or sometimes with physical signs, such as facial sensory or motor impairment, and can result from cerebrovascular disease, disseminated sclerosis, infections such as HIV infection, space-occupying lesions such as neoplasms or aneurysms, or lesions that may irritate the trigeminal nerve roots along the pons, or the tracts more centrally in the CNS.

CLINICAL FEATURES

In both ITN and STN, the pain is unilateral and follows the sensory distribution of cranial nerve V, typically radiating to the maxillary (V2) or mandibular (V3) area (**Fig. 52.2**).

TN has the following main characteristics as based on definitions of the International Headache Society and International Association for the Study of Pain:

- Paroxysmal attacks of facial pain that last a few seconds to <2 min; occurring especially in the morning, rarely at night.
- Pain has at least four of the following characteristics:
  - a unilateral distribution along one or more divisions of the trigeminal nerve
  - a sudden intense, sharp superficial, stabbing or burning quality
  - the pain intensity is severe
  - precipitation from trigger areas or by certain daily activities, such as eating, talking, washing the face, shaving or cleaning the teeth
  - the patient is usually entirely asymptomatic between paroxysms, but some patients experience a dull ache at other times.
- The attacks are stereotyped in the individual patient.
- There is no neurological deficit in ITN but STN needs to be excluded by history, physical examination, imaging and special investigations when necessary. There is also an increased risk of cerebrovascular events in patients with TN, so blood pressure assessment is indicated.

A less common form of the disorder, called 'atypical trigeminal neuralgia', may cause less intense, constant, dull burning or aching pain, sometimes with occasional electric-shock-like stabs, usually unilaterally, but some patients experience pain on both sides. Patients with atypical trigeminal neuralgia may occasionally be developing mixed connective tissue disease (MCTD). Other differential diagnoses include the trigeminal autonomic cephalgias (Ch. 17).

DIAGNOSIS

Trigeminal sensory testing is important to elicit deficits, bilateral involvement of the trigeminal nerve, and abnormal trigeminal reflexes associated with an increased risk of STN which must be excluded (**Algorithm 52.1**) by:

- History.
- Examination, including careful neurological assessment, especially of the cranial nerves – particularly the trigeminal nerve and those closely related to the trigeminal (i.e. cranial nerves VI, VII and VIII).
- Investigations, including (**Table 52.1**):
  - imaging: by radiography, MRI or CT to exclude cerebral space-occupying or demyelinating lesions. Imaging identifies structural causes for TN in up to 15% of patients. Many specialists recommend elective MRI for all patients to exclude an uncommon mass lesion or aberrant vessel compressing the trigeminal nerve roots, or demyelination, and it is mandatory if any atypical features or neurological features are present, and in patients under 50 years. There is insufficient evidence to support or refute the usefulness of MRI to identify neurovascular compression of the trigeminal nerve but fusion MRI with multiplanar reconstruction, MR angiography (MRA) or MR cisternography can detect vascular indentation and can predict the presence of symptoms in patients
  - blood tests: e.g. possibly ESR, CRP or PV to exclude vasculitides, anti-RNP antibodies for MCTD, and serology for Lyme disease or, rarely, HIV.

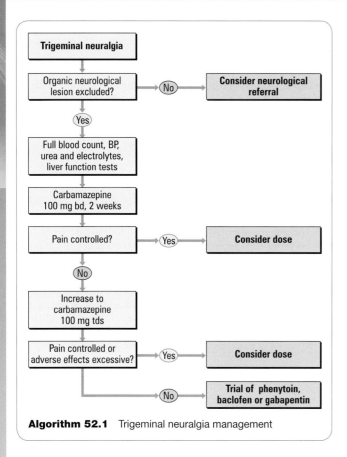

Algorithm 52.1 Trigeminal neuralgia management

Table 52.2 Regimens that might be helpful in management of patient suspected of having trigeminal neuralgia

Regimen	Use in primary care	Use in secondary care (intractable pain)
Beneficial	Carbamazepine	Peripheral neurosurgery (temporary relief)
Likely to be beneficial	Oxcarbazine Lamotrigen Baclofen	Microvascular decompression Gamma knife radiofrequency thermocoagulation of trigeminal Gasserian ganglion
Unproven effectiveness	Acupuncture Antidepressants Clonazepam Gabapentin Pregabalin Sumatriptan Tizanidine Topiramate Valproate Ziconotide Transcutaneous electrical nerve stimulation (TENS)	

Table 52.1 Aids that might be helpful in diagnosis/prognosis/management in some patients suspected of having trigeminal neuralgia*

In most cases	In some cases
Neurological opinion	Tooth/jaw/sinus/skull radiography
MRI/CT	Serum ferritin, vitamin B$_{12}$ and
Full blood picture**	corrected whole blood folate levels
Blood pressure**	Serology (Lyme disease, HIV)
Urea and electrolytes**	ANA
Liver function tests**	ESR
	HLA-B1502, if Asian/Chinese

*See text for details and glossary for abbreviations.
**For monitoring carbamazepine adverse effects.

Generally, ITN is diagnosed from the typical history, a negative neurological exam, a negative MRI and investigations, together with a positive response to a trial of the anticonvulsant carbamazepine.

TREATMENT (see also Chs 4 and 5)

- Patient information is an important aspect in management.
- Patients with TN are best seen at an early stage by a specialist in order to confirm the diagnosis and initiate treatment.
- ITN is often an intermittent disease with apparent remissions for months or years, but recurrence is common and very often the pain spreads to involve a wider area over time and the intervals between episodes tend to shorten. Few patients have spontaneous remission. Thus active treatment is usually indicated (**Table 52.2**), typically being medication.

Medical treatment

Medical treatment is successful for >80% of patients, the preferred treatments being anticonvulsant drugs, muscle relaxants or neuroleptic agents. The American Academy of Neurology and the European Federation of Neurological Societies recommend carbamazepine (stronger evidence) or oxcarbazepine (better tolerability) as first-line treatments. Carbamazepine, an anticonvulsant which is related to the tricyclic antidepressants, is the choice anticonvulsant in most instances (Ch. 5), and:

- prevents attacks of neuralgia in 60% of patients
- is not an analgesic and, if given when an attack starts, will not relieve the pain; rather it must be given continuously prophylactically for long periods
- is typically given in 100 mg doses twice daily for 2 weeks initially, then three times daily, increasing by 100 mg every 3 days to a maximum of 1000 mg/day. Most patients respond to 200–400 mg carbamazepine three times daily
- must be used carefully and under strict medical surveillance, and never in patients who are HLA-B1502, if Asian/Chinese because of the risk of erythema multiforme (Ch. 42)
- is contraindicated in pregnancy as it is teratogenic
- dosage control can be effected by blood monitoring
- dose should be increased to control the pain, while at the same time avoiding ataxia and other adverse effects.

May cause adverse effects in up to one-third of patients, which include mainly:

- ataxia
- drowsiness

- visual disturbance
- headache
- gastrointestinal effects
- facial dyskinesias
- folate deficiency
- hypertension.

Can cause other less common, but potentially serious, adverse effects, which include:

- rashes, sometimes severe and exfoliative, though rarely life-threatening
- pancytopenia or rarely leukopenia, which is idiosyncratic but typically occurs within the first 3 months of treatment.

Requires monitoring of patients, which should include:

- balance (disturbed – ataxia): this tends to be the feature that limits the dose of carbamazepine
- blood pressure (may increase): patients must have a baseline test and then blood pressure estimations for 3 months, then 6-monthly
- blood tests: electrolytes (sodium levels may be reduced – hyponatraemia); patients must have a baseline test and then monthly tests of urea and electrolytes; liver function (may be impaired; patients must have a baseline test and then liver function tests (bilirubin, transaminases) for 3 months, then 6-monthly); bone marrow function (red and white cells and/or platelets may be depressed; patients must have a baseline and then monthly tests of red and white cell and platelet numbers, and corrected whole blood folate levels)
- may interact with cimetidine and isoniazid, potentiates lithium and interferes with oral contraceptives.

Should carbamazepine provide inadequate pain relief, or if adverse effects are intolerable, the synergistic combination of carbamazepine with lamotrigine or baclofen may provide relief. Long acting local analgesic injections as peripheral blocks (e.g. ropivacaine – an amide which is less cardiotoxic than bupivacaine) may be of additional value.

If these regimens fail to control trigeminal neuralgia, a neurological opinion is in order. Meanwhile, phenytoin or other choices which may be effective are shown in **Table 52.2**.

Some patients report having reduced or relieved pain by means of alternative medical therapies, such as acupuncture, chiropractic adjustment, self-hypnosis or meditation. Some agents, such as proparacaine eyedrops, once considered of value, have no proven beneficial effect.

For patients refractory to medical treatments, or where adverse effects are intolerable, surgery may be needed.

Neurosurgical treatment

Gasserian ganglion percutaneous techniques, gamma knife surgery and microvascular decompression are the most promising options but patients may elect to try peripheral surgery first:

- Peripheral surgery: which involves deliberately interrupting nerve conduction in a division or branch of the trigeminal nerve, and may bring temporary relief of analgesia for some months and without permanent anaesthesia. These procedures include:
  - injections, usually of long-acting analgesics such as ropivacaine, or of streptomycin, alcohol or glycerol, around the mandibular or infraorbital foramen
  - local cryosurgery
  - chemical peripheral neurectomy of a trigeminal nerve division, using alcohol or phenol
  - radiofrequency thermocoagulation.
- Intracranial surgery open surgical procedures include posterior cranial fossa procedures, which are successful in providing instant and prolonged pain relief, but with possible morbidity and even mortality. Microvascular decompression of the trigeminal root (MVD) is currently the gold-standard method – repositioning the artery that supposedly irritates the trigeminal nerve as it emerges from the brain stem – since it gives the longest duration of pain control and is not followed by anaesthesia, paraesthesiae or pain as in some other neurosurgical procedures.
- Percutaneous approaches to trigeminal gangliolysis by heating, compressing, or chemicals are considered to have less associated risk and less cost than do open procedures. They can be done by inserting a needle into the skull through the face. Radiofrequency lesioning (RFL; percutaneous radiofrequency trigeminal gangliolysis (PRTG)) is the most commonly performed of these procedures. Percutaneous Fogarty balloon microcompression (PBM) and percutaneous retrogasserian glycerol rhizotomy (PRGR) are also used. Pain is exchanged for anaesthesia (and, therefore, a risk of damage to the cornea) and, sometimes, continuous anaesthesia, but with pain (anaesthesia dolorosa).
- Stereotactic gamma knife radiosurgery: the least invasive treatment, with the fewest adverse effects, offering a high rate of pain control of approximately 80% and with a low risk of facial paraesthesia, and a low pain recurrence rate. Its potential disadvantages include the use of radiation and the fact that benefit often takes 6 weeks or more to be considered successful.

For older patients, radiofrequency thermocoagulation of the Gasserian ganglion is recommended. In younger patients, the first choice is typically microvascular decompression.

FOLLOW-UP OF PATIENTS

Long-term follow-up as shared care is usually appropriate but if the pain falls out of medical control, or the patient has already had surgical intervention, secondary care is more appropriate.

TRIGEMINAL AUTONOMIC CEPHALGIAS

(See Ch. 17)

OTHER NEURALGIAS

RAEDER PARATRIGEMINAL NEURALGIA

Severe persistent pain in and around the eye with an associated Horner syndrome (see Ch. 56) is often caused by a lesion at the base of the skull and requires neurological attention.

GLOSSOPHARYNGEAL NEURALGIA

Glossopharyngeal neuralgia is much less common than trigeminal neuralgia. The pain is of a similar nature, but affects the throat and ear, and is typically triggered by swallowing or coughing. Occasionally, glossopharyngeal neuralgia is secondary to lesions (often tumours) in the posterior cranial fossa or jugular foramen (jugular foramen syndrome) and there are then often lesions of the vagus (X) and accessory (XI) nerves. Carbamazepine is usually less effective treatment than for trigeminal neuralgia and adequate relief of pain can be difficult, though gabapentin may be effective.

HERPETIC AND POST-HERPETIC NEURALGIA

Herpes zoster (shingles) is often preceded and accompanied by neuralgia (Ch. 43). Neuralgia may also persist after the rash has resolved. Pain in the trigeminal region may follow an attack of zoster, especially in older patients. In half those patients the pain resolves within 2 months but in others it may continue for up to 2 years or longer. Post-herpetic neuralgia is defined by the International Headache Society as pain developing during the acute phase of herpes zoster and persisting >6 months thereafter. Spontaneous improvement may follow, however, after about 18–36 months in some patients.

Post-herpetic neuralgia causes continuous burning pain that may be so intolerable that suicide can become a risk. Few analgesics relieve post-herpetic neuralgia, and treatment is difficult, but there may be relief using:

- gabapentin
- antidepressants (amitriptyline, desipramine or maprotiline)
- oxycodone

- carbamazepine (see above)
- topical capsaicin 0.025% or lidocaine
- transcutaneous electrical nerve stimulation (TENS – which increases beta endorphin and met-enkephalin).

In acute zoster, a regimen of 1000 mg of valaciclovir hydrochloride 3 times a day for 7 days plus gabapentin at an initial dose of 300 mg/day may be effective in ameliorating zoster and reducing post-herpetic neuralgia.

PATIENT INFORMATION SHEET

Trigeminal neuralgia

▼ Please read this information sheet. If you have any questions, particularly about the treatment or potential side-effects, please ask your doctor.
- This is an uncommon disorder.
- The cause is unknown, but involves spontaneous activity of pain nerves.
- It is not inherited.
- It is not known to be infectious.
- Similar symptoms may be seen in some neurological conditions (which we will exclude).
- There are usually no long-term consequences.
- X-rays, scans and blood tests may be required.
- Symptoms may be controlled, but not cured, by drugs with an anticonvulsant action.
- Uncontrolled pain may be treated by freezing the nerve, or surgery.

USEFUL WEBSITES

American Pain Foundation: http://www.painfoundation.org/

The Facial Pain Association: http://www.fpa-support.org/

PubMed Health, Trigeminal neuralgia. http://www.ncbi.nlm.nih.gov/pubmedhealth/PMH0001751/

FURTHER READING

Cha, J., Kim, S.T., Kim, H.J., et al., 2011. Trigeminal neuralgia: Assessment with T2 VISTA and FLAIR VISTA fusion imaging. Eur. Radiol. 21 (12), 2633–2639.

Chakravarthi, P.S., Ghanta, R., Kattimani, V., 2011. Microvascular decompression treatment for trigeminal neuralgia. J. Craniofac. Surg. 22 (3), 894–898.

Cruccu, G., Gronseth, G., Alksne, J., et al., 2008. AAN-EFNS guidelines on trigeminal neuralgia management. Eur. J. Neurol. 15 (10), 1013–1028.

de Siqueira, S.R., da Nobrega, J.C., de Siqueira, J.T., Teixeira, M.J., 2006. Frequency of postoperative complications after balloon compression for idiopathic trigeminal neuralgia: prospective study. Oral Surg. Oral Med. Oral Pathol. Oral Radiol. Endod. 102 (5), e39–e45.

Edlich, R.F., Winters, K.L., Britt, L., Long 3rd, W.B., 2006. Trigeminal neuralgia. J. Long Term Eff. Med. Implants 16 (2), 185–192.

Gaul, C., Hastreiter, P., Duncker, A., Naraghi, R., 2011. Diagnosis and neurosurgical treatment of glossopharyngeal neuralgia: clinical findings and 3-D visualization of neurovascular compression in 19 consecutive patients. J. Headache Pain 12 (5), 527–534.

Gorgulho, A.A., De Salles, A.A., 2006. Impact of radiosurgery on the surgical treatment of trigeminal neuralgia. Surg. Neurol. 66 (4), 350–356.

Gronseth, G., Cruccu, G., Alksne, J., 2008. Practice parameter: the diagnostic evaluation and treatment of trigeminal neuralgia (an evidence-based review): report of the Quality Standards Subcommittee of the American Academy of Neurology and the European

Federation of Neurological Societies. Neurology 71 (15), 1183–1190.

He, L., Wu, B., Zhou, M., 2006. Non-antiepileptic drugs for trigeminal neuralgia. Cochrane Database Syst. Rev 19 (3) CD004029.

Hojaili, B., Barland, P., 2006. Trigeminal neuralgia as the first manifestation of mixed connective tissue disorder. J. Clin. Rheumatol. 12 (3), 145–147.

Jorns, T.P., Zakrzewska, J.M., 2007. Evidence-based approach to the medical management of trigeminal neuralgia. Br. J. Neurosurg. 21 (3), 253–261.

Kanai, A., Suzuki, A., Osawa, S., Hoka, S., 2006. Sumatriptan alleviates pain in patients with trigeminal neuralgia. Clin. J. Pain 22 (8), 677–680.

Karibe, H., Goddard, G., McNeill, C., Shih, S.T., 2011. Comparison of patients with orofacial pain of different diagnostic categories. Cranio 29 (2), 138–143.

Kunkel, R.S., 2006. Headaches in older patients: special problems and concerns. Cleve. Clin. J. Med. 73 (10), 922–928.

Lacerda Leal, P.R., Amédée Roch, J., Hermier, M., et al., 2011. Structural abnormalities of the trigeminal root revealed by diffusion tensor imaging in patients with trigeminal neuralgia caused by neurovascular compression: a prospective, double-blind, controlled study. Pain 152 (10), 2357–2364.

Lapolla, W., Digiorgio, C., Haitz, K., et al., 2011. Incidence of postherpetic neuralgia after combination treatment with gabapentin and valacyclovir in patients with acute herpes zoster: open-label study. Arch. Dermatol. 147 (8), 901–907.

Larsen, A., Piepgras, D., Chyatte, D., Rizzolo, D., 2011. Trigeminal neuralgia: diagnosis and medical and surgical management. JAAPA 24 (7), 20–25.

Lemos, L., Fontes, R., Flores, S., et al., 2010. Effectiveness of the association between carbamazepine and peripheral analgesic block with ropivacaine for the treatment of trigeminal neuralgia. J. Pain Res. 3, 201–212.

Lewis, M.A.O., Sankar, V., De Laat, A., Benoliel, R., 2007. Oral Surg. Oral Med. Oral Pathol. Oral Radiol. Endod 103, S32.e1–S32.e24.

Liu, H., Li, H., Xu, M., et al., 2010. A systematic review on acupuncture for trigeminal neuralgia. Altern. Ther. Health Med. 16 (6), 30–35.

Marchettini, P., Formaglio, F., Lacerenza, M., 2006. Pain as heralding symptom in disseminated sclerosis. Neurol. Sci. 27 (Suppl. 4), s294–s296.

McMonagle, B., Connor, S., Gleeson, M., 2011. Venous haemangioma of the mandibular division of the trigeminal nerve. J. Laryngol. Otol. 28, 1–2.

Meyer, R.A., Bagheri, S.C., 2011. Clinical evaluation of peripheral trigeminal nerve injuries. Atlas Oral Maxillofac. Surg. Clin. North Am. 19 (1), 15–33.

Michiels, W.B., McGlthlen, G.L., Platt, B.J., Grigsby, E.J., Trigeminal neuralgia relief with intrathecal ziconotide. Clin. J. Pain 27 (4), 352–354.

Obermann, M., 2010. Treatment options in trigeminal neuralgia. Ther. Adv. Neurol. Disord. 3 (2), 107–115.

Obermann, M., Katsarava, Z., 2009. Update on trigeminal neuralgia. Expert Rev. Neurother. 9 (3), 323–329.

Ordás, C.M., Cuadrado, M.L., Simal, P., et al., 2011. Wallenberg's syndrome and symptomatic trigeminal neuralgia. J. Headache Pain. 12 (3), 377–380.

Pan, S.L., Chen, L.S., Yen, M.F., et al., 2011. Increased risk of stroke after trigeminal neuralgia - a population-based follow-up study. Cephalalgia 31 (8), 937–942.

Prajsnar, A., Balak, N., Walter, G.F., et al., 2011. Recurrent paraganglioma of Meckel's cave: Case report and a review of anatomic origin of paragangliomas. Surg. Neurol. Int. 2, 45.

Regis, J., Metellus, P., Hayashi, M., et al., 2006. Prospective controlled trial of gamma knife surgery for essential trigeminal neuralgia. J. Neurosurg. 104 (6), 913–924.

Rogers, C.L., Shetter, A.G., Fiedler, J.A., et al., 2000. Gamma knife radiosurgery for trigeminal neuralgia: the initial experience of the Barrow neurological institute. Int. J. Radiat. Oncol. Biol. Phys. 47, 1013–1019.

Rughani, A.I., Dumont, T.M., Lin, C.T., et al., 2011. Safety of microvascular decompression for trigeminal neuralgia in the elderly. J. Neurosurg. 115 (2), 202–209.

Simms, H.N., Honey, C.R., 2011. The importance of autonomic symptoms in trigeminal neuralgia. J. Neurosurg. 115 (2), 210–216.

Sindou, M., Leston, J., Howeidy, T., et al., 2006. Microvascular decompression for primary Trigeminal Neuralgia (typical or atypical). Long-term effectiveness on pain; prospective study with survival analysis in a consecutive series of 362 patients. Acta Neurochir. (Wien) 148, 1235–1245.

Tanigawa, T., Sasaki, H., Kaneda, M., et al., 2012. Lacrimal dacryostenosis with severe facial pain misdiagnosed as trigeminal neuralgia. Auris Nasus Larynx. 39 (2), 233–235.

Thorsen, S.W., Lumsden, S.G., 1997. Trigeminal neuralgia: sudden and long-term remission with transcutaneous electrical nerve stimulation. J. Manipulative Physiol. Ther. 20 (6), 415–419.

Trescot, A.M., 2003. Cryoanalgesia in interventional pain management. Pain Physician 6 (3), 345–360.

van Kleef, M., van Genderen, W.E., Narouze, S., et al., 2009. Trigeminal neuralgia. 1. Pain Pract 9 (4), 252–259.

Viana, M., Glastonbury, C.M., Sprenger, T., Goadsby, P.J., 2011. Trigeminal neuropathic pain in a patient with progressive facial hemiatrophy (Parry-Romberg syndrome). Arch. Neurol. 68 (7), 938–943.

Xu, S.J., Zhang, W.H., Chen, T., et al., 2006. Neuronavigator-guided percutaneous radiofrequency thermocoagulation in the treatment of intractable trigeminal neuralgia. Chin. Med. J. (Engl) 119 (18), 1528–1535.

Yang, M., Zhou, M., He, L., Chen, N., Zakrzewska, J.M., 2011. Non antiepileptic drugs for trigeminal neuralgia. Cochrane Database Syst. Rev (1) CD004029.

Zakrzewska, J.M., 2010. Assessment and treatment of trigeminal neuralgia. Br. J. Hosp. Med. (Lond) 71 (9), 490–494.

Zakrzewska, J.M., Lopez, B.C., 2006. Trigeminal neuralgia. Clin. Evid. 15, 1827–1835.

Zakrzewska, J.M., McMillan, R., 2011. Trigeminal neuralgia: the diagnosis and management of this excruciating and poorly understood facial pain. Postgrad. Med. J. 87 (1028), 410–416.

RELEVANT SYSTEMIC DISORDERS

First do no harm.

Hippocrates

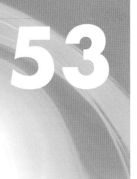

53

Human immunodeficiency virus infection

Key Points

- HIV is a lethal retrovirus infection transmitted by blood and body fluids
- HIV damages a subset of cells (CD4$^+$ cells) leading to severe T-helper cell immune defects
- Defences against fungi, viruses, mycobacteria and parasites are especially impaired
- Clinical disease (HIV disease) manifests after a long latency – with tumours, infections and other features
- Common manifestations are Kaposi sarcoma and lymphomas; infections with herpesviruses and papillomaviruses, candidosis and cryptococcosis, tuberculosis, and toxoplasmosis
- Acquired immune deficiency syndrome (AIDS) is the term used when the CD4 T lymphocyte count falls <200 cells/mL
- Antiretroviral therapy (ART) can prolong life in HIV/AIDS but can cause cardiac and many other adverse effects

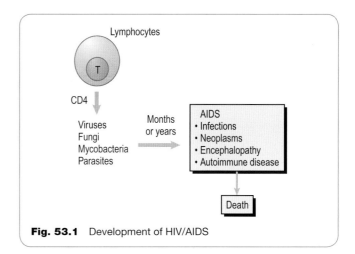

Fig. 53.1 Development of HIV/AIDS

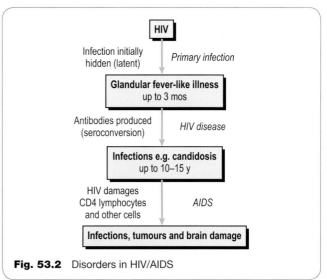

Fig. 53.2 Disorders in HIV/AIDS

INTRODUCTION

This is a potentially lethal condition. Infection with the RNA retroviruses known as human immunodeficiency viruses (HIV) – formerly termed 'human T lymphotrophic virus III' (HTL-III) – produces HIV infection which eventually damages T lymphocytes, especially those that are CD4$^+$, thus causing HIV disease and ultimately the acquired immune deficiency syndrome (AIDS). In healthy persons aged 5 years and older, with normally functioning immune systems, the CD4$^+$ T-cell counts usually range from 500–1500 cells/mL. These immunocytes are crucial to host defences against fungi, viruses, mycobacteria and parasites.

HIV predisposes to infection with fungi, viruses, mycobacteria and/or parasites, and the appearance of clinical diseases, at which time the condition is termed 'HIV disease'. This then progresses over time to AIDS, defined as a CD4$^+$ T-lymphocyte count at or <200 cells/mL in the presence of HIV infection. Premature death follows (**Figs 53.1** and **53.2**) though current anti-retroviral treatment (ART) can prolong life.

INCIDENCE

AIDS was first recognized in the USA in the early 1980s in the male gay populations, although the infection has subsequently been recognized to have existed in Africa some decades before then, at least in the 1950s. The causal virus proved to be a retrovirus, termed initially human T lymphotropic virus III (HTLV-III), and subsequently renamed HIV. The epidemic has spread worldwide in all sections of the community, largely in resource-poor groups so that, in the developing world HIV/AIDS is a leading cause of death in young people.

AGE

Worldwide, sexually active adults continue to be the age group mainly affected, predominantly heterosexuals but men who have sex with men are often infected (usually >15%). The number of cases in older adults is rising and in children continues to rise, largely through the increasing prevalence of infection in pregnant females.

GENDER

Worldwide there is little if any difference in gender affected by HIV.

GEOGRAPHIC

The HIV epidemic:

- appears to have originated from an epicentre in sub-Saharan Africa, probably Zaire and Cameroon
- rate of increase has slowed in most parts of the developed world
- worldwide has spread mainly via heterosexual sex, although the incidence is still especially high in men who have sex with men (MSM)
- in the Commonwealth of Independent States (CIS) (former Russian empire) and Asia is of major concern
- is not infrequently accompanied by infection with other blood-borne agents (e.g. hepatitis viruses) and/or sexually shared infections (e.g. syphilis), and/or tuberculosis which is increasingly multi-drug resistant (MDR-TB).

PREDISPOSING FACTORS AND TRANSMISSION

HIV is present in tissues and body fluids (including blood and saliva) of HIV-infected persons, transmitted mostly where the viral load is high and transmitted:

- Readily through sharing needles and/or syringes (primarily for recreational drug injection).
- Commonly by unprotected sexual intercourse with an infected person. The risk of transmission via various sexual practices varies; anal intercourse is more risky than vaginal; and genital intercourse is more risky than orogenital or oroanal sex. Transmission by recipient oral sex is far lower (estimated at 0.04% per act) than is transmission by recipient anal sex (0.82% per act).
- Sometimes to babies born to HIV-infected women, before or during birth – or through breastfeeding after birth.
- Less commonly (and now very rarely in countries where blood is screened for HIV), through transfusions of infected blood or blood clotting factors, or transplants.
- Rarely in the healthcare setting, by being stuck with needles or other sharps containing HIV-infected blood (needlestick injuries) or, less frequently, after infected blood has entered a worker's open cut or a mucous membrane (e.g. the mouth, eyes or inside of the nose).
- Rarely by saliva, presumably because of protection from salivary:
  - SLIP1 (secretory leukocyte protease 1)
  - peroxidases
  - thrombospondin-1
  - human beta defensins (HBD-2 and 3)
  - salivary chemokines CCL2, CCL4, CCL5 and CCL11 increase in HIV-exposed uninfected individuals, and may have a protective effect.

Barrier precautions are highly effective at preventing transmission in all social and work situations, except for needlestick injuries. Transmission is best prevented by:

- **A**bstinence
- **B**e faithful
- **C**ondom always.

AETIOLOGY AND PATHOGENESIS

- There are two main HIV viruses responsible for HIV infection and several strains of each, but little difference between them in terms of pathogenesis, manifestations of infection, treatment or prognosis:
  - HIV-1 is by far the most common worldwide
  - HIV-2 has spread from West Africa mainly.
- Most HIV infections are initiated at mucosal sites, including the oral mucosa. HIV RNA, proviral DNA, and infected cells are detected in the oral mucosa and saliva of infected individuals. The oral mucosa is not permissive for efficient HIV replication and therefore may differ in susceptibility to infection when compared to other mucosal sites. HIV exposure through oral sex appears sufficient to induce systemic HIV-specific CD4$^+$ and CD8$^+$ T-cell immune responses in some uninfected individuals HIV-specific T-cell responses in HIV-exposed uninfected individuals include HIV-Gag or Nef-specific T-cell responses. Serum neutralizing anti HIV-1 activity also develops but it is unclear whether such responses are protective, or are merely evidence of exposure.
- Infection with HIV infects cells with CD4 receptors. Though these are largely CD4$^+$ T-helper lymphocytes, brain glial cells are also CD4$^+$ and thus become dysfunctional and die. The declining CD4 cell count (and there is a falling ratio of CD4/CD8 cells) thus results in progressive immune deficiency, and also encephalopathy and dementia.
- As T-cell-mediated immune protection diminishes, patients become predisposed to infection with fungi, viruses, mycobacteria and parasites.
- Infections arise from commensal organisms (i.e. organisms that in the immunocompetent host cause no or little obvious harm) which become opportunistic pathogens, or from exogenous pathogens.
- Opportunistic pathogens include Candida species and other fungi, and some herpesviruses – especially herpes simplex virus (HSV), varicella zoster virus (VZV), Epstein–Barr virus (EBV), cytomegalovirus (CMV) and human herpesvirus-8 (HHV-8). Some viruses may cause neoplasms; HHV-8 causes Kaposi sarcoma (hence it is called KS HV), EBV causes lymphomas and some human papilloma viruses (HPV) may cause cervical, anal and oropharyngeal carcinomas.
- Exogenous pathogens encountered depends on the environment but include especially some mycoses such as *Pneumocystis carinii (jiroveci)*, cryptococcus and histoplasmosis; tuberculosis and atypical mycobacteria, such as *Mycobacterium avium-intercellulare*; as well as parasites such as cryptosporidia, *Toxoplasma gondii* and Leishmania.

CLINICAL FEATURES

ACUTE HIV INFECTION

Acute HIV infection passes unrecognized in the majority since features are so non-specific. In one-third to one-half of those infected, during the 4–7-week period of rapid viral replication immediately following exposure, there can be fever, malaise, lymphadenopathy, myalgia and other features closely mimicking glandular fever. Seroconversion and a broad HIV-1 specific immune response occur, usually within 30–50 days. High levels of HIV RNA are present in the blood.

CONTINUING HIV INFECTION

Following acute infection, HIV remains within the body, unlike many other infections that the host can combat. There follows an asymptomatic and variable period, often of years, when the virus is latent. There is a massive viraemia with wide dissemination of HIV in the blood to lymphoid organs, but the resulting immune response only partially suppresses HIV, and some virus survives, leading to the gradual loss of CD4+ T cells and progressive deterioration of immune function. There may be persistent generalised lymphadenopathy.

HIV DISEASE

HIV disease (symptomatic HIV infection) manifests as the CD4+ T cell count progressively declines over a period which may extend over 5–15 years or more, and the person starts to manifest:

- Infections: the most important infections are *Pneumocystis carinii* pneumonia (PCP), candidosis (**Fig. 53.3**), cryptococcosis, herpesviruses (especially HSV, VZV, EBV and CMV) and parasites, such as toxoplasmosis and Leishmaniasis. Tuberculosis is increasing in HIV-infected persons in whom it may involve mycobacteria resistant to a range of antitubercular drugs (multi-drug-resistant tuberculosis: MDR-TB or extended drug resistant tuberculosis: XR-TB).
- Neoplasms: most of which are malignant, appear to be virally related and include Kaposi sarcoma associated with KSHV (Ch. 43; **Figs 53.4** and **53.5**), lymphomas associated with EBV, and cervical or anal carcinomas associated with HPV.

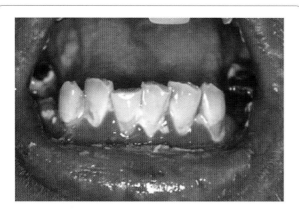

Fig. 53.3 Candidosis in AIDS

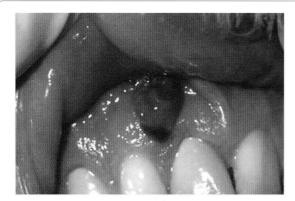

Fig. 53.4 Kaposi sarcoma in AIDS

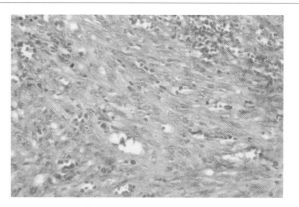

Fig. 53.5 Kaposi sarcoma histopathology

- Neuropsychiatric disease: which may include dementia and other cerebral syndromes. A degenerative neurological condition characterized by loss of coordination, mood swings, loss of inhibitions and widespread cognitive dysfunction, is the most common CNS complication.
- General deterioration with anorexia, diarrhoea, wasting ('slim disease'), premature ageing and autoimmune phenomena, such as thrombocytopenia.

AIDS

AIDS is the most severe manifestation of HIV infection. The US Centers for Disease Control and Prevention (CDC) list numerous opportunistic infections and neoplasms that, in the presence of HIV infection, constitute an AIDS diagnosis. These criteria include a CD4+ T-cell count ≤200 cells/mL in the presence of HIV infection (summarized in **Table 53.1**) and categorizes adults on the basis of CD4+ T-lymphocyte counts and clinical conditions associated with HIV infection, as follows.

The CD4 counts are defined as:

- Category 1: ≥500 cells/mL
- Category 2: 200–499 cells/mL
- Category 3: <200 cells/mL.

The clinical categories of HIV infection are defined as:

- Category A: (HIV infection)
  - asymptomatic HIV infection
  - persistent generalized lymphadenopathy (PGL)
  - acute (primary) HIV infection with accompanying illness or history of acute HIV infection.
- Category B: (HIV disease)
  - bacillary angiomatosis (epithelioid angiomatosis)
  - candidosis, oropharyngeal (thrush)
  - candidosis, vulvovaginal
  - cervical dysplasia
  - constitutional symptoms, such as fever (38.5°C) or diarrhoea
  - hairy leukoplakia, oral
  - herpes zoster (shingles)
  - idiopathic thrombocytopenic purpura
  - listeriosis
  - pelvic inflammatory disease
  - peripheral neuropathy.

Table 53.1 CDC classification of HIV and AIDS

CD4 count (cells/mL) (category)	Acute HIV infection, asymptomatic or PGL (A)	Symptoms and signs of progressive HIV infection, not AIDS (B)	AIDS (C)
≥500 (1)	A1	B1	C1
200–499 (2)	A2	B2	C2
<200 (3)	A3	B3	C3

- Category C: (AIDS)
  - candidosis, bronchi, trachea, or lungs
  - candidosis, oesophageal
  - cervical cancer, invasive
  - coccidioidomycosis, disseminated or extrapulmonary
  - cryptococcosis, extrapulmonary
  - cryptosporidiosis, chronic intestinal
  - cytomegalovirus disease
  - cytomegalovirus retinitis
  - encephalopathy, HIV-related
  - herpes simplex: chronic ulcer(s); or bronchitis, pneumonitis, or esophagitis
  - histoplasmosis, disseminated or extrapulmonary
  - isosporiasis, chronic intestinal
  - Kaposi sarcoma
  - lymphoma, Burkitt
  - lymphoma, immunoblastic
  - lymphoma, primary, of brain
  - *Mycobacterium avium* complex or *M. kansasii*, disseminated or extrapulmonary
  - *Mycobacterium tuberculosis*, any site (pulmonary or extrapulmonary)
  - *Mycobacterium*, other species, disseminated or extrapulmonary
  - *Pneumocystis carinii* (now *jiroveci*) pneumonia (PCP)
  - pneumonia, recurrent
  - progressive multifocal leukoencephalopathy
  - *Salmonella septicemia*, recurrent
  - toxoplasmosis of brain
  - wasting syndrome due to HIV ('slim disease').

PROGNOSIS

The prognosis of HIV/AIDS has almost invariably been poor and death virtually inevitable, although there are rare patients who show remarkable genetic resistance. Antiretroviral agents that have been developed that can significantly slow the progression of HIV disease so now affected people can survive for many years.

DIAGNOSIS OF HIV INFECTION

Considerable compassion is required in the diagnosis of such a catastrophic infection as HIV, since it impacts on virtually all aspects of the person's life as well as that of their family and others, eventually resulting in unpleasant, painful and incapacitating illnesses and their treatment. Confidentiality must be maintained at all times and the patient's consent and views always sought, including when considering informing other healthcare workers of any details about the person involved. There must always be appropriate counselling:

- HIV testing is discussed in Ch. 3. HIV infection at the very early stage may manifest no detectable antibody production and thus, at this time, the test for serum HIV antibodies alone (serotesting) can be falsely negative.

MANAGEMENT OF HIV DISEASE

Few, if any, patients have spontaneous remission and, thus, treatment is almost invariably indicated although, in rare cases, the disease progresses very slowly and may only at a very late stage manifest with serious complications. Patient information is an important aspect in management.

There has been remarkable progress in improving the quality and duration of life of HIV-infected persons because of:

- better education of patients and health professionals
- better recognition of opportunistic disease processes
- better therapy for acute and chronic complications
- the introduction of effective chemoprophylaxis; trimethoprim-sulfamethoxazole in particular reduces not only the incidence of PCP, but also of toxoplasmosis and bacterial infections
- the development of a range of antiretroviral therapies (ART) and their use now in early infection. Protease inhibitors are used together with reverse transcriptase inhibitors as highly active antiretroviral therapy (HAART) (see Ch. 5) which has significantly reduced the incidence of most infections and extended life substantially even to the 70's. However, some infections, such as herpes zoster and HPV-induced warts have increased. However, many drugs are liable to fairly severe adverse reactions and, perhaps more significantly, viral resistance has arisen (see Ch. 5). Combination antiretroviral therapy (CART) has increased life expectancy but also cardiac complications. In the era of CART, drug adverse effects may cause more morbidity than AIDS. There is some controversy as to the increase in cardiac disease and myocardial infarction, and as to the importance of prophylaxis of infections.

Effective and safe vaccines against HIV, however, are still in their infancy.

IMMUNE RECONSTITUTION INFLAMMATORY SYNDROME

The immune reconstitution inflammatory syndrome (IRIS) is a paradoxical immunoinflammatory reaction (brought about by improved immune status following ART) which can be serious, even fatal. IRIS initiation and progression seem to be linked to an increased CD4+ T-helper and CD8+ T-suppressor cell count and reduction in T-regs, with exaggerated cytokine release. Though few individuals starting ART are likely to experience IRIS, AIDS patients are more at risk if they are put on ART for the first time, or if they have recently been treated for an opportunistic infection. IRIS manifests with features that often resemble an AIDS-defining illness or other condition seen in people with HIV/AIDS.

CLINICAL FEATURES

The clinical presentation of IRIS is usually atypical. The manifestations depend on the trigger antigen, which can be an infective agent (viable or nonviable), a host antigen, or a tumour antigen. The range of common conditions that can occur or be exacerbated in IRIS are shown in **Table 53.2**; oral lesions are discussed below.

DIAGNOSIS

IRIS lesions may have atypical presentations but the diagnosis is usually made by astute clinicians, aware of the possibility of IRIS.

TREATMENT (see also Chs 4 and 5)

Most IRIS is self-limiting, but since a few cases can be overwhelming and even life-threatening, early recognition is important. Treatment is usually to continue the anti-HIV regimen and to give antimicrobials to treat infections and systemic corticosteroids to temporarily suppress the inflammatory process.

OROFACIAL LESIONS IN HIV/AIDS

Oral features of HIV/AIDS reflect the T-cell immune defect and are, thus, mainly the consequence of fungal or viral or sometimes mycobacterial or parasitic infections (**Tables 53.1–53.3** and **Box 53.1**):

- The most common are candidosis (candidiasis) and hairy leukoplakia. These are significantly associated with heterosexual route of HIV transmission.
- Necrotizing gingivitis, accelerated periodontitis, Kaposi sarcoma, lymphomas, salivary gland disease, ulcers of various infective aetiologies and other lesions may also be seen.

Table 53.2 Manifestations of immune reconstitution syndrome (IRIS)

Known infections	Other conditions
Cryptococcus	Aphthous-like ulcers
Cytomegalovirus	Castleman disease (Ch. 56)
Hepatitis viruses	Eosinophilic folliculitis
Herpes simplex virus lesions	Graves disease
	Myopathy
Herpes zoster	Non-Hodgkin lymphoma (NHL)
Histoplasmosis	Progressive multifocal
Kaposi sarcoma herpesvirus (KSHV)	leukoencephalopathy
	Sarcoidosis
Leprosy	Systemic lupus erythematosus (SLE)
Mycobacterium avium	
Papillomavirus	
Pneumocystis carinii	
Tuberculosis	

- These oral diseases have a number of common features, namely that generally they are:
  - not absolutely specific for HIV/AIDS, but are more a manifestation of the immune defect; thus similar lesions can be seen in other immune defects
  - generally more likely to manifest as the CD4 cell count falls to low levels
  - more likely to be seen where the oral hygiene is poor
  - more likely where there is also malnutrition
  - more likely if the patient smokes tobacco
  - often controlled, at least temporarily, by antiretroviral treatment (however, some lesions – such as zoster and warts – have increased since the advent of ART; see below).

Oral lesions may:

- indicate HIV infection that is previously undiagnosed
- be used in staging and therapy decisions
- cause the patient pain or aesthetic problems
- increase the liability for HIV transmission.

HIV-RELATED ORAL CANDIDOSIS

Oral levels of *C. albicans* and other yeasts are increased in HIV infection, and infection is common. Oral candidosis is:

- the most common opportunistic infection in HIV-infected persons
- often the initial manifestation of symptomatic HIV infection
- seen at some point in at least 90% of HIV-infected patients
- seen in all groups at risk, especially HIV-infected intravenous drug users.

Oral candidosis is related to:

- the immune defect; in general, the frequency of isolation of *Candida* species increases with increasing severity of HIV disease and with lower CD4 and/or CD4/CD8 ratios. T cells from HIV-infected patients also produce low interferon (IFN)-gamma, and there is a non-protective Th0/Th2 response to *C. albicans* antigen
- *C. albicans* from HIV + people which have an ectophosphatase activity significantly higher than the other isolates and show greater adhesion to epithelial cells and thus may contribute to establishment of candidosis
- hyposalivation and other salivary changes in HIV infection, such as reduced calprotectin, IgA, lactoferrin and anti-*Candida* antibodies
- smoking
- antimicrobial use.

Aetiology and pathogenesis

- Yeasts colonize the mouths of about 85% of HIV-infected persons.
- CD4 lymphocytes are deficient in the cellular infiltrate of candidal lesions in HIV infection. Salivary histatin-5 concentrations are also significantly lower.
- *Candida albicans* causes >85% of oral candidosis, but up to 35 strains have been found.
- The strain of *Candida* usually remains constant. Recurrence is usually caused by a persistent strain, but occasionally a different strain appears and there may be sexual reinfection.

Table 53.3 Orofacial lesions in HIV/AIDS

Type of disorder		Examples	Manifestations
Infection	Viral	Herpes simplex	Ulceration
		Herpes varicella zoster	Ulceration and pain
		Cytomegalovirus	Ulceration
		Epstein–Barr virus	Ulceration, lymphoma, hairy leukoplakia
		Kaposi sarcoma herpesvirus (KSHV)	Kaposi sarcoma
		Human papillomaviruses	Papillomas or warts
		Molluscum contagiosum	Papules
	Fungal	Candida	White or red lesions, ulceration or lump
		Cryptococcus neoformans	
		Geotrichium candidum	
		Histoplasma capsulatum	
		Mucoracea	
		Aspergillus	
	Bacterial	Mycobacterium tuberculosis	Ulceration or lump
		Non-tuberculous mycobacteria	
		Escherichia coli	
		Klebsiella pneumoniae	
		Actinomyces israelii	
		Bartonella (Rochalimaea) henselae and quintana	Epithelioid angiomatosis
		Periodontal flora	See text
	Protozoal	Leishmania	Ulceration or lump
Autoimmune		Aphthous-like ulcers	
		HIV salivary gland disease	
		Thrombocytopenia	
Other		Facial palsy	
		Trigeminal neuralgia	
		Taste disturbance	
		Exfoliative cheilitis	
		Hyperpigmentation	

BOX 53.1 Classification of oral lesions in HIV disease

Group I: Lesions strongly associated with HIV infection
- Candidosis:
  - erythematous
  - hyperplastic
  - thrush
- Hairy leukoplakia (EBV)
- HIV gingivitis
- Necrotizing ulcerative gingivitis
- HIV periodontitis
- Kaposi sarcoma
- Non-Hodgkin lymphoma

Group II: Lesions less commonly associated with HIV infection
- Atypical ulceration (oropharyngeal)

- Idiopathic thrombocytopenic purpura
- Salivary gland diseases:
  - dry mouth
  - unilateral or bilateral swelling of major salivary glands
- Viral infections (other than EBV):
  - cytomegalovirus
  - herpes simplex virus
  - human papilloma virus (warty-like lesions): condyloma acuminatum, focal epithelial hyperplasia and verruca vulgaris
  - varicella-zoster virus: herpes zoster and varicella

Group III: Lesions possibly associated with HIV infection
- A miscellany of rare diseases

- *C. albicans* isolates from HIV-infected persons may show increased:
  - adherence to oral epithelial cells
  - hyphal formation with epithelial invasion
  - aspartyl proteinase secretion
  - resistance to antifungal drugs, especially amphotericin, itraconazole and fluconazole, even despite no previous exposure.

- *C. albicans* serotypes change with the progression of HIV disease from the A predominant biotype to serotype B, although the latter is found especially in homosexual men, irrespective of their HIV serostatus.
- Serotype B in particular appears resistant to fluconazole, although itraconazole, voriconazole and posaconazole may still be active.

- About 15% of candidosis in HIV disease is due to non-*albicans* species, including:
  - *C. kruseii*
  - *C. tropicalis*
  - *C. parapsilosis*
  - *C. lambica*
  - *C. kefyr*
  - *C. geotrichium*
  - *Torulopsis glabrata*
  - *Saccharomyces cerevisiae.*
- Infections with non-*albicans* species are increasing, coincident with increasing use of prolonged antifungal therapy.
- *C. krusei* and *T. glabrata* particularly are becoming a problem since they are less likely to respond to fluconazole.
- New species closely related to *C. krusei*, such as *C. inconspicua,* are emerging and often fluconazole-resistant.
- New organisms, such as *C. dubliniensis*, related to *C. albicans*, have appeared, but at least at present remain largely fluconazole-sensitive.
- Up to 25% of HIV-infected patients with candidosis have infection by *C. albicans* plus other species.

Clinical features (see also Ch. 39)

Thrush (pseudomembranous candidosis) is one of the most obvious oral lesions in HIV infection and tends to be associated with lower CD4 counts, typically <200 cells/mL (see **Fig. 53.3**).

Other types of candidosis may also be seen, especially:

- erythematous; indeed, this form of candidosis may be a common early oral manifestation of HIV infection and presents as pink or red macular lesions, typically on the palate and dorsum of tongue and often mixed with white lesions (**Fig. 53.6**)
- angular stomatitis (cheilitis)
- median rhomboid glossitis
- hyperplastic candidosis.

Diagnosis

This is mainly clinical, supported by investigations discussed in Ch. 39.

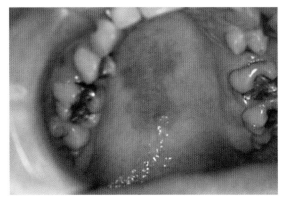

Fig. 53.6 Erythematous candidosis in HIV disease; a typical site is the vault of the palate in a 'fingerprint' pattern

Treatment (see also Chs 4 and 5)

Early treatment of oral candidosis in HIV disease is warranted, not only because of the discomfort, but also because foci may act as reservoirs for spread, particularly to the oesophagus:

- Predisposing factors, such as smoking and hyposalivation should be managed first.
- Antiretroviral and protease inhibitor treatment of HIV infection may aid resolution. Non-nucleoside reverse transcriptase inhibitors (NNRTI) regimens appear to be most effective in decreasing candidosis, consistent with current therapeutic guidelines, which recommend NNRTI-based therapy as the treatment of choice for initial ART.
- Antifungals; topical therapy of candidosis with gentian violet, nystatin, or clotrimazole is often successful initially within about 14 days, but relapses are common and these agents are not always palatable, or accepted by children. Failures are mainly attributable to underlying immunodeficiency and poor patient compliance due to:
  - polypharmacy
  - gastrointestinal upset
  - unpalatable taste of some agents
  - drug intolerance.
- Topical chlorhexidine is typically of minimal significant benefit in candidosis but triclosan may be beneficial. Gentian violet, lemon juice and lemon grass (*Cymbopogon citratus*) are other possible therapies.
- Antifungal prophylaxis should also be considered. Antifungal resistance is now a significant clinical problem in HIV-infected persons, especially in intravenous drug users, even in patients who have received no fluconazole, since resistance may be transferred and fluconazole-resistant species may be transmitted between patients. Azole resistance appears to arise because of changes in fungal enzymes or permeability. Risk factors include:
  - severe immune defect
  - previous fluconazole use, especially intermittent or low-dose therapy. Fortunately, there may still be clinical response to fluconazole in fluconazole-resistant candidosis, and amphotericin, ketoconazole, itraconazole, voriconazole, and posaconazole may remain clinically effective. Therapy in fluconazole-resistant cases, therefore, includes: topical amphotericin or higher oral doses of fluconazole (200–600 mg/day), fluconazole suspension as an oral rinse, ketoconazole (400 mg/day) or itraconazole (200–400 mg/day). Voriconazole, posaconazole or caspofungin may be indicated.

HAIRY LEUKOPLAKIA

Hairy leukoplakia (HL) is a common, corrugated (or 'hairy') white lesion usually seen on the tongue mainly in HIV/AIDS and other immunocompromising states.

Hairy leukoplakia:

- may be associated with EBV
- typically affects the lateral margins of the tongue (**Figs 53.7** and **53.8**)
- produces a white lesion that is not removed by wiping with a gauze
- is not known to be premalignant
- is a predictor of bad prognosis
- may be associated with lymphoma elsewhere.

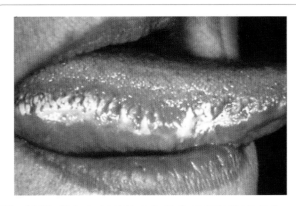

Fig. 53.7 Hairy leukoplakia is typically symptomless and bilateral on tongue margins

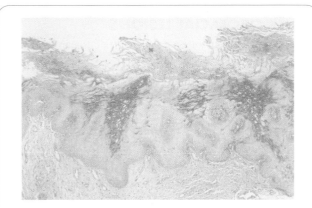

Fig. 53.8 Hairy leukoplakia histopathology

Diagnosis is largely clinical, supported by proof of EBV and usually HIV testing. Treatment is not often required, but the condition often resolves with aciclovir or other agents active against EBV, or with antiretroviral agents.

KAPOSI SARCOMA

Kaposi sarcoma (KS):

- arises from endothelial cells
- has been called 'gay cancer' by some since it is transmitted sexually especially to MSM, and seen rarely in HIV-infected children or haemophiliacs
- is caused by a newly identified virus KSHV, which is transmitted sexually, often as a co-infection with HIV. Like all herpesviruses this is a DNA virus, seen more commonly where hygiene is poor, and remains latent after infection. It is found in saliva
- presents initially as asymptomatic red, blue or purple macules
- progresses to papules, nodules or ulcers and may become painful
- is most common around the face (especially on the nose) and mouth
- occurs especially at the hard/soft palate junction or the anterior maxillary gingivae (see **Fig. 53.4**).

Diagnosis of KS must be supported by biopsy examination (see **Fig. 53.5**), since a clinically and histologically similar but

distinct lesion caused by the bacterium *Bartonella* (*Rochalimaea*) *henselae* or *quintana* can cause a lesion, epithelioid angiomatosis, that responds well to antibiotics. Management of oral KS is often with intralesional injections of vinblastine, or systemic chemotherapy. KS responds badly to irradiation. Rapidly progressive facial lymphoedema developing concurrently with, or immediately after rapid enlargement of oral KS may herald impending demise.

LYMPHOMAS

Lymphomas are seen increasingly in AIDS and are often:

- non-Hodgkin lymphomas (NHL)
- part of widespread disease
- seen in the maxillary gingivae/fauces (**Fig. 53.9**)
- lymphomas occurring more specifically in HIV-positive patients include a rare entity, namely 'plasmablastic lymphoma' (PBL) of the oral cavity. PBL is an aggressive variant of diffuse large B-cell lymphoma. Oral PBLs are strongly associated with HIV infection, with plasmablastic morphologic features without plasmacytic differentiation, and lacking CD20 expression. There is a good early responses to chemotherapy, but high relapse rates and poor prognosis, though better overall survival compared with patients with extraoral PBLs. Extraoral PBLs occur in patients with underlying non-HIV-related immunosuppression and universally demonstrate plasmacytic differentiation
- associated with EBV (NHL) or KSHV (plasmablastic lymphomas)
- fairly resistant to therapy.

Diagnosis must be confirmed by biopsy examination. Management is with chemotherapy.

GINGIVAL AND PERIODONTAL DISEASE

Necrotizing ulcerative gingivitis (**Fig. 53.10**) and periodontitis can be features of HIV infection, and typically these:

- occur disproportionately to the level of oral hygiene and plaque control
- are painful
- are localized
- cause rapid alveolar bone loss.

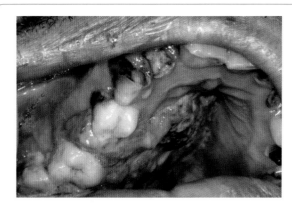

Fig. 53.9 Lymphoma in AIDS

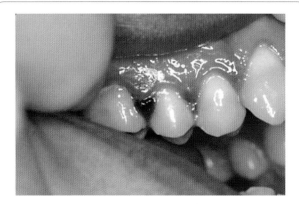

Fig. 53.10 Necrotizing gingivitis in AIDS

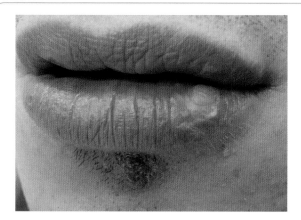

Fig. 53.11 HPV and HSV infections in AIDS

Diagnosis is clinical. The possibility of HIV/AIDS is heightened where there are additional suggestive lesions or where there is clear high risk of HIV infection, such as in an intravenous drug user. Management is with improved oral hygiene, debridement, chlorhexidine and sometimes metronidazole.

MOUTH ULCERS

Mouth ulcers may appear in HIV disease, but are, of course, common lesions in many non-HIV-infected persons. Ulcers may be unrelated to the HIV infection, or may be related to:

- aphthous-type ulcers, especially of the major type
- neoplasms, such as Kaposi sarcoma or lymphoma
- opportunistic pathogens, such as the herpesviruses (herpes simplex, varicella zoster, EBV, CMV), fungi (e.g. histoplasmosis or cryptococcosis), mycobacteria (e.g. tuberculosis or non-tuberculous mycobacteria (NTM)) or protozoa (e.g. leishmaniasis)
- drug use.

Ulcers may be part of widespread disease, such as disseminated cytomegalovirus infection, disseminated cryptococcosis or disseminated lymphoma, and thus the advice of a physician can be helpful if not mandatory. Diagnosis can be difficult and biopsy with microbial DNA studies may well be indicated.

Management depends on the aetiology, but chlorhexidine and topical analgesics can be helpful. Antimicrobials or other specific therapies are often indicated to control the lesions, depending on the cause. Granulocyte colony stimulating factors or thalidomide may be helpful in aphthous-like ulceration (Ch. 5).

SALIVARY CONDITIONS

- Parotitis and hyposalivation (HIV-salivary gland disease; HIV-SGD) are seen particularly in HIV-infected children. HIV-SGD, a hallmark of diffuse infiltrative lymphocytosis syndrome may have a BK virus pathogenesis. Cystic salivary lesions are increasingly recognized.
- Factors significantly associated with both hyposalivation and xerostomia include; sex, stage of HIV infection, risk group of HIV infection, systemic disease, and medication use.

OTHER OROFACIAL LESIONS

A wide spectrum of other orofacial lesions can be seen in HIV/AIDS, including the following:

- Cervical lymph node enlargement, as part of persistent generalized lymphadenopathy.
- Chronic sinusitis, which may be related to bacterial or, increasingly, fungal pathogens, such as aspergillosis or zygomycosis.
- HSV infections (**Fig. 53.11**).
- HPV infections, in particular genital warts (condyloma acuminata) in or around the mouth (**Fig. 53.11**). Persistent HPV infection is very frequent in HIV-positive men who have sex with men and these seem to have more frequent penile and oral HPV-associated diseases. Concurrent oral and anogenital HPV infection appears to be uncommon. Two manifestations of HPV that may be on the rise are HPV-32-associated oral warts and HPV-16-associated oral cancers.
- Cranial neuropathies, such as facial palsy, pain or sensory loss.

OROFACIAL CONSEQUENCES OF ANTIRETROVIRAL THERAPY (see also Ch. 5)

Use of ART may long-term be associated with:

- reduced risks of having orofacial pain, dryness (though some studies have shown no effect on salivary function), some lesions such as candidosis and periodontal pockets
- increased risk of having oral warts, hyposalivation, erythema multiforme, toxic epidermal necrolysis, lichenoid reactions, exfoliative cheilitis, ulceration, paraesthesia, and parotid swelling and potentially an increased risk later of oral squamous cell carcinoma. HPV-associated oral warts have a prevalence of 0.5% in the general population, occur in up to 5% of HIV-seropositive subjects, and in up to 23% of HIV-seropositive subjects on ART
- IRIS and orofacial lesions: especially candidosis but also herpes labialis, necrotizing periodontitis, hairy leukoplakia, zoster, Kaposi sarcoma and HPV lesions. Other oral lesions in IRIS of uncertain aetiopathogenesis include parotid swelling, hyposalivation and ulceration.

USEFUL WEBSITES

CDC National Prevention Information Network: http://www.cdcnpin.org/
www.hiv-druginteractions.org

MedicineNet.com, Human Immunodeficiency Virus (HIV Management). http://www.medicinenet.com/human_immunodeficiency_virus_hiv_aids/article.htm

FURTHER READING

Baccaglini, L., Atkinson, J.C., Patton, L.L., Glick, M., 2007. Management of oral lesions in HIV-positive patients. Oral Surg. Oral Med. Oral Pathol. Oral Radiol. Endod. 103, S50.e1–S50.e23.

Beyari, M.M., Hodgson, T.A., Cook, R.D., et al., 2003. Multiple human herpesvirus 8 infection. J. Infect. Dis. 188, 678–689.

Beyari, M.M., Hodgson, T.A., Kondowe, W., et al., 2004. Herpesvirus 8 virus (Kaposi's sarcoma-associated herpesvirus) in urine: monotypy and compartmentalization. J. Clin. Microbiol. 42, 3313–3316.

Beyari, M.M., Hodgson, T.A., Kondowe, W., et al., 2005. Inter- and intra-person cytomegalovirus infection in Malawian families. J. Med. Virol. 75, 575–582.

Bhayat, A., Yengopal, V., Rudolph, M., 2010. Predictive value of group I oral lesions for HIV infection. Oral Surg. Oral Med. Oral Pathol. Oral Radiol. Endod. 109 (5), 720–723.

Blignaut, E., Patton, L.L., Nittayananta, W., et al., 2006. (A3) HIV Phenotypes, oral lesions, and management of HIV-related disease. Adv. Dent. Res. 19 (1), 122–129.

Bonifaz, A., Vázquez-González, D., Macías, B., et al., 2010. Oral geotrichosis: report of 12 cases. J. Oral Sci. 52 (3), 477–483.

Boy, S.C., van Heerden, M.B., Wolfaardt, M., et al., 2009. An investigation of the role of oral epithelial cells and Langerhans cells as possible HIV viral reservoirs. J. Oral Pathol. Med 38 (1), 114–119.

Cameron, J.E., Hagensee, M.E., 2008. Oral HPV complications in HIV-infected patients. Curr. HIV/AIDS Rep. 5 (3), 126–131.

Capoluongo, E., Moretto, D., Giglio, A., et al., 2000. Heterogeneity of oral isolates of Candida albicans in HIV-positive patients: correlation between candidal carriage, karyotype and disease stage. J. Med. Microbiol. 49, 985–991.

Casiglia, J.W., Woo, S., 2000. Oral manifestations of HIV infection. Clin. Dermatol. 18, 541–551.

Castillo, J.J., Reagan, J.L., 2011. Plasmablastic lymphoma: a systematic review. Scientific World J 11, 687–696.

Ceballos-Salobrena, A., Gaitan-Cepeda, L.A., Ceballos-Garcia, L., et al., 2000. Oral lesions in HIV/AIDS patients undergoing highly active antiretroviral treatment including protease inhibitors: a new face of oral AIDS? AIDS Patient Care – Sex. Trans. Dis 14, 627–635.

Chaiyachati, K., Cinti, S.K., Kauffman, C.A., Riddell, J., 2008. HIV-infected patients with anal carcinoma who subsequently developed oral squamous cell carcinoma: report of 2 cases. J. Int. Assoc. Physicians AIDS Care (Chic) 7 (6), 306–310.

Chapple, I.L., Hamburger, J., 2000. The significance of oral health in HIV disease. Sex. Transm. Infect. 76, 236–243.

Dios, P.D., Ocampo, A., Miralles, C., et al., 2000. Changing prevalence of human immunodeficiency virus-associated oral lesions. Oral Surg. Oral Med. Oral Pathol. Oral Radiol. Endod. 90, 403–404.

Dios, P.D., Scully, C., 2002. Adverse effects of antiretroviral therapies: focus on orofacial effects. Expert Opin. Drug Saf. 1, 304–317.

dos Santos Pinheiro, R., França, T.T., Ribeiro, C.M., et al., Oral manifestations in human immunodeficiency virus infected children in highly active antiretroviral therapy era. J. Oral Pathol. Med. 38 (8), 613–622.

Epstein, J.B., 2007. Oral malignancies associated with HIV. J. Can. Dent. Assoc. 73 (10), 953–956.

Feller, L., Khammissa, R.A., Wood, N.H., et al., 2010. Facial lymphoedema as an indicator of terminal disease in oral HIV-associated Kaposi sarcoma. SADJ 65 (1), 14, 16–18.

Feller, L., Khammissa, R.A., Wood, N.H., et al., 2011. HPV-associated oral warts. SADJ 66 (2), 82–85.

Francischini, E., Martins, F.M., Braz-Silva, P.H., et al., 2010. HIV-associated oral plasmablastic lymphoma and role of adherence to highly active antiretroviral therapy. Int. J. STD AIDS 21 (1), 68–70.

Gaitan Cepeda, L.A., Ceballos Salobreña, A., López Ortega, K., et al., 2008. Oral lesions and immune reconstitution syndrome in HIV +/AIDS patients receiving highly active antiretroviral therapy. Epidemiological evidence. Med. Oral Patol. Oral Cir. Bucal 13 (2), E85–E93.

Giacaman, R.A., Asrani, A.C., Gebhard, K.H., et al., 2008. Porphyromonas gingivalis induces CCR5-dependent transfer of infectious HIV-1 from oral keratinocytes to permissive cells. Retrovirology 5, 29.

Gileva, O., Sazhina, M., Gileva, E., et al., 2004. Spectrum of oral manifestations of HIV/AIDS in the Perm region (Russia) and identification of self-induced ulceronecrotic lingual lesions. Med. Oral 9, 212–215.

Gonçalves, L.S., Souto, R., Colombo, A.P., 2009. Detection of Helicobacter pylori, Enterococcus faccalis, and Pseudomonas aeruginosa in the subgingival biofilm of HIV-infected subjects undergoing HAART with chronic periodontitis. Eur. J. Clin. Microbiol. Infect. Dis. 28 (11), 1335–1342.

González, O.A., Ebersole, J.L., Huang, C.B., 2009. Oral infectious diseases: a potential risk factor for HIV virus recrudescence? Oral Dis. 15 (5), 313–327.

Greenspan, D., Canchola, A.J., MacPhail, L.A., et al., 2001. Effect of highly active antiretroviral therapy on frequency of oral warts. Lancet 357, 1411–1412.

Griffin, E., Krantz, E., Selke, S., et al., 2008. Oral mucosal reactivation rates of herpesviruses among HIV-1 seropositive persons. J. Med. Virol. 80 (7), 1153–1159.

Hansra, D., Montague, N., Stefanovic, A., et al., 2010. Oral and extraoral plasmablastic lymphoma: similarities and differences in clinicopathologic characteristics. Am. J. Clin. Pathol. 134 (5), 710–719.

Hasselrot, K., Bratt, G., Duvefelt, K., et al., 2010. HIV-1 exposed uninfected men who have sex with men have increased levels of salivary CC-chemokines associated with sexual behavior. AIDS 24 (10), 1569–1575.

Hasselrot, K., Bratt, G., Hirbod, T., et al., 2010. Orally exposed uninfected individuals have systemic anti-HIV responses associating with partners' viral load. AIDS 24 (1), 35–43.

Hasselrot, K., Säberg, P., Hirbod, T., et al., 2009. Oral HIV-exposure elicits mucosal HIV-neutralizing antibodies in uninfected men who have sex with men. AIDS 23 (3), 329–333.

Jainkittivong, A., Lin, A.L., Johnson, D.A., et al., 2009. Salivary secretion, mucin concentrations and Candida carriage in HIV-infected patients. Oral Dis. 15 (3), 229–234.

Jensen, L., Jensen, A.V., Praygod, G., et al., 2010. Infrequent detection of Pneumocystis jirovecii by PCR in oral wash specimens from TB patients with or without HIV and healthy contacts in Tanzania. BMC Infect. Dis. 10, 140.

Jurevic, R.J., Traboulsi, R.S., Mukherjee, P.K., et al., 2011. Oral HIV/AIDS Research Alliance Mycology Focus group. Identification of gentian violet concentration that does not stain oral mucosa, possesses anti-candidal activity and is well tolerated. Eur. J. Clin. Microbiol. Infect. Dis. 30 (5), 629–633.

Kreuter, A., Wieland, U., 2009. Human papillomavirus-associated diseases in HIV-infected men who have sex with men. Curr. Opin. Infect. Dis. 22 (2), 109–114.

Leao, J.C., Kumar, N., McLean, K.A., et al., 2000. Effect of human immunodeficiency virus-1 protease inhibitors on the clearance of human herpesvirus 8 from blood of human immunodeficiency virus-1-infected patients. J. Med. Virol. 62, 416–420.

Magalhaes, M.G., Bueno, D.F., Serra, E., et al., 2001. Oral manifestations of HIV positive children. J. Clin. Pediatr. Dent. 25, 103–106.

Malamud, D., Abrams, W.R., Barber, C.A., et al., 2011. Antiviral activities in human saliva. Adv. Dent. Res. 23 (1), 34–37.

Mark, K.E., Wald, A., Magaret, A.S., et al., 2010. Rapidly cleared episodes of oral and anogenital herpes simplex virus shedding in HIV-infected adults. J. Acquir. Immune Defic. Syndr. 54 (5), 482–488.

Mbopi-Keou, F.X., Belec, L., Teo, C.G., et al., 2002. Synergism between HIV and other viruses in the mouth. Lancet Infect. Dis. 2, 416–424.

Mbopi-Keou, F.X., Legoff, J., Picketty, C., et al., 2004. Salivary production of IgA and IgG to human herpes virus 8 latent and lytic antigens by patients in whom Kaposi's sarcoma has regressed. AIDS 18, 338–340.

Menon, T., Herrera, M., Periasamy, S., et al., 2010. Oral candidiasis caused by Kodamaea ohmeri in a HIV patient in Chennai, India. Mycoses 53 (5), 458–459.

Mindel, A., Tenant-Flowers, M., 2001. ABC of AIDS: natural history and management of early HIV infection. BMJ 322, 1290–1293.

Mittal, M., 2009. AIDS in children – epidemiology, clinical course, oral manifestations and management. J. Clin. Pediatr. Dent. 34 (2), 95–102.

Moayedi, S., 2010. Head, neck and ophthalmologic manifestations of HIV in the emergency department. Emerg. Med. Clin. North Am. 28 (2), 265–271.

Mulu, A., Diro, E., Tekleselassie, H., et al., 2010. Effect of Ethiopian multiflora honey on fluconazole-resistant Candida species isolated from the oral cavity of AIDS patients. Int. J. STD AIDS 21 (11), 741–745.

Nair, R.G., Owotade, F.J., Leao, J.C., et al., 2011. Coinfections associated with human immunodeficiency virus infection: workshop 1A. Adv. Dent. Res. 23 (1), 97–100.

Namakoola, I., Wakeham, K., Parkes-Ratanshi, R., et al., 2010. Use of nail and oral pigmentation to determine ART eligibility among HIV-infected Ugandan adults. Trop. Med. Int. Health 15 (2), 259–262.

Niedermeier, A., Kovnerystyy, O., Braun-Falco, M., 2010. Syphilis in the context of HIV-infection - a complex disease. Dtsch. Med. Wochenschr. 135 (28–29), 1423–1426.

Nittayananta, W., Chanowanna, N., Winn, T., 2010. Mode of HIV transmission associated with risk of oral lesions in HIV-infected subjects in Thailand. J. Oral Pathol. Med. 39 (2), 195–200.

Nittayananta, W., DeRouen, T., Arirachakaran, P., et al., 2008. A randomized clinical trial of chlorhexidine in the maintenance of oral candidiasis-free period in HIV infection. Oral Dis. 14, 665–670.

Nittayananta, W., DeRouen, T.A., Arirachakaran, P., et al., 2008. A randomized clinical trial of chlorhexidine in the maintenance of oral candidiasis-free period in HIV infection. Oral Dis. 14 (7), 665–670.

Nittayananta, W., Talungchit, S., Jaruratanasirikul, S., et al., 2010. Effects of long-term use of HAART on oral health status of HIV-infected subjects. J. Oral Pathol. Med. 39 (5), 397–406.

Ortega, K.L., Ceballos-Salobreña, A., Gaitán-Cepeda, L.A., Magalhães, M.G., 2008. Oral manifestations after immune reconstitution in HIV patients on HAART. Int. J. STD AIDS 19 (5), 305–308.

Ortega, K.L., Vale, D.A., Magalhães, M.H., 2009. Impact of PI and NNRTI HAART-based therapy on oral lesions of Brazilian HIV-infected patients. J. Oral Pathol. Med. 38 (6), 489–494.

Owotade, F., Shiboski, C., Poole, L., et al., 2008. Prevalence of oral disease among adults with primary HIV infection. Oral Dis. 14, 497–499.

Palefsky, J., 2009. Human papillomavirus-related disease in people with HIV. Curr. Opin. HIV AIDS 4 (1), 52–56.

Papagatsia, Z., Jones, J., Morgan, P., Tappuni, A.R., 2009. Oral Kaposi sarcoma: a case of immune reconstitution inflammatory syndrome. Oral Surg. Oral Med. Oral Pathol. Oral Radiol. Endod. 108 (1), 70–75.

Patel, M., Shackleton, J.A., Coogan, M.M., Galpin, J., 2008. Antifungal effect of mouth rinses on oral Candida counts and salivary flow in treatment-naïve HIV-infected patients. AIDS Patient Care STDS 22 (8), 613–618.

Patel, M., Shackleton, J.T., Coogan, M.M., 2006. Effect of antifungal treatment on the prevalence of yeasts in HIV-infected subjects. J. Med. Microbiol. 55 (Pt 9), 1279–1284.

Patton, L.L., 2000. Sensitivity, specificity, and positive predictive value of oral opportunistic infections in adults with HIV/AIDS as markers of immune suppression and viral burden. Oral Surg. Oral Med. Oral Pathol. Oral Radiol. Endod. 90, 182–188.

Patton, L.L., McKaig, R., Strauss, R., et al., 2000. Changing prevalence of oral manifestations of human immunodeficiency virus in the era of protease inhibitor therapy. Oral Surg. Oral Med. Oral Pathol. Oral Radiol. Endod. 89, 299–304.

Patton, L.L., Ranganathan, K., Naidoo, S., et al., 2011. Oral lesions, HIV phenotypes, and management of HIV-related disease: Workshop 4A. Adv. Dent. Res. 23 (1), 112–116.

Pérez, C.L., Hasselrot, K., Bratt, G., et al., 2010. Induction of systemic HIV-1-specific cellular immune responses by oral exposure in the uninfected partner of discordant couples. AIDS 24 (7), 969–974.

Pienaar, E.D., Young, T., Holmes, H., 2006. Interventions for the prevention and management of oropharyngeal candidiasis associated with HIV infection in adults and children. Cochrane Database Syst. Rev. 19 (3), CD003940.

Plantinga, T.S., Hamza, O.J., Willment, J.A., et al., 2010. Genetic variation of innate immune genes in HIV-infected African patients with or without oropharyngeal candidiasis. J. Acquir. Immune Defic. Syndr. 55 (1), 87–94.

Portela, M.B., Kneipp, L.F., Ribeiro de Souza, I.P., et al., 2010. Ectophosphatase activity in Candida albicans influences fungal adhesion: study between HIV-positive and HIV-negative isolates. Oral Dis. 16 (5), 431–437.

Ramirez-Amador, V., Nittayananta, W., Magalhães, M., et al., 2011. Clinical markers of immunodeficiency and mechanism of immune reconstitution inflammatory syndrome and highly active antiretroviral therapy on HIV: workshop 3A. Adv. Dent. Res. 23 (1), 165–171.

Rohrmus, B., Thoma-Greber, E.M., Bogner, J.R., et al., 2000. Outlook in oral and cutaneous Kaposi's sarcoma. Lancet 356, 2160.

Schmidt-Westhausen, A.M., Priepke, F., Bergmann, F.J., et al., 2000. Decline in the rate of oral opportunistic infections following introduction of highly active antiretroviral therapy. J. Oral Pathol. Med. 29, 336–341.

Schorling, S.R., Kortinga, H.C., Froschb, M., et al., 2000. The role of Candida dubliniensis in oral candidiasis in human immunodeficiency virus-infected individuals. Crit. Rev. Microbiol. 26, 59–68.

Scully, C., Dios, P.D., 2001. HIV topic update; adverse orofacial reactions to antiretroviral therapies. Oral Dis. 7, 205–210.

Scully, C., Greenspan, J., 2006. Human immunodeficiency virus (HIV) transmission in dentistry. J. Dent. Res. 85, 794–800.

Scully, C., Porter, S., 2000. HIV topic update: oro-genital transmission of HIV. Oral Dis. 6, 92–98.

Scully, C., Watt-Smith, P., Dios, P., Giangrande, P.L.F., 2002. Complications in HIV-infected and non-HIV-infected hemophiliacs and other patients after oral surgery. Int. J. Oral Maxillofac. Surg. 31, 634–640.

Shiboski, C.H., Patton, L.L., Webster-Cyriaque, J.Y., et al., 2009. Oral HIV/AIDS Research Alliance, Subcommittee of the AIDS Clinical Trial Group. The Oral HIV/AIDS Research Alliance: updated case definitions of oral disease endpoints. J. Oral Pathol. Med. 38 (6), 481–488.

Syrjänen, S., 2011. Human papillomavirus infection and its association with HIV. Adv. Dent. Res. 23 (1), 84–89.

Tappuni, A.R., Immune reconstitution inflammatory syndrome. Adv. Dent. Res. 23 (1), 90–96.

Termine, N., Giovannelli, L., Matranga, D., et al., 2011. Oral human papillomavirus infection in women with cervical HPV infection: new data from an Italian cohort and a metanalysis of the literature. Oral Oncol. 47 (4), 244–250.

Thompson 3rd, G.R., Patel, P.K., Kirkpatrick, W.R., et al., 2010. Oropharyngeal candidiasis in the era of antiretroviral therapy. Oral Surg. Oral Med. Oral Pathol. Oral Radiol. Endod. 109 (4), 488–495.

Torres, S.R., Garzino-Demo, A., Meiller, T.F., et al., 2009. Salivary histatin-5 and oral fungal colonisation in HIV + individuals. Mycoses 52 (1), 11–15.

Tsang, C.S., Samaranayake, L.P., 2000. Oral yeasts and coliforms in HIV-infected individuals in Hong Kong. Mycoses 43, 303–308.

Tsang, C., Samaranayake, L., 2010. Immune reconstitution inflammatory syndrome after highly active antiretroviral therapy: a review. Oral Dis. 16, 248–256.

Tugizov, S.M., Webster-Cyriaque, J.Y., Syrianen, S., et al., 2011. Mechanisms of viral infections associated with HIV: workshop 2B. Adv. Dent. Res. 23 (1), 130–136.

Vultaggio, A., Lombardelli, L., Giudizi, M.G., et al., 2008. T cells specific for Candida albicans antigens and producing type 2 cytokines in lesional mucosa of untreated HIV-infected patients with pseudomembranous oropharyngeal candidiasis. Microbes Infect. 10 (2), 166–174.

Wadhwa, A., Kaur, R., Bhalla, P., 2010. Saccharomyces cerevisiae as a cause of oral thrush & diarrhoea in an HIV/ AIDS patient. Trop. Gastroenterol. 31 (3), 227–228.

Weinberg, A., Naglik, J.R., Kohli, A., et al., 2011. Innate immunity including epithelial and nonspecific host factors: workshop 1B. Adv. Dent. Res. 23 (1), 122–129.

Wright, S.C., Maree, J.E., Sibanyoni, M., 2009. Treatment of oral thrush in HIV/AIDS patients with lemon juice and lemon grass (Cymbopogon citratus) and gentian violet. Phytomedicine 16 (2–3), 118–124.

Wu, L., Cheng, J., Maruyama, S., et al., 2009. Lymphoepithelial cyst of the parotid gland: its possible histopathogenesis based on clinicopathologic analysis of 64 cases. Hum. Pathol. 40 (5), 683–692.

Xavier, S.D., Bussoloti Filho, I., de Carvalho, J.M., et al., 2009. Prevalence of human papillomavirus (HPV) DNA in oral mucosa of men with anogenital HPV infection. Oral Surg. Oral Med. Oral Pathol. Oral Radiol. Endod. 108 (5), 732–737.

Zapata, W., Rodriguez, B., Weber, J., et al., 2008. Increased levels of human beta-defensins mRNA in sexually HIV-1 exposed but uninfected individuals. Curr. HIV Res. 6 (6), 531–538.

Iatrogenic disease

INTRODUCTION

A number of medical and surgical treatments and dental interventions (**Table 54.1**) can result in iatrogenic (from the Greek *iatros* = doctor) diseases affecting various orofacial tissues and/or oral healthcare. A surprisingly wide range of infections, materials and drugs can affect the orofacial tissues on occasion and the astute diagnostician will always search the literature for such possibilities.

The most dramatic effects of iatrogenic disease however, are usually seen in cancer and transplant patients especially in those treated with radiotherapy to the head and neck region; in patients on cytotoxic chemotherapeutic agents; in patients on immunosuppressive therapy; or in those on combinations of these regimens.

IATROGENIC INFECTIONS

Fortunately, iatrogenic infections apart from opportunistic infections, are uncommon in the practice of oral medicine. Opportunistic infections, such as candidosis and herpesvirus infections, are common in immunocompromised patients, or those treated with some agents causing hyposalivation, antimicrobials, and some topical corticosteroid and other agents. Tuberculosis is an increasing issue in immunocompromised people, and people on immunosuppressive drugs including those treated with biologic agents (Ch. 5). The blood-borne agents such as hepatitis viruses, HIV, syphilis and prions should not be transmitted if standard infection control procedures are implemented. Hospital acquired infections have thus far not been a major issue in oral medicine (**Table 54.2**).

DRUG ADVERSE REACTIONS

It is important for the clinician to take a comprehensive drug history and always consider whether a drug may behind the clinical problem in question, since drugs can sometimes give rise to a range of adverse orofacial manifestations (**Table 54.3**), particularly salivary changes – notably hyposalivation, but also other features. Amongst the most common and important reactions and drugs implicated are:

- Hyposalivation: antidepressants, antihypertensives, antihistamines and anticholinergics.
- Swelling of gingiva: calcium channel blockers, ciclosporin and phenytoin.
- Swelling of lips/face: ACE inhibitors, aspirin and penicillins.
- Erythema multiforme: allopurinol, barbiturates, NSAIDs and protease inhibitors.
- Lichenoid lesions: antimalarials, beta-blockers, NSAIDs, phenothiazines and sulfonylureas.
- Ulceration/mucositis: barbiturates, cytotoxic agents (e.g. 5-fluorouracil, doxorubicin, and methotrexate), nicorandil, nonsteroidal antiinflammatory drugs (NSAIDs), sulfonamides and tetracyclines.
- Hyperpigmentation: antimalarials, cytotoxic agents, minocycline and zidovudine.
- Bruxism: ecstasy.
- Osteochemonecrosis: bisphosphonates.

The osteochemonecrosis resulting from bisphosphonates; adverse effects from recreational drugs; and opportunistic infections secondary to cytotoxic chemotherapy and increased prevalence of dysplastic and malignant lip and oral lesions in immunosuppressed patients and those using photosensitisers such as antihypertensive drugs are discussed below and in Ch. 31. Other possible reactions are shown in **Tables 54.4–54.31**.

OSTEOCHEMONECROSIS

Bisphosphonates (BP) are drugs used to prevent osteoporosis and bone resorption in, for example, metastatic malignant disease. Bisphosphonates are intravenously used (IV-BPs) for treatment of hypercalcaemia of malignancy, as well as prevention of skeletal-related events (SREs) and reduction of bone pain in cancer patients with osteolytic lesions. They are most commonly used in patients with multiple myeloma, breast, prostate, and lung cancers. Oral BPs are used mainly for prophylaxis of osteoporosis, and so are widely prescribed.

Table 54.1 Iatrogenic orofacial disease

Cause	Specifics	Disorders
Cancer treatments	See text	
Dental appliances	Dentures/obturators	Denture-related stomatitis
		Angular stomatitis
		Denture-induced hyperplasia
		Traumatic ulceration
		Caries
	Orthodontic appliances*	Traumatic ulceration
		Stomatitis
		Pain
		Root resorption
		Decalcification
		Caries
Dental interventions	Cross-infection	Various agents
	Local analgesic injections	Transient diplopia
		Transient facial palsy
		Nerve damage
		Haematoma
		Trismus
		Infection
	Tissue damage	Mainly soft tissue haematomas, lacerations or ulceration
	Tissue infection	Various
	Inhaled foreign bodies	Respiratory obstruction or infection
	Swallowed foreign bodies	Typically pass without consequence
	Foreign body in tissues	Granulomatous reaction
	Air in tissues	Surgical emphysema
	Psychological sequelae	Dental anxiety
		Dental phobia
Dental materials	Amalgam	Amalgam tattoo
		Lichenoid reactions
	Other materials	Foreign body gingivitis
	Corrosives	Burns
	Allergens	Angioedema
Drugs	See Tables 54.3–54.31	Wide range of disorders
Immunosuppressive treatments	See text	
Restorative dental procedures	Damage to teeth or soft tissues	Fracture or trauma
		Root perforation
	Pulp damage	Non-vital teeth
		Dental abscess
		Odontogenic infections
	Endodontic material extrusion	Nerve damage
		Sinus infection
		Osteochemonecrosis
	Endodontic instrument breakage	Endodontic failure
Surgery	Infection	Localized osteitis (dry socket)
		Osteomyelitis
		Bisphosphonate osteonecrosis
		Osteoradionecrosis
	Nerve injury	Sensory loss
		Facial palsy
	Bone fracture	Alveolar bone or jaw fracture

*Although some TMJ pain-dysfunction has been attributed to orthodontic treatment no reliable evidence is available.
**Suggestedly implicated in Alzheimer disease but no reliable evidence available.

Table 54.2 Some relevant iatrogenic infections

Infection	Examples	Comments
Fungi	Candida species	Implicated in candidosis and some cases of angular cheilitis and denture-related stomatitis Implicated in orofacial infections mainly in immunocompromised patients
	Deep mycoses	Implicated in orofacial infections mainly in immunocompromised patients
Bloodborne viruses	Hepatitis B	Immunization indicated for clinical personnel
	Hepatitis C	Implicated in some cases of lichenoid reactions and sicca syndrome
	HIV	See Ch. 53
Other viruses	Herpesviruses	See Ch. 43
Bacteria	Various	Wound infections
	Staphylococcus aureus	Implicated in some cases of angular cheilitis, sialadenitis, osteomyelitis, lymphadenitis and other infections
	Meticillin-resistant Staphylococcus aureus (MRSA)	May be community- (CA-MRSA) or hospital-acquired (HA-MRSA)
	Vancomycin-resistant Staphylococcus aureus (VRSA)	May also be resistant to meropenem and imipenem
	Mycobacterium tuberculosis and non-tuberculous mycobacterioses	A serious issue in immunocompromised people Implicated in some cases of ulceration and cervical lymphadenopathy
Prions	Creutzfeldt-Jakob and new variant Creutzfeldt–Jakob disease	Infectious agent composed of protein in a misfolded form, highly resistant to sterilization

Bisphosphonates were recognized from a series of case reports to be responsible for osteochemonecrosis of the jaw (bisphosphonate-related osteonecrosis of the jaw (BRONJ)) – defined as 'exposed necrotic bone appearing in the jaws of patients treated by BPs never irradiated in the head and neck area and that has persisted for >8 weeks'. BRONJ was very similar to the 'phossy jaw' reported in previous centuries as a result of occupational exposure to red phosphorus in makers of matches.

Most cases (>90%) of BRONJ have been in patients with cancer who received IV-BPs, in particular the nitrogen-containing BPs pamidronate and zoledronate, the cumulative incidence ranging from 1:10 to 1:1000 but the risk from oral BPs is far lower (<1:10 000). In addition, nitrogen-containing BPs induce mucosal cell damage and impede wound healing.

Aetiology and pathogenesis

BPs act especially by blocking the osteoclast HMG-CoA reductase (mevalonate) path, inhibiting the cell activities, as well as directly inhibiting osteogenesis in bone-healing. BPs remain in bone and exert these effects for many years or even decades. Risk factors for BRONJ include systemic and local factors (**Table 54.32**), especially tooth extraction.

Clinical features

BRONJ primarily affects the mandibular alveolar bone/mylohyoid ridge area, and features may include any or all of the following:

- exposed bone
- loose teeth
- foul discharge
- pain
- fistulae.

Lamina dura sclerosis or loss, and periodontal ligament space widening may be early manifestations.

Prevention

Prevention of BRONJ is fundamental, since no cure is known, and should include:

- Risk assessment.
- Patient counselling about risks.
- Avoiding elective oral surgery: including extractions or endosseous implant placement, or carrying out the treatment well before commencing BPs, or after a 6-month drug holiday.
- Preventive measures (dental screening, all dental work done at least 6 weeks before starting BPs) can produce a three-fold reduction of BRONJ related to zoledronate in myeloma patients. One protocol suggested to prevent BRONJ includes the raising of a flap before tooth extraction associated with a broad-spectrum antibiotic started three days before, and advancing the flap for primary closure.
- Serum collagen telopeptide (CTX) levels: a reliable index of bone turnover rates might predict BRONJ risk but this is controversial. Perhaps CTX monitoring could help determine the best timing for a 'drug holiday'.

Diagnosis

BRONJ diagnosis is mostly from a history of BP therapy and typical clinical symptoms. Because BRONJ has a variety on appearances on imaging, the diagnosis cannot be made from imaging alone though periapical and panoramic radiographs serve for initial screening. CT and MRI provide a more comprehensive evaluation. Bone scans can show abnormal radionuclide uptake 10–14 days before radiographic changes are seen on conventional films. Tetracycline bone fluorescence has recently been used to visualize margins of osteonecrosis more precisely: fluorescence–guided bone resection might improve the surgical therapy of BRONJ.

Table 54.3 Main adverse drug effects in the orofacial region

Effects		Examples	See Table
Salivary changes	Hyposalivation	Tricyclic antidepressants	54.4
	Salivary gland swelling or pain	Antihypertensives	54.5
	Sialorrhoea	Anticholinesterases	54.6
Halitosis	Halitosis	Disulfiram	54.7
Taste disturbances	Taste acuity loss (hypogeusia) or distortion (dysgeusia)	Protease inhibitors	54.8
Mucosal	Burns	Caustics, such as lime Cocaine Aspirin Potassium tablets Pancreatic supplements Trichloracetic acid Hydrogen peroxide Sodium lauryl sulfate,	
	Aphthous-like ulceration	Cytotoxic agents Immunosuppressive agents Nicorandil NSAIDS	54.9
	Mucositis	Cytotoxic drugs especially methotrexate, 5-fluorouracil, doxorubicin, melphalan, mercaptopurine or bleomycin	54.9
	Candidosis	Corticosteriods Antibiotics	54.10
	Contact stomatitis or stomatitis venenata Granulomas Cosmetic fillers	Antibiotics	54.11
	Lichenoid eruptions	Antimalarials Beta blockers NSAIDs Phenothiazines Sulfonylureas	54.12
	Erythema multiforme	Allopurinol Carbamazepine Barbiturates NSAIDs Protease inhibitors	54.15
	Pemphigoid	Furosemide	54.13
	Pemphigus	Rifampicin	54.14
	Lupus-like (lupoid) disorders	Hydralazine	54.16
	Discolouration and pigmentation	Amalgam Betel Chlorhexidine Crack cocaine Heavy metal salts Imatinib Tobacco	54.17
Cheilitis	Contact cheilitis	Protease inhibitors Retinoids	54.18
Swellings	Gingival enlargement	Calcium channel blockers Ciclosporin Phenytoin	54.19
	Angioedema	ACE inhibitors Aspirin Penicillins	54.20

Table 54.3 Main adverse drug effects in the orofacial region—Cont'd

Effects		Examples	See Table
Neurological	Neuropathies	Protease inhibitors	54.21
	Abnormal facial movements	Dopa Metoclopramide Phenothiazines	54.22
	Pain	ACE inhibitors Vinca alkaloids	54.23
	Burning sensation	ACE inhibitors Protease inhibitors	54.24
	Bruxism Trismus	Ecstacy Metoclopramide	54.25
Lymph nodes	Swelling	Carbamazepine Phenytoin	54.26
Tooth	Jaw development	Cytotoxic agents Phenytoin	54.27
	Hypersensitivity	Hydrogen peroxide or carbamide peroxide	54.28
	Damage	Tetracyclines	54.29
	Discolouration (**Fig. 54.1**)	Tetracyclines	54.30
Bone	Osteochemonecrosis	Bisphosphonates	54.31

Table 54.4 Drug-related hyposalivation

Drugs most commonly implicated	Drugs occasionally implicated
Alpha receptor antagonists for treatment of urinary retention Anticholinergics Antidepressants (serotonin agonists, or noradrenaline and/or serotonin re-uptake blockers) Antipsychotics such as phenothiazines Atropinics Diuretics Muscarinic receptor antagonists for treatment of overactive bladder Protease inhibitors Radioiodine	Amphetamines Antihistamines Antihypertensive agents Antimigraine agents Appetite suppressants Benzhexol Benzodiazepines, hypnotics, opioids and drugs of abuse Benztropine Biperiden Bronchodilators Bupropion Clonidine Cyclobenzaprine Cytokines Cytotoxics Decongestants and 'cold cures' Dideoxyinosine Diuretics Fenfluramine Fluoxetine Ganglion-blocking agents Histamine 2 antagonists and proton pump inhibitors Interleukin-2 Ipratropium Isotretinoin Leva-dopa Lithium Monoamine oxidase Omeprazole Opiates Orphenadrine Phenothiazines Propantheline Retinoids Selegiline Skeletal muscle relaxants Thiabendazole

Table 54.5 Drug-related salivary gland swelling or pain

Drugs most commonly implicated	Drugs occasionally implicated
Antihypertensives Chlorhexidine Cytotoxics Iodides	Antithyroid agents Bretylium Cimetidine Clonidine Clozapine Deoxycycline Famotidine Ganglion-blocking agents Insulin Interferon Isoprenaline Methyldopa Naproxen Nifedipine Nitrofurantoin Oxyphenbutazone Phenothiazines Phenylbutazone Phenytoin Ranitidine Ritodrine Sulfonamides Trimepramine

Management

Treatment is usually conservative alone when the disease presents at an early stage; a more surgical approach is supported at a later stage, or in refractory cases. Hyperbaric oxygen may be a possible adjunctive therapy.

RECREATIONAL DRUGS

Although not causing iatrogenic disease, a range of recreational drugs can damage the orofacial region (**Table 54.33**)

Table 54.6 Drug-related sialorrhoea/hypersalivation

Drugs most commonly implicated	Drugs occasionally implicated
Anticholinesterases	Alprazolam
Clozapine	Amiodarone
	Buprenorphine
	Buspirone
	Clonazepam
	Diazoxide
	Ethionamide
	Gentamicin
	Guanethidine
	Haloperidol
	Imipenem/cilastatin
	Iodides
	Kanamycin
	Ketamine
	Lamotrigine
	Leva-Dopa
	Mefenamic acid
	Mercurials
	Nicardipine
	Niridazole
	Nitrazepam
	Pentoxifylline
	Remoxipride
	Risperidone
	Rivastigmine
	Tacrine
	Tobramycin
	Triptorelin
	Venlafaxine
	Zaleplon

Table 54.8 Drug-related taste abnormalities

Drugs most commonly implicated	Drugs occasionally implicated
Antithyroids	Acarbose
Aurothiomalate	Acetazolamide
Aztreonam	Amitryptiline
Baclofen	Aspirin
Biguanides	Atrovastatin
Calcitonin	Ceftirizine
Captopril	Cisplatin
Cilazapril	Clidinium
Metronidazole	Clomipramine
Penicillamine	Cocaine
Protease inhibitors	Diazoxide
	Dicyclomine
	Enalapril
	Etidronate
	Fluoxetine
	Fluvoxamine
	Histone deacetylase inhibitors
	Imatinib
	Indometacin
	Isotretinoin
	Leva-dopa
	Losartan
	Pentamidine
	Phenytoin
	Propantheline
	Rifabutin
	Rivastigmine
	Sorafenib
	Spironolactone
	Topiramate
	Venlafaxine

Table 54.7 Drug-related halitosis

Drugs most commonly implicated	Drugs occasionally implicated
Drugs causing hyposalivation	Dimethyl sulfoxide (DMSO)
	Disulfiram
	Isorbide dinitrate

Table 54.9 Drug-related oral ulceration

Drugs most commonly implicated	Drugs occasionally implicated
Cytotoxics	Alendronate
Immunosuppressive agents	Aurothiomalate
Nicorandil	Aztreonam
NSAIDs, e.g. Indometacin	Captopril
	Clarithromycin
	Cocaine
	Dapsone
	Emepromium
	Everolimus
	Gold
	Interferons
	Isoprenaline
	Losartan
	Mycophenolate mofetil
	Naproxen
	Olanzapine
	Pancreatin
	Penicillamine
	Phenindione
	Phenylbutazone
	Phenytoin
	Potassium chloride
	Proguanil
	Protease inhibitors
	Sertraline
	Sirolimus
	Spironolactone
	Sulfonamides
	Tetracyclines

CANCER THERAPY AND COMPLICATIONS

See Ch. 31 and **Table 54.34**.

CANCER PAIN

Pain may be associated with tissue invasion, or cancer therapies, and is best managed pharmacologically with oral, rectal, transdermal, subcutaneous, or intravenous administration of NSAIDs, opioids and adjuvant drugs. Failing these, interventions that may be required include:

- Peripheral nerve blocks:
  - maxillary
  - mandibular
  - glossopharyngeal.
- Ganglion blocks:
  - sphenopalatine
  - trigeminal
  - stellate.

Table 54.10 Drug-related oral candidosis

Drugs most commonly implicated	Drugs occasionally implicated
Broad-spectrum antimicrobials	–
Corticosteroids	
Cytotoxics	
Drugs causing hyposalivation	
Immunosuppressives	

Table 54.11 Drug-related contact stomatitis (stomatitis venenata)

Drugs most commonly implicated	Drugs occasionally implicated
Anaesthetics	Chewing gum
Antibiotics	Cosmetics
Antiseptics	Dental materials
Barbiturates	
Dentifrices	
Mouthwashes	
Phenacetin	
Sulfonamides	
Tetracyclines	

Table 54.12 Drug-related lichenoid reactions

Drugs most commonly implicated	Drugs occasionally implicated
Antihypertensives	ACE inhibitors
Antimalarials	Amiphenazole
NSAIDs	Beta blockers
	Captopril
	Carbamazepine
	Carbimazole
	Chloroquine
	Chlorpropamide
	Cimetidine
	Clofibrate
	Daclizumab
	Dapsone
	Dipyridamole
	Ethionamide
	Gaunoclor
	Gold
	Griseofulvin
	Labetalol
	Lincomycin
	Lithium
	Mepacrine
	Mercury (amalgam)
	Metformin
	Methyldopa
	Metronidazole
	Niridazole
	Oxprenolol
	Para-aminosalicylate
	Penicillamine
	Phenindione
	Phenothiazines
	Practolol
	Propranolol
	Prothionamide
	Quinidine
	Quinine
	Streptomycin
	Sulfonamides
	Tetracycline
	Thiazides
	Tolbutamide
	Triprolidine

Table 54.13 Drug-related pemphigoid-like reactions

Drugs most commonly implicated	Drugs occasionally implicated
Furosemide	Captopril
Penicillamine	Clonidine
NSAIDs	Sulfonamides

Table 54.14 Drug-related pemphigus-like reactions

Drugs most commonly implicated	Drugs occasionally implicated
Diclofenac	Captopril
Penicillamine	Cephalexin
Rifampicin	Ethambutol
	Glibenclamide
	Ibuprofen
	Penicillamine
	Practolol

Table 54.15 Drug-related erythema multiforme (and Stevens–Johnson syndrome and toxic epidermal necrolysis)

Drugs most commonly implicated	Drugs occasionally implicated
Allopurinol	Adalimumab
Anticonvulsants	Bupropion
Barbiturates	Candesartan
Carbamazepine	Busulphan
Co-trimoxazole Hydantoins	Cephalosporins
NSAIDs	Chlorpropamide
Penicillin	Clindamycin
Phenytoin	Codeine
Sulfonamides	Ethambutol
	Furosemide
	Gold
	Metformin
	Minoxidil
	Oestrogens
	Phenothiazines
	Phenylbutazone
	Progestogens
	Protease inhibitors
	Quinolones
	Rifampicin
	Tetracyclines
	Tolbutamide
	Vancomycin
	Verapamil

Table 54.16 Drug-related lupoid reactions

Drugs most commonly implicated	Drugs occasionally implicated
Hydralazine	Ethosuximide
Procainamide	Gold
	Griseofulvin
	Isoniazid
	Methyldopa
	Para-aminosalicylate
	Penicillin
	Phenothiazines
	Phenytoin
	Streptomycin
	Sulfonamides
	Tetracyclines

Table 54.17 Drug-related oral mucosal pigmentation

Drugs most commonly implicated	Drugs occasionally implicated
Amalgam	ACTH
Chlorhexidine	Amiodarone
Smoking/tobacco	Amodiaquine
	Anticonvulsants
	Arsenic
	Betel
	Bismuth
	Bromine
	Busulphan
	Chlorhexidine
	Chloroquine
	Clofazimine
	Coal
	Copper
	Cyclophosphamide
	Doxorubicin
	Gold
	Heroin
	Hydroxycarbamide
	Hydroxychloroquine
	Imatinib mesylate
	Iron
	Ketoconazole
	Lead
	Manganese
	Menthol
	Mepacrine
	Methyldopa
	Minocycline
	Oral contraceptives
	Palifermin
	Phenolphthalein
	Phenothiazines
	Quinacrine
	Quinidine
	Silver
	Thallium
	Tin
	Vanadium
	Zidovudine

Table 54.18 Drug-related cheilitis

Drugs most commonly implicated	Drugs occasionally implicated
Etretinate	Atrovastatin
Indinavir	Busulphan
Isotretinoin	Clofazimine
Protease inhibitors	Clomipramine
Vitamin A	Cyancobalamin
	Gold
	Methyldopa
	Psoralens
	Streptomycin
	Sulfasalazine
	Tetracycline

Table 54.19 Drug induced gingival overgrowth (DIGO)

Drugs most commonly implicated	Drugs occasionally implicated
Amlodipine	Amphetamines
Ciclosporin	Cotrimoxazole
Diltiazem	Erythromycin
Felodipine	Ethosuximide
Lacidipine	Ketoconazole
Nifedipine	Lamotrigine
Oral contraceptives	Lithium
Phenytoin	Phenobarbitone
Verapamil	Primidone
	Sertraline
	Topiramate
	Valproate
	Vigabatrin

Table 54.20 Drug-related angio-oedema

Drugs most commonly implicated	Drugs occasionally implicated
ACE inhibitors	Angiotensin II antagonists
Aspirin	Antidepressants
Penicillin	Bupropion
Sulfonamides	Clindamycin
	COX-II inhibitors
	Droperidol
	Mianserin
	NSAIDs
	Proton pump inhibitors
	Statins
	SSRIs
	Vaccines

Table 54.21 Drug-related trigeminal paraesthesia or hypoaesthesia

Drugs most commonly implicated	Drugs occasionally implicated
Acetazolamide	Amitryptiline
Articaine	Chlorpropamide
Labetalol	Colistin
Protease inhibitors	Ergotamine
Vincristine	Gonadotropin-releasing hormone analogues
	Hydralazine
	Interferon alpha
	Isoniazid
	Mefloquine
	Methotrexate
	Methysergide
	Monoamine oxidase inhibitors
	Nalidixic acid
	Nicotinic acid
	Nitrofurantoin
	Pentamidine
	Phenytoin
	Prilocaine
	Propofol
	Propranolol
	Stilbamidine
	Streptomycin
	Sulfonylureas
	Sulthiame
	Tolbutamide
	Tricyclics
	Trilostane

Table 54.22 Drug-related involuntary facial movements

Drugs most commonly implicated	Drugs occasionally implicated
L-dopa	Butyrophenones
Metoclopramide	Carbamazepine
Phenothiazines	Ecstacy
	Lithium
	Methamphetamine
	Methyldopa
	Metirosine
	Phenytoin
	Tricyclic antidepressants
	Trifluoroperazine

Table 54.23 Drug-related orofacial pain

Drugs most commonly implicated	Drugs occasionally implicated
ACE inhibitors	Benztropine
Nitrites	Biperidin
Vinca alkaloids	Griseofulvin
	Lithium
	Penicillins
	Phenothiazines
	Stilbamidine
	Ticarcillin
	Vitamin A

Table 54.24 Drug-related burning mouth

Drugs most commonly implicated	Drugs occasionally implicated
Cytotoxic drugs	Antidepressants
ACE inhibitors	Clonazepam
HRT	
Protease inhibitors	
Proton pump inhibitors	

Table 54.25 Drug-related bruxism or trismus

Drugs most commonly implicated	Drugs occasionally implicated
Ecstacy	Duloxetin
	Fluoxetine
	Metoclopramide
	Phenothiazines
	Pregabalin
	Propofol
	Suxamethonium
	Tricyclic antidepressants

Table 54.26 Drug induced gingival hypersensitivity

Drugs most commonly implicated	Drugs occasionally implicated
Allopurinol	Abacavir
Carbamazepine	Atenolol
Lamotrogine	Azathioprine
Phenobarbitone	Captopril
Phenytoin	Dapsone
Sulfasalazine	Diltiazem
Sulfonamides	Gold salts
	Isoniazid
	Mexiletine
	Minocycline
	Nevirapine
	Oxicam
	Trimethoprim

Table 54.27 Drugs used in pregnancy that may induce cleft palate

Drugs most commonly implicated	Drugs occasionally implicated
Alcohol	Antihypertensives
Anticonvulsants	Corticosteroids
Cocaine	Cytotoxic agents
Fluconazole	Thalidomide
Heroin	
Phenytoin	
Retinoids	
Tobacco	
Topiramate	

Table 54.28 Drugs that may induce tooth hypersenstitivity

Drug	Examples
Tooth whiteners	Carbamide peroxide
	Hydrogen peroxide

- Central neuraxial techniques:
  - intraventricular opiates
  - intrathecal pump.
- Surgical complications.

Despite careful planning, surgical complications can still arise, though the impact can be minimized by vigilance.

CANCER SURGERY. POST-OPERATIVELY

PAIN

Post-operative pain is usually present for at least 24 h. Severe pain may need to be controlled by opioids (Ch. 5).

Table 54.29 Drugs that may lead to tooth structure damage

Drug	Examples	Possible damage to tooth structure
Sugar-containing oral (liquid) medication	Various	Caries
Drugs that result in decreased salivary secretion (hyposalivation)	See **Table 54.4**	Caries
Drugs with a low pH	Aspirin, antiasthmatic drugs	Erosion
Drugs causing gastro-oesophageal reflux	Theophylline, anticholinergics, progesterone, calcium channel blockers, antiasthmatics	Erosion
Drugs inducing bruxism	Dopamine agonists, dopamine antagonists, tricyclic antidepressants, selective serotonin reuptake inhibitors, alcohol, cocaine, amphetamines	Attrition
Drugs used for internal tooth bleaching	Hydrogen peroxide and sodium perborate	Cervical root resorption
Drugs used for treatment of childhood cancers	Cytotoxic agents	Abnormal dental development
Anticonvulsants	Phenytoin	Abnormal dental development
Fluorides	Any	Fluorosis

Table 54.30 Drug-related extrinsic tooth discolouration

Drugs most commonly implicated	Drugs occasionally implicated
Chlorhexidine	Antibiotics
Ciprofloxacin	Clarithromycin
Fluorides	Enalapril
Iron	Essential oil
Tetracyclines	Etidronate
	Fosinopril
	Imipenem
	Lisinopril
	Metronidazole
	Penicillin
	Pentamidine
	Perindopril
	Propafenone
	Quinapril
	Ramipril
	Terbinafine
	Trandolopril
	Zopiclone

Table 54.31 Drug-related osteonecrosis

Drugs most commonly implicated	Drugs occasionally implicated
Bisphosphonates	Denosumab
	Bevacizumab
	Sunitinib

Table 54.32 Risk factors for osteochemonecrosis

Systemic risk factors	Local risk factors
Duration of BP exposure i.v. administration Potent nitrogen-containing BPs (i.e. zoledronate, pamidronate and ibandronate) Smoking Diabetes mellitus Rheumatoid arthritis CYP2C8 gene diversity or reduced interleukin-17 Possibly chemotherapeutic agents, thalidomide, or bortezomib Denosumab (monoclonal antibody for treating osteoporosis)	Dental extractions: increase risk at least 16-fold and up to 44-fold Denture wearing: an almost 5-fold increased risk for patients taking zoledronate and also wearing dentures Periodontal disease: as a risk factor remains controversial

OEDEMA

Postoperative oedema depends largely on the extent of surgery but can be reduced by:

- minimizing the trauma, duration and extent of the operation
- using corticosteroids (e.g. 4–8 mg dexamethasone i.v.)
- nursing patient in head-up position.

If post-operative swelling may compromise the airway, a prophylactic tracheostomy should be considered

TRISMUS

Trismus can also be reduced by minimizing trauma.

Table 54.33 Maxillofacial consequences of use of specific recreational drugs

Drug	Possible complications
Alcohol	Leukoplakia, carcinoma, tooth erosion, glossitis/oral ulcers/angular stomatitis from malnutrition, sialosis, foetal alcohol syndrome
Amphetamine	Picking at the face, bruxism, hyposalivation and increased caries incidence 'Meth mouth' is the term given to the neglect and poor oral hygiene seen in methamphetamine users
Barbiturates	Facial pain, bullous reactions
Betel	Submucous fibrosis, leukoplakia, carcinoma
Cannabis	White lesions (burns), hyposalivation, possible leukoplakia, carcinoma
Cocaine	Temporarily numbness of lips and tongue, gingival erosions, dry mouth, bruxism dental erosion Caries and periodontal disease, especially acute necrotizing gingivitis, are more frequent Cocaine may precipitate cluster headaches Oronasal fistulae
Ecstasy	Tooth clenching, bruxism, TMJ dysfunction, dry mouth, attrition, dental erosion, mucosal burns or ulceration, circumoral paraesthesiae and periodontitis
Khat	Leukoplakia, carcinoma
Nicotine	Due to tobacco: leukoplakia, carcinoma, dry socket, necrotizing gingivitis, periodontitis, impaired wound healing and implant success
Opiates	Hyposalivation
Solvents	Perioral dermatitis, foetal gasoline/petrol syndrome

Table 54.34 Orofacial complications of cancer therapy

Therapy	Oral complications
Radiotherapy	Pain, mucositis, hyposalivation, candidosis, caries, sialadenitis, osteoradionecrosis, fibrosis
Chemotherapy	Pain, mucositis, hyposalivation, candidosis, herpesviruses, neuropathy
Surgery	Pain, neuropathy, disfigurement, impaired speech and swallowing Scarring Carotid blow-out (haemorrhage), chyle leakage, salivary leakage

INFECTION

Wound infection can produce significant pain, swelling, restricted function and poor cosmetic results and will likely prolong hospitalization. Infections are most likely:

- in males;
- in advanced tumours
- after extensive surgery
- after tissue transplantation
- where oral healthcare is poor.

The diagnosis of infection is usually as, at about 3–7 days after operation, the wound appears inflamed, swollen and tender. There may be pus and pyrexia. Infection under neck flaps is particularly dangerous as the internal carotid artery may be eroded (see below 'carotid blow-out'). Infections may settle spontaneously within a few days, but pus or a swab should be taken to identify the organism and test sensitivity to antibiotics. If the wound is not draining but is fluctuant, one or more sutures should be removed, sinus forceps inserted and gently opened to allow pus drainage.

FLAP COMPLICATIONS

Micro-surgical flap transfers are usually lengthy, technically demanding and therefore physiologically traumatic operations capable of potentially major complications such as myocardial infarction, stroke and death. Contra-indications for flap procedures therefore include significant co-morbidities. Advanced age is not necessarily a contraindication, nor is a well-controlled severe medical co-morbidity.

Post-operative staff must be familiar with the general care of hydration, filling pressures, urine output, body temperature and pain. Pain should be well controlled to prevent anxiety. Anticoagulation (e.g. Dextran 40, heparin, or aspirin) may be needed, that in turn leads to vasoconstriction. Flap vitality should be monitored by regular and frequent clinical examination for the first 48 h (flap colour, skin turgor, refill and needle test–which should result in the oozing of bright red blood up to a minute after the needle is withdrawn). Others use monitoring techniques such as Doppler ultrasound, temperature monitoring, pulse oximetry or near infrared spectroscopy. If the flap vascularity is suspected to be compromised, hypotension must be excluded, the patient repositioned to relieve any pedicle obstruction, haematoma excluded and compressive dressings or tight sutures removed. If these simple manoeuvres fail, the flap must be re-explored immediately.

EATING PROBLEMS

Patients should be weighed regularly. Dieticians should be consulted. Nutrition may need supplemented:

- enterally by naso-gastric (NG) or orogastric tube, percutaneous endoscopic gastostomy (PEG) or radiologically-inserted gastrostomy (RIG). Continuous infusion of a liquid feed is preferred, since intermittent feeding may cause diarrhoea
- parenterally, i.e. via an i.v. catheter (central line) in the subclavian or jugular veins (total parenteral nutrition; TPN). A central line is a silicone rubber skin-tunnelled central venous catheter (e.g. Hickman® or Groshong®).

If a central line is necessary, urea, electrolytes and liver function must then be monitored.

RARER COMPLICATIONS
Vascular complications

Sacrifice of the common or internal carotid arteries can produce some of the most serious complications seen in head and neck surgery. When internal carotid artery resection is planned, balloon-test occlusion with hypotensive challenge reliably assesses the risk. In bilateral neck dissections where one internal jugular vein (IJV) is preserved, post-operative imaging shows thrombosis in up to 30%. If both IJVs are to be transected then conduits in the external venous system should be preserved wherever possible. Bilateral internal jugular vein (IJV) ligation may produce raised intra-cranial pressure (ICP) along with secondary hypertension (Cushing reflex). The rise in ICP commonly requires aggressive treatment – hyperventilation, fluid restriction, corticosteroids and mannitol.

Carotid blow-out is more likely where the patient has had radiotherapy, damage to the artery during surgery and salivary fistulae and is associated with over 60% morbidity and 50% mortality. If it is anticipated that the carotid artery will be exposed, the vessels should be covered, e.g. dermal graft, fascia lata or levator scapulae muscle flap. If impending blow-out is suspected (e.g. as suggested by a sentinel bleed), stent-grafts may be preferred over emergency open carotid artery ligation (which may well be complicated by neurological sequelae such as hemiplegia, hemi-anaesthesia, aphasia and dysarthria).

Air embolism is rare but potentially lethal and most commonly follows damage to the IVJ during surgery. Large air emboli produce sudden falls in end-tidal carbon dioxide and blood pressure and, in severe cases air can be aspirated from the right side of the heart. A pre-cordial Doppler probe may detect a characteristic murmur. Pressure should be applied to the affected vein and the patient placed in the Trendelenburg head down position and rotated to the left. Hyperbaric oxygen is the ultimate and effective treatment.

Seroma

Seroma is the accumulation of serous fluid under large flaps, and appears as a large fluctuant swelling that is neither warm nor tender. Seromas may have to be drained several times using large syringes and needles or cannulae. Moderate pressure dressings should then be applied.

Sialocele

Sialocele is a swelling due to leakage of saliva occasionally appearing over the area of the parotid following partial parotidectomy. Sialoceles usually settle spontaneously with time, but may need to be managed in a manner similar to seromas. A hyoscine transdermal patch may be helpful.

Frey syndrome

This may follow damage in the parotid region by trauma, submandibular gland surgery, neck dissection, or carotid endarterectomy, and is characterized by skin redness and sweating after eating or thinking or talking about food. Testing with lemon or a positive starch-iodine test can be diagnostic. Treatments include topical hyoscine or intradermal botulinum toxoid.

Chyle leak

Chyle leak arises from damage to the chyle duct, often only identified when feeding is begun. Management approaches include nutritional, surgical and pharmacological therapy.

Nerve damage

The spinal accessory nerve to the trapezius muscle if damaged can cause significantly shoulder disability. Other nerves also at risk include the vagus, lingual, hypoglossal and marginal mandibular branch of the facial nerves. Transection of the vagus nerve can result in intra-operative cardiac problems. Transient neuropraxia to the phrenic branch of the vagus often manifests post-operatively with changes on plain radiography but, if a severe pulmonary problem exists, especially with concurrent pectoris major flat harvest, respiration may be compromised. Bilateral phrenic nerve palsies may necessitate periods of prolonged mechanical ventilation. The sympathetic trunk is also at risk of injury, but subsequent Horner syndrome is rare.

Pneumothorax

Pneumothorax may occur when surgery is low in the neck particularly if the lung apex is high. Pleural tears should be closed and their integrity tested by hyper-inflating the lung, placing the patient in the Trendelenburg position and irrigating the area to observe bubbles. Imaging can determine the need for open drainage.

Radiation toxicities

Radiotherapy (RT) damages mucosa after 12 exposures, skin after 21 and also damages endothelium after 60. RT damages only cells undergoing mitosis – such as epithelium. Bone cells only undergo mitosis after trauma.

RT can cause a range of adverse effects (**Table 54.35**). Some–notably mucositis and hyposalivation – arise almost immediately and are predictable, whilst others appear later and unpredictably. Mucositis, dysphagia, xerostomia, dermatitis and pain – significantly impair QoL, as do hyposalivation (up to 90% incidence) and grade 3 (severe) dysphagia (up to 30%).

Late RT toxicity is permanent and also may include:

- jaw osteoradionecrosis
- sensori-neural hearing loss
- skin fibrosis
- laryngeal cartilage necrosis
- cervical atherosclerosis.

Table 54.35 Oral complications of radiotherapy and management

Complication	Management
Candidosis	Nystatin suspension 100 000 IU/mL as mouthwash four times daily Fluconazole suspension, itraconazole liquid or posaconazole suspension if immunocompromised
Caries	Daily topical fluoride applications; high fluoride toothpastes; ACP Avoid sugary diet
Dental hypersensitivity	Fluoride applications/mouthwashes
Hyposalivation	Saliva substitute (mouth wetting agents)* Frequent ice cubes, popsicles or sips of water Sialogogues, e.g. pilocarpine or cevimeline
Mucositis	Prophylaxis: Amifostine 200 mg/m² /day Betamethasone mouthwash four times daily from the day before radiotherapy, throughout the course Opiates such as buprenorphine for analgesia
Osteoradionecrosis	Avoid by atraumatic extractions under antibiotic cover, with primary wound closure Planned pre-radiotherapy extractions or extractions within 3 months of radiotherapy
Sialadenitis	Antimicrobials
Taste loss	Consider zinc sulphate
Tooth and jaw maldevelopment	–
Trismus	Jaw-opening exercises three times daily

*Artificial saliva (e.g. methylcellulose) or mucin. ACP, amorphous calcium phosphate.

Table 54.36 Minimizing oral complications of radiotherapy

Method	Regime	Comments
Minimize radiation dose	Ipsilateral irradiation Positioning devices Shielding	
	Conformational field planning	Intensity modulated radiotherapy (IMRT) or image guided radiotherapy (IGRT)
	Helical tomotherapy	Hi-art
	Gland repositioning	Invasive
Medical protection	Sialoprotective agents	Pilocarpine Amifostine
Emergent therapies	Salivary gland transplantation Salivary gland cell replacement	Minimally invasive salivary gland transfer (MIST) Stem cell or bone marrow cell transplantation

Mucositis can lead to a number of problems, including:

- significantly interfering with quality of life
- acting as a portal for septicaemia, especially streptococcal, sometimes with lethal consequences
- extending hospitalization
- increasing costs of care.

Mucositis can be reduced by (**Tables 54.35** and **54.36**):

- minimizing doses and field of radiation
- using mucosa-sparing blocks
- using amifostine before therapy
- avoiding chemo-radiotherapy
- betamethasone mouthwashes.
- using new radiation techniques

The time to healing depends on the radiation dose intensity, but is usually complete within 3 weeks after the end of treatment. Tobacco smoking delays resolution.

Treatment (see also Chs 4 and 5) includes:

- Opioids, such as morphine and hydromorphone.
- Avoiding irritants (smoking, spirits or spicy foods).
- Good oral hygiene.
- Topical analgesics used prior to meals to help combat pain and dysphagia, such as:
  - benzydamine hydrochloride
  - 2% lidocaine (lignocaine) mouthwash
  - aspirin.

There are many other preparations used, often variants on the 'magic mouthwash' (viscous lidocaine, diphenhydramine, bismuth salicylate and a corticosteroid).

HYPOSALIVATION

Hyposalivation (**Fig. 54.3**) predisposes to caries (**Fig. 54.4**), candidosis and bacterial acute ascending sialadenitis (**Fig. 54.5**) (see Ch. 15) and is discussed also in Ch. 31. Changes may be:

- quantitative (dry mouth or hyposalivation)
- qualitative (pH falls; buffering capacity decreases; electrolytes change).

IMMEDIATE COMPLICATIONS
MUCOSITIS

RT it is most often administered in small fractions over several weeks and to a localized area. Radiation-induced mucositis is invariable within the radiated field of mucosa and typically begins at cumulative doses of about 15 Gy (i.e. after around 10 days) and reaches full severity at 30 Gy, persisting for weeks or months Tissues such as the soft palate, and the lateral borders and ventral surface of the tongue and floor of the mouth which have a good vascular supply or a higher cell turnover rate are more susceptible to radiation mucositis. Risk factors for radiation mucositis apart from the radiation dose and fractionation include:

- concurrent chemotherapy
- younger age
- alcohol
- poor oral hygiene
- dental disease.

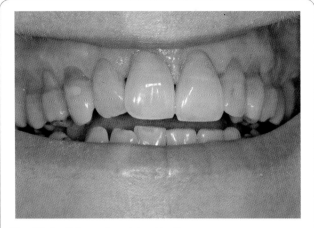

Fig. 54.1 Tetracycline stained teeth

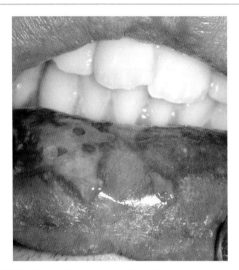

Fig. 54.2 Mucositis presents with widespread erosions in cancer therapy

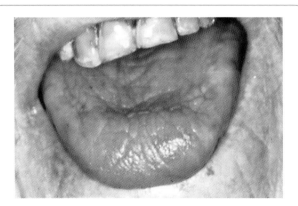

Fig. 54.3 Hyposalivation after head and neck irradiation treatment

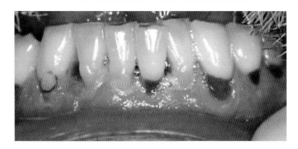

Fig. 54.4 Radiation caries - common after radiotherapy involving the salivary glands

Factors predisposing to salivary changes include:

- radiation
- dose
- fraction size and number of exposures
- type
- salivary gland
- function before RT
- volume irradiated.

Hyposalivation can be reduced by (**Tables 54.35** and **54.36**):

- minimizing doses and field of radiation
- using parotid-sparing techniques such as IMRT (Intensity Modulated RT)
- using amifostine or pilocarpine before therapy
- avoiding chemo-radiotherapy.

Emergent therapies are on the horizon, including salivary stem cell transplantation.

Loss of taste is due to taste bud damage or hyposalivation.

Caries can rapidly progress and affect areas usually not pre-disposed, such as incisal edges, smooth surfaces, and the lower incisor as well as other areas.

Candidosis is an issue for oral cancer patients because of hyposal-ivation, treatment-related immunosuppression, frequent use of antibiotics and sometimes of cytotoxic drugs. The diet may also favour *Candida* colonization, if fermentable carbohydrates are frequently consumed. The wearing of dental prostheses or obturators also predisposes. **Table 54.37** gives guidelines for the prevention and management of oral candidosis.

Sialadenitis may follow irradiation and cytostatic drugs and, in turn, may lead to irreversible hyposalivation which, with poor general health, renders cancer patients liable to ascending infective (bacterial) sialadenitis,, mainly involv-ing *Streptococcus viridans* and *Staphylococcus aureus* (often penicillin-resistant), ascending from the oral cavity. The management of sialadenitis often means hospitaliza-tion of the patient and includes:

- analgesia and prompt treatment with amoxicillin (flu-cloxacillin or amoxicillin/clavulanate if staphylococci and not allergic to penicillin; erythromycin or azithromy-cin in penicillin allergy)
- surgical drainage if there is fluctuation
- hydration
- salivation stimulation by use of chewing gum or sialogogues.

Trismus arises usually because of reduced vascularity from the endarteritis obliterans following radiotherapy (**Fig. 54.6**)

Table 54.37 Prevention and management of candidosis (candidiasis) in patients with oral cancer

Prevention	Treatment
Oral hygiene instruction Professional tooth cleaning at individually assessed intervals Dental prostheses and other reconstructive structures must be kept clean by mechanical brushing at least twice daily (chlorhexidine or commercial chemical cleaning preparations are also recommended for cleaning removable dental prostheses) In prevention of recurrent *Candida* infections, antifungal agents (see below) may be used for one week every 2–6 weeks Mouth wetting agents are recommended	Infection verified by culture samples and sensitivity testing Systemic antifungal medication avoided, if possible, because of potential selection of resistant strains Topical antifungal agents are treatment of first choice (e.g. nystatin, miconazole) for 5–6 weeks Alternatively, or in addition, non-alcohol containing chlorhexidine (1 mg/mL) mouth rinses twice daily for two weeks Dental prostheses should be treated to avoid recurrent *Candida* infections

Adapted from Meurman and Scully 2012.

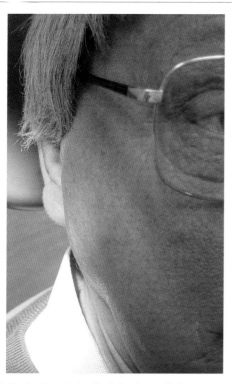

Fig. 54.5 Acute sialadenitis following radiotherapy

leading to fibrosis in the muscles of mastication and surrounding tissues. The trismus may also result from scar tissue from surgery, nerve damage, tumour infiltration or a combination of factors. RT that affects the TMJ, or the masticatory muscles, is most likely to cause trismus. Tumours related to this type of radiation include nasopharyngeal, base of tongue, salivary gland, and cancers of the maxilla or mandible. Trismus is most likely when the RT is in excess of 60 Gy, and when the patient has been previously irradiated. Radiation-induced trismus may begin toward the end of RT, or at any time during the subsequent 12 months, and tends to increase slowly over several weeks or months (see Ch. 23).

Osteoradionecrosis (ORN) is potentially the most serious complication. ORN follows endarteritis obliterans from RT in high doses involving the oral cavity, maxilla, mandible and salivary glands. ORN is defined as exposed irradiated bone tissue that fails to heal over a period of 3 months without a residual or recurrent tumour.

Aetiology and pathogenesis

- The mandible, a compact bone with high density and poor vascularity, is more prone than the maxilla to ORN.
- ORN risk is greatest:
  - when radiation dose exceeds 60 Gy
  - from 10 days before, to several years after radiotherapy, maximal at 3–12 months
  - in the malnourished or immunoincompetent.
- The initiating factor is often trauma, such as tooth extraction, or oral infection or ulceration from a dental appliance.

The pathogenesis of ORN is not completely understood but it appears in hypoxic, hypovascular and hypocellular tissue, where there is tissue breakdown leading to a non-healing wound. ORN as a radiation-induced fibroatrophic mechanism, involves free radical formation, endothelial dysfunction, inflammation, microvascular thrombosis, fibrosis and remodeling, and finally bone and tissue necrosis.
Risk factors for ORN include:

- Radiation related factors: e.g. total dose, photon energy, brachytherapy, field size, fractionation. With IMRT, only small partial volumes of the jaw are exposed to high radiation doses, so this may translate into a reduction of ORN.
- Trauma and surgery: risk is increased when tooth extractions are performed *after* RT, but there appears little increased risk when extractions are performed before. There is no infection, but teeth in the field of irradiation might be the portal of entry for microorganisms. About 50% of ORN are 'spontaneous' and appear without a history of previous tooth removal. The single most important factor associated with ORN development is mandibular surgery.
- Drug use: alcohol and tobacco are risk factors for ORN. In contrast, corticosteroids or anticoagulants used before or after RT reduce the risk of ORN.
- Genetics: the development of ORN may be related to the presence of the T variant allele at -509 within the transforming growth factor (TGF-β1) gene.

Clinical features

Presentation of ORN is of exposed bone in an irradiated mouth, with or without external sinuses, pain and pathological fracture.

Table 54.38 Emergent ORN treatments

Physical	Chemical
Ultrasound	Bone morphogenetic proteins
Distraction osteogenesis	Fibroblast growth factors
Hyperbaric oxygen therapy	Alpha tocopherol
	Pentoxifylline

Table 54.39 Oral complications of chemotherapy and management

Complication	Management
Bleeding	Local haemostasis
Mucositis	Prophylaxis (see **Table 54.41** for growth factors): Oral cooling using ice chips 30 min for 5-Fluorouracil 20 min for Edatrexate
Pain	Opioids, e.g. buprenorphine Benzydamine hydrochloride used prior to meals 2% lidocaine (lignocaine) solution mouthwash
Tooth maldevelopment	-
Taste disturbances	See Ch. 22
Candidosis	Nystatin suspension 100 000 IU/mL as mouth wash four times daily Fluconazole if immunocompromised

Modified from Rubenstein et al., 2004.

Management

Treatment is by long-term antimicrobials, especially tetracycline (which has high bone penetration), and local cleansing. Conservative management is preferred, not least since most patients have undergone major surgery before ORN arises and, as a consequence usually wish to avoid additional jaw surgery. Up to 60% of early and localized cases of ORN resolve with medication and wound care alone. Pentoxifylline (PTX), an antioxidant methylxanthine derivative with an anti-tumour necrosis factor α effect, administered for 6 months or a combination of PTX and alpha tocopherol (vitamin E), another antioxidant, significantly accelerates healing. Myocutaneous flaps and microvascular free bone flaps can be used to restore mandibular continuity and also bring non- irradiated soft tissue coverage with an intact blood supply.

Other emergent treatments are shown in **Table 54.38**. The role of hyperbaric oxygen (HBO) therapy is controversial.

Prevention of ORN

ORN is three times higher in dentate than in edentulous patients, which has led to a strategy of preventive extractions of all decayed and periodontally compromised teeth before jaw RT. However, since caries and periodontal disease are so common, there is controversy regarding whether such teeth should *always* be removed. Patients about to be treated with RT do need intensive preventive dental treatment but it is now generally accepted that teeth that really need to be extracted before RT are only those within the high-dose field that are unrestorable or have advanced periodontal involvement. The extractions must be done *before* RT, and patients who required multiple dental extractions or extensive surgical extractions, or both, can be given eight weeks of pentoxifylline 400 mg twice daily with tocopherol 1000 IU, starting a week before the procedure, as prophylaxis.

ONCOGENESIS: Irradiation for retinoblastoma, can lead to the development of jaw osteosarcoma.
DISTURBED DEVELOPMENT: RT can cause maldevelopment of jaws and teeth in children.
CAROTID ARTERIOSCLEROSIS: RT can accelerate or initiate this.

CHEMOTHERAPY TOXICITIES

The oral adverse effects of chemotherapy (CTX) can include mainly (**Table 54.39**):

- mucositis: which may affect some two-thirds of patients
- infections: especially candidal, herpesviruses and human papillomaviruses (Chs 39 and 43)
- pain: related to mucositis or infections, or to drugs such as vinca alkaloids and doxorubicin

- bleeding: thrombocytopenia increases the liability to gingival and oral bleeding
- hyposalivation (Ch. 8)
- taste disturbances (Ch. 22): some cytotoxic agents can be responsible, such as histone acetylase inhibitors (vorinostat; romidepsin)
- tooth maldevelopment.

MUCOSITIS

Unlike the case with radiotherapy, chemotherapy is usually administered over a short time, so the injury to mucosae tends to be acute but affects the whole gastrointestinal tract. CTX appears to cause injury to the mucosal barrier, with activation of the NF-kB pathway and release of cytokines such as TNF alpha, IL-1 and IL-6.

Most patients on high-dose CTX develop severe oral mucositis which usually appears within 4–7 days after initiation of treatment and peaks within 2 weeks. Mucositis is seen especially with CTX using:

- cisplatin
- etoposide
- melphalan;

but is also seen with:

- anthracyclines (bleomycin, dactinomycin, daunorubicin, doxorubicin, epirubicin, idarubicin, mitomycin, mitoxantrone)
- antimetabolites (cytarabine, fluorouracil, floxuridine, methotrexate, thioguanine)
- antimitotics (taxanes, e.g. docetaxel and paclitaxel; vinca alkaloids, e.g. vinblastine and vindesine);

and less with:

- asparaginase
- carmustine.

The damage induced by CTX is a complex phenomenon that affects both epithelium and lamina propria. There are several stages in mucositis:

- Initiation: the production of reactive oxygen species, direct cellular damage.
- Activation of transcription factors (e.g. nuclear factor-κB; NF-κB) leading to a local increase in pro-inflammatory cytokines (e.g. interleukin (IL)-6, and tumour necrosis factor (TNF)).
- Feedback mechanisms result in amplification and acceleration of the process, which finally leads to ulceration.
- Following cessation of the process, there is healing.

The oral microflora is considered to play only a secondary role in the pathogenesis of mucositis.

Mucositis can arise as a consequence of the:

- direct effect of the interventive regimen on cell division
- oral infections that may ensue
- release of cytokines (such as interleukin-1 and tumour necrosis factor-α)
- aggravation by trauma.

Risk factors for CTX mucositis include:

- age
- body mass index
- female gender
- salivary function
- poor oral health
- mucosal trauma
- co-morbidities (e.g. diabetes mellitus, impaired renal function).

Genetic determinants including genes that:

- regulate the availability of active chemotherapy drug metabolites (e.g. folate-metabolizing enzymes may help to identify patients at greater risk for methotrexate toxicity; dihydropyrimidine dehydrogenase (DPYD) variants may identify those at risk with fluorouracil)
- are involved in the direct cell response to the drug
- are associated with the expression of inflammatory mediators.

Clinical features

Mucositis typically presents as widespread erythema, ulceration, swelling, and atrophy. Since CTX-induced damage affects the entire alimentary tract mucosae, terms such as alimentary mucositis and mucosal barrier injury are also then appropriately used. Mucositis presents with:

- pain
- erythema
- ulceration (**Fig. 54.2**)
- sometimes bleeding.

Diagnosis

Lesions in the cancer patient that can complicate the diagnosis of mucositis include:

- Fungal and viral infections; ulcerations induced by herpesviruses for example can confuse, but differs clinically from mucositis in that they may also involve the tongue dorsum, the gingivae and the hard palate.

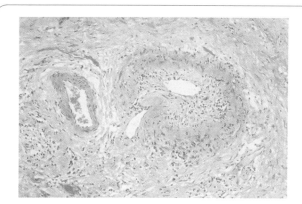

Fig. 54.6 Radiation-induced endarteritis obliterans

- Acute graft-versus-host disease (aGVHD) after haematopoietic stem cell transplant (HSCT: bone marrow transplant) may present as lichenoid lesions, desquamation and ulceration that may be difficult to distinguish from mucositis.
- Neutropenic ulcers in myelosuppressed patients, are usually well-defined and painful. Typically, microbiological tests are then negative.

Diagnosis of mucositis is clinical and it is helpful to score the degree in order to monitor progression and therapy. A number of instruments are available to evaluate the observable, subjective and functional dimensions of oral mucositis (e.g. World Health Organization, National Cancer Institute Common Terminology Criteria for Adverse Events, or Eilers' Oral Assessment Guide for a more comprehensive oral assessment).

Clinician-based scorings of toxicities often fail to coincide with targeted mucosal evaluation or patients' reporting of symptoms. For example, while incidence of oral mucositis reported by oncologists was about 15% in patients receiving CTX for colorectal cancer, over 70% of the patients being treated reported significant mouth or throat soreness. (**Table 54.40**).

QoL

Many patients report oral mucositis as the most debilitating and troublesome adverse effect of cancer therapy, and that opioid analgesics do not always adequately relieve pain, but instead lead to other issues such as dry mouth and constipation. Mucositis is also associated with poorer treatment outcomes and increased financial burdens, a longer hospital stay, and an increased use of narcotics and nutritional support. In some patients, mainly those undergoing myeloablative haematopoietic stem cell transplant (HSCT, or bone marrow transplant), mucositis predisposes to fever and infections, and occasionally mortality.

Table 54.40	WHO mucositis scale
Grade	**Clinical features**
0	–
1	Soreness/erythema
2	Erythema and ulcers – but able to eat solids
3	Ulcers – but requires liquid diet
4	Oral alimentation not possible

Treatment (see also Chs 4 and 5)

Fortunately, although there are few randomized controlled studies, and the available prophylactic and therapeutic strategies are limited, discomfort from mucositis can be reduced as shown in **Table 54.41**. Patients on chemotherapy may also suffer a range of other problems (**Box 54.1**).

Since infections may be associated, appropriate diagnosis and antimicrobial agents must be considered. Fungal or bacterial infections may be seen particularly in either CTX- (or RT-) induced mucositis.

Interventions which have some proven success with some evidence base include:

- excellent oral care, including pre-treatment dental evaluation
- oral cryotherapy using ice popsicles
- exposure to soft laser
- systemic administration of keratinocyte growth factor (palifermin), FDA-approved for use in patients with haematologic malignancies receiving myelotoxic therapy requiring haematopoietic stem cell support. In this group of patients, it reduces the number of days suffering from mucositis, with no special adverse effects other than an occasional rash. A single dose of palifermin before each cycle reduced the incidence and severity of mucositis from doxorubicin used to treat sarcomas, the drug was generally well tolerated, but most patients experienced thickening of oral mucosae.

> **BOX 54.1 Systemic adverse effects possible in patients on chemotherapy**
>
> - Cardiotoxicity
> - Renal failure
> - Pulmonary fibrosis
> - Myelosuppression
> - Alopecia
> - Nausea
> - Vomiting
> - Diarrhoea
> - Cystitis
> - Sterility
> - Myalgia
> - Neuropathy ('hand and foot syndrome')
> - Local reactions
> - Phlebitis

Interventions which show some statistically significant evidence of a benefit, also include aloe vera, amifostine, granulocyte-colony stimulating factor (G-CSF), intravenous glutamine, honey, sucralfate and polymixin/tobramycin/amphotericin (PTA) antibiotic pastille/paste. There are many other preparations used, often variants on the 'magic mouthwash' (viscous lidocaine, diphenhydramine, bismuth salicylate and a corticosteroid).

Table 54.41 Evidence-based clinical practice guidelines for care of patients with mucositis

Protocol	Intent	Patient groups
Oral care protocols	To prevent oral disease	All patients
Patient-controlled analgesia with morphine	To treat mucositis pain	Especially in haematopoietic stem cell transplantation (HSCT)
Radiotherapy: prevention		
Midline radiation blocks three-dimensional RT	To prevent or ameliorate mucositis	RT to head and neck
Benzydamine	To prevent or ameliorate mucositis	RT to head and neck
Chlorhexidine	*Not be used* to prevent or ameliorate mucositis	RT to head and neck
Sucralfate		
Antimicrobials		
Standard-dose chemotherapy prevention		
Oral cryotherapy 20–30 min	To prevent or ameliorate mucositis	Patients treated with bolus doses of edatrexate or 5-fluorouracil (5-fu)
Aciclovir	*Not to be used* to prevent or ameliorate or treat established mucositis	Standard-dose chemotherapy
Chlorhexidine		
High dose chemotherapy with or without total body irradiation plus haematopoietic cell transplantation: prevention		
Keratinocyte growth factor-1 (palifermin) in a dose of 60 µg/kg/day for 3 days prior to conditioning treatment and for 3 days post-transplant	Prevent or ameliorate mucositis	Patients with haematological Malignancies receiving high-dose chemotherapy and total body irradiation with autologous stem cell transplant
Cryotherapy	Prevent or ameliorate mucositis	Patients receiving high-dose melphalan HSCT
Pentoxifylline or GM-CSF mouthwashes	*Not to be used* to prevent or ameliorate mucositis	
Low-level laser therapy (LLLT)	Prevent or ameliorate mucositis and pain	Patients receiving high-dose chemotherapy or chemoradiotherapy before HSCT

Adapted from Keefe et al, 2007.

Emergent agents being trialled for the amelioration of the suffering of mucositis include buprenorphine transdermal patches for analgesia, and agents designed to enhance resolution– supplements (e.g. glutamine, zinc sulphate), enzymes involved in the detoxification of reactive oxygen species (e.g. glutathione-S-transferase) and antimicrobial peptides. The traditional Chinese medicine Rhodiola algida has been reportedly beneficial. In addition, approaches aimed at modifying overexpression of pro-inflammatory cytokines offer promise.

IMMUNOSUPPRESSION AND COMPLICATIONS

Immunosuppressive therapy is used especially to suppress:

- rejection in transplant recipients (bone marrow, kidney, liver, pancreas, heart and heart–lung); these are the most severely immunocompromised patients
- autoimmune disorders
- connective tissue diseases
- some malignant tumours, especially lymphoproliferative neoplasms.

A variety of drugs are used to induce immunosuppression, especially corticosteroids and calcineurin antagonists (such as ciclosporin, tacrolimus and sirolimus). Drugs such as azathioprine, cyclophosphamide and chlorambucil are cytotoxic to a range of cells, including some immunocytes, and are, therefore, also used for immunosuppression (Ch. 5). A range of orofacial effects can arise (**Box 54.2**), especially infections and malignant neoplasms.

INFECTIONS

Patients on immunosuppressive agents are at risk from oral infections, which may be opportunistic (involving microorganisms that are normally commensal) or may involve exogenous pathogens, and can include:

- Fungal infections:
  - candidosis (see Ch. 39)
  - *Aspergillus* spp. may infect the paranasal sinuses, palate or other sites by direct extension and haematogenously. Diagnosis is by demonstration of hyphae in a smear, serology and biopsy. Intravenous amphotericin may be effective
  - mucormycosis (zygomycosis: phycomycosis) is infection by *Mucor* or *Rhizopus* spp., mainly of the paranasal sinuses and nose of immunosuppressed or poorly controlled diabetic or leukaemic patients. Diagnosis is by biopsy and culture: treatment is by control of underlying disease, debridement and intravenous amphotericin
  - mycobacterioses.
- Herpetic infections (Ch. 43).
- Odontogenic infections, which are potentially life threatening in the immunosuppressed patient, and broad-spectrum

cover is needed (such as penicillin plus gentamicin). Partially erupted third molars are a potential source of infection.

Patients may also be at risk from attempts at treatment; thus, for example, broad-spectrum antibiotics used to control bacterial infections increase the hazard of fungal infections. Patients are often on ciclosporin and antihypertensive agents, and are at risk of drug-related gingival swelling from ciclosporin and from calcium channel blockers (Ch. 12). The swelling appears to be greater with the combination of ciclosporin-nifedipine than with ciclosporin-amlodipine or ciclosporin only.

NEOPLASMS

Neoplasms, at least some of which are virally related, may also be a risk in chronic immunosuppression including:

- Kaposi sarcoma
- lymphoproliferative syndromes (post-transplant lymphoproliferative disease: PTLD), which may appear late – even many years after transplantation – and range from hyperplastic-appearing lesions to non-Hodgkin lymphoma or multiple myeloma. Reduction in immunosuppressives can often reverse PTLD. Surgical resection, cytotoxics, anti-CD21 and anti-CD24 antibodies, interferon-alpha and rituximab have been effectively used for treatment
- squamous cell carcinomas of the skin and of the lip.

TRANSPLANTATION AND COMPLICATIONS

Orofacial complications can follow transplantation of solid organs or bone marrow (human precursor cell transplantation (HPCT) or haematopoietic stem cell transplantation (HSCT)) – largely as a consequence of the immunosuppression used.

SOLID ORGAN TRANSPLANTATION

Immunosuppressive therapy is universally used after organ transplantation, with the potential problems outlined above.

Patients who have had organ transplantation are additionally predisposed to:

- acute angioedema
- pyogenic granulomas, commonly affect the gingiva, the lip or the tongue
- mucosal lesions similar to orofacial granulomatosis. Long-standing oral mucosal lesions in solid organ- (liver) transplanted children have been described as multiple spherical nodules on the dorsum of the tongue, which later on displayed a fissured appearance. Most patients also presented with mucosal tags or ridges and swollen lips similar to those found in orofacial granulomatosis (Ch. 46). In addition, most patients had a clinical history of immediate-onset food-induced allergic reactions, including transient angioedema
- oral malignant neoplasms (carcinomas, lymphomas and Kaposi sarcoma).

HAEMATOPOIETIC STEM CELL TRANSPLANTATION

HSCT is increasingly used to treat:

- congenital metabolic diseases
- congenital immune diseases

> **BOX 54.2 Orofacial effects possible in patients on immunosuppressive therapy**
>
> - infections
> - neoplasms
> - other effects, e.g. ciclosporin-induced gingival swelling

- haematological malignancies (aplastic anaemia, leukaemias, lymphomas)
- solid malignancies.

The procedure of HSCT involves the recipient receiving:

- ablation of bone marrow cells by high-dose CTX with drugs such as cyclophosphamide
- total (whole) body irradiation (TBI)
- transfusion of bone marrow aspirate from a donor who has been stimulated with growth factors.

This regimen results in:

- profound immunosuppression until the donor bone marrow graft takes and, therefore, patients must be isolated to reduce the risk of infections
- graft-versus-host disease (GVHD) which arises in about 60% of cases can produce further immune defects and is potentially lethal
- lymphoproliferative syndromes (post-transplant lymphoproliferative disorder (PTLD)) and lymphomas (see above) in rare patients.

ORAL COMPLICATIONS OF HSCT

Oral complications are common in HSCT and can be a major cause of morbidity from the effects of the underlying disease, chemo- or radiotherapy, or GVHD and include:

- Graft-versus-host disease (GVHD) (see below).
- Mucositis: this typically begins around 5 days post-HSCT, but by around 9–14 days post-HSCT basal cells regenerate and it resolves. Apart from the measures discussed above to minimize mucositis, it may be ameliorated by use of glutamine and interleukin-11
- Ulceration: mainly a consequence of granulocytopenia, this resolves by around 9–14 days post-HSCT, when the neutrophils rise >500 cells/mL.
- Infections: superficial infections are frequent and can involve a wide range of microorganisms, mainly:
  - herpes simplex virus (HSV): about 60% of patients secrete HSV orally within 50 days, and many have lesions, such as ulcers
  - cytomegalovirus (CMV): about 60% of patients secrete CMV between days 30 and 150 and lesions, such as ulcers, may result
  - varicella-zoster virus (VZV): 40% are infected within 6 months and 80% develop zoster
  - Epstein–Barr virus (EBV): about 60% secrete EBV and, although uncommon, hairy leukoplakia or lymphoproliferative disease may result
  - human papilloma viruses (HPV): can cause extensive warty lesions over the 3–8 months post transplant
  - candidosis: carriage and oral lesions are almost invariable in the absence of prophylactic antifungal therapy
  - mucormycosis: a rare, but serious complication
  - bacterial septicaemia is less common, but 25–75% of septicaemias arise from the oral cavity involving viridans *Streptococci*, *Enterococci*, *Leptotrichia buccalis* and Gram-negative organisms.
- Hyposalivation.
- Bleeding.

- Dental maldevelopment: most children undergoing HSCT have disturbed tooth development, including missing teeth, shortened roots, and arrested root development.
- Malignant neoplasms: most patients develop genetic instability in their oral mucosa and oral malignant disease occasionally arises even after 5–10 years after HSCT. In half the cases, the tongue is the primary location, followed by the salivary gland and the neoplasms may have more aggressive behaviour with poorer prognosis.

GRAFT-VERSUS-HOST DISEASE (GVHD)

GVHD can arise after an immunocompetent graft is administered, with viable and functional immune cells, provided that the recipient is immunologically disparate – histoincompatible- and immunocompromised and therefore unable to inactivate or destroy the transplanted cells. HSCT transfers T lymphocytes which perceive host tissues as antigenically foreign via HLA and other antigens, and mount an immune attack on the host, the transferred T cells producing cytokines, including TNK alpha and IFN-gamma (IFNγ). There is a positive associations between IL-6 and oral GVHD severity and erythema, as well as the positive trend with oral ulceration.

Acute GVHD appears between 10 and 100 days post transplant, and is seen in about 60% of transplant survivors.

Chronic GVHD occurs after 100 days post-HSCT and affects around 50% of patients after HSCT, may follow acute GVHD, or may arise *ab initio*.

Acute GVHD

Acute GVHD affects mainly the liver, gastrointestinal tract and mucocutaneous tissues, and can be lethal and so prophylactic immunosuppressive therapy using methotrexate and ciclosporin is usually used for the first 100 days post-HSCT. The oral manifestations of acute GVHD are difficult or impossible to differentiate from chemotherapy-induced mucositis and consist of:

- painful mucosal desquamation and ulceration. Erythema and ulceration are most pronounced at 7–11 days after HSCT, and may be associated with obvious infection. Small white lesions affect the buccal and lingual mucosa early on, but clear by day 14. The ventrum of the tongue, buccal and labial mucosa and gingiva may be affected
- cheilitis
- hyposalivation; most significant in the first 14 days after transplantation and a consequence of drug treatment and/or irradiation
- infections; candidosis, HSV stomatitis (occasionally zoster), CMV, protozoal and Gram-positive bacterial infections
- purpura and bleeding.

Acute GVHD is treated with high-dose immunosuppressive therapy.

Chronic GVHD

Chronic GVHD is severe and involves multiple organs, mainly the liver, gastrointestinal tract, eyes and skin including, in 80% of cases, oral lesions including:

- generalized mucosal erythema
- lichenoid lesions (**Fig. 54.7**)
- ulceration

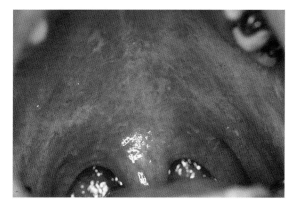

Fig. 54.7 Lichenoid lesions in graft-versus-host disease

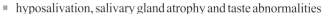

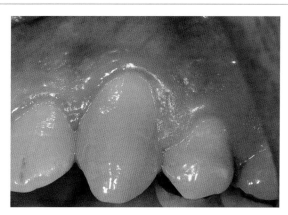

Fig. 54.8 Very early lesions of ciclosporin-induced gingival swelling appearing on the interdental papillae

- hyposalivation, salivary gland atrophy and taste abnormalities
- infections, especially candidosis
- hairy leukoplakia
- sclerodermatous syndrome
- ciclosporin-induced gingival swelling (**Fig. 54.8**).

Chronic GVHD is treated with high-dose immunosuppressive therapy.

Diagnosis of GVHD

Diagnosis is from the history and clinical features and a mucosal or labial salivary gland biopsy, which shows mononuclear cell infiltrates. The National Institutes of Health (NIH) scale is available for scoring oral cGVHD.

Management of GVHD

Management of oral lesions is best with use of:

- oral hygiene measures
- analgesics (morphine or hydromorphone)
- topical azathioprine or ciclosporin
- non-alcoholic chlorhexidine mouth rinses
- nystatin or fluconazole suspension
- pilocarpine
- xylitol chewing gum
- artificial saliva (mouth wetting agents)
- growth factors.

USEFUL WEBSITES

Drugs.com, Drug Side Effects. http://www.drugs.com/sfx/
MedicineNet.com, Chemotherapy and Cancer Treatment, Coping with Side Effects. http://www.medicinenet.com/script/main/art.asp?articlekey=21716

Medscape, Oral Manifestations of Drug Reactions. http://emedicine.medscape.com/article/1080772
Wikipedia, Iatrogenesis. http://en.wikipedia.org/wiki/Iatrogenesis

FURTHER READING

Abdollahi, M., Radfar, M., 2003. A review of drug-induced oral reactions. J. Contemp. Dent. Pract. 15, 10–31.

Al Akhrass, F., Debiane, L., Abdallah, L., et al., 2011. Palatal mucormycosis in patients with hematologic malignancy and stem cell transplantation. Med. Mycol. 49 (4), 400–405.

Albert, M.H., Becker, B., Schuster, F.R., 2007. Oral graft vs. host disease in children–treatment with topical tacrolimus ointment. Pediatr. Transplant. 11 (3), 306–311.

Anees, M.M., Reich, A., Hirschberg, L., et al., 2011. Enhanced enzymatic activity of Candida species responsible for oral candidiasis in renal transplant recipients. Mycoses 54 (4), 337–344.

Bagan, J.V., Jimenez, Y., Murillo, J., et al., 2006. Jaw osteonecrosis associated with bisphosphonates: multiple exposed areas and its relationship to teeth extractions. Study of 20 cases. Oral Oncol 42, 327–329.

Bagan, J.V., Murillo, J., Jimenez, Y., et al., 2005. Avascular jaw osteonecrosis in association with

cancer chemotherapy: series of 10 cases. J. Oral Med. Pathol. 34, 120–123.

Bagan, J.V., Thongprasom, K., Scully, C., 2004. Adverse oral reactions associated with the Cox-2 inhibitor rofecoxib. Oral Dis. 10, 401–403.

Basić-Jukić, N., Bubić-Filipi, L., Prgomet, D., et al., 2010. Head and neck malignancies in Croatian renal transplant recipients. Bosn. J. Basic Med. Sci. 10 (Suppl. 1), S37–S39.

Bensadoun, R.J., Patton, L.L., Lalla, R.V., Epstein, J.B., 2011. Oropharyngeal candidiasis in head and neck cancer patients treated with radiation: update 2011. Support Care Cancer 19 (6), 737–744.

Bensadoun, R.J., Riesenbeck, D., Lockhart, P.B., et al., 2010. A systematic review of trismus induced by cancer therapies in head and neck cancer patients. Support Care Cancer 18 (8), 1033–1038.

Brand, H.S., Bots, C.P., Raber-Durlacher, J.E., 2009. Xerostomia and chronic oral complications among patients treated with haematopoietic stem cell transplantation. Br. Dent. J. 207 (9), E17; discussion 428-9.

Bruce, A.J., Subtil, A., Rogers 3rd, R.S., Castro, L.A., 2006. Monomorphic Epstein–Barr virus (EBV)-associated large B-cell posttransplant lymphoproliferative disorder presenting as a tongue ulcer in a pancreatic transplant patient. Oral Surg. Oral Med. Oral Pathol. Oral Radiol. Endod. 102 (4), e24–e28.

Clarkson, J.E., Worthington, H.V., Furness, S., et al., 2010. Interventions for treating oral mucositis for patients with cancer receiving treatment. Cochrane Database Syst. Rev. (8), CD001973.

Condò, R., Maturo, P., Perugia, C., Docimo, R., 2011. Oral lesions in paediatric patients with graft-versus-host disease. Eur. J. Paediatr. Dent. 12 (1), 50–54.

Coppes, R.P., Stokman, M.A., 2011. Stem cells and the repair of radiation-induced salivary gland damage. Oral Dis. 17 (2), 143–153.

Correia-Silva, J., Bruna-Romero, O., Resende, R., et al., 2010. Saliva as a source of HCMV DNA in allogeneic stem cell transplantation patients. Oral Dis. 16, 210–216.

Cutler, C., Li, S., Kim, H.T., et al., 2005. Mucositis after allogeneic hematopoietic stem cell transplantation: a cohort study of methotrexate- and non-methotrexate-containing graft-versus-host disease prophylaxis regimens. Biol. Blood Marrow Transplant. 11 (5), 383–388.

Dahllöf, G., Wondimu, B., Barr-Agholme, M., et al., 2011. Xerostomia in children and adolescents after stem cell transplantation conditioned with total body irradiation or busulfan. Oral Oncol. 47 (9), 915–919.

Defabianis, P., Braida, S., Guagnano, R., 2010. 180-day screening study for predicting the risk factors for developing acute oral Graft-versus-Host disease in paediatric patients subjected to allogenic haematopoietic stem cells transplantation. Eur. J. Paediatr. Dent. 11 (1), 31–34.

Deng, Z., Kiyuna, A., Hasegawa, M., et al., 2010. Oral candidiasis in patients receiving radiation therapy for head and neck cancer. Otolaryngol. Head Neck Surg. 143 (2), 242–247.

Dijkstra, P.U., Kalk, W.W., Roodenburg, J.L., 2004. Trismus in head and neck oncology: a systematic review. Oral Oncol. 40 (9), 879–889.

Dirschnabel, A.J., Martins Ade, S., Dantas, S.A., et al., 2011. Clinical oral findings in dialysis and kidney-transplant patients. Quintessence Int. 42 (2), 127–133.

Diz Dios, P., Scully, C., 2012. Cancer of the mouth for the dental team; comprehending the condition, causes, controversies, control and consequences 13. Pain. Dent. 391, 65–67.

Duerr, M., Glander, P., Diekmann, F., et al., 2010. Increased incidence of angioedema with ACE inhibitors in combination with mTOR inhibitors in kidney transplant recipients. Clin. J. Am. Soc. Nephrol. 5 (4), 703–708.

Elad, S., Wexler, A., Garfunkel, A.A., et al., 2006. Oral candidiasis prevention in transplantation patients: a comparative study. Clin. Transplant. 20 (3), 318–324.

Elad, S., Zadik, Y., Zeevi, I., et al., 2010. Oral cancer in patients after hematopoietic stem-cell transplantation: long-term follow-up suggests an increased risk for recurrence. Transplantation 90 (11), 1243–1244.

Elad, S., Zeevi, I., Or, R., et al., 2010. Validation of the National Institutes of Health (NIH) scale for oral chronic graft-versus-host disease (cGVHD). Biol. Blood Marrow Transplant. 16 (1), 62–69.

Epstein, J.B., Gorsky, M., Epstein, M.S., et al., 2001. Topical azathioprine in the treatment of immune-mediated chronic oral inflammatory conditions. Oral Surg. 91, 56–61.

Esquiche León, J., Takahama Júnior, A., Vassallo, J., et al., 2011. EBV-Associated Polymorphic Posttransplant Lymphoproliferative Disorder Presenting as Gingival Ulcers. Int. J. Surg. Pathol. 19 (2), 241–246.

Fall-Dickson, J.M., Mitchell, S.A., Marden, S., et al., 2010. Oral symptom intensity, health-related quality of life, and correlative salivary cytokines in adult survivors of hematopoietic stem cell with oral chronic graft-versus-host disease. Biol. Blood Marrow Transplant 16 (7), 948–956.

Fiske, J., Lewis, D., 2001. Guidelines for the oral management of oncology patients requiring radiotherapy, chemotherapy and bone marrow transplantation. J. Disability Oral Health 2, 3–14.

Furness, S., Glenny, A.M., Worthington, H.V., et al., 2010. Interventions for the treatment of oral cavity and oropharyngeal cancer: chemotherapy. Cochrane Database Syst. Rev. (9), CD006386. Update in: Cochrane Database Syst. Rev. 4:CD006386.

Furness, S., Glenny, A.M., Worthington, H.V., et al., 2011. Interventions for the treatment of oral cavity and oropharyngeal cancer: chemotherapy. Cochrane Database Syst. Rev. (4), CD006386.

Glenny, A.M., Furness, S., Worthington, H.V., et al., 2010. Interventions for the treatment of oral cavity and oropharyngeal cancer: radiotherapy. Cochrane Database Syst. Rev. (12), CD006387.

Gligorov, J., Bastit, L., Gervais, H., et al., 2011. Prevalence and treatment management of oropharyngeal candidiasis in cancer patients: results of the French CANDIDOSCOPE study. Int. J. Radiat. Oncol. Biol. Phys. 80 (2), 532–539.

Güleç, A.T., Haberal, M., 2010. Lip and oral mucosal lesions in 100 renal transplant recipients. J. Am. Acad. Dermatol. 62 (1), 96–101.

Hernández, G., Arriba, L., Jiménez, C., et al., 2003. Rapid progression from oral leukoplakia to carcinoma in an immunosuppressed liver transplant recipient. Oral Oncol. 39 (1), 87–90.

Imanguli, M.M., Alevizos, I., Brown, R., et al., 2008. Oral graft-versus-host disease. Oral Dis 14, 396–412.

Imanguli, M.M., Atkinson, J.C., Mitchell, S.A., et al., 2010. Salivary gland involvement in chronic graft-versus-host disease: prevalence, clinical significance, and recommendations for evaluation. Biol. Blood Marrow Transplant. 16 (10), 1362–1369.

Imanguli, M.M., Pavletic, S.Z., Guadagnini, J.P., 2006. Chronic graft versus host disease of oral mucosa: review of available therapies. Oral Surg. Oral Med. Oral Pathol. Oral Radiol. Endod. 101 (2), 175–183.

Jen, Y.M., Lin, Y.C., Wang, Y.B., Wu, D.M., 2006. Dramatic and prolonged decrease of whole salivary secretion in nasopharyngeal carcinoma patients treated with radiotherapy. Oral Surg. Oral Med. Oral Pathol. Oral Radiol. Endod. 101 (3), 322–327.

Johnson, J., van As-Brooks, C.J., Fagerberg-Mohlin, B., Finizia, C., 2010. Trismus in head and neck cancer patients in Sweden: incidence and risk factors. Med. Sci. Monit 16 (6), CR278–CR282.

Joshi, V., Scully, C., 2012. Cancer of the mouth for the dental team; comprehending the condition, causes, controversies, control and consequences 18. Dental management. Dent. Update (In Press).

Kalavrezos, N., Scully, C., 2012. Cancer of the mouth for the dental team; comprehending the condition, causes, controversies, control and consequences 10. Surgical management of oral cancer. Dent. Update (In Press).

Kav, S., Aslan, O., Tekin, F., et al., 2009. Quality of life and difficulties of patients encountered after autologous stem cell transplantation. J. BUON 14 (4), 673–680.

Keefe, D.M., Schubert, M.M., Elting, L.S., et al., 2007. 2007 Updated clinical practice guidelines for the prevention and treatment of mucositis. Cancer 109 (5), 820–831.

Kerawala, C.J., Scully, C., 2012. Cancer of the mouth for the dental team; comprehending the condition, causes, controversies, control and consequences 11. Surgical complications and adverse effects. Dent. Update (In Press).

Khan, F.M., Sy, S., Louie, P., et al., 2010. Genomic instability after allogeneic hematopoietic cell transplantation is frequent in oral mucosa, particularly in patients with a history of chronic graft-versus-host disease, and rare in nasal mucosa. Blood 116 (10), 1803–1806.

Kojima, T., Kanemaru, S.I., Hirano, S., et al., 2011. Regeneration of radiation damaged salivary glands with adipose-derived stromal cells. Laryngoscope 121 (9), 1864–1869.

Kruse, A.L., Grätz, K.W., 2009. Oral carcinoma after hematopoietic stem cell transplantation–a new classification based on a literature review over 30 years. Head Neck Oncol. 1, 29.

Lalla, R.V., Latortue, M.C., Hong, C.H., et al., 2010. A systematic review of oral fungal infections in patients receiving cancer therapy. Support Care Cancer 18 (8), 985–992.

Lee, R., Slevin, N., 2011. Inconsistencies in the care of head and neck cancer patients experiencing trismus. Eur. J. Oncol. Nurs. 15 (4), 364.

Lew, J., Smith, J., 2007. Mucosal graft-vs-host disease. Oral Dis 13, 519–529.

Lin, C.Y., Chang, F.H., Chen, C.Y., et al., 2011. Cell therapy for salivary gland regeneration. J. Dent. Res. 90 (3), 341–346.

Loo, W.T., Jin, L.J., Chow, L.W., et al., 2010. Rhodiola algida improves chemotherapy-induced oral mucositis in breast cancer patients. Expert Opin. Investig. Drugs 19 (Suppl. 1), S91–S100.

López-Pintor, R., Hernández, G., De Arriba, L., De Andrés, A., 2010. Comparison of oral lesion prevalence in renal transplant patients under immunosuppressive therapy and healthy controls. Oral Dis. 16, 89–95.

López-Pintor, R.M., Hernández, G., de Arriba, L., 2009. Oral ulcers during the course of cytomegalovirus infection in renal transplant recipients. Transplant Proc. 41 (6), 2419–2421.

López-Pintor, R.M., Hernández, G., de Arriba, L., et al., 2009. Amlodipine and nifedipine used with cyclosporine induce different effects on gingival enlargement. Transplant Proc. 41 (6), 2351–2353.

López-Pintor, R.M., Hernández, G., de Arriba, L., de Andrés, A., 2010. Comparison of oral lesion prevalence in renal transplant patients under immunosuppressive therapy and healthy controls. Oral Dis. 16 (1), 89–95.

Lyons, A.J., West, C.M., Risk, J.M., et al., 2012. Osteoradionecrosis in Head-and-Neck Cancer Has a Distinct Genotype-Dependent Cause. Int. J. Radiat. Oncol. Biol. Phys. 82, 1479–1484.

Madrid, M., Scully, C., 2012. Cancer of the mouth for the dental team; comprehending the condition, causes, controversies, control and consequences 17. Osteonecrosis. Dent. 39, 377–379.

Maldonado, N.I., Cabanillas, F., Jaffe, E.S., et al., 2011. Successful treatment of a patient with Epstein-Barr virus-positive B-cell lymphoproliferative disorder resembling post-transplant lymphoproliferative disorder using single-agent rituximab. J. Clin. Oncol. 29 (22), e658–e660.

Mann, P.A., McNicholas, P.M., Chau, A.S., et al., 2009. Impact of antifungal prophylaxis on colonization and azole susceptibility of Candida species. Antimicrob. Agents Chemother. 53 (12), 5026–5034.

Marx, R.E., 2006. Oral and intravenous bisphosphonate-induced osteonecrosis of the jaws. Quintessence Publishers, London.

Mawardi, H., Elad, S., Correa, M.E., et al., 2011. Oral epithelial dysplasia and squamous cell carcinoma following allogeneic hematopoietic stem cell transplantation: clinical presentation and treatment outcomes. Bone Marrow Transplant. 46 (6), 884–891.

Mawardi, H., Pavlakis, M., Mandelbrot, D., Woo, S.B., 2010. Sirolimus oral ulcer with Cedecea davisae superinfection. Transpl. Infect. Dis. 12 (5), 446–450.

Mawardi, H., Stevenson, K., Gokani, B., et al., 2010. Combined topical dexamethasone/tacrolimus therapy for management of oral chronic GVHD. Bone Marrow Transplant. 45 (6), 1062–1067.

Meier, J.K., Wolff, D., Pavletic, S., et al., 2011. Oral chronic graft-versus-host disease: report from the International Consensus Conference on clinical practice in cGVHD. Clin. Oral Investig. 15 (2), 127–139.

Meurman, J.H., Scully, C., 2012. Cancer of the mouth for the dental team; comprehending the condition, causes, controversies, control and consequences 16. Infections. Dent. 39, 298–299.

Montebugnoli, L., Gissi, D.B., Marchetti, C., Foschini, M.P., 2011. Multiple squamous cell carcinomas of the oral cavity in a young patient with graft-versus-host disease following allogenic bone marrow transplantation. Int. J. Oral Maxillofac. Surg. 40 (5), 556–558.

Mosel, D., Bauer, R., Lynch, D., Hwang, S., 2011. Oral complications in the treatment of cancer patients. Oral Dis. 17 (6), 550–559.

Nihtinen, A., Anttila, V.J., Richardson, M., et al., 2010. Invasive Aspergillus infections in allo-SCT recipients: environmental sampling, nasal and oral colonization and galactomannan testing. Bone Marrow Transplant. 45 (2), 333–338.

Nutting, C.M., Scully, C., 2012. Cancer of the mouth for the dental team; comprehending the condition, causes, controversies, control and consequences 12. Radiotherapy and chemotherapy. Dent. 38, 717–719.

Ohman, D., Björk, Y., Bratel, J., et al., 2010. Partially erupted third molars as a potential source of infection in patients receiving peripheral stem cell transplantation for malignant diseases: a retrospective study. Eur. J. Oral Sci. 118 (1), 53–58.

Olczak-Kowalczyk, D., Pawłowska, J., Garczewska, B., et al., 2010. Oral candidiasis in immunosuppressed children and young adults after liver or kidney transplantation. Pediatr. Dent. 32 (3), 189–194.

Pettis, Polimeni A, Berloco, P.B., Scully, C., 2012. Orofacial diseases in solid organ and hematopoietic stem cell transplant recipients. Oral DiseasesMar3 Epub.

Plantinga, T.S., van der Velden, W.J., Ferwerda, B., et al., 2009. Early stop polymorphism in human DECTIN-1 is associated with increased candida colonization in hematopoietic stem cell transplant recipients. Clin. Infect. Dis. 49 (5), 724–732.

Ponticelli, C., Bencini, P.L., 2011. Nonneoplastic mucocutaneous lesions in organ transplant recipients. Transpl. Int. 24 (11), 1041–1050.

Porter, S.R., Scully, C., 2000. Adverse drug reactions in the mouth. Clin. Dermatol 18, 525–532.

Porter, S.R., Scully, C., 2012. Cancer of the mouth for the dental team; comprehending the condition, causes, controversies, control and consequences 15. Salivary and taste complications. Dent. 39, 225–227.

Porter, S.R., Scully, C., Hegarty, A., 2004. An update of the etiology and management of xerostomia. Oral Surg. Oral Med. Oral Pathol. Oral Radiol. Endod. 97, 28–46.

Raber-Durlacher, J.E., Scully, C., 2012. Cancer of the mouth for the dental team; comprehending the condition, causes, controversies, control and consequences 14. Mucositis. Dent. 39, 145–147.

Redding, S.W., Bailey, C.W., Lopez-Ribot, J.L., et al., 2001. Candida dubliniensis in radiation-induced oropharyngeal candidiasis. Oral Surg. Oral Med. Oral Pathol. Oral Radiol. Endod. 91, 659–662.

Rogers, S.N., Scully, C., 2012. Cancer of the mouth for the dental team; comprehending the condition, causes, controversies, control and consequences 9. Quality of life. Dent. 38, 497–499.

Rubenstein, E.B., Peterson, D.E., Schubert, M., et al., 2004. Clinical practice guidelines for the prevention and treatment of cancer therapy-induced oral and gastrointestinal mucositis. Cancer 100 (Suppl. 9), 2026–2046.

Ruggiero, S.L., Fantasia, J., Carlson, E., 2006. Bisphosphonate-related osteonecrosis of the jaw: background and guidelines for diagnosis, staging and management. Oral Surg. Oral Med. Oral Pathol. Oral Radiol. Endod. 102 (4), 433–441.

Saalman, R., Sundell, S., Kullberg-Lindh, C., et al., 2010. Long-standing oral mucosal lesions in solid organ-transplanted children-a novel clinical entity. Transplantation 89 (5), 606–611.

Saif, I., Adkins, A., Kewley, V., et al., 2011. Routine and emergency management guidelines for the dental patient with renal disease and kidney transplant. Part 1. Dent. Update 38 (3), 179–182, 185–186.

Sato, J., Goto, J., Harahashi, A., et al., 2011. Oral health care reduces the risk of postoperative surgical site infection in inpatients with oral squamous cell carcinoma. Support Care Cancer 19 (3), 409–416.

Schelenz, S., Abdallah, S., Gray, G., et al., 2011. Epidemiology of oral yeast colonization and infection in patients with hematological malignancies, head neck and solid tumors. J. Oral Pathol. Med. 40 (1), 83–89.

Scott, B., D'Souza, J., Perinparajah, N., et al., 2011. Longitudinal evaluation of restricted mouth opening (trismus) in patients following primary surgery for oral and oropharyngeal squamous cell carcinoma. Br. J. Oral Maxillofac. Surg. 49 (2), 106–111.

Scully, C., 2003. Drug effects on salivary glands; dry mouth. Oral Dis. 9, 165–176.

Scully, C., Bagan, J.V., 2004. Adverse drug reactions in the orofacial region. Crit. Rev. Oral Biol. Med. 15, 221–239.

Scully, C., Bagan, J.V., 2010. Oral Cancer. In Davies AN, Epstein JB. Oral Complications of Cancer and its managment OUP. Oxford, pp53–64.

Scully, C., Epstein, J., Sonis, S., 2003. Oral mucositis: A challenging complication of radiotherapy, chemotherapy, and radiochemotherapy: Part 1, pathogenesis and prophylaxis of mucositis. Head Neck 25, 1057–1070.

Scully, C., Epstein, J., Sonis, S., 2004. Oral mucositis; A challenging complication of radiotherapy, chemotherapy, and radiochemotherapy: Part 2, diagnosis and management of mucositis. Head Neck 26, 77–84.

Scully, C., Sonis, S., Diz Dios, P., 2006. Oral mucositis. Oral Dis. 12, 229–241.

Ship, J.A., Vissink, A., Challacombe, S.J., 2007. Use of prophylactic antifungals in the immunocompromised host. Oral Surg. Oral Med. Oral Pathol. Oral Radiol. Endod. 103, S6.e1–S6.e14.

Sonis, S., 2010. New thoughts on the initiation of mucositis. Oral Dis. 16, 597–600.

Spolidorio, L.C., Spolidorio, D.M., Massucato, E.M., et al., 2006. Oral health in renal transplant recipients administered cyclosporin A or tacrolimus. Oral Dis. 12 (3), 309–314.

Stachiw, N., Hornig, J., Gillespie, M.B., 2010. Minimally-invasive submandibular transfer (MIST) for prevention of radiation-induced xerostomia. Laryngoscope 120 (Suppl. 4), S184.

Stiff, P., 2001. Mucositis associated with stem cell transplantation: current status and innovative approaches to management. Bone Marrow Transpl. 27 (Suppl. 2), S3–S11.

Swinnen, L., 2001. Post-transplant lymphoproliferative disorders: implications for acquired immunodeficiency syndrome-associated malignancies. J. Natl. Cancer Inst. Monogr. 28, 38–43.

Tran, S.D., Redman, R.S., Barrett, A.J., et al., 2011. Microchimerism in salivary glands after blood- and marrow-derived stem cell transplantation. Biol. Blood Marrow Transplant. 17 (3), 429–433.

Tran, S.D., Sumita, Y., Khalili, S., 2011. Bone marrow-derived cells: A potential approach for the treatment of xerostomia. Int. J. Biochem. Cell Biol. 43 (1), 5–9.

Tredwin, C., Scully, C., Bagan, J.V., 2005. Drug-induced dental disorders. Adv. Drug. Reaction Bull. 232, 891–894.

Tredwin, C., Scully, C., Bagan, J.V., 2005. Drug-induced disorders of teeth. J. Dent. Res. 84, 596–602.

Vadhan-Raj, S., Trent, J., Patel, S., et al., 2010. Single-dose palifermin prevents severe oral mucositis during multicycle chemotherapy in patients with cancer: a randomized trial. Ann. Intern. Med. 153 (6), 358–367.

van der Pas-van Voskuilen, I.G., Veerkamp, J.S., Bresters, D., et al., 2010. Tooth development disturbances following haematopoietic stem cell transplantation. Ned. Tijdschr. Tandheelkd. 117 (6), 331–335.

Vissink, A., Mitchell, J.B., Baum, B.J., et al., 2010. Clinical management of salivary gland hypofunction and xerostomia in head-and-neck cancer patients: successes and barriers. Int. J. Radiat. Oncol. Biol. Phys. 78 (4), 983–991.

Vokurka, S., Skardova, J., Karas, M., et al., 2010. Oropharyngeal mucositis pain treatment with transdermal buprenorphine in patients after allogeneic stem cell transplantation. J. Pain Symptom Manage. 39 (6), e4–e6.

Watkins, B., Pouliot, K., Fey, E., et al., 2010. Attenuation of radiation- and chemoradiation-induced mucositis using gamma-d-glutamyl-l-tryptophan (SCV-07). Oral Dis. 16, 655–660.

Weber, C., Dommerich, S., Pau, H.W., Kramp, B., 2010. Limited mouth opening after primary therapy of head and neck cancer. Oral Maxillofac. Surg. 14 (3), 169–173.

Worthington, H.V., Clarkson, J.E., Bryan, G., 2011. Interventions for preventing oral mucositis for patients with cancer receiving treatment. Cochrane Database Syst. Rev. (4), CD000978.

Worthington, H.V., Clarkson, J.E., Bryan, G., et al., 2010. Interventions for preventing oral mucositis for patients with cancer receiving treatment. Cochrane Database Syst. Rev. (12), CD000978.

55 Oral manifestations of disorders of specific systems

This chapter annotates the orofacial manifestations of disorders of specific systems: further details can be found elsewhere in this book.

BOX 55.1 Cardiovascular disease

Angina pectoris
- Pain referred to jaw rarely
- Ulceration caused by nicorandil

Anticoagulants
- Bleeding tendency

Giant cell arteritis (cranial or temporal arteritis)
- Pain usually over the temple
- Rarely, tongue pain or ischaemic necrosis

Hereditary haemorrhagic telangiectasia
- Telangiectasias that may bleed profusely

Hypertension (problems caused by some antihypertensive agents)
- Dry mouth
- Gingival swelling (nifedipine)

- Lichenoid lesions (methyldopa, ACE inhibitors)
- Angioedema (ACE inhibitors)
- Burning mouth (ACE inhibitors)
- Lip cancer

Ischaemic heart disease
- Arterial calcifications on orthopantomogram
- Possibly periodontitis

Polyarteritis nodosa
- Ulcers

Shunts: right to left (e.g. Fallot tetralogy)
- Cyanosis
- Delayed tooth eruption

BOX 55.2 Connective tissue disease

Any connective tissue disease
- Sjögren syndrome
- Lymph node enlargement
- Facial sensory loss

Ehlers–Danlos syndrome
- Temporomandibular joint hypermobility
- Pulp stones
- Periodontitis rarely

Felty syndrome
- Temporomandibular arthritis
- Sjögren syndrome
- Drug reactions (e.g. lichenoid)
- Ulcers

Lupus erythematosus
- White lesions
- Ulcers
- Sjögren syndrome

Mixed connective tissue disease
- Ulceration

- Pain
- Sjögren syndrome

Rheumatoid arthritis
- Temporomandibular arthritis
- Sjögren syndrome
- Drug reactions (e.g. lichenoid)

Still syndrome
- Temporomandibular arthritis
- Sjögren syndrome
- Ankylosis

Systemic sclerosis
- Stiffness of lips, tongue, etc.
- Trismus
- Telangiectasia
- Sjögren syndrome
- Periodontal ligament widened on radiography
- Mandibular resorption
- Oral cancer

BOX 55.3 Endocrine conditions

Acromegaly
- Spaced teeth
- Mandibular prognathism
- Macroglossia

Diabetes mellitus
- Periodontal disease, accelerated
- Hyposalivation
- Candidosis
- Sialosis
- Lichen planus
- Oral cancer

Gigantism
- Spaced teeth
- Mandibular prognathism
- Macroglossia
- Megadontia

Hyperparathyroidism
- Giant cell granulomas
- Loss of lamina dura
- Osteitis fibrosa cystica, rarely

Hypoadrenocorticism
- Mucosal hyperpigmentation

Hypoparathyroidism (congenital)
- Dental hypoplasia
- May be chronic candidosis if there is associated immune defect

Hypopituitarism (congenital)
- Microdontia
- Retarded tooth eruption

Hypothyroidism (congenital)
- Macroglossia
- Retarded tooth eruption

Menopause
- Osteoporosis

Precocious puberty
- Accelerated tooth eruption (fibrous dysplasia in Albright syndrome)

Pregnancy
- Gingivitis
- Epulis

BOX 55.4 Gastrointestinal disorders

Chronic pancreatitis
- Sialosis
- IgG4 syndrome

Coeliac disease
- Ulcers
- Glossitis
- Angular stomatitis
- Dental hypoplasia in severely affected children

Crohn disease
- Facial or lip swelling
- Mucosal tags
- Gingival hyperplasia
- Cobblestoning of mucosa
- Ulcers
- Glossitis
- Angular stomatitis
- Cervical lymphadenopathy

Cystic fibrosis
- Salivary gland swelling

Gardner syndrome (familial colonic polyps)
- Osteomas

Gastric regurgitation
- Tooth erosion
- Halitosis

Malabsorption syndromes
- Ulcers
- Glossitis
- Angular stomatitis
- Sialosis

Patterson–Kelly syndrome
- Oral cancer

Pancreatic cancer
- Periodontitis

Pernicious anaemia
- Ulcers
- Glossitis
- Angular stomatitis

Peutz–Jeghers syndrome (small intestinal polyps)
- Melanosis

BOX 55.5 **Haematological disorders and immune defects**

Aplastic anaemia
- Ulcers
- Bleeding tendency

Graft-versus-host disease
- Lichenoid lesions
- Dry mouth

Haematinic – iron, folic acid or vitamin B_{12} deficiency
- Burning mouth sensation
- Glossitis
- Ulcers
- Angular cheilitis

Haemolytic disease of newborn
- Pigmentation
- Rarely, enamel defects

Haemopoietic stem cell transplantation
- Ulcers
- Mucositis
- Hyposalivation
- Graft-versus-host disease

Hypereosinophilic syndrome
- Ulceration

Hypoplasminogenaemia
- Gingival swelling and ulceration

Leukaemia
- Infections
- Ulcers
- Bleeding tendency
- Gingival swelling in myelomonocytic leukaemia
- Cervical lymph node enlargement
- Labial sensory loss

Leukocyte defects
- Infections, especially herpetic and candidal
- Ulcers

Lymphoma
- Infections
- Ulcers
- Swelling
- Cervical lymph node enlargement

Multiple myeloma
- Bone pain
- Tooth mobility
- Amyloid

Myelodysplastic syndrome
- Ulcers
- Labial sensory changes

Sickle cell anaemia
- Jaw deformities caused by marrow expansion
- Rarely, osteomyelitis or pain

Thalassaemia major
- Jaw deformities caused by marrow expansion

Thrombocytopenia
- Bleeding tendency
- Purpura

Immunodeficiencies
- See below for HIV

Ataxia telangiectasia
- Recurrent sinusitis
- Ulceration
- Facial and oral telangiectasia

- Cervical lymphomas
- Mask-like facial expression

Chédiak–Higashi syndrome
- Cervical lymph node enlargement
- Ulceration
- Periodontitis

Chronic benign neutropenia
- Ulceration
- Severe periodontitis

Chronic granulomatous disease
- Cervical lymph node enlargement and suppuration
- Candidosis (including CMC)
- Enamel hypoplasia
- Acute gingivitis
- Ulceration

Cyclic neutropenia
- Ulceration
- Severe periodontitis
- Eczematous lesions of the face

Common variable immunodeficiency
- Recurrent sinusitis
- Candidosis (including CMC)

Di George syndrome (CATCH22)
- Abnormal facies
- Candidosis (including CMC)
- Viral infections
- Bifid uvula
- Dental hypoplasia

Haim–Munk syndrome
- Periodontitis

Hereditary angioedema
- Swellings of face, mouth and pharynx

Job syndrome
- Abnormal facies

Lazy leukocyte syndrome
- Periodontitis
- Candidosis (including CMC)

Papillon–Lefevre syndrome
- Periodontitis

Selective IgA deficiency
- Tonsillar hyperplasia
- Ulceration
- Viral infections
- Parotitis

Severe combined immunodeficiency (SCID)
- Candidosis (including CMC)
- Viral infections
- Ulceration
- Absent tonsils
- Recurrent sinusitis

Sex-linked agammaglobulinaemia
- Cervical lymph node enlargement
- Ulceration
- Recurrent sinusitis
- Absent tonsils

Wiskott–Aldrich syndrome
- Candidosis
- Viral infections
- Purpura

BOX 55.6   Immunological disorders

See also connective tissue disorders, and skin diseases.

Angioedema
- Facial swelling

Behçet syndrome
- Ulcers

Graft-versus-host disease
- Lichenoid lesions
- Sicca syndrome
- Infections

Kawasaki disease (mucocutaneous lymph node syndrome)
- Cervical lymph node enlargement
- Sore tongue
- Cheilitis

Langerhans histiocytoses (histiocytosis X)
- Loosening of teeth
- Jaw radiolucencies

Myasthenia gravis and other myopathies
- Facial weakness
- Lingual weakness
- Dysarthria

Reiter syndrome (reactive arthritis)
- Ulcers
- Lesions like erythema migrans

Sarcoidosis
- Hyposalivation
- Salivary gland swelling
- Heerfordt syndrome (parotid swelling, lacrimal swelling, facial palsy)
- Sjögren syndrome
- Oral swellings

Sweet syndrome
- Ulcers

Wegener granulomatosis
- Gingival swellings
- Ulcers

BOX 55.7   Infectious diseases

Aspergillosis
- Antral infections

Candidosis
- White lesions
- Red lesions
- Angular stomatitis

Cat-scratch disease
- Lymph node enlargement

Coxsackie viruses
- Ulcers in herpangina and in hand, foot and mouth disease

Cryptococcosis
- Ulcers

Cytomegalovirus
- Ulcers
- Sialadenitis

ECHO viruses
- Ulcers in herpangina and in hand, foot and mouth disease

Epstein–Barr virus (in infectious mononucleosis)
- Sore throat
- Tonsillar exudate
- Palatal petechiae
- Cervical lymph node enlargement
- Ulcers
- Lymphoma
- Sialadenitis
- Recurrent parotitis, possibly in children
- Facial palsy

Gonorrhoea
- Pharyngitis
- Gingivitis
- Temporomandibular arthritis

Hepatitis C (see Box 55.8)

Herpes simplex
- Ulcers in primary infection
- Gingivitis in primary infection
- Vesicles on lips in recurrence (rarely, oral ulcers)
- Lymph node enlargement
- Facial palsy
- Erythema multiforme

Herpes zoster-varicella
- Ulcers in chicken pox, or in zoster of trigeminal maxillary or mandibular divisions
- Pain in maxillary or mandibular zoster
- Facial palsy in Ramsay–Hunt syndrome of zoster of the geniculate ganglion

Human herpesvirus-8
- Kaposi sarcoma

Histoplasmosis
- Ulcers

HIV (human immunodeficiency virus causing AIDS)
- Lymph node enlargement
- Infections, particularly herpetic and candidal
- Ulcers
- Kaposi sarcoma
- Lymphoma
- Hairy leukoplakia
- Parotitis
- Hyposalivation
- Periodontitis
- Cranial nerve lesions
- Purpura

Leprosy
- Cranial nerve palsies

BOX 55.7 Infectious diseases—Cont'd

Lyme disease
- Facial palsy
- Facial sensory loss
- Facial pain

Measles
- Koplik's spots

Mucormycosis
- Antral infections

Mumps
- Salivary gland swelling

Papilloma viruses
- Warts
- Papillomas
- Condyloma acuminata
- Focal epithelial hyperplasia

Paracoccidioidomycosis
- Ulcers

Rubella
- Palatal petechiae
- Dental hypoplasia in congenital rubella

Syphilis
- Chancre
- Mucous patches
- Ulcers
- Gumma
- Pain from neurosyphilis
- Leukoplakia
- Lymph node enlargement
- Hutchinson teeth in congenital syphilis

Toxoplasmosis
- Cervical lymph node enlargement

Tuberculosis (including atypical mycobacteria)
- Ulcers rarely
- Cervical lymph node enlargement

BOX 55.8 Liver disorders

Alcoholic cirrhosis
- Bleeding tendency
- Sialosis

Biliary atresia
- Dental hypoplasia
- Pigmented teeth

Chronic active hepatitis
- Lichen planus

Hepatitis C
- Salivary swelling and hyposalivation
- Lichen planus

Jaundice
- Bleeding tendency
- Jaundice

Kernicterus
- Dental hypoplasia
- Pigmented teeth

Primary biliary cirrhosis
- Sjögren syndrome
- Lichen planus

Transplants
- Infections
- Neoplasms
- Gingival swelling

BOX 55.9 Metabolic disorders

Amyloidosis
- Macroglossia
- Purpura
- Salivary swelling
- Hyposalivation

Erythropoietic porphyria
- Reddish teeth
- Bullae/erosions
- Dental hypoplasia

Folic acid deficiency
- Burning mouth

- Ulcers
- Glossitis
- Angular cheilitis

Haemochromatosis
- Salivary swelling
- Hyposalivation

Hypophosphataemia
- Dental hypoplasia
- Large pulp chambers

Hypophosphatasia
- Loosening and loss of teeth (hypoplastic cementum)

BOX 55.9 Metabolic disorders—Cont'd

Iron deficiency
- Burning mouth
- Ulcers
- Glossitis
- Angular cheilitis

Lesch–Nyhan syndrome (congenital hyperuricaemia)
- Self-mutilation

Mucopolysaccharidosis
- Spaced teeth
- Retarded tooth eruption
- Temporomandibular joint anomalies
- Enamel defects
- Cystic lesions

Neimann–Pick disease
- Retarded tooth eruption
- Loosening of teeth
- Mucosal pigmentation

Rickets (vitamin D dependent)
- Dental hypoplasia
- Large pulp chambers

Scurvy
- Gingival swelling
- Purpura
- Ulcers

Tangier disease
- Orange tonsillar deposits

Trimethylaminuria
- Halitosis

Vitamin B_{12} deficiency
- Burning mouth
- Ulcers
- Glossitis
- Angular cheilitis

BOX 55.10 Neurological disorders

Alzheimer disease
- Hyposalivation
- Impaired oral hygiene

Bulbar palsy
- Fasciculation of tongue

Cerebral palsy
- Spastic tongue
- Dysarthria
- Attrition
- Drooling

Cerebrovascular disease
- Facial palsy
- Facial sensory loss
- Drooling

Choreoathetosis
- Green staining of teeth in kernicterus

Disseminated sclerosis
- Pain
- Sensory loss
- Facial palsy
- Taste changes

Down syndrome
- Delayed tooth eruption
- Macroglossia
- Scrotal tongue
- Maxillary hypoplasia
- Anterior open bite

- Hypodontia
- Periodontal disease
- Cheilitis
- Drooling

Dysautonomias
- Drooling or dry mouth

Epilepsy
- Trauma to teeth/jaws/mucosa
- Gingival swelling if on phenytoin

Facial palsy
- Palsy and poor natural cleansing of mouth on same side

Neurosyphilis
- Pain rarely
- Dysarthria
- Tremor of tongue

Parkinsonism
- Drooling
- Tremor of tongue

Riley–Day syndrome
- Self-mutilation
- Prominent fungiform papillae
- Salivary swelling
- Sialorrhoea/drooling

Stroke
- Periodontitis

Trigeminal neuralgia
- Pain

BOX 55.11 Mental health disorders

Any disorder
- Pain
- Impaired oral hygiene
- Periodontal disease
- Caries

Anorexia nervosa
- Tooth erosion
- Sialosis

Anxiety states
- Dry mouth
- Cheek biting
- Bruxism

Bulimia
- Tooth erosion

Depression, hypochondriasis and various psychoses
- Dry mouth
- Discharges
- Pain
- Disturbed taste

- Disturbed sensation
- Artefactual ulcers
- Exfoliative cheilitis
- Bruxism
- Burning mouth

Drug abuse
- Oral burns
- Bruxism
- Oral neglect
- HIV/AIDS

Munchausen syndrome
- Self-mutilation
- Feigned dental disease

BOX 55.12 Genitourinary disorders

Chronic kidney disease
- Hyposalivation
- Halitosis/taste disturbance
- Leukoplakia
- Dental hypoplasia in children
- Renal osteodystrophy
- Bleeding tendency
- Angioedema

Dialysis
- Hyposalivation
- Sialadenitis

Nephrotic syndrome
- Dental hypoplasia

Post-renal transplantation
- Infections, particularly herpetic and candidal
- Bleeding tendency
- Gingival swelling if on ciclosporin or nifedipine
- Leukoplakia and carcinoma

Renal rickets (vitamin D resistant)
- Delayed tooth eruption
- Dental hypoplasia
- Enlarged pulp

Urethroplasty
- Post-operative complications from oral mucosal grafting

BOX 55.13 Respiratory disorders

Asthma
- Candidosis
- Caries

Bronchiectasis
- Dry mouth
- Malodour

Chronic obstructive airways diseases
- Cyanosis

Kartagener syndrome
- Sinusitis

Pneumonia
- Periodontitis

BOX 55.14   Skeletal disorders

Cherubism
- Jaw swellings

Cleidocranial dysostosis (dysplasia)
- Delayed tooth eruption
- Multiple supernumerary teeth
- Dentigerous cysts
- Short tooth roots

Craniofacial dysostosis (Crouzon syndrome)
- Maxillary hypoplasia
- Cleft palate

Fibrous dysplasia
- Expansive jaw lesions

Mandibulofacial dysostosis (Treacher–Collins syndrome)
- Cleft palate
- Mandibular hypoplasia

Osteogenesis imperfecta
- Dentinogenesis imperfecta in some

Osteopetrosis (Albers–Schonberg disease)
- Cranial neuropathies
- Delayed tooth eruption
- Osteomyelitis after tooth extractions

Osteoporosis
- Jaw osteoporosis
- Bisphosphonate osteochemonecrosis

Paget disease
- Expansive jaw lesions
- Hypercementosis
- Osteomyelitis rarely after tooth extractions
- Post-extraction bleeding

BOX 55.15   Skin diseases

Acanthosis nigricans
- Papillomas

Chronic bullous disease of childhood
- Ulcers
- Blisters, rarely
- Desquamative gingivitis

Chronic mucocutaneous candidosis
- Chronic candidosis

Darier's disease
- White lesions

Dermatitis herpetiformis
- Ulcers
- Blisters, rarely
- Desquamative gingivitis

Ectodermal dysplasia
- Hypodontia
- Dental anomalies (peg-shaped teeth)
- Hyposalivation

Ellis–van Creveld syndrome (chondroectodermal dysplasia)
- Multiple fraeni
- Short roots
- Hypodontia

Epidermolysis bullosa
- Blisters
- Erosions

- Scarring
- Dental hypoplasia

Erythema multiforme
- Ulcers
- Blood-stained crusting of lips

Lichen planus
- White lesions
- Red lesions
- Erosions
- Desquamative gingivitis

Linear IgA disease
- Ulcers
- Blisters, rarely
- Desquamative gingivitis

Pemphigoid
- Blisters
- Ulcers
- Desquamative gingivitis

Pemphigus
- Ulcers
- Blisters, rarely
- Desquamative gingivitis

Psoriasis
- White lesions
- Lesions like erythema migrans

Toxic epidermal necrolysis
- Ulcers

USEFUL WEBSITES

Emedicine.com, Oral Manifestations of Systemic
Disorders. http://emedicine.medscape.com/
article/1081029

FURTHER READING

Almeida, O.D.P., Scully, C., 2002. Fungal infections of the mouth. Brazilian J. Oral Sci. 1, 19–26.

Gómez-Moreno, G., Cutando, A., Arana, C., Scully, C., 2005. Hereditary blood coagulation disorders. Management and dental treatment. J. Dent. Res. 84, 978–985.

Hegarty, A.M., Barrett, A.W., Scully, C., 2004. Pyostomatitis vegetans. Clin. Exp. Dermatol. 28, 1–7.

Machuca, G., Rodríguez, S., Martínez, M., et al., 2005. Descriptive study about the influence of general health and socio-cultural variables on the periodontal health of early menopausal patients. Periodontology 2, 75–84.

Scully, C., 2001. Gastroenterological diseases and the mouth. Practitioner 245, 215–222.

Scully, C., Gokbuget, A.Y., Allen, C., et al., 2001. Oral manifestations indicative of plasminogen deficiency (hypoplasminogenemia). Oral Surg. Oral Med. Oral Pathol. 91, 344–347.

Scully, C., Roberts, G., Shotts, R., 2001. The mouth in heart disease. Practitioner 245, 432–437.

Scully, C., Shotts, R., 2001. The mouth in neurological disorders. Practitioner 245, 539–549.

Scully, C., 2001. The mouth in dermatological disorders. Practitioner 245, 942–952.

Scully, C., Kumar, N., 2002. Dentistry for those requiring special care. Prim. Dent. Care 10, 17–22.

Shotts, R., Scully, C., 2002. How to identify and deal with tongue problems. Pulse 62, 73–76.

Scully, C., Wolff, A., 2002. Oral surgery in patients on anticoagulant therapy. Oral Surg. Oral Med. Oral Pathol. Oral Radiol. Endod. 94, 57–64.

Scully, C., Diz Dios, P., Shotts, R., 2004. Oral health care in patients with the most important medically compromising conditions; 1. platelet disorders. CPD Dentistry 5, 3–7.

Scully, C., Diz Dios, P., Shotts, R., 2004. Oral health care in patients with the most important medically compromising conditions; 2. congenital coagulation disorders. CPD Dentistry 5, 8–11.

Scully, C., Diz Dios, P., Shotts, R., 2004. Oral health care in patients with the most important medically compromising conditions; 3. anticoagulated patients. CPD Dentistry 5, 47–49.

Scully, C., Diz Dios, P., Shotts, R., 2004. Oral health care in patients with the most important medically compromising conditions; 4. patients with cardiovascular problems. CPD Dentistry 5, 50–55.

Scully, C., Diz Dios, P., Shotts, R., 2004. Oral health care in patients with the most important medically compromising conditions; 5. patients at risk for endocarditis. CPD Dentistry 5, 75–79.

Scully, C., Diz Dios, P., Shotts, R., 2004. Oral health care in patients with the most important medically compromising conditions; 6. patients undergoing radiotherapy. CPD Dentistry 6, 80–84.

Scully, C., Diz Dios, P., Shotts, R., 2005. Oral health care in patients with the most important medically

compromising conditions; 7. patients undergoing chemotherapy. CPD Dentistry 6, 3–6.

Scully, C., Diz Dios, P., Shotts, R., 2005. Oral health care in patients with the most important medically compromising conditions; 8. diabetes mellitus. CPD Dentistry 6, 7–11.

Scully, C., Chaudhry, S., 2006. Aspects of Human Disease 1. Atheroma and coronary artery (ischaemic heart) disease. Dent. Update 33, 251.

Scully, C., Chaudhry, S., 2006. Aspects of Human Disease 2. Angina pectoris. Dent. Update 33, 317.

Scully, C., Chaudhry, S., 2006. Aspects of Human Disease 3. Myocardial infarction. Dent. Update 33, 381.

Scully, C., Chaudhry, S., 2006. Aspects of Human Disease 4. Hypertension. Dent. Update 33, 443.

Scully, C., Chaudhry, S., 2006. Aspects of Human Disease 5. Infective endocarditis. Dent. Update 33, 509.

Scully, C., Chaudhry, S., 2006. Aspects of Human Disease 6. Congenital heart disease. Dent. Update 33, 573.

Scully, C., Van Bruggen, W., Dios, P.D., et al., 2002. Down syndrome; lip lesions and *Candida albicans*. Br. J. Dermatol. 147, 37–40.

Scully, C., Cawson, R.A., 2005. Medical problems in dentistry, fifth ed. Churchill Livingstone, Edinburgh.

Scully, C., Diz Dios, P., Kumar, D., 2007. Special care in dentistry. In: Handbook of oral healthcare. Churchill Livingstone, Edinburgh.

EPONYMOUS AND OTHER CONDITIONS

What the mind does not know, the eyes do not see (and the ears do not hear).
Hindu saying

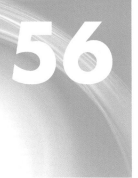

This chapter includes synopses of several eponymous conditions relevant to oral medicine, presented alphabetically.

Abrikossof tumour Granular cell myoblastoma (tumour).

Addison disease (hypoadrenocorticism) Adrenocortical destruction, reduced cortisol, and subsequent increased release of pituitary adrenocorticotrophic hormone (ACTH). A rare disease of young or middle-aged females, the usual cause is autoimmune hypoadrenalism, rarely, tuberculosis, histoplasmosis (sometimes in HIV/AIDS) or carcinomatosis. Weight loss, weakness, and hypotension, with brown hyperpigmentation, especially in sites usually pigmented (areolae and genitals) or traumatized, in flexures, on the gingiva, and at the occlusal line are seen. Diagnosis is from low blood pressure, low plasma electrolyte and cortisol levels and impaired response to ACTH stimulation (Synacthen test). Management is fludrocortisone plus corticosteroids.

Adies (Holmes–Adie) pupil A benign condition. One pupil is dilated and reacts only very slowly to light or convergence together with loss of knee or ankle jerks.

Albers-Schonberg disease Osteopetrosis (p. 405).

Albright syndrome (McCune–Albright syndrome) Polyostotic fibrous dysplasia with skin pigmentation and an endocrine abnormality (usually precocious puberty in girls).

Allgrove syndrome – Triple-A syndrome (AAA), or Achalasia–Addisonianism–Alacrimia syndrome A genetic defect due to mutations in the *AAAS* gene, which codes for a WD-repeat protein termed ALADIN which may cause hyposalivation but the main problems are progressive adrenocorticohypofunction, lack of tears, achalasia, hypotension and hyperpigmentation.

Alstrom syndrome Congenital nerve deafness and retinitis pigmentosa.

Apert syndrome Autosomal dominant craniofacial synostosis, which includes facial dysmorphology, limb (hands and feet) defects, and learning disability.

Argyll–Robinson pupils Small, irregular, unequal pupils which fail to react to light, but do react to accommodation. Characteristically caused by neurosyphilis, may also be seen in diabetes, disseminated sclerosis or other conditions.

Arnold–Chiari syndrome A congenital malformation in which the brainstem and cerebellum are longer than normal and protrude into the spinal canal.

Ascher syndrome (Ascher-Laffer syndrome) Congenital double lip with blepharoclasia and thyroid goitre.

Avellis syndrome A unilateral paralysis of the larynx and palate.

Bannayan–Riley–Ruvalcaba syndrome A rare autosomal dominant disorder related to Cowden syndrome, affecting chromosome 10q and the PTEN (phosphatase and tensin homologue) gene, characterized by excessive growth before and after birth. The head is large (macrocephaly) and often long and narrow (scaphocephaly); normal intelligence or mild learning disability; pigmented macules on penis, tongue polyps and/or subcutaneous hamartomas.

Battle sign Bruising over the mastoid bone – sign of a basilar skull fracture.

Becker syndrome Severe muscular dystrophy that results in progressive weakness of limb and breathing muscles.

Beckwith–Wiedemann syndrome Congenital gigantism, and omphalocoele or umbilical hernia.

Beeson sign Myalgia, facial oedema and fever in trichinosis.

Behçet syndrome 'Adamantiades syndrome' (see Ch. 36).

Bell palsy The common lower motor neurone facial palsy (see Ch. 37).

Bell sign Seen in lower motor neurone facial palsy, when the eye rolls upward on attempted closure.

Bence–Jones protein Immunoglobulin light chains which spill over into the urine (Bence–Jones proteinuria) when there is overproduction of γ-globulins in myelomatosis.

Biemond syndrome Congenital obesity and hypogonadism.

Binder syndrome Congenital maxillonasal dysplasia, and absent or hypoplastic frontal sinuses.

Blackfan–Diamond syndrome Congenital red cell aplasia.

Block–Sulzberger disease (incontinentia pigmenti) Congenital hyperpigmented skin lesions, skeletal defects, learning disability and hypodontia.

Bloom syndrome Congenital telangiectasia, depigmentation and short stature.

Bohn nodules Keratin-filled cysts derived from palatal salivary gland structures scattered all over the palate, especially at the junction of the hard and soft palate.

Book syndrome Autosomal dominant condition of palm and sole hyperhidrosis, hypodontia and premature whitening of hair.

Bourneville disease (epiloia, tuberous sclerosis) Autosomal dominant; two loci – one on 9q34 and one on 16p13. A phakomatosis, there are fibromas at the nail bases (subungual fibromas); hamartomas in brain, kidneys and heart; and nodules in the nasolabial fold (adenoma sebaceum), plus pitting enamel hypoplasia.

Bruton syndrome Sex-linked hypoimmunoglobulinaemia, cervical lymph node enlargement, oral ulceration, recurrent sinusitis, absent tonsils.

Burkitt lymphoma Caused by Epstein–Barr virus, most common in children in sub-Saharan African endemic malaria areas, especially Uganda and Kenya, characterized by lymphomatous deposits in many tissues, especially the jaws (in 50% of patients). Responds well to chemotherapy.

Byar–Jurkiewicz syndrome Gingival fibromatosis, hypertrichosis, giant fibroadenomas of the breast, and kyphosis.

Cannon disease Congenital white sponge naevus.

Carabelli cusp Congenital additional palatal cusp on upper molars.

Carney syndrome Autosomal dominant syndrome of myxomas, spotty lip pigmentation and endocrine overactivity (often Cushing syndrome). Cardiac myxomas cause death or serious disability in a quarter of affected patients.

Castleman disease A rare disorder characterized by benign tumours in lymph node tissue throughout the body (i.e. systemic disease (plasma cell type)).

Chediak–Higashi syndrome A congenital immune defect in which neutrophils have large inclusions. Juvenile periodontitis and early tooth loss, plus oral ulceration.

Christmas disease Blood clotting factor IX defect.

Chvostek sign Tapping the skin over the facial nerve elicits involuntary twitching of the muscles of the upper lip or ipsilateral side of face – a sign of hypocalcaemia.

Clutton joints Symmetrical hydrarthrosis of knees in congential syphilis, appearing around puberty.

Cockayne syndrome Premature ageing, dwarfism, deafness and neuropathy.

Coffin–Lawry syndrome Congenital osteocartilaginous anomalies and learning disability.

Coffin–Siris syndrome Congenital defective neutrophil function, susceptibility to infection and skin pigmentation.

Cohen syndrome Autosomal recessive syndrome of alveolar bone loss, neutropenia, learning disability and obesity.

Costen syndrome Outmoded term relating to facial pain, otalgia and occlusal abnormalities, replaced by 'temporomandibular pain–dysfunction syndrome'.

Cowden syndrome Autosomal dominant disorder affecting PTEN (phosphatase and tensin homologue) gene, congenital multiple hamartomas with oral papillomatosis and risk of breast and thyroid cancer.

Coxsackie virus Named after a town in New York state, Coxsackie viruses are many, and can cause herpangina, hand, foot and mouth disease, and other illnesses.

CREST syndrome Calcinosis, Raynaud disease, oesophageal involvement, sclerodactyly and telangiectasia (see scleroderma).

Crohn disease (See orofacial granulomatosis: OFG). A chronic inflammatory idiopathic granulomatous disorder that may be caused by *Mycobacterium avium* subspecies *paratuberculosis*. Mutations in the CARD15 gene (NOD2 gene) are also implicated. About 20% have a blood relative with some form of inflammatory bowel disease.

Cronkhite–Canada syndrome Hypogeusia followed by diarrhoea, and ectodermal changes including alopecia, nail dystrophy and skin and buccal melanotic hyperpigmentation. Colonic polyps may be present.

Cross syndrome Athetosis, learning disability, gingival fibromatosis and hypopigmentation.

Crouzon syndrome Autosomal-dominant premature fusion of cranial sutures, midface hypoplasia and proptosis.

Curry–Jones syndrome Unilateral coronal synostosis and microphthalmia, plagiocephaly, craniofacial asymmetry, iris coloboma, broad thumbs, hand syndactyly, foot polydactyly, skin lesions, gastrointestinal abnormalities and developmental delay.

Cushing syndrome Moon face with buffalo hump, hirsutism and hypertension due to an ACTH-producing pituitary adenoma.

Darier disease (Darier–White disease) An autosomal-dominant skin disorder with follicular hyperkeratosis, and sometime white oral papules.

Destombes–Rosai–Dorfman syndrome Rosai–Dorfman syndrome.

Di George syndrome A third branchial arch defect related to a chromosome 22 anomaly (CATCH22 syndrome) causing immunodeficiency; cardiac, thyroid and parathyroid defects.

Down syndrome (trisomy 21) The commonest recognizable congenital chromosomal anomaly. Patients are of short stature with characteristic brachycephaly, midface retrusion and upward sloping palpebral fissures (Mongoloid slant). Learning disability and dental anomalies and periodontitis are common.

Duhring disease Dermatitis herpetiformis.

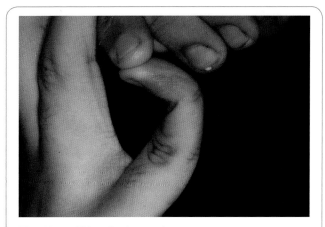

Fig. 56.1 Ehlers-Danlos syndrome

Eagle syndrome An elongated styloid process associated with dysphagia and pain on chewing, and on turning the head towards the affected side.

ECHO viruses Enteric cytopathogenic human orphan viruses.

Ehlers–Danlos syndrome A group of congenital collagen disorders (autosomal dominant, autosomal recessive, or X-linked), with altered mechanical properties of skin, joints, ligaments and blood vessels. Phenotypes vary depending upon which collagen type is affected. EDS is characterized by hyperflexible joints, hyperextensible skin, bleeding and bruising, and mitral incompetence. Patients can bend the thumb right back (**Fig. 56.1**) and may be able to touch the tip of their nose with their tongue. Recurrent dislocation of the temporomandibular joint may be seen. Dental anomalies include deep-fissured premolars and molars, dentinal abnormalities, such as shortened deformed roots, and multiple large pulp stones. Ten types were described: in types IV, VIII and IX there is severe early onset periodontal disease with loss of permanent teeth. Type III genotypes show resistance to local analgesia.

Ellis–van Creveld syndrome Also known as 'chondroectodermal dysplasia'. This syndrome mapped to chromosome 4p consists of congenital polydactyly, dwarfism, ectodermal dysplasia, hypodontia and hypoplastic teeth and multiple fraenae.

Epstein–Barr virus A herpesvirus implicated in infectious mononucleosis, hairy leukoplakia, nasopharyngeal carcinoma and some lymphomas.

Epstein pearls Cystic keratin-filled nodules derived from entrapped epithelial remnants along the line of fusion along the midpalatine raphe.

Ewing tumour A primary malignant neoplasm of undifferentiated bone mesenchymal cells, extremely aggressive, expands rapidly, invades the soft tissues, and metastasizes early. Characteristically affects children and young adults, particularly males, but is rare in the jaws. Radiographically it has either a sunray or an onion-peel appearance due to deposition of new bone in layers. Microscopy shows sheets of uniform small round cells, with scanty, indistinct cytoplasm which contain glycogen. Treatment is chemo-radiotherapy, with a 5-year survival rate of over 50%.

Fabry disease Angiokeratoma corporis diffusum universale. An X-linked recessive error of glycosphingolipid metabolism with angiokeratomas on scrotum, hypertension, fever, renal disease and risk of myocardial infarction.

Fallot tetralogy The combination of a ventricular septal defect (VSD) with pulmonary stenosis, the aorta 'overriding' the VSD and right ventricular hypertrophy.

Fanconi anaemia Congenital anaemia, abnormal radii and risk of oral carcinoma and leukaemia.

Felty syndrome Rheumatoid arthritis and neutropenia.

Filatov disease Infectious mononucleosis.

Fitzgerald–Gardner syndrome Gardner syndrome

Foix–Chavany–Marie syndrome Bilateral anterior opercular syndrome, is a paralysis of the face and pharynx with anarthria, drooling, and general weakness in the face, caused by bilateral damage to the brain operculum, usually from a stroke, trauma or infection, and causing no limb paralysis and not interfering with involuntary movement such as smiling, chewing or blinking eyes.

Fordyce disease (Fordyce spots) See Ch. 24.

Frey syndrome Gustatory sweating and flushing after trauma to skin overlying a salivary gland due to crossover of sympathetic and parasympathetic innervation to the gland and skin.

Froehlich syndrome Congenital obesity, hypogonadism, and risk of learning disability and open bite.

Gardner syndrome Familial adenomatous polyposis (FAP), formerly termed familial polyposis coli (FPC). An autosomal dominant condition caused by mutation in *APC* tumour suppressor gene on chromosome 5. Intestinal polyps have a 100% risk of undergoing malignant transformation, so early identification of disease is critical. Gardner described the occurrence of FAP with extracolonic manifestations of desmoids, osteomas and epidermoid cysts. Unerupted and supernumerary teeth may be present. Multifocal pigmented lesions of the fundus of the eye are seen in 80%.

Garré osteomyelitis This is proliferative periostitis (p. 405).

Gasserian ganglion The trigeminal ganglion.

Gaucher disease The most common genetic disease affecting Ashkenazi Jewish people of Eastern European ancestry, leading to a specific deficiency of the enzyme glucocerebrosidase and lipid-storage disorder. It may cause dry mouth.

Gilles de la Tourette syndrome Coprolalia (utterance of obscenities).

Goldenhar syndrome A variant of congenital hemifacial microsomia, presenting with microtia (small ears), agenesis of the mandibular ramus and condyle, vertebral abnormalities and epibulbar dermoids.

Goltz syndrome (focal dermal hypoplasia) An X-linked disorder with multiple mesenchymal defects, skin lesions, and oral warts and dental defects.

Gorlin–Goltz syndrome (Gorlin syndrome; multiple basal cell naevi syndrome; naevoid basal cell carcinoma syndrome (NBCCS)). An autosomal-dominant trait related to chromosome 9q22.3-q31 and associated with *patch* gene mutations and deletions. The syndrome consists of multiple basal cell carcinomas (BCC), keratocystic odontogenic tumours (KCOTs), vertebral and rib anomalies and temporoparietal bossing with broad nasal root, calcification of the falx cerebri and abnormal sella turcica. Jaw cysts are indistinguishable from other KCOTs and are treated similarly. Diagnosis is suggested by major criteria – positive family history; more than one BCC; KCOTs (first sign in 75%); palmar or plantar pits; or calcified falx cerebri. Minor criteria include congenital skeletal anomalies: bifid, fused, splayed or missing ribs; or bifid, wedged or fused vertebrae; occipitofrontal circumference over 97th percentile, with frontal bossing; cardiac or ovarian fibromas; medulloblastoma; lymphomesenteric cysts; and congenital malformations, such as cleft lip and/or palate, polydactyly, congenital ocular anomaly (cataract, microphthalmos, coloboma).

Graves disease Hyperthyroidism with ophthalmopathy and exophthalmos.

Grinspan syndrome Lichen planus, diabetes and hypertension (probably actually due to lichenoid reactions to antihypertensive and antidiabetic drugs).

Guillain–Barré syndrome Acute infective polyneuritis; facial palsy may be seen.

Hailey–Hailey disease Autosomal-dominant, benign familial pemphigus presenting in the second or third decade with skin and oral blisters and vegetations.

Haim–Munk syndrome Similar to Papillon–Lefevre syndrome, plus pyogenic skin infections, arachnodactyly, acro-osteolysis, onychogryphosis and pes planus.

Hajdu–Cheney syndrome Rare connective tissue disorder, featuring ulcerating lesions on the palms and soles, accompanied by softening and destruction of bones (acro-osteolysis). Abnormal development of bones, joints and teeth also occurs.

Hallerman–Streiff syndrome Congenital cranial anomalies, microophthalmia, cataracts, mandibular hypoplasia and abnormal temporomandibular joint.

Hand–Schüller–Christian disease Langerhans histiocytosis.

Hansen disease Leprosy.

Heck disease (focal epithelial hyperplasia) Papillomas caused by human papilloma viruses 13 or 32, seen especially in ethnic groups such as American Indians and Inuits.

Heerfordt syndrome Sarcoidosis associated with lacrimal and salivary swelling, uveitis and fever (uveoparotid fever) and facial palsy.

Henoch–Schonlein purpura Allergic purpura, which may cause oral petechiae.

Hermansky–Pudlak syndrome Congenital albinism and bleeding tendency.

Hodgkin disease Lymphoma that affects particularly males in middle age. Progressive lymphoid tissue involvement, often begins in the neck with enlarged, discrete and rubbery lymph nodes. Drinking alcohol may cause pain in affected lymph nodes. Pain, fever, night sweats, weight loss, malaise, bone pain and pruritus are common. Treatment by chemotherapy and radiotherapy is remarkably successful.

Horner syndrome This is caused by interruption of sympathetic nerve fibres peripherally as a result, for example, of trauma to the neck, or lung cancer infiltrating the superior cervical sympathetic ganglion, and comprises, usually, unilateral:

- miosis (pupil constriction)
- ptosis (drooping of the upper eyelid)
- loss of sweating of the ipsilateral face
- apparent enophthalmos (retruded eyeball).

Horton cephalgia Migrainous neuralgia.

Hughes syndrome Anti-phospholipid syndrome: blood hypercoagulability leads to deep vein thrombosis, stroke (CVEs), coronary thrombosis and pregnancy complications.

Hunterian chancre Syphilitic primary chancre.

Hurler syndrome Congenital mucopolysaccharidosis causing growth failure, learning disability, large head, frontal bossing, hypertelorism, coarse facial features (gargoylism) macroglossia (**Fig. 56.2**) and mandibular radiolucencies.

Hutchinson–Gilford syndrome Progeria (see Werner syndrome).

Hutchinson teeth Screwdriver-shaped incisor teeth in congenital syphilis.

Hutchinson triad Hutchinson teeth, interstitial keratitis and deafness.

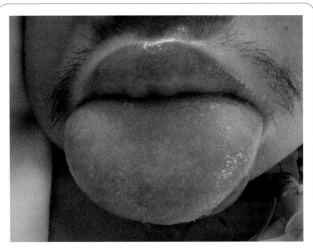

Fig. 56.2 Macroglossia in mucopolysaccharidosis

Imerslund–Grasbeck syndrome Juvenile pernicious anaemia

Jackson–Lawler syndrome A type of pachyonychia congenita with no oral leukoplakia, but neonatal teeth and early loss of secondary teeth.

Jadarsohn–Lewandowski syndrome Pachyonychia congenita.

Job syndrome Hyper-IgE syndrome.

Jones syndrome Curry–Jones syndrome.

Kaposi sarcoma (KS) A malignant neoplasm of endothelial cells caused by human herpesvirus 8, seen especially in HIV/AIDS or immunosuppressed patients.

Kartagener syndrome Primary ciliary dyskinesia (PCD). Congenital dextrocardia, immunodeficiency, sinusitis and recurrent respiratory infections (and male infertility).

Kawasaki disease (mucocutaneous lymph node syndrome) Fever, cheilitis, lymphadenopathy, desquamation of hands and feet, and cardiac lesions in periodic epidemics with geographic spread, suggest an infectious aetiology. Management includes gamma globulin and aspirin and long-term anticoagulation.

Kikuchi–Fujimoto disease A self-limiting idiopathic illness of pyrexia, neutropenia and cervical lymphadenopathy in young Asian women. Can be confused histologically and clinically with lymphoma or systemic lupus erythematosus.

Kimura disease A chronic idiopathic inflammatory condition presenting with a painless, slowly enlarging soft tissue mass (or masses), associated lymphadenopathy and peripheral eosinophilia; 85% of cases are seen in males.

Klinefelter syndrome A chromosome abnormality in men, causing hypogonadism.

Klippel–Feil anomaly Congenital association of cervical vertebrae fusion and short neck, low-lying posterior hairline, syringomyelia and other neurological anomalies, and sometimes unilateral renal agenesis and cardiac anomalies.

Koplik spots Small white spots on the buccal mucosa during measles prodrome.

Kuttner tumour Salivary swelling in IgG4 syndrome

Kveim test An outdated skin test for sarcoidosis.

Laband syndrome (Zimmerman–Laband syndrome) A form of hereditary gingival fibromatosis with skeletal anomalies and large digits.

Langerhans cell histiocytoses (histiocytosis X) Rare neoplasms arising from Langerhans cells (dendritic intraepithelial macrophage-like cells). Swelling and gingival ulceration, particularly in molar region, are common and teeth may loosen and exfoliate. Failure of healing of a socket, or the appearance of a pathological fracture may be presenting features. The spectrum includes the following:

- Solitary eosinophilic granuloma of bone: usually benign with osteolytic lesion only and seen in adults. There is sometimes gross periodontal destruction.
- Multifocal eosinophilic granuloma (Hand–Schuller–Christian disease): a more malignant form in children and young adults characterized by osteolytic lesions and sometimes diabetes insipidus and proptosis.
- Letterer–Siwe disease: the most malignant form; seen in infants and characterized by failure to thrive, fever, hepatosplenomegaly and skeletal osteolytic lesions that may cause pain, swelling and loosening of teeth.

Differentiate from other osteolytic disorders, especially carcinomatosis and myelomatosis. Diagnose by radiography and biopsy: foamy macrophages (Birbeck granules may be seen by EM), eosinophils and bone destruction. Surgery used to manage solitary lesions; radiotherapy/chemotherapy for multifocal disease.

Larsen syndrome A mainly autosomal recessive condition, consisting of cleft palate, flattened facies, multiple congenital dislocations and deformities of the feet.

Laurence–Moon–Biedl syndrome Congenital retinitis pigmentosa, obesity, polydactyly, learning disability and blindness.

Laugier–Hunziker syndrome (Laugier–Hunziker–Baran syndrome) Labial and oral mucosal brown to black pigmented macules and nail hyperpigmentation.

Lemierre syndrome Throat infection is followed by identified potentially lethal anaerobic septicaemia – postanginal septicaemia with metastatic abscesses – most commonly in the lung, due to the anaerobe *Fusobacterium necrophorum.*

Leopard syndrome (cardiocutaneous lentiginosis syndrome) LEOPARD syndrome and Noonan syndrome are allelic disorders caused by different mutations in *PTPN11*, a gene encoding the protein tyrosine phosphatase SHP-2 located at chromosome 12q24.1. It consists of:

- lentigines (multiple)
- electrocardiographic conduction abnormalities
- ocular hypertelorism
- pulmonary stenosis
- abnormalities of genitalia
- retardation of growth
- deafness.

Lesch–Nyhan syndrome Congenital defect of purine metabolism causing learning disability, choreoathetoid cerebral palsy and aggressive self-mutilation.

Letterer–Siwe disease Langerhans histiocytosis.

Lewar disease (pulse granuloma) A hard mass in the lower buccal sulcus indented or ulcerated by a denture flange. Hyaline bodies seen subperiosteally on histology are vegetable leguminous pulses, which provoke a foreign body reaction. Vegetable matter becomes embedded under the mucosa following tooth extraction or from denture pressure. Treatment is by curettage.

Loeys-Dietz syndrome A recently-discovered AD syndrome features similar to Marfan syndrome with bifid uvala but related to transforming growth factor gene.

Lowe syndrome (cerebrohepatorenal syndrome) Congenital hypotonia and flexion contractures.

Ludwig angina Infection of sublingual and submandibular fascial spaces.

Lyell disease (toxic epidermal necrolysis) Originally described in relation to staphylococcal infection (see p. 408).

Lyme disease Infection with *Borrelia burgdorferi* from deer ticks, causing rashes, fever, arthropathy and facial palsy. First recognized in the town of Lyme, Connecticut, USA, but prevalent worldwide. CDC recommendations for serologic diagnosis are to screen with a polyvalent ELISA test or C6 peptide antibodies and confirm equivocal and positive results with western blot assay.

Maffucci syndrome Multiple enchondromas, haemangiomas (often in the tongue), and risk of malignant chondrosarcomas.

MAGIC syndrome Mouth and genital ulcers and interstitial chondritis. A variant of Behçet syndrome.

Mantoux test Skin test for delayed-type hypersensitivity reaction to bacillus Calmette Guerin (BCG; for tuberculosis).

Marcus Gunn syndrome Jaw-winking syndrome (eyelid winks during chewing), with ptosis.

Marfan syndrome An autosomal-dominant condition linked to chromosome 15 in FBN1 gene, which codes for fibrillin-1, essential for the formation of elastic fibres. Reduced levels of fibrillin-1 allow transforming growth factor (TGFβ) to damage heart and lungs. Prevalent among basketball and volleyball players, patients are tall, thin and with arachnodactyly (long, thin spider-like hands). There may be spontaneous pneumothorax, lens dislocation, aortic regurgitation or dissecting aneurysms, mitral valve prolapse, and palate is occasionally cleft or with bifid uvula. Joint laxity is common and TMJ may dislocate. Multiple dental cysts are less common oral complications. Can be confused with Loeys–Dietz syndrome, caused by mutations in the TGFβ receptor genes TGFβR1 and TGFβR2.

Marie–Sainton syndrome Cleidocranial dysplasia.

Melkersson–Rosenthal syndrome The rare association of facial swelling (usually granulomatous cheilitis), with facial palsy and fissured tongue.

Miescher cheilitis Oligosymptomatic labial granulomatosis or Crohn disease.

Mikulicz disease Salivary gland and lacrimal gland swelling, often related to IgG4 syndrome.

Mikulicz syndrome Salivary gland and lacrimal gland swelling related to malignant disease.

Mikulicz ulcer Minor aphthous ulceration.

Moebius syndrome A complex congenital anomaly involving multiple cranial nerves, affecting mainly the abducens and facial nerves, and often associated with limb anomalies. Muscle transplantation has been used to address the lack of facial animation, lack of lower lip support and speech difficulties.

Moon molars Hypoplastic molars from congenital syphilis.

Munchausen syndrome The fabrication of stories by the patient, aimed at the patient receiving operative intervention.

Murray syndrome Multiple hyaline dermal tumours, gingival fibromatosis and recurrent infections.

Murray–Puretic–Drescher syndrome (juvenile hyaline fibromatosis) A rare autosomal recessive disease characterized by cutaneous nodules, especially around the head and neck and often involving the lips. The effects increase with age and also include joint contractures, gingival swelling and osteolytic lesions.

Nelson syndrome A rare condition with hyperpigmentation caused by ACTH overproduction in response to adrenalectomy, used for breast cancer.

Neumann bipolar aphthosis The association of recurrent aphthae with genital ulceration; probably this is a stage in the development of Behçet syndrome.

Nikolsky sign A term meaning blistering, or the extension of a blister, on gentle pressure (seen mainly in pemphigus and pemphigoid).

Non-Hodgkin lymphomas (NHL) More common than Hodgkin disease and generally with a poorer prognosis, and a predilection for the gastrointestinal tract and central nervous system. Enlargement of cervical lymph nodes is often the first sign, but NHL may occur in the gingivae or faucial region; a recognized complication of HIV/AIDS and may be Epstein–Barr virus related.

Noonan syndrome (see also Leopard syndrome, Ch. 57) Congenital short stature and webbed neck, sometimes with cardiac anomalies, pulmonary stenosis and cherubism.

Ollier syndrome Multiple enchondromas.

Osler–Rendu–Weber disease (hereditary haemorrhagic telangiectasia; HHT) An autosomal-dominant disorder where telangiectases are present orally, periorally and in the nose, gastrointestinal tract and occasionally on the palms. Telangiectases may bleed, and cryosurgery or laser treatment may be needed (**Fig. 56.3**).

Paget disease of bone A bone disorder characterized by the total disorganization of bone remodelling

Papillon–Lefevre syndrome A congenital condition mapped to chromosome 11q with a defect in the polymorphonuclear leukocyte lysosomal enzyme cathepsin c, causing palmoplantar hyperkeratosis and juvenile periodontitis, which affects both dentitions, and immunodeficiency. Acitretin may correct the defective CD3-induced T lymphocyte activation.

Parrot nodes Frontal bossing in congenital syphilis.

Parry-Romberg syndrome Progressive hemifacial atrophy.

Paterson–Kelly–Brown syndrome (Plummer–Vinson syndrome) The association of dysphagia (due to a post-cricoid web of *Candida* which is premalignant), microcytic hypochromic anaemia, koilonychia (spoon-shaped nails) and angular cheilitis (secondary to the anaemia).

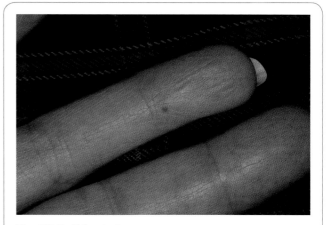

Fig. 56.3 Telangiectases

Paul–Bunell test (Paul–Bunell–Davidson or Forssman antibody test) A serological test for heterophile antibodies in infectious mononucleosis (glandular fever).

Peutz–Jeghers syndrome An autosomal-dominant condition due to a chromosome 19p *STK11/LKB1* (serine/threonine kinase 11) often associated with gene mutation mutations in LKB1. It consists of circumoral melanosis and intestinal polyposis. Oral brown or black macules appear in infancy and affect especially the lips and buccal mucosa and may be seen on extremities and abdomen. The intestinal polyposis may cause intussusception or other types of obstruction. Almost 50% of patients develop and die from some type of cancer by age 57 years – often extra-intestinal cancers.

Pfeiffer disease Infectious mononucleosis.

Pierre–Robin syndrome Congenital micrognathia, cleft palate and glossoptosis.

Pindborg tumour Calcifying epithelial odontogenic tumour.

Plummer–Vinson syndrome Patterson–Kelly–Brown syndrome.

Popischill–Feyrter aphthae A term used for palatal ulceration in neonates.

Prader–Willi syndrome Congenital obesity, hypogonadism, learning disability, diabetes and dental defects.

Quincke oedema Angioedema.

Ramon syndrome Cherubism, arthritis, epilepsy, gingival fibromatosis, hypertrichosis and learning disability.

Ramsay–Hunt syndrome A lower motor neurone facial palsy due to herpes zoster of the geniculate ganglion of the seventh nerve. Presents with vesicles in the ipsilateral pharynx, external auditory canal and on the face.

Rapp–Hodgkin syndrome Ectodermal dysplasia, kinky hair, cleft lip/palate, popliteal pterygium and ectrodactyly.

Raynaud syndrome A vascular spasm in response to cooling, seen in the digits in connective tissue disorders.

Reiter syndrome The association of arthritis, urethritis and balanitis, and conjunctivitis, found mainly in men with HLA-B27 and a high incidence of sexually transmitted infections (mainly Chlamydia). Reiter syndrome is the most common cause of arthritis in young men. A postdysenteric form is more common in women, often after infection with *Shigella flexneri*, *Salmonella typhimurium*, *Yersinia enterocolitica*, *Campylobacter jejuni*, or *Chlamydia trachomatis*. Oral lesions are circinate papules on the palate and elsewhere. Skin lesions resemble psoriasis on the palms and soles (keratoderma blennorhagica). Treatment is with NSAIDs.

Rett syndrome Congenital bruxism and hand-wringing, often with learning disability.

Rieger syndrome Congenital ocular anomalies, iridal hypoplasia, glaucoma and blindness, maxillary hypoplasia and dental hypoplasia with oligo- and microdontia.

Riga-Fede disease TUGSE (traumatic ulcerative granuloma with stromal eosinophilia).

Riley–Day syndrome Inherited familial dysautonomia; sympathetic dysfunction, salivary swelling, sialorrhoea and self-mutilation, seen particularly in Ashkenazi Jews.

Romberg syndrome (hemifacial atrophy) Progressive atrophy of the soft tissues usually of half the face, associated with contralateral Jacksonian epilepsy and trigeminal neuralgia. It starts in the first decade and lasts about 3 years before it becomes quiescent.

Rosai–Dorfmann syndrome Sinus histiocytosis with massive lymphadenopathy or Destombes–Rosai–Dorfman syndrome. A benign, non-Langerhans cell, histiocytic proliferative disorder that primarily affects lymph nodes.

Rothmund–Thomson syndrome Congenital poikiloderma, hypogonadism, dwarfism, cataracts and microdontia.

Rubinstein–Taybi syndrome (broad thumb–great toe syndrome) Short stature with a small head size, and developmental delay. The most striking physical feature is broad, sometimes angulated thumbs and first toes. Facial features include a prominent beaked nose and down-slanting eyes. Undescended testes occur in males.

Rutherfurd syndrome Corneal dystrophy, neurosensory hearing loss, gingival fibromatosis and delayed tooth eruption.

Ruvalcaba–Myrhe–Smith syndrome Bannayan–Riley–Ruvalcaba syndrome.

Sabin–Feldmann test Serological test for toxoplasmosis.

Saethre–Chotzen syndrome An autosomal-dominant craniosynostosis associated with cleft palate as well as other disturbances of the facial skeleton and extremities.

Saxon test A simple, reproducible, cheap test for hyposalivation, which involves chewing on a weighed sterile sponge for 2 min and then re-weighing the sponge. Normal subjects produce at least 2.75 g of saliva in 2 min.

Schmidt syndrome Autoimmune polyendocrinopathy; congenital hypoadrenocorticism, hypoparathyroidism, diabetes and malabsorption, with candidosis.

Schmincke-Regaud tumour A lymphoeithelial carcinoma usually at the base of tongue.

Schwannoma (see p. 403).

Seckel syndrome Congenital microcephaly, learning disability, zygomatic and mandibular hypoplasia.

Simpson–Golabi–Behmel syndrome X-linked dysplasia gigantism, with tissue overgrowth leading to coarse ('bulldog-like') face with protruding jaw and tongue, and wide nasal bridge, and an increased risk of Wilm tumour and neuroblastoma.

Sipple syndrome Multiple endocrine neoplasia (MEN) type 3 (MEN 3; sometimes called 2b) affecting several endocrine glands with multiple mucosal neuromas, phaeochromocytoma and medullary thyroid carcinoma (calcitonin levels raised).

Sjögren–Larsson syndrome Congenital ichthyosis, learning disability, cerebral palsy and indifference to pain.

Sjögren syndrome See Ch. 50.

Sluder syndrome Migrainous neuralgia.

Smith–Lemli–Opitz syndrome Congenital short stature, learning disability, syndactyly, urogenital and maxillary anomalies.

Stafne bone cavity An ectopic inclusion of salivary tissue in the mandible, often from the submandibular gland. Radiography shows a cystic radiolucency. No treatment is indicated, but if a diagnosis cannot be confirmed by sialography, or if serial radiographs show an increase in cavity size, exploratory surgery is indicated.

Stevens–Johnson syndrome See Ch. 42.

Still syndrome Juvenile rheumatoid arthritis.

Sturge–Weber syndrome (encephalotrigeminal angiomatosis) A congenital hamartomatous angioma of the upper face (naevus flammeus), oral mucosa and underlying bone (with hemihypertrophy of bone and accelerated eruption of associated teeth), extending intracranially to cause convulsions, and contralateral hemiplegia and intracerebral calcifications, and sometimes learning disability.

Sutton ulcers Major aphthae.

Sweet syndrome Acute neutrophilic dermatosis with erythematous, well-demarcated skin papules and plaques; red mucosal lesions and ulcers, often associated with malignant disease or induced by drugs. Treatment is with systemic corticosteroids.

Takayasu disease Pulseless aorta and large arteries.

Thibierge–Weissenbach syndrome The CREST syndrome.

TORCH syndrome Toxoplasmosis, other infections, rubella, cytomegalovirus, herpes simplex induced foetal abnormalities.

Treacher–Collins syndrome (mandibulofacial dysostosis) Autosomal-dominant first branchial arch defect with downward sloping (anti-mongoloid slant) palpebral fissures, hypoplastic malar complexes, mandibular retrognathia, deformed pinnas, hypoplastic sinuses, eye colobomas, and middle and inner ear hypoplasia (deafness).

Trotter syndrome Acquired unilateral deafness, pain in the mandibular (third) division of the trigeminal nerve, ipsilateral palatal immobility, and trismus due to invasion of the nasopharynx and the trigeminal nerve by a malignant tumour. *Pterygopalatine fossa syndrome* is a similar condition, where the first and second divisions of the trigeminal nerve are affected.

Turner syndrome Complete or partial deletion of the X chromosome. Affects females only, with short stature, low hairline, web neck, broad chest and widely spaced nipples, increased carrying angle of the elbows and non-functioning ovaries. Occasionally cherubism is found.

Turner tooth Hypoplastic tooth due to damage to the developing tooth germ.

Tzanck cells Abnormal epithelial squames in pemphigus or herpetic infections.

Urbach–Wiethe disease Lipoid proteinosis and hyalinosis cutis et mucosae.

Von Recklinghausen disease Multiple neurofibromas with skin pigmentation, skeletal abnormalities and central nervous system involvement.

Von Willebrand disease Common bleeding disorder caused by defective blood clotting factor VIII and platelet dysfunction.

Waardenburg syndrome Congenital heterochromia iridis (different coloured eyes), deafness, and white forelock, with prognathism.

Waldeyer ring Lymphoid tissue surrounding the entrance to the oropharynx (tonsils and adenoids).

Wallenberg syndrome Posterior inferior cerebellar artery occlusion leading to lateral medullary syndrome.

Warthin tumour Benign salivary gland neoplasm – adenolymphoma or papillary cystadenoma lymphomatosum.

Wegener granulomatosis Idiopathic disseminated malignant granulomatosis. A rare, idiopathic disorder of necrotizing granulomatosis. Initially affecting the respiratory tract, arteritis affects small vessels in lungs, kidneys, eyes, skin, muscles, joints and mouth and is potentially lethal. A painless progressive swelling of the gingiva in a previously healthy mouth, particularly associated with swollen inflamed papillae with a fairly characteristic 'strawberry-like' appearance, should arouse suspicion (**Fig. 56.4**). Diagnosis is supported by biopsy, imaging and anti-neutrophil cytoplasmic antigens (ANCA), anaemia, elevated ESR, CRP or PV and white blood cell and platelet counts. Management is antimicrobials, cytotoxic agents or radiotherapy.

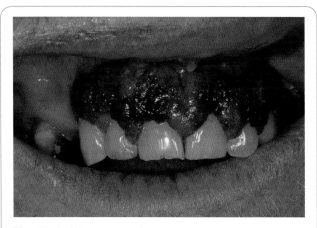

Fig. 56.4 Wegener granulomatosis

Werner syndrome Congenital alopecia, dwarfism, senility, early atherosclerosis, delayed tooth eruption and mandibular hypoplasia.

Whipple disease A rare potentially lethal bacterial infection with *Tropheryma whippelii* that infects the small bowel to cause malabsorption, but may affect immune system, heart, lungs, brain, joints, and eyes.

William syndrome Genetic disorder characterized by mild learning disability, unique personality characteristics, distinctive facial features and cardiovascular disease (elastin arteriopathy). A range of connective tissue abnormalities is observed and hypercalcaemia and/or hypercalciuria are common.

Wilson syndrome (hepatolenticular degeneration) Disorder of copper metabolism leading to hepatic disease; renal disease; spasticity; tremor and mental problems.

Wiskott–Aldrich syndrome X-linked recessive immunodeficiency with thrombocytopenia, infections, eczema (TIE syndrome) and lymphoreticular malignancies.

Witkop disease Hereditary benign intraepithelial dyskeratosis – seen mainly in parts of the USA.

Zimmerman–Laband syndrome Laband syndrome.
Zinsser-Cole-Engelmann syndrome Dyskeratosis congenita.

FURTHER READING

Barnes, L., Eveson, J.W., Reichart, P., Sidransky, D., 2005. WHO classification of tumours; pathology and genetics – head and neck tumours. IARC, Lyon.

Scully, C., Langdon, J.D., Evans, J.H., 2009. A marathon of eponyms: 1 Albers-Schonberg disease (osteopetrosis). Oral Dis. 15, 246–247.

Scully, C., Langdon, J.D., Evans, J.H., 2009. A marathon of eponyms: 2 Bell palsy (idiopathic facial palsy). Oral Dis. 15, 307–308.

Scully, C., Langdon, J.D., Evans, J.H., 2009. A marathon of eponyms: 3 Crouzon syndrome. Oral Dis. 15, 367–368.

Scully, C., Langdon, J.D., Evans, J.H., 2009. A marathon of eponyms: 4 Down syndrome. Oral Dis. 15, 434–436.

Scully, C., Langdon, J.D., Evans, J.H., 2009. A marathon of eponyms: 5 Ehlers-Danlos syndrome. Oral Dis. 15, 517–518.

Scully, C., Langdon, J.D., Evans, J.H., 2009. A marathon of eponyms: 6 Frey syndrome (gustatory sweating). Oral Dis. 15, 608–609.

Scully, C., Langdon, J.D., Evans, J.H., 2010. A marathon of eponyms: 7 Gorlin-Goltz syndrome (naevoid basal cell carcinoma syndrome). Oral Dis. 16, 117–118.

Scully, C., Langdon, J.D., Evans, J.H., 2010. A marathon of eponyms: 8 Hodgkin disease or lymphoma. Oral Dis. 16, 217–218.

Scully, C., Langdon, J.D., Evans, J.H., 2010. A marathon of eponyms: 9 Imerslund-Grasbeck syndrome (Juvenile pernicious anaemia). Oral Dis. 16, 219–220.

Scully, C., Langdon, J.D., Evans, J.H., 2010. A marathon of eponyms: 10 Jadassohn-Lewandosky syndrome (pachyonychia congenita). Oral Dis. 16, 310–311.

Scully, C., Langdon, J.D., Evans, J.H., 2010. A marathon of eponyms: 11 Kaposi sarcoma. Oral Dis. 16, 402–403.

Scully, C., Langdon, J.D., Evans, J.H., 2010. A marathon of eponyms: 12 Ludwig angina. Oral Dis. 16, 496–497.

Scully, C., Langdon, J.D., Evans, J.H., 2010. A marathon of eponyms: 13 Melkersson-Rosenthal syndrome. Oral Dis. 16, 707–708.

Scully, C., Langdon, J.D., Evans, J.H., 2010. A marathon of eponyms: 14 Noonan syndrome. Oral Dis. 16, 839–840.

Scully, C., Langdon, J.D., Evans, J.H., 2011. A marathon of eponyms: 15 Osler-Rendu-Weber disease. Oral Dis. 17, 125–127.

Scully, C., Langdon, J.D., Evans, J.H., 2011. A marathon of eponyms: 16 Paget disease of bone. Oral Dis. 17, 238–243.

Scully, C., Langdon, J.D., Evans, J.H., 2011. A marathon of eponyms: 17 Quincke oedema (angioedema). Oral Dis. 17, 342–344.

Scully, C., Langdon, J.D., Evans, J.H., 2011. A marathon of eponyms: 18 Robin sequence. Oral Dis. 17, 443–444.

Scully, C., Langdon, J.D., Evans, J.H., 2011. A marathon of eponyms: 19 Sjögren syndrome. Oral Dis. 17, 538–540.

Scully, C., Langdon, J.D., Evans, J.H., 2011. A marathon of eponyms: 20 Treacher Collins syndrome. Oral Dis. 17, 619–620.

Scully, C., Langdon, J.D., Evans, J.H., 2011. A marathon of eponyms: 21 Urbach-Wiethe disease. Oral Dis. 17, 729–730.

Scully, C., Langdon, J.D., Evans, J.H., 2012. A marathon of eponyms: 22 Virchow node. Oral Dis. 18, 107–108.

Scully, C., Langdon, J.D., Evans, J.H., 2012. A marathon of eponyms: 23 Wegener granulomatosis. Oral Dis. 18, 214–216.

Scully, C., Langdon, J.D., Evans, J.H., 2012. A marathon of eponyms: 24 Xmas (Christmas) disease. Oral Dis. 18, 315–316.

Scully, C., Langdon, J.D., Evans, J.H., 2012. A marathon of eponyms: 25 Yersiniosis. Oral Dis. 18, 417–419.

Scully, C., Langdon, J.D., Evans, J.H., 2012. A marathon of eponyms: 26 Zinsser-Cole-Engelmann syndrome. Oral Dis. 18 (5), 522–523.

Other conditions

This chapter includes synopses of a number of conditions relevant to oral medicine, not appearing elsewhere. These are presented alphabetically. If a specific condition is not found here, please refer to the index, since it may well be located elsewhere in the book.

Acanthosis nigricans A rare paraneoplastic condition where papillomatous oral lesions are seen often in patients with internal malignancy.

Acatalasia Autosomal recessive defect in the enzyme catalase, which normally removes reactive oxygen species, such as hydrogen peroxide, from tissues. Severe periodontal destruction and oral ulceration can result.

Achondroplasia (chondrodystrophia fetalis) An autosomal dominant condition in which endochondral ossification is reduced. The most common form of short-limbed dwarfism – patients have disproportionately short limbs, bowed legs, kyphosis, prominent buttocks and abdomen, and trident hands with short fingers. The skull is relatively large, having prominent frontal, occipital and parietal bones. The middle third of the face can be hypoplastic with nasal bridge depressed and a class III type malocclusion. The foramen magnum is often narrow and spinal cord compression can occur. Joints can be of limited mobility and the pelvic inlet narrow.

Acrodermatitis enteropathica A rare genetic disorder of zinc metabolism causing mouth ulceration and candidosis, rash around orifices, and alopecia.

Actinic prurigo (AP) A chronic, pruritic skin disease caused by an abnormal reaction to sunlight.

Actinomycosis A rare infection with *Actinomyces israelii*, below the mandibular angle (not lymph nodes) that may follow jaw fracture or tooth extraction. Prolonged therapy, usually with penicillin, is indicated.

Acute necrotizing (ulcerative) gingivitis A non-contagious anaerobic gingival infection associated with overwhelming proliferation of *Borrelia vincentii* and fusiform bacteria. Predisposing factors include smoking, viral respiratory infections and immune defects, such as in HIV/AIDS. Uncommon, except in resource-poor groups, this typically affects adolescents and young adults, especially in institutions, armed forces, etc., or people with HIV/AIDS.

Characteristic features include severe gingival soreness, profuse bleeding, halitosis and a bad taste. Interdental papillae are ulcerated with necrotic slough. Malaise, fever and/or cervical lymph node enlargement (unlike herpetic stomatitis) are rare. Cancrum oris (noma) is a very rare complication, usually in debilitated children. (p. 404)

Diagnosis is usually clinical. Smear for fusospirochaetal bacteria and leukocytes; blood picture occasionally. Differentiate from acute leukaemia or herpetic stomatitis. Manage by oral debridement, metronidazole (penicillin if pregnant) and oral hygiene.

Amelogenesis imperfecta A rare genetic defect of enamel formation due to mutations in AMELX, ENAM, and MMP20 genes, with a wide variety of patterns. All teeth are equally affected, as are other family members. Diagnosis is from clinical features (**Fig. 57.1, Table 57.1**).

Fluorosis, tetracycline staining, dentinogenesis imperfecta and oculodentodigital dysplasia may need to be differentiated. Management requires restorative dental care.

Amyloidosis The deposition in tissues of amyloid – an eosinophilic hyaline material, with a fibrillar structure on ultramicroscopy. Amyloid can be identified via Congo red stain under fluorescent or polarized light, thioflavine T stain under fluorescent light, or immunoreactivity with antibodies for immunoglobulin light chains.

Primary (including myeloma-associated) amyloidosis: associated with deposits of immunoglobulin light chains. Manifestations include macroglossia and oral petechiae or blood-filled bullae (secondary purpura).

Secondary amyloidosis: seen mainly in rheumatoid arthritis and ulcerative colitis, rarely affects the mouth, and is associated with deposits of AA proteins.

Diagnose from biopsy; blood picture; raised ESR, CRP or PV and marrow biopsy; serum proteins and electrophoresis; urinalysis (Bence–Jones proteinuria; Ch. 56); skeletal survey for myeloma. Manage by chemotherapy (melphalan, corticosteroids or fluoxymesterone).

Angina bullosa haemorrhagica (localized oral purpura) Blood blisters in the mouth or pharynx, mainly on soft palate, seen in absence of any immunological or platelet-associated cause. Seen mainly in older people, the aetiology is unclear, though there are occasional associations with use of steroid inhalers. There is rapid onset, with breakdown of the blister in a day or two to an ulcer. Diagnose from clinical features, although it may be necessary to confirm haemostasis is normal; and rarely to biopsy to exclude pemphigoid. Manage by reassurance. Topical analgesics may provide symptomatic relief.

Angiomas See haemangiomas.

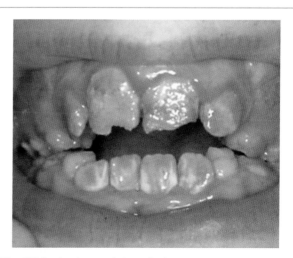

Fig. 57.1 Amelogenesis imperfecta

Table 57.1 Amelogenesis imperfecta

Type	1	2	3	4
Name	Hypoplastic	Hypocalcified	Hypomaturation	Hypomaturation with taurodontism
Defect	Matrix	Calcification	Maturation	Mixed – between types 1 and 3
Enamel thickness and colour	Thin, hard, pitted or grooved	Normal thickness, softer and liable to attrition Discoloured white to brownish-yellow, and darkening with age	Normal thickness, softer and liable to attrition	Variable
Radiographic features	Normal enamel density	Enamel similar to dentine		
Inheritance	AD, AR or x	AD or AR	AD, AR or x	AD

AD = autosomal Dominant, AR= autosomal recessive, X = X-linked

Angiomyoma A rare benign hamartoma involving blood vessels and muscle.

Ankyloglossia (tongue-tie) An uncommon genetic condition which results in the lingual fraenum anchoring the tongue tip, restricting tongue protrusion and lateral movements. Oral cleansing (but not speech) is impaired. Differentiate from tethering by scarring. Management is surgery (fraenectomy) if severe.

Branchial cyst A lymphoepithelial cyst that may arise from enclavement of salivary tissue in a lymph node, or from the cervical sinus. It usually becomes apparent in the third decade. It requires excision.

Bullous pemphigoid An autoimmune disease usually with widespread crops of tense, fluid-filled blisters on the skin. The diagnosis is confirmed by biopsy. Bullous pemphigoid is treated with prednisolone (enteric-coated).

Caries Dental caries can occur on any tooth surface exposed to the oral environment, but not surfaces retained within bone. There are four factors in the aetiology: a tooth surface (enamel or dentine); cariogenic (or potentially caries-causing) bacteria in dental plaque; fermentable carbohydrates; and time. The specific bacterial species believed to cause caries include *Streptococcus mutans* and *Lactobacilli*. Particularly for root caries, the most closely associated bacteria are *Lactobacillus acidophilus*, *Actinomyces viscosus*, *Nocardia* spp., and *Strep. mutans*. Sugars (sucrose, glucose, fructose) are metabolized to acetic, lactic, formic and succinic acids. Different individuals are susceptible to different degrees depending on tooth shape, oral hygiene, and the flow and buffering capacity of their saliva.

Carotid body tumour A slow-growing, but malignant neoplasm of chromaffin cells that both invades locally and metastasizes. It presents as a mass over the internal carotid artery and transmits the carotid pulsation. It must be resected.

CATCH22 Stands for **c**ardiac abnormality, **a**bnormal facies, **T**-cell deficit due to thymic hypoplasia, **c**left palate, and **h**ypocalcaemia due to hypoparathyroidism, caused by a chromosome **22** defect.

Cheek biting (morsicatio buccarum) Common and seen in adults mainly, especially anxious patients, and those with other psychologically related disorders, e.g. temporomandibular pain–dysfunction syndrome, it is also rarely caused by self-mutilation, seen in psychiatric disorders, learning disability, Lesch-Nyhan syndrome (Ch. 56) and some rare syndromes with insensitivity to pain. Abrasion of the superficial epithelium leaves whitish fragments on reddish background. The lesions are invariably restricted to the lower labial mucosa and/or buccal mucosa near the occlusal line on one or both sides.

Chemical burns Can be caused by various chemicals or drugs; notably aspirin put in the sulcus to try to relieve toothache, or cocaine. A white lesion with sloughing mucosa is seen. Diagnosis is by history and clinical features.

Chikungunya fever A mosquito-borne arboviral illness similar to dengue fever; causes arthralgia and mouth ulceration

Chondroma A benign tumour, rare in the jaws. The anterior maxilla, mandibular symphysis and the coronoid and condylar processes are the most common sites. Chondromas are typically found in the older patient and form slow-growing, painless masses. Provided surgical excision of these masses is complete, recurrence is unlikely.

Chondrosarcomas These tend to affect the older patient and, although isolated cases arise from chondromas, most arise *de novo*. The behaviour is very unpredictable, but many grow rapidly and produce extensive local destruction. Radical surgery, the only means of eradicating the tumour, can be difficult as the edges may not be apparent clinically or radiographically. Multiple local recurrence is common and the prognosis is worse than for osteosarcoma.

Chorea Consists of a writhing movement of continuous abrupt and intermittent movements that flow randomly from one part of the body to another. Chorea may affect the head and neck, especially in tardive dyskinesia. This is usually a late (hence tardive) complication manifesting as non-random, focal patterned or stereotyped movement induced by dopamine receptor blocking drugs, such as metoclopramide, phenothiazines or butyrophenones, and is somewhat similar to oromandibular dystonia. Senile chorea, including edentulous dyskinesia or orodyskinesia, is found in 16% of the edentulous.

Chronic ulcerative stomatitis This is similar to erosive lichen planus, with ulcers and erosions affecting mainly the buccal or lingual mucosae, but sometimes the gingivae. The lesions and clinically normal mucosa have a distinct pattern of a particulate stratified squamous-epithelium-specific (SES) antinuclear antibody (ANA) on direct immunofluorescent examination of perilesional tissue, and patients can have circulating ANA. Hydroxychloroquine is effective therapy.

Cleidocranial dysplasia (dysostosis) A rare autosomal dominant condition, or mutation. Clinical features include exaggerated transverse diameter of cranium, delayed fontanelle closure, multiple wormian bones, frontal and parietal bossing, depressed nasal bridge, maxillary hypoplasia, underdeveloped paranasal sinuses, high arched palate (? cleft), delayed or failed tooth eruption, multiple supernumerary teeth, dentigerous cysts, aplastic or hypoplastic clavicles (shoulders can be approximated), short stature and other skeletal anomalies.

Diagnosis is from the family history and ability to bring together the shoulders; jaw, skull and skeletal radiography.

Management is to leave unerupted teeth alone unless there are complications. Eruption of permanent teeth is retarded and dentigerous cysts are frequently found. Supernumerary teeth are common in cleidocranial dysplasia, especially in the anterior mandible. The crowns of the teeth are normal, but the roots can be short, thin and lack acellular cement. Surgery is often necessary.

Coeliac disease Coeliac disease is a reaction to gluten, ingestion of which activates immune cells in the small intestine, which trigger inflammation and local damage, disrupting food absorption. Untreated coeliac patients lose weight, develop deficiency syndromes such as anaemia, and experience symptoms such as diarrhoea. Dental hypoplasia and oral ulceration may result. Diagnosis is confirmed by malabsorption, blood tissue transglutaminase antibodies and villous atrophy on jejunal biopsy. Gluten is found in wheat, barley and rye, which means that many dietary staples, such as bread, many breakfast cereals and foods like pizza and pasta, can no longer be eaten.

Congenital epulis A rare reactive process seen on the alveolus of a neonate.

Constricted pupils Constricted pupils (miosis) can be caused by sympathetic nerve lesions, cholinergic drugs (e.g. pilocarpine or neostigmine) or opiates (heroin, etc.). Thus, heroin addicts may be recognized by 'pin-point pupils'. Raised intracranial pressure is the most important cause of pupil constriction and is noted when the pupil also becomes non-reactive owing to pressure on the oculomotor nerve. It may occur after head injury, intracranial haemorrhage or brain tumour.

CREST syndrome Calcinosis, Raynaud disease, oesophageal involvement, sclerodactyly and telangiectasia (see scleroderma, p. 406).

Cri-du-chat syndrome Short arm of chromosome 5 deletion, resulting in microcephaly, hypertelorism, and laryngeal hypoplasia causing a characteristic shrill cry.

Crystal deposition diseases ('gout') A term used to encompass diseases that produce crystals in joints (e.g. gout, chondrocalcinosis, secondary gout caused by cytotoxic therapy) including the temporomandibular joint. Gout itself is an uncommon disorder of metabolism in which excessive levels of uric acid in the blood and other body fluids crystallize out in synovial fluid causing acute inflammation. The patient complains of a painful, swollen joint and 'pan-meniscal crepitation' is elicited on movement. Acute attacks are often preceded by a 'binge' of dietary or alcohol excess or 'starvation', trauma or unusual physical exercise, surgery or systemic illness. In chronic gout, tophi are frequently felt in the cartilage of the pinna of the ear. Diagnosis is clinical, but usually confirmed by a leukocytosis, raised ESR, CRP or PV raised serum urate level and aspiration biopsy for examination under polarizing light for crystals of urate (or pyrophosphate in pseudo-gout). Imaging is not often particularly helpful, since the appearance resembles osteoarthritis. Treatment must not be restricted just to the local treatment of the TMJ. NSAIDs should be started. Colchicine is effective. Gout is usually treated prophylactically with allopurinol. Dietary advice and weight control are also important.

Cyst A pathological cavity having liquid, semi-liquid or gaseous contents. It is frequently, but not always, lined with epithelium. Cysts of the jaws mostly arise from odontogenic epithelium, and are relatively common lesions (Ch. 45). Non-odontogenic developmental cysts are uncommon and were said to form from entrapment of epithelium during the fusion of embryological processes, but this embryological concept has now been discarded. The lining of these cysts is either stratified squamous epithelium or pseudostratified ciliated columnar (respiratory) epithelium. Non-odontogenic cysts include the following:

- *Nasopalatine or incisive canal cysts:* derived from the vestigial oronasal ducts. They may occur either within the nasopalatine canal, or in the soft tissues of the palate at the opening of the canal, grow slowly, and may discharge into the mouth giving a salty taste. Radiological examination shows a well-defined, rounded ovoid or occasionally heart-shaped defect in the anterior maxilla. Nasopalatine cysts must be distinguished from a normal large anterior palatine fossa which may be up to 7 mm in diameter, and from radicular cysts associated with the maxillary incisors. These cysts should be enucleated and seldom recur.

- *Nasolabial cysts:* soft tissue cysts found within the nasolabial fold. They are lined by respiratory epithelium, and if allowed to grow may distort the upper lip and alar base. Treatment is by simple excision.

Cystic hygroma A developmental anomaly of lymphatics presenting as a swelling of the neck seen before the age of 2 years. It may extend into the mediastinum and/or tongue. Cystic hygroma is usually surgically removed.

Dentinogenesis imperfecta A rare autosomal-dominant disorder in which the dentine is abnormal in structure and, hence, translucent (**Fig. 57.2**), and poorly attached to enamel. All teeth are affected, but primary teeth are more severely affected than permanent teeth. In the permanent dentition the teeth that develop first are generally more severely affected than those that develop later. The teeth:

- are translucent
- may vary in colour from grey to blue or brown
- enamel is poorly adherent to the abnormal underlying dentine and easily chips and wears
- crowns are bulbous with pronounced cervical constriction and the roots are short
- fracture easily (there is progressive obliteration of pulp chambers and root canals with secondary dentine)
- periapical radiolucencies are not uncommon.

There are three types of dentinogenesis imperfecta:

- Type I (associated with osteogenesis imperfecta): most severe in deciduous dentition; bone fractures; blue sclerae; progressive deafness; caused by mutations in one of several genes.
- Type II (hereditary opalescent dentine): defect equal in both dentitions; caused by mutations in the DSPP gene. A few families with type II have progressive hearing loss in addition to dental abnormalities.
- Type III (Brandywine type – first identified in Brandywine, Maryland, USA): associated with occasional shell teeth and multiple pulpal exposures; caused by mutations in the DSPP gene.

Differentiate mainly from amelogenesis imperfecta, tetracycline staining and dentine dysplasia. Management is by restorative dental care.

Dermatitis herpetiformis An uncommon chronic skin disorder associated often with gluten-sensitive enteropathy, affecting mainly middle-aged males. Symmetrical papulovesicular eruptions on extensor surfaces. Oral lesions of vesicles and/or desquamative gingivitis, similar to pemphigoid typically follow skin lesions. Biopsy of perilesional tissue, with histological and immunostaining examination are essential to diagnosis, showing IgA deposits at the papillae. Jejunal biopsy often indicated. Dapsone is the main therapy – sulfamethoxypyridazine and sulfasalazine are alternatives. A gluten-free diet can minimize disease activity and can reduce or avoid the need for drugs.

Dermatomyositis A rare autoimmune disorder that occasionally presents with oral ulcers and erythema of the tongue, palate or gingivae.

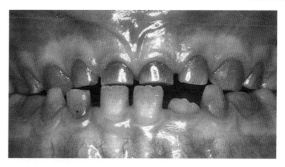

Fig. 57.2 Dentinogenesis imperfecta

Dermoid cyst A rare developmental cyst that presents as a doughy painless swelling in the midline floor of mouth and needs to be differentiated from ranula and cystic hygroma. Diagnosis is by aspiration, but there is a risk of infection. Management is by surgical removal.

Desquamative gingivitis A fairly common problem in which the gingivae show chronic desquamation and is a term that denotes a particular clinical picture and not a diagnosis in itself. Many of the patients are middle-aged women. Desquamative gingivitis is mainly a manifestation of:

- mucocutaneous disorders, usually. Most gingival involvement in the vesiculobullous or skin diseases (dermatoses) is related to lichen planus or pemphigoid, but pemphigus, dermatitis herpetiformis, linear IgA disease, chronic ulcerative stomatitis and other conditions may need to be excluded. Most of these conditions are acquired, but a few are congenital with a strong hereditary predisposition, such as epidermolysis bullosa
- chemical damage, such as reactions to sodium lauryl sulphate in toothpastes
- allergic responses
- drugs
- psoriasis
- pyostomatitis vegetans.

Some patients make no complaint, but others complain of persistent gingival soreness, worse when eating spices, or acidic foods, such as tomatoes or citrus fruits. Most patients are seen only when vesicles and bullae have broken down to leave desquamation, and the clinical appearance is thus of erythematous gingivae, mainly labially, the erythema and loss of stippling extending apically from the gingival margins to the alveolar mucosae. The desquamation may vary from mild almost insignificant small patches to widespread erythema with a glazed appearance. In addition to a full history and examination, biopsy examination and histopathological and immunological investigations are frequently indicated. Conditions which should be excluded include:

- reactions to mouthwashes, chewing gum, medications and dental materials
- candidosis
- lupus erythematosus
- plasma cell gingivitis
- Crohn disease, sarcoidosis and orofacial granulomatosis
- leukaemias
- factitial (self-induced) lesions.

The treatment of desquamative gingivitis consists of:

- improving the oral hygiene
- minimizing irritation of the lesions
- specific therapies for the underlying disease where available
- local or systemic immunosuppressive or dapsone therapy, notably corticosteroids.

Corticosteroid creams used overnight in a soft polythene splint may help.

Dilated pupils (mydriasis) Can be caused by parasympathetic lesions affecting the third nerve, Holmes–Adie syndrome (Ch. 56), Horner syndrome (Ch. 56), anticholinergic drugs (e.g. atropine or similar drugs), sympathomimetic drugs (e.g. adrenaline, cocaine). Users of cocaine or crack cocaine may thus have dilated pupils.

Drug addiction (illegal drug use) This is increasingly common, particularly in urban areas. Addicts in need of a 'fix' will often falsely complain of severe pain or injury. Disturbed behaviour in a drug addict may be caused by withdrawal symptoms and the patient may need compulsory detention. If an addict is admitted to the ward, contact a licensed psychiatrist for heroin or cocaine to be given for addicts. The most serious problems in the management of addicts include:

- overdose
- withdrawal effects
- behavioural problems (including theft)
- violence
- hepatitis
- HIV infection
- other infections
- oral lesions typically are those of these conditions or neglect of hygiene.

Dysarthria (disordered speech) Normal speech involves a complex series of muscles, particularly the muscles of respiration, larynx, pharynx, palate, tongue and lips and, like all voluntary muscle activity, is under control from higher centres, both pyramidal and extrapyramidal. The act of speaking is a highly coordinated sequence involving articulation and phonation under direct control of the vagus, glossopharyngeal, hypoglossal and facial nerves. Conditions affecting the tongue, palate, pharynx, larynx or these nerves or their central connections, or sensory nerves, can lead to disturbed speech. However, speech also involves a wide range of acquired skills, deficiencies of which impede interpersonal communication irrespective of any other impairment in language usage.

Deranged speech can be due commonly to drugs (including alcohol), CNS disorders as in learning disabilities, cerebral palsy, parkinsonism, delirium or dementia; loss of voice due to laryngeal disease or paralysis (dysphonia); or defects in articulation because of paralysis, rigidity, tissue loss or scarring, or involuntary movements of tongue or palate. The most common oral cause of dysarthria is immobility of the tongue after a lingual block local analgesic injection, trauma to the tongue, scarring, diseases affecting the tongue (such as carcinoma) or foreign bodies (such as in oral piercing). Spastic dysarthria is usually caused by cerebrovascular disease affecting the motor cortex (causing pseudobulbar palsy), extrapyramidal disease, such as parkinsonism, or drugs, such as phenothiazines; basal ganglia disease causes choreic dysarthria; cerebellar disease causes ataxic dysarthria. Alcohol also has this effect. Paralytic dysarthria is less common, but may be caused by medulla oblongata disease (bulbar palsy), cranial nerve lesions affecting nerves VII, IX, X, XI or XII, myopathies, such as myasthenia gravis. Patients with persistent dysarthria should be referred for a neurological opinion.

Dyskinesias Abnormal movements of the tongue or facial muscles, sometimes with abnormal jaw movements, bruxism or dysphagia. Involuntary tongue protrusion and retraction, and facial grimacing are common dyskinesias. They differ from dystonias mainly in that muscle spasm is less prominent, but they may be difficult to differentiate clinically. They are usually caused by extrapyramidal disease, such as athetosis, or drugs. Most dyskinesias resolve within 4 weeks of stopping any causal medication. If not, treat with anti-parkinsonian drugs (e.g. benzhexol), baclofen, benzodiazepines, dopamine depletors (reserpine or tetrabenazine), calcium channel blockers, clozapine, buspirone, α-adrenergic agonists, vitamin E or botulinum toxoid.

Dysphasias Disturbances of language use (or aphasias), and may be caused by brain disease, such as stroke or after head injury, in which there is loss of production and comprehension of speech and language.

Dystonias A group of uncommon neurological diseases characterized by abnormal movements, such as sustained and patterned contractions producing abnormal postures, repetitive twisting or squeezing.

Epidermolysis bullosa A rare genetically-determined disorder related to a defect in the epidermolysis bullosa antigen in the epithelial basal lamina, leading to blistering after trauma, and scarring, which may cause severe disability, such as limb deformities, microstomia, ankyloglossia and trismus. Enamel hypoplasia may be seen. Diagnosis is from the family history and a biopsy to exclude other blistering diseases. Management includes careful attention to oral hygiene. Trauma should be minimized, and drugs such as phenytoin may help reduce the blistering.

Epidermolysis bullosa acquisita A rare non-inherited chronic mechanobullous disease characterized by autoantibodies directed against type

VII collagen. Clinically, bullae are frequently induced after mechanical irritation. The diagnosis should be made on the history, clinical features, histopathological, direct and indirect immunofluorescent examination. Biopsy of perilesional tissue, with histological and immunostaining examination are essential to the diagnosis. Topical corticosteroids effectively control gingival lesions. Systemic corticosteroids alone or in association with immunosuppressive agents and dapsone are suggested treatments.

Exfoliative cheilitis (tic de levres) An uncommon condition affecting the lip vermilion, characterized by continuous production and desquamation of unsightly, keratin scales which, when removed, leave a normal lip beneath (**Fig. 57.3**). The aetiology is unknown, but some cases may be factitious.

Familial holoprosencephaly Congenital malformation of the forebrain and midface: microphthalmia, hypopituitarism and hypertelorism.

Fibro-osseous lesions A group of disorders of unknown aetiology, composed of fibrous and ossified tissue. The main disorders include Paget disease of bone, fibrous dysplasia and cherubism and the ossifying fibroma.

Fissured lip Lip fissures may appear especially where there is exposure to adverse environments (**Fig. 57.4**), or where the lip swells as in Down syndrome (Ch. 56) or cheilitis granulomatosa (Ch. 46).

Fissured (plicated or scrotal) tongue An extremely common genetic condition, the dorsum has deep irregular fissures, but is normally papillated (**Fig. 57.5**). A fissured tongue may also be seen in Down syndrome or Melkersson–Rosenthal syndrome (Ch. 56). There are associations with erythema migrans in particular. The diagnosis is usually clear cut. The lobulated tongue of Sjögren syndrome (Ch. 50) must be differentiated.

Fluorosis The condition of enamel defects caused by high levels of fluoride. High levels in drinking water are uncommon in the developed world, but are particularly common in parts of the Middle East, India and Africa. Fluorosis affects many teeth:

- *Mildest form:* white flecks or spotting or diffuse cloudiness.
- *More severe form:* yellow-brown or darker patches.
- *Most severe form:* yellow-brown or darker patches, sometimes with pitting (**Fig. 57.6**).

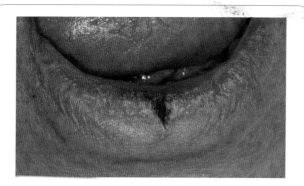

Fig. 57.4 Fissured lip

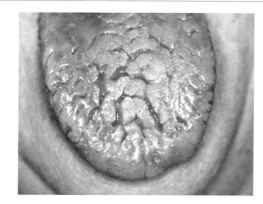

Fig. 57.5 Fissured tongue

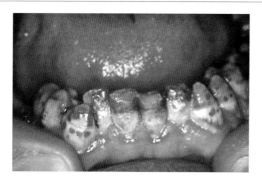

Fig. 57.6 Severe fluorosis

Diagnosis is from history, clinical appearance and data about fluoride content of drinking water. It is necessary to differentiate from amelogenesis imperfecta and tetracycline staining. Management of severe forms is by the use of veneers or crowns.

Foliate papillitis The foliate papillae are found on the posterolateral border of the tongue, at the junction of the anterior two-thirds with the posterior third. The size and shape of the foliate papillae are variable and occasionally they swell if irritated mechanically or if there is an upper respiratory infection, and this is termed 'foliate papillitis'. Located at a site of high predilection for lingual cancer, they may give rise to unnecessary concern about cancer.

Furred tongue Coating of the tongue is quite commonly seen in healthy adults, particularly in edentulous patients, those who are on a soft, non-abrasive diet, those with poor oral hygiene, or those who are fasting. The coating in these instances appears to be of

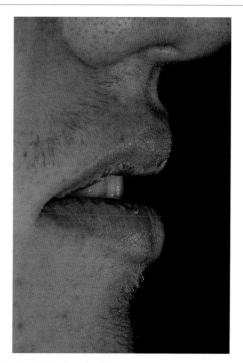

Fig. 57.3 Exfoliative cheilitis

epithelial, food and microbial debris, which collects since it is not mechanically removed. Indeed, the tongue is the main reservoir of some microorganisms, such as *Candida albicans* and some *Streptococci*. The tongue may be coated with off-white debris in many illnesses, particularly febrile diseases, hyposalivation and ill patients – especially those with poor oral hygiene or who are dehydrated. The history is important to exclude a congenital or hereditary cause of a white lesion or candidosis. The clinical appearances may strongly suggest the diagnosis, but investigations are often required if the white lesion does not scrape away from the mucosa with a gauze. Biopsy may then rarely be indicated. Treatment is of the underlying cause.

Geotrichosis An uncommon opportunistic oral infection caused by *Geotrichum candidum*. Oral geotrichosis shows three clinical varieties: pseudomembranous (75%), hyperplastic, and palatine ulcer. It is treated as oral candidosis.

Gingival bleeding This is usually explained by the presence of gingivitis. However, unexplained bleeding can be due to thrombocytopenia (e.g. in leukaemia, HIV disease, idiopathic thrombocytopenic purpura, myelodysplastic syndromes) or occasionally warfarin, other drugs or blood clotting defects.

Glossitis The term given when the tongue is sore or, more appropriately, when the dorsum of tongue becomes depapillated and red. Causes include anaemia, vitamin or iron (haematinic) deficiency, chemotherapy or radiation therapy, or infection, such as candidosis. Glossitis in haematinic deficiency states, is seen mainly in:

- malabsorption states
- pernicious anaemia
- chronic bleeding from the gastrointestinal or genitourinary tract
- vegans
- dietary faddists
- resource-poor circumstances (deficiencies of vitamins of the B group other than B_{12} are an occasional cause of glossitis, mainly seen in chronic alcoholics or in those with malabsorption or starvation).

The tongue may appear completely normal or there may be:

- linear or patchy red lesions: especially in vitamin B_{12} deficiency.
- depapillation with erythema: in deficiencies of iron, folic acid or B vitamins lingual depapillation begins at the tip and margins of the dorsum, but later involves the whole dorsum (bald tongue).

Various other patterns are described, in deficiencies of:

- riboflavin: papillae enlarge initially, but are later lost
- niacin: red, swollen, enlarged 'beefy' tongue
- pyridoxine: swollen, purplish tongue.

There may also be:

- pallor
- burning mouth syndrome
- ulceration
- angular stomatitis.

Differentiate from erythema migrans, lichen planus and acute candidosis. As sore tongue can be the initial symptom of iron, folate or vitamin B_{12} deficiency and can precede any haemoglobin fall, a full blood picture with assays of iron (serum ferritin), vitamin B and folate are essential. Biopsy is rarely indicated. Replacement therapy should be instituted after the underlying cause is established and rectified.

Glossopharyngeal neuralgia A rare condition in which pain with all the characteristics of trigeminal neuralgia is experienced in the posterior tongue, fauces, pharynx and sometimes beneath the angle of the mandible. Treatment is with carbamazepine or, in intractable cases, posterior fossa neurosurgery.

Glycogen storage diseases Inborn errors of metabolism. Type 1B results in neutropenia and periodontal destruction.

Gonorrhoea Infection with *Neisseria gonorrhoea* in the mouth is uncommon or rarely recognized. Pharyngitis may occur after orogenital or oroanal contact. Swab for culture and sensitivity. Treat with amoxicillin or ciprofloxacin.

Granular cell myoblastoma (granular cell tumour) A fairly common hamartoma, the origin of which is unclear. Presents as a pedunculated or occasionally sessile swelling on the gingivae, tongue, buccal mucosa or lip. It should be excised. Histology shows a pseudo-epitheliomatous appearance, but it is benign.

Haemangiopericytoma A rare tumour arising from pericytes; there are benign and malignant forms.

Haemochromatosis An inborn error of iron overload which may cause diabetes, cardiomyopathy and mucocutaneous brown pigmentation or salivary swelling One of the most common metabolic errors, manifesting mainly in males, iron is excessively absorbed and deposits in tissues, causing hyperpigmentation, diabetes, hypogonadism, cirrhosis and cardiomyopathy.

Haemophilia Haemophilia A: deficiency of blood clotting factor VIII. Haemophilia B: Christmas disease (Ch. 56). Haemophilia C: von Willebrand disease (Ch. 56).

Hairy leukoplakia HIV-infected and other severely immunocompromised patients may develop white oral lesions with a vertically corrugated or 'hairy' surface ('hairy leukoplakia') which usually affects the lateral margins or dorsum of tongue. Epstein–Barr virus may be implicated (Ch. 53).

Hand, foot and mouth disease A common Coxsackie virus (Ch. 56) infection (usually A16; rarely A5 or A10), with an incubation of 2–6 days occuring in small epidemics, in children. Clinical features include oral ulcers resembling herpetic stomatitis, but affecting labial and buccal mucosa, no gingivitis, mild fever, malaise, anorexia, rash (red papules that evolve to superficial vesicles in a few days, found mainly on palms and soles). Diagnose from the clinical features. Serology is confirmatory, but rarely required. Differentiate from herpetic stomatitis, chickenpox. Management is symptomatic (see herpes simplex, Ch. 43).

Hemifacial spasm A spasm of the angle of the mouth or the eyelid, worse towards evening. Usually idiopathic, it may be caused by a vascular anomaly affecting the vertebrobasilar vessels (dolichoectasia) causing pressure on the facial nerve. Some cases herald a cerebellopontine angle lesion or other lesion irritating the facial nerve. CT or MRI are indicated. Botulinum toxin injections into the affected muscles may give relief. Anticholinergics, phenytoin, carbamazepine or benzodiazepines may help. Rarely are myectomy or microvascular decompression indicated. Hemimasticatory spasm is similar, but affects the masticatory muscles and may be associated with progressive hemifacial atrophy. It also often responds to botulinum toxin.

Herpangina A Coxsackie virus infection (A7, A9, A16; B1, B2, B3, B4 or B5) or echovirus (9 or 17) with an incubation period of 2–6 days. Clinical features include oropharyngeal ulcers, no gingivitis, cervical lymphadenitis (moderate), fever, malaise, irritability, anorexia, vomiting, but no rash. Diagnose from clinical features. Serology (theoretically) is confirmatory. Differentiate from herpetic stomatitis and chickenpox. Manage symptomatically.

Holoprosencephaly A common developmental defect affecting the neural crest cells populating the frontonasal mass and the forebrain, with the associated appearance of midface defects.

Hypercementosis This may be idiopathic or arise in:

- occlusal trauma
- an overerupted non-opposed tooth
- periapical infection
- Paget disease
- acromegaly.

Hypereosinophilic syndrome A multisystem disorder in which there can be oral ulceration and sinusitis, characterized by a high blood eosinophil count ($>1.5 \times 10^9$/L) for >6 months. Categorized under the idiopathic group of eosinophilias, the lymphocytic form is characterized by T-lymphocyte clonality, IL-5 production, and a possible progression to T-cell lymphoma. Oral lesions are more frequently associated with the myeloproliferative form, characterized by an increased risk of developing myeloid malignancies. Patients may be asymptomatic or severely unwell and can present with generalized non-specific features such as fatigue, night sweats and pruritus; diarrhoea; urticaria; thrombocytopenia; cardiomyopathy and a range of other complications. Diagnosis is supported by raised ESR, abnormal LFTs, abnormal ECG and chest radiography showing pleural effusions. Treatment is with corticosteroids, interferon or emergent monoclonals such as imatinib.

Hyperparathyroidism *Primary hyperparathyroidism* – usually due to a parathyroid adenoma, carcinoma or hyperplasia of parathyroid tissue or ectopic production of parathyroid hormone (PTH) (e.g. by tumours of lung or kidney). May also rarely occur in association with adenomas of other endocrine glands (the multiple endocrine adenoma syndromes). Serum calcium levels are raised, as usually is the alkaline phosphatase. Phosphate levels are reduced. The clinical features are the direct result of either excess PTH or calcium, and particularly include renal stones, bone lesions, polyuria and abdominal pain ('stones, bones and abdominal groans'). Anorexia and psychoses are not uncommon:

- *Secondary hyperparathyroidism:* usually the consequence of renal disease in which low serum calcium as a consequence of impaired renal production of dihydroxycholecalciferol induces increased parathyroid activity, and eventually hyperplasia of the parathyroid glands. Secondary hyperparathyroidism may also follow malabsorption syndromes. Calcium levels are usually normal or low.
- *Tertiary hyperparathyroidism:* a consequence of chronic overstimulation of the gland in secondary hyperparathyroidism, which rarely leads to neoplastic change in the parathyroids, which then escape the normal control of serum calcium.

Oral manifestations of hyperparathyroidism include reduced bone density (the outlines of the maxillary antrum, inferior dental canal and inferior border of the mandible can become less distinct), loss of the lamina dura, root resorption and radiolucencies (particularly of the mandible). The radiolucent lesions are either areas of high osteoclastic activity or giant cell lesions. The giant cell lesions can present intraorally as epulides. Hyperparathyroidism is managed by excision of the neoplastic or hyperplastic parathyroid tissue. In the secondary and tertiary disorders, treatment of the underlying disorder is also required.

Hypodontia A reduction in the number of teeth. The teeth most commonly missing are third molars and maxillary lateral incisors, followed by mandibular and maxillary second premolars. It may be associated with microdontia. If >6 teeth missing, the term oligodontia is sometimes used. Anodontia is total absence of the dentition. A genetic trait, ectodermal dysplasia should be considered.

Hypoglossal nerve lesions LMN lesions of the twelfth cranial nerve lead to unilateral tongue weakness, wasting and fasciculation. When protruded the tongue deviates towards the weaker side. Bilateral supranuclear (UMN) twelfth nerve lesions produce slow, limited tongue movements; the tongue is stiff and cannot be protruded far, and fasciculation is absent. Causes of lesions may be within the brainstem (infarction, syringobulbia, motor neurone disease or poliomyelitis; at the skull base (jugular and anterior condylar foramina) causes include trauma and tumours (nasopharyngeal carcinoma, glomus tumour or neurofibroma) and within the neck and nasopharynx trauma or tumours (nasopharyngeal carcinoma, metastases) or polyneuropathy.

Hypoparathyroidism Usually caused by damage to, or loss of, parathyroid tissue during neck surgery (e.g. thyroidectomy). It may also arise rarely as a familial disorder (idiopathic hypoparathyroidism) or very rarely as a consequence of *in utero* damage when it is associated with cellular immunodeficiency (CATCH 22 syndrome: p. 396). The major clinical features are related to the low serum calcium levels. Tetany (hyperexcitability of muscles) is the most obvious and disturbing feature and can lead to laryngeal spasm. Hypoparathyroidism frequently causes paraesthesia about the mouth. Tapping the skin over the facial nerve can elicit involuntary twitching of the muscles of the upper lip

or ipsilateral side of face (Chvostek sign). Hypoparathyroidism can cause enamel hypoplasia of developing teeth and delayed tooth eruption. Treat with hydroxycholecalciferol.

Pseudohypoparathyroidism is a rare condition in which PTH is secreted normally, but the tissue receptors are unresponsive. The features are similar to those of hypoparathyroidism, plus a tendency to short stature and small fingers, but no dental manifestations.

Hypophosphatasia A rare genetic defect in alkaline phosphatase, causing cemental aplasia or hypoplasia and tooth mobility and early loss. Serum alkaline phosphatase is decreased with increased vitamin B6 and increased urinary phosphoethanolamine.

Hypoplasminogenaemia A rare genetic defect in plasminogen. Manifestations include swollen, painless, nodular and ulcerated gingivae covered with a yellowish-pink pseudomembrane, and ligneous conjunctivitis.

Idiopathic bone necrosis An unusual disorder in which a small portion of bone, typically of the mylohyoid ridge, undergoes spontaneous necrosis and sequestration with pain and ulceration.

Impetigo contagiosa A highly contagious skin infection with streptococci (group A). Uncommon, and seen mainly in underprivileged children (aged 2–6 years), lesions spread by touch to several areas. Clinical features include papules which change into vesicles surrounded by erythema then multiple pustules with golden crusts. Regional lymphadenitis is sometimes seen, but systemic symptoms are rare. Diagnosis is clinical together with culture of pus. On lips, herpes labialis is the prime differential diagnosis, but other vesiculobullous diseases should also be excluded. Management is with antibiotics. If there is no systemic toxicity, use chlortetracycline cream. If there are systemic symptoms, oral flucloxacillin should be used. *Staphylococcus aureus* phage type 71 causes bullous impetigo, a severe form with fever.

IMMP is a distinct condition Isolated mucocutaneous melanotic pigmentation (IMMP) similar to Peutz–Jegher syndrome but with no mutations in LKB1 though associated with various malignant neoplasms in women (Ch. 56).

Juvenile hyaline fibromatosis A hereditary condition which may involve the gingiva, with swelling and a prominent PAS-positive matrix of chondroitin sulfate.

Leiomyoma A rare benign tumour from smooth muscle.

Leukaemia A malignant proliferation of leukocytes. Common oral manifestations in leukaemia include lymphadenopathy, bleeding, petechiae, gingival swelling, ulceration. Other findings include sensory changes (particularly of the lower lip), extrusion of teeth, painful swellings over the mandible, parotid swelling (Mikulicz syndrome Ch. 56), fungal infections, and predisposition to herpesvirus lesions. Diagnose by a blood film, white cell count (raised), differential count (shows blasts), platelet count (reduced) and bone marrow biopsy. Treat mainly by chemotherapy. Oral hygiene should be carefully maintained with chlorhexidine mouth rinses and a soft toothbrush. Prophylactic antifungal and antiviral therapy is also indicated. Many chemotherapeutic agents can cause oral ulceration. Methotrexate is a major offender, but ulceration may be prevented or ameliorated by concomitant intravenous administration of folinic acid ('leucovorin rescue') or topical folinic acid (see Ch. 54). There are several types of leukaemia:

- *Acute lymphoblastic leukaemia* (ALL). The most common leukaemia of childhood, it has a peak incidence at 3–5 years of age. Malignant lymphoblasts proliferate and infiltrate the viscera, skin and central nervous system. Marrow infiltration causes granulocytopenia (predisposing to infections), thrombocytopenia (causing a bleeding tendency) and anaemia ('there is no leukaemia without anaemia').
- *Acute myeloblastic leukaemia* (AML). The most common acute leukaemia of adults. Features are similar to acute lymphoblastic leukaemia, but central nervous system involvement is rare.

- *Chronic lymphocytic leukaemia* (CLL). The most common chronic leukaemia. It mainly affects the older patient. Some patients are asymptomatic, while in others there is fever, weight loss, anorexia, haemorrhage and infections. Lymph node enlargement is early and may be detected in the neck. CLL may need no treatment.
- *Chronic myeloid leukaemia* (CML). This is characterized by proliferation of myeloid cells in the bone marrow, peripheral blood and other tissues, and mainly affects those over 40 years of age. Splenomegaly and hepatomegaly are common. Anaemia, weight loss and joint pains are not uncommon. The prognosis is variable, but sooner or later there is transformation to an acute phase similar to AML (blast crisis).

Leukocyte adhesion deficiency (LAD) Autosomal recessive defect in beta integrins (Mac-1 or P150,95), impeding polymorphonuclear leukocyte adhesion and migration. Presents with infections and juvenile periodontitis.

Leukopenia This may result from viral infections (especially HIV), drugs, irradiation, or can be idiopathic. There is a predisposition to infections, and persistent ulcers lacking an inflammatory halo. Diagnose by a full blood picture and bone marrow biopsy. Manage by improving oral hygiene; antimicrobials as necessary.

Linear IgA disease and chronic bullous dermatosis of childhood These are subepithelial immune blistering diseases in which there is linear deposition of IgA autoantibodies at the epithelial basement membrane zone:

- *Linear IgA disease* (adults): oral lesions that mimic mucous membrane pemphigus, in particular oral vesicles and ulcers.
- *Chronic bullous dermatosis* (childhood): similar oral lesions and sometimes scarring.

Diagnosis is by biopsy of perilesional tissue, with histological and immunostaining. Most patients respond to high-dose prednisolone (enteric-coated), dapsone or sulfonamides.

Lingual varicosities A fairly common condition of older people in which distended blood vessels are seen on the tongue ventrum **(Fig. 57.7)**. No treatment necessary.

Lipoma A rare benign tumour of adipose tissue, presenting as a slow-growing, yellowish, soft, semifluctuant, painless mass usually in the buccal mucosa. Diagnose by biopsy; manage by excision.

'Loose bodies' Hydroxyapatite crystal deposits within the temporomandibular joint space may be seen in osteochondritis dissecans (1–3 'loose bodies'); osteoarthritis (1–10 'loose bodies'); chip fracture of the articular surface (1–3 'loose bodies'); or synovial chondromatosis (50–500 'loose bodies'); and can cause pain. If the pain does not respond to conservative treatment, joint exploration may be needed.

Lupus erythematosus A rare autoimmune disease seen usually in females. The aetiology is unclear, but drugs, hormones and viruses may contribute in genetically predisposed persons:

- Discoid lupus erythematosus (DLE): oral lesions are seen in up to 25% of those with cutaneous DLE, mainly in the buccal mucosa, gingiva and lip. Characteristic features include central erythema, white spots or papules, radiating white striae at margins and peripheral telangiectasia.

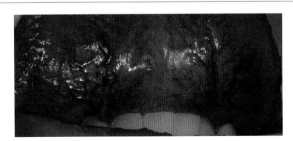

Fig. 57.7 Lingual (sub-lingual) varices

- Systemic lupus erythematosus (SLE): oral lesions like those in DLE, but usually more severe ulceration. SLE may also be associated with Sjögren syndrome and, rarely, temporomandibular joint arthritis.
- Diagnose by biopsy, blood picture and autoantibodies, especially crithidial (double-stranded DNA). Antinuclear factors are present in SLE, not in DLE. Biopsy shows the lupus band test with basement membrane zone deposits of IgG/IgM. Differentiate from lichen planus, leukoplakia (keratosis), galvanic-induced white lesions and carcinoma. Management includes:
- DLE: topical corticosteroids, cryosurgery or excision of localized lesions; there is a small predisposition to carcinoma.
- SLE: systemic corticosteroids, azathioprine, chloroquine or gold.

Lymphomas (See also Burkitt lymphoma, Hodgkin disease and non-Hodgkin lymphoma Ch. 56.) Malignant tumours that originate in lymph nodes and lymphoid tissue.

Malignant melanoma A malignant tumour of melanocytes. usually presenting as a heavily pigmented (occasionally non-pigmented) macule or, later, a nodule or ulcer. It may spread across several cm. The palate is most frequently affected, with spread to regional lymph nodes and then bloodstream. To differentiate naevi and other pigmented lesions, diagnosis is by wide excision biopsy. However, if melanoma clinically is a significant possibility, the patient should be referred for immediate surgery.

Masseteric hypertrophy May result from repeated jaw clenching or bruxism.

Measles A common childhood exanthem, caused by measles virus, with an incubation of 7–14 days. Features include Koplik spots (Ch. 56), rash (maculopapular), conjunctivitis, runny nose, cough, fever, malaise and anorexia. Diagnose from clinical features; a rising antibody titre is confirmatory. Differentiate from thrush and Fordyce spots (not in children). Management is symptomatic.

Meth mouth A term that applies to teeth affected by problems that can include caries, attrition, cracks and erosion attributed to heavy methamphetamine use caused by a combination of drug-induced hyposalivation, poor oral hygiene, frequent consumption of carbonated beverages, and tooth grinding and clenching.

Mixed connective tissue disease Characterized by anti-RNP autoantibodies, this may present with hyposalivation, trigeminal neuropathy, oral ulceration or Sjögren syndrome.

Multiple endocrine adenoma (MEN) syndrome There are three main types:

- MEN 1: parathyroid tumours, pancreatic tumours, and pituitary tumours.
- MEN 2a: medullary thyroid cancers (MTC), phaeochromocytoma, and parathyroid tumours.
- MEN 2b: medullary thyroid cancers, phaeochromocytoma and neuromas.

There are specific genetic causes for each of the three types and any particular MEN family will have only one type of MEN.

Muscular dystrophies Genetic myopathies which may cause facial muscle weakness:

- Facioscapular humeral muscular dystrophy: an autosomal-dominant condition, which progresses slowly. A dull-looking face which has no expression in conversation and can only just straighten the lips for a smile is characteristic, especially if seen with absence of blinking. As the name implies, the shoulders and upper part of the arms are also involved.
- Dystrophia myotonica: an autosomal-dominant condition. The first muscles involved are the sternomastoids and facial muscles, but the muscles of mastication may also become involved, with progress to other muscle groups. Myotonic features are seen early and followed by muscle wasting. Other features are premature baldness, cataracts, testicular atrophy and cardiomyopathy.

Myasthenia gravis An autoimmune disorder with defective neuromuscular transmission, which may first present as weakness of ocular movement or even facial movement.

Myelodysplastic syndrome A spectrum of essentially preleukaemic states. Can cause oral ulceration.

Myeloma A plasma cell tumour. Typically progresses to myelomatosis, but can present as:

- soft-tissue myeloma
- solitary osseous myeloma
- multiple myeloma (myelomatosis) – a disease mainly of middle-aged and older people, and sometimes related to exposure to ionizing radiation or petroleum products. The initial feature is abnormal serum immunoglobulins, occasionally detectable by chance, raised ESR, rouleaux formation or high plasma viscosity, or serum protein investigations. Years may elapse before discrete, punched-out radiolucent osteolytic lesions appear, especially in the skull and jaws. When the jaws are involved there may be pain, paraesthesia or anaesthesia, loosening of teeth and pathological fracture. Anaemia, weakness and weight loss are manifestations of advanced disease. A few patients also develop amyloidosis. Neoplastic proliferation of plasma cells in the bone marrow and their release of cytokines, such as interleukin-1, ultimately causes hypercalcaemia, renal failure, suppression of haemopoiesis and many other secondary effects. The abnormal immunoglobulins have defective antibody activity, and thus infections occur, and there may be plasma hyperviscosity with a clotting or bleeding tendency and neurological sequelae.

Diagnosis depends on showing:

- a monoclonal immunoglobulin peak on serum electrophoresis
- spillover of light chains into the urine (Bence–Jones proteinuria Ch. 56)
- plasma cell neoplasia on marrow biopsy
- osteolytic lesions on skeletal radiographs or by bone scanning.

Management is by radiotherapy and cytotoxic chemotherapy.

Myositis ossificans A rare idiopathic condition in which muscles ossify. Occasionally the same reaction follows trauma to muscle. Radiographs tend to show the calcifications and alkaline phosphatase levels are markedly raised.

Myxoma Rare in the oral cavity, this can arise in bone or soft tissue and, although benign, is aggressive and difficult to eradicate because it tends to infiltrate normal tissue.

Nasopharyngeal carcinoma Appears to be EBV-related, is common in Inuits and Chinese. The commonest features are a blocked nose, unilateral deafness, cervical lymphadenopathy. Trotter syndrome (Ch. 56) may occur. Treatment is usually chemo-radiotherapy.

Necrotizing sialometaplasia A rare condition in which there is ulceration, usually in a smoker in the palate, which heals spontaneously over several weeks. Associated with salivary gland infarction, histology can be confusing, since it has an appearance resembling neoplasia (pseudoepitheliomatous hyperplasia).

Nerve sheath tumours Neoplasms arising from a nerve or showing nerve sheath differentiation. Benign and malignant variants. Several distinct benign subtypes are recognized, including Schwannoma (neurilemoma, neurinoma), neurofibroma and perineurioma:

- *Schwannomas:* (see below)
- *Neurofibromas:* unencapsulated tumours composed of spindle cells in a fibromyxoid stroma
- *Perineuriomas:* arise in soft tissues or nerves, and are composed of cells with elongated bipolar cytoplasmic processes arranged in whorls or a storiform pattern. The neoplastic cells express vimentin and epithelial membrane antigen, but are negative for S-100 protein, desmin, muscle-specific actin, and CD34
- Most malignant NSTs arise from Schwann cells, and approximately two-thirds are associated with neurofibromas

Neurilemmoma (Schwannoma) A rare benign encapsulated neoplasm of neurilemmal cells of the nerve axonal sheath with distinct Antoni A and B components, hyaline vessel walls, and nuclear palisading. Tumour cells are strongly immunopositive for S-100 protein. Presents as a slowly enlarging painless mass, usually in the tongue, sometimes with facial pain and/or atrophy of the muscles of mastication. Facial nerve Schwannomas can cause facial palsy or compressive hearing loss resulting from ossicular interference and sensorineural hearing loss due to effects on cochlear nerve in the internal auditory canal. Can present with vestibular symptoms resulting from compression of the vestibular nerve; sensorineural hearing loss, tinnitus and disequilibrium. Schwannomas that arise from the glossopharyngeal, vagus or accessory nerves can be in the jugular foramen and present with variable cerebellar and acoustic symptoms, or can cause glossopharyngeal dysfunction (e.g. hoarseness, difficulty swallowing) and/or spinal accessory symptoms (e.g. trapezius atrophy). Schwannomas involving the oculomotor, trochlear and abducens nerves are rare, but can include palsy of the affected muscle and ipsilateral cavernous sinus symptoms if the mass is in the sinus. Hypoglossal Schwannomas can present with ipsilateral deviation of the tongue, possibly with associated hemiatrophy.

Neurofibromas (See Von Recklinghausen disease Ch. 56) Neurofibromas occasionally undergo sarcomatous change. Mucosal 'neurofibromas' (plexiform neuromas) may be seen in multiple endocrine neoplasia type III syndrome (with medullary carcinoma of the thyroid). Management is by excision. Neurofibromatosis type 2 (NF2) is also called the multiple inherited Schwannomas, meningiomas and ependymomas (MISME) syndrome. Diagnosis is by biopsy.

Noma (cancrum oris; gangrenous stomatitis) Gangrene that may follow acute ulcerative gingivitis in malnourished, debilitated, or severely immunocompromised patients. Anaerobes, particularly *Bacteroides* (*Porphyromonas*) species, *Fusobacterium necrophorum* (an animal pathogen), *Prevotella intermedia*, Actinomyces and alpha haemolytic streptococci, have been implicated. In cases following ANUG, *Streptococcus anginosus* and *Abiotrophia* spp. are the predominant species. In early noma, predominant species include *Ochrobactrum anthropi*, *Stenotrophomonas maltophilia*, an uncharacterized species of *Dialister*, and an uncultivated phylotype of *Leptotrichia*. A range of species or phylotypes are found in advanced noma, including *Propionibacterium acnes*, *Staphylococcus* spp., *Stenotrophomonas maltophilia*, *Ochrobactrum anthropi*, *Achromobacter* spp., *Afipia* spp., *Brevundimonas diminuta*, *Capnocytophaga* spp., *Cardiobacterium* spp., *Eikenella corrodens*, *Fusobacterium* spp., *Gemella haemoylsans*, and *Neisseria* spp. Phylotypes unique to noma infections include those in the genera *Eubacterium*, *Flavobacterium*, *Kocuria*, *Microbacterium*, and *Porphyromonas* and the related *Streptococcus salivarius* and genera *Sphingomonas* and *Treponema*. Spreading necrosis penetrates the buccal mucosa, leading to gangrene and an orocutaneous fistula and scarring. Diagnosis is clinical; an immune defect should always be excluded. Management includes improving nutrition, systemic antibiotics (clindamycin, penicillin, tetracyclines or metronidazole) and plastic surgery.

Orofacial–digital syndromes A group of inherited conditions manifesting with cleft lip and other facial anomalies, tongue clefts and multiple fraenae. Various dental defects, lingual and gingival nodules may be seen.

Ossifying fibroma This has features both of a developmental anomaly and a neoplasm. It presents as a painless, localized slow-growing, hard swelling of the jaw which radiographically is a well-defined radiolucency with a thin sclerotic margin containing irregular opaque masses. Histological examination shows little or no distinction between ossifying fibroma and fibrous dysplasia, except perhaps that a cellular, homogeneous calcified material is usually more obvious in ossifying fibroma. Distinction between ossifying fibroma and fibrous dysplasia, therefore, relies heavily on the localized nature and slow growth pattern of the ossifying fibroma. Surgical enucleation is curative.

Osteitis deformans Paget disease (Ch. 56).

405

Osteochondroma (osteocartilaginous exostosis) Arises from the epiphyseal region of bone as cartilage-capped bony outgrowths, usually in children. Lesions may be solitary, or multiple in the syndrome of hereditary multiple exostoses. In the jaws the most common site is the coronoid process. Solitary lesions are entirely benign, but in patients with multiple osteochondromas there is a significant risk of malignant change.

Osteogenesis imperfecta (brittle bone syndrome; fragilitas ossium) A group of at least four types of inherited bone disorder characterized by excessive bone fragility and a number of extra-skeletal connective tissue disorders. Affected children may have multiple rib fractures (giving a 'beaded' radiographic appearance) and shortened concertina-like long bones. The skull is soft, with multiple wormian bones. Fracture of limb bones following mild injury is the most common skeletal problem. Patients are usually of short stature, with grossly deformed limbs and deformities of the spine and trunk and often cannot walk. Some have dentinogenesis imperfecta.

Blue sclera occur in up to 90% of all patients. Deafness is common due to defective sound conduction through the external and middle ear. Hormones (calcitonin), vitamins (e.g. vitamin C or D), fluoride and flavonoids are of little value and surgical intervention for skeletal deformities is usually needed.

Osteomyelitis This literally means 'inflammation of the bone marrow', although sometimes the subperiosteal bone is mainly affected. Acute osteomyelitis primarily affects the mandible, usually affects adults and is essentially an osteolytic, destructive process, but an osteoblastic response is typical of sclerosing osteomyelitis. In children, proliferative periostitis may occur. Bacteria can spread to bone:

- from local odontogenic infections (the commonest cause)
- from other adjacent structures (e.g. otitis media, tonsillitis, suppurative sialadenitis)
- haematogenous spread of organisms (this is rare in relation to the jaws).

When osteomyelitis of the mandible does occur, it may be a sign of an underlying debilitating disease, such as diabetes mellitus, an immune defect, or the effects of alcoholism: alternatively, it may be related to reduced vascularity, such as after irradiation or in rare conditions like Paget disease or osteopetrosis. *Staphylococcus aureus* is the commonest organism causing osteomyelitis in the jaws, but streptococci (both α- and β-haemolytic) and anaerobic organisms (e.g. *Bacteroides* and *Peptostreptococci* species) are occasionally implicated.

In acute osteomyelitis the organisms excite acute inflammation in the medullary bone and the consequent oedema and exudation causes pus to be forced under pressure through the medullary bone. The pressure causes thrombosis of intrabony vessels (i.e. the inferior dental artery), reducing the vascular supply to the bone, which then necroses. Eventually pus bursts through the cortical plate to drain via sinuses in the skin or mucosa. Where pus penetrates the cortex it may spread subperiosteally, stripping the periosteum and, thus, further reducing the blood supply. Necrotic bone becomes sequestrae surrounded by pus and these either spontaneously discharge or remain and perpetuate infection. The periosteum lays down new bone to form an involucrum encasing the infected and sequestrated bone. The involucrum, although perforated by sinuses, may prevent sequestra from being shed. Finally, if little new bone is formed, a pathological fracture may occur. Mandibular osteomyelitis presents with a deep-seated, boring pain and swelling. Teeth in the affected segment are mobile and tender to percussion, and pus oozes from the gingival crevices. Once pus penetrates the cortical plate the pain improves and discharge appears. Labial anaesthesia is a characteristic feature because of pressure on the inferior alveolar nerve. The patient is often febrile and toxic with enlarged regional lymph nodes. Diagnosis is clinical, supported by imaging which, in established cases, shows marked bony destruction and sequestration but, since the changes are seen only after there has been significant decalcification of bone, early cases may not be detected and, in these, isotope bone scanning using technetium

diphosphonate may show increased uptake. There is a leukocytosis with neutrophilia, and a raised ESR, CRP or PV . Treatment is by antibiotic therapy and usually drainage. Penicillin is the drug of choice, but many staphylococci are now penicillin-resistant, and for these infections, flucloxacillin or fusidic acid may be used. Lincomycin and clindamycin also give high bone levels, but, because of a high incidence of pseudo-membranous colitis, are now regarded as second-line drugs. Metronidazole gives good bone levels and is indicated where anaerobic infection is suspected. Drainage of established pus follows the same guidelines used for other infections. When dead bone is exposed in the mouth, it can often be left to sequestrate without surgical interference, but sequestrectomy should be undertaken if the separated dead bone fails to discharge and decortication of the mandible may be needed in order to allow this and drainage.

Hyperbaric oxygen is an effective adjunct for recalcitrant osteomyelitis, especially where anaerobic organisms are involved:

- *Acute maxillary osteomyelitis:* this is seen rarely, and usually in infants, presumably because the lack of development of the antrum at this age makes the maxilla a dense bone.
- Chronic osteomyelitis: this presents with intermittent pain and swelling, relieved by the discharge of pus through longstanding sinuses. Bone destruction is localized and often a single sequestrum may be the source of chronic infection. Removal of the sequestrum and curettage of the associated granulation tissue usually produces complete resolution.
- *Focal sclerosing osteomyelitis*: this is usually asymptomatic and is revealed as an incidental radiographic finding. Most common in young adults, it is usually associated with apical infection of a mandibular molar. Radiographically there is a dense, radio-opaque area of sclerotic bone related to the tooth apical area, caused by formation of endosteal bone. This appears to be a response to low-grade infection in a highly immune host. Following tooth extraction the infection usually resolves (but the area of sclerotic bone often remains).
- *Diffuse sclerosing osteomyelitis*: a sclerotic endosteal reaction that, like focal sclerosing osteomyelitis, appears to be a response to low-grade infection. However, the area of bone involved is widespread and it sometimes involves most of the mandible or occasionally the maxilla. Sometimes the infection arises in an abnormally osteosclerotic mandible, such as in Paget disease, osteopetrosis or fibrous dysplasia. Intermittent swelling, pain and discharge of pus may persist for years. Management is difficult because of the extensive nature of the disease process. Long-term antibiotics, curettage and limited sequestrectomy all have their place.
- *Proliferative periostitis (Garré osteomyelitis)*: This is more common in children than adults. The cellular osteogenic periosteum of the child responds to low-grade infection, such as apical infection of a lower first molar tooth, by proliferation and deposition of subperiosteal new bone. The subperiosteal bone may be deposited in layers, producing an onion-skin appearance radiologically, which can simulate Ewing sarcoma. The endosteal bone, however, may appear to be completely normal, but in severe cases also appears moth-eaten radiologically. Removal of the infective source is usually followed by complete resolution, although subsequent bone remodelling can take a considerable time.

Osteonecrosis of jaws (ONJ) ONJ, or osteochemonecrosis, can arise in people who have used bisphosphonates. Intravenous bisphosphonates, such as Pamidronate (Aredia) and Zoledronate (Zometa), are a particular high risk, but even oral bisphosphonates used for >3 years are a risk. ONJ usually presents after dental treatment, especially surgery, with painful, exposed and necrotic bone, primarily of the alveolar bone of the mandible. Therefore, it is best to avoid elective oral surgery, including endosseous implant placement, or the treatment should be carried out well before commencing bisphosphonates. Therapy is primarily supportive, involving nutritional support along with superficial debridement and oral saline irrigation. Antibiotics are indicated only for definite secondary infection. Necrotic bone requires resection. Vascularized free tissue transfer provides an immediate reconstruction option with a shortened treatment course.

Osteoradionecrosis (ORN) This can arise in people who have been irradiated in the region of the jaws (Ch. 54). It presents similarly to ONJ. It can be spontaneous, but it most commonly results from tissue injury, especially surgery. Therapy is as for ONJ, plus hyperbaric oxygen.

Osteopetrosis (marble bone disease; Albers–Schonberg disease) Bone disease characterized by increased bone density with replacement of normal medullary bone by irregular avascular bone. Marrow is replaced by bone, and thus extramedullary sites such as the liver, spleen and lymph nodes develop haemopoietic function. Osteopetrosis is inherited in an autosomal-dominant or recessive manner. Patients with the autosomal-dominant form of osteopetrosis have good general health and a normal lifespan. There is no effective treatment for the recessive form: regular blood transfusions, corticosteroids and splenectomy may correct the anaemia; cranial nerve decompression may be necessary and, if hydrocephalus develops, ventricular shunts may be required. However, most affected children die in the first decade of life, usually as a consequence of overwhelming infection or haemorrhage. The jaws, particularly the maxillae, are thickened and sclerotic and the paranasal sinuses are often reduced in size. Recurrent sinusitis and cranial nerve palsies (especially II, III, V, VII and VIII) are other orofacial problems of osteopetrosis. Children with the recessive form of osteopetrosis may have teeth with hypoplastic enamel, shortened roots and an increased susceptibility to caries. Eruption of teeth can be delayed or absent. Pathological fracture is common. As a consequence of the sclerotic bone, dental extractions can be difficult and the mandible also liable to fracture. The reduced vascularity of bone predisposes to postextraction osteomyelitis.

Osteoporosis A fairly common condition, characterized by the loss of both the organic matrix and the mineralized components of bone, although serum biochemistry is normal. The most common cause of osteoporosis is ageing, especially in females (hormonal), but drugs (especially corticosteroids) and several other disorders can also increase the rate of bone loss. The main clinical problem of osteoporosis is fracture of either the neck of femur or collapse of vertebral bodies. Osteoporosis has no notable oral manifestations, but may affect the jaws and predispose to fracture or periodontal bone loss. Osteoporosis is managed by treatment of the underlying disorder (where possible) and by use of stimulators of osteogenesis (fluoride, phosphate, sex hormones or parathyroid hormone) or inhibitors of bone resorption (e.g. calcium, vitamin D, bisphosphonates). The bisphosphonates predispose to osteonecrosis of the jaws.

Osteosarcoma An aggressive malignant neoplasm which typically affects young patients. Males are affected twice as frequently as females. Only rarely are the mandible or maxilla affected. The aetiology is largely unknown, although about 3% of patients with osteosarcomas have a history of irradiation for other lesions. It should be noted that there is another peak incidence of osteosarcoma in the over-50s, which probably represents the small but significant malignant change in patients with pre-existing Paget disease. Osteosarcomas are classified as either sclerosing or osteolytic, depending on the degree of bone formation or destruction, and may be predominantly medullary or subperiosteal. A rare subtype called a *parosteal or juxtacortical osteosarcoma*, grows from the superficial surface of the bone and is relatively well differentiated. This variant grows much more slowly than the conventional osteosarcoma and metastasizes late. A characteristic feature of osteosarcoma is the 'sunray' appearance on radiography. In the jaws, symmetrical widening of the periodontal ligament in associated teeth may be an early sign. Although the prognosis for osteosarcomas of the jaws is marginally better than for those of the long bones, the outlook is usually poor.

Pachyderma oralis White sponge naevus.

Pachyonychia congenita A rare, usually autosomal-dominant syndrome, in which the main clinical sign is onychodystrophy of all finger and toe nails. There may be oral white lesions.

Papillomas The most common benign soft tissue neoplasms; usually caused by human papilloma virus (HPV) infections. Commonly asymptomatic, a papilloma is a pedunculated lesion, either pink or white if hyperkeratinized, on the palate, tongue or other sites. Diagnosis is confirmed by biopsy (**Fig. 57.8**). Management is with topical podophyllin or intralesional α-interferon, imiquimod or surgery.

Paraneoplastic pemphigus This is associated mainly with non-Hodgkin lymphoma, chronic lymphoid leukaemia, sarcomas, thymomas or Castleman disease. There are serum autoantibodies reacting with transitional epithelium, and lichenoid features on biopsy, with intra- and subepithelial clefting, and IgG and C3 deposits. Antibodies are directed against desmosomes and hemidesmosomes, especially against desmoplakin or BP1. Clinical features include severe stomatitis and cheilitis in all cases, conjunctival lesions, genital lesions, and polymorphous skin eruption on the trunk, palms and soles.

Periodic fever, aphthae, pharyngitis and adenopathy (PFAPA) An unusual cause of mouth ulceration (with the other features) in children, which appears to respond to cimetidine. There is a disorder of innate immunity with environmentally triggered activation of complement and IL-1β/-18.

Phakomatoses The term given to a range of disorders affecting ectoderm, with neurological manifestations and sometimes with learning disability, which include: Sturge–Weber syndrome, Von Recklinghausen neurofibromatosis, ataxia telangiectasia and tuberous sclerosis (epiloia; Bourneville disease: Ch. 56).

Pharyngeal pouch A rare pulsion diverticulum that appears because of a potential weakness in the pharyngeal muscles. Dysphagia characterized by regurgitation of food results and may cause aspiration into the lungs.

Porphyrias A group of rare disorders of porphyrin metabolism:

- *Erythropoietic porphyria* may cause reddish discolouration of both dentitions, hirsutism, and skin blisters.
- *Hepatic porphyria* predisposes to mouth blisters (and is a contraindication to use of intravenous barbiturates).

Pregnancy gingivitis An exacerbation of chronic gingivitis by pregnancy. Common mainly after the second month of pregnancy, pregnancy gingivitis presents with erythema, swelling and liability to bleed. Occasionally, a proliferative response at the site of a particularly dense plaque accumulation leads to a pregnancy epulis (pyogenic granuloma). This is a soft, red or occasionally firm swelling of the dental papilla. It may be asymptomatic unless traumatized by biting or toothbrushing. Oral hygiene should be improved. If asymptomatic, an epulis should be left alone – it may regress after parturition. If symptomatic, excision biopsy is indicated.

Progeria (Werner syndrome) A collagen abnormality causing dwarfism, premature ageing and a characteristic facial appearance due to

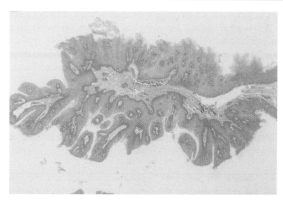

Fig. 57.8 Papilloma

a disproportionately small face with mandibular retrognathia and a beak-like nose. Death occurs usually in the mid-teens.

Pseudoxanthoma elasticum An autosomal-recessive condition of progressive calcification of elastic tissue in the retina, skin, cardiovascular system, and oral lesions of yellow plaques, somewhat resembling Fordyce spots.

Psoriasis Psoriasis of the oral mucosa is rare and is characterized by erythema, white or greyish plaques, and lesions similar to erythema migrans. Gingival involvement in the form of desquamative gingivitis may rarely be seen. Biopsy, with histological and immunostaining are essential to the diagnosis. Topical corticosteroids may be helpful in these cases.

Pyostomatitis vegetans Oral condition characterized by miliary pustules and ulcers or erosions affecting the gingivae, particularly labially, and the buccal, labial, lingual or palatal mucosae, typically associated with, and following the onset of, inflammatory bowel disease. Biopsy of perilesional tissue, with histological and immunostaining examination are essential to the diagnosis. The oral lesions may respond at least partially to topical corticosteroids. The underlying disease should be treated, typically with dapsone, systemic corticosteroids, sulphasalazine, azathioprine or sulphamethoxypyridazine. Some patients report benefit from zinc supplementation. Lesions may resolve following colectomy.

Radiolucencies Radiolucent lesions in the jaws may be due to cysts, infection, neoplasms arising in bone and metastatic neoplasms, bone disease (hyperparathyroidism, hypophosphatasia, cherubism; fibrous dysplasia; osteoporosis; osteonecrosis) and bone marrow expansion (haemolytic anaemias) or odontogenic cysts or tumours.

Radio-opacities Radio-opaque lesions in the jaws may be due to unexpected teeth, foreign bodies, bone disease (osteomyelitis; fibrous dysplasia; Paget disease (Ch. 56) Gardner syndrome (Ch. 56) osteopetrosis; neoplasms arising in bone and metastatic neoplasms especially from the prostate) or odontogenic lesions such as odontomes, hypercementosis, and calcifying odontogenic tumour.

Rickets and osteomalacia Bone diseases characterized by a decrease in the mineral, but not organic, content of bone. Unmineralized osteoid is present in large amounts, but there is a deficiency of mature mineralized bone. The term 'rickets' is used when the disorder affects children (when bones are still growing), the term 'osteomalacia' when adults are affected. The most common cause of rickets and osteomalacia in the western world is a deficiency of vitamin D, which can arise from dietary deficiency of vitamin D, gastrointestinal disease or in disorders of vitamin D metabolism. Dietary deficiency of vitamin D is still seen in older reclusive patients and in Asians living in Northern Europe on a poor diet which also contains phytates (such as in chapatis), since these inhibit calcium absorption from the gut, especially if they have little sun exposure in purdah. Vitamin D is normally synthesized in skin stimulated by sunlight. Renal disease impairs the conversion of vitamin D to dihydroxycholecalciferol and consequently can lead to 'renal rickets'. Rickets is clinically characterized by a spectrum of bony deformities, which range from mild bowing of the long bones of the legs to gross skeletal deformity and dwarfism. Osteomalacia causes generalized bone pain and tenderness, vertebral collapse, pelvic deformities and myopathy. Correction of any underlying clinical disorder is required and supplements of one of the metabolites of cholecalciferol are the usual lines of therapy for osteomalacia and rickets.

Rubella A highly infectious viral disease that causes cervical lymphadenopathy, a macular rash starting on the face and behind the ears, mild fever, sore throat and, occasionally, palatal petechiae. Transplacental infection of the foetus may cause high-tone deafness, learning disability, blindness, cardiac defects or death.

Salivary fistula An abnormal communication between the gland or ducts and skin or mucous membrane. Internal fistulae are uncommon and asymptomatic. Trauma to the major glands or duct may (rarely) cause a persistent external fistula that is unpleasant and may lead to infection. Surgical repair is then indicated.

Scleroderma An uncommon idiopathic connective tissue disease seen mainly in middle-aged females. Clinical features include oral telangiectases, restricted mouth opening with microstomia, pale fibrotic 'chicken' tongue and a widened periodontal space on radiography, but the teeth are not mobile. Diffuse scleroderma is clinically characterized by skin thickening involving the face, neck, trunk, and proximal upper and lower extremities, as well as significant internal organ involvement, including the lungs, heart, gastrointestinal tract, and kidney, and is classically associated with antitopoisomerase-I antibodies (anti-topo-I or anti-Scl-70) and the absence of anticentromere antibodies (ACA). Limited scleroderma involves skin thickening in the face, neck, and distal extremities, with frequent development of isolated pulmonary hypertension and ischamic digital loss, characterized by ACA. The CREST syndrome (calcinosis, Raynaud syndrome (Ch. 56), oesophageal lesions, sclerodactyly, telangiectasia) is a rare variant. Overlap syndromes, such as mixed connective tissue disease (MCTD), with features of systemic lupus erythematosus (SLE), polymyositis (PM), rheumatoid arthritis (RA), and scleroderma are associated with anti-U1-small nuclear ribonucleoprotein particle (U1-snRNP) antibodies. Diagnosis is from clinical features, histopathology and autoantibodies. Management is often with penicillamine.

Scurvy Vitamin C (ascorbic acid) deficiency. Arises when no fresh fruit or vegetables are eaten for a long period. Diffusely swollen, boggy, and purplish gingivae with purpura and haemorrhage are seen. Diagnosis is from leukaemia mainly from the dietary history, clinical features, blood film and white cell ascorbic acid. Management is with vitamin C.

Solitary bone cysts Lesions that occur most commonly in the long bones, they may also be found occasionally in the jaws. Their cause is speculative, but they may arise after trauma to the bone when an intramedullary haematoma forms and then degenerates rather than healing. Haemorrhagic bone cysts are generally painless and expansion is uncommon, the lesions usually being coincidentally discovered during radiographic examination. They are seen most often in the posterior body of the mandible in young persons. Clear or blood-stained fluid may be found within the bony cavity, but preoperative aspiration may at times not yield any product. Radiologically there is a well-defined translucency with a scalloped appearance around the apices of the teeth, which are vital. Surgery is undertaken in order to make a definitive diagnosis. There is no detectable cyst lining and sometimes only a thin fibrous membrane. Curettage produces bone fragments and connective tissue sometimes with granulation tissue. However, such surgical opening of the cavity usually leads to spontaneous resolution.

Subepithelial immune blistering diseases These include pemphigoid variants, dermatitis herpetiformis, acquired epidermolysis bullosa, linear IgA disease and chronic bullous disease of childhood.

Superior vena cava obstruction Obstruction of cardiac venous return, usually by lung cancer, may produce oedema and cyanosis of face, neck and arms.

Surgical emphysema Escape of air into the tissues, usually after using an air rotor to section a tooth for removal, may give rise to diffuse swelling, which characteristically is painless, but gives rise to crepitus on palpation.

Syphilis A sexually transmitted infection caused by *Treponema pallidum*. Other treponematoses, including yaws, bejel and pinta, are rare in the developed world:

- *Congenital syphilis*: this manifests with frontal bossing, saddle nose, Hutchinsonian incisors, Moon or mulberry molars and rhagades. Learning disability, interstitial keratitis, deafness, sabre tibiae and Clutton joints may be seen (Ch. 56).
- *Acquired syphilis*: predominantly an infection of the sexually promiscuous (prostitutes, men who have sex with men, travellers, armed forces). Diagnosis is by direct smear of primary and secondary stage lesions. Serology becomes positive late in the primary stage. Penicillin by injection (or erythromycin or tetracycline). Incubation period 9–90 days.

- *Primary syphilis (Hunterian or hard chancre)*: this is a small papule which develops into a large painless indurated ulcer, with regional lymphadenitis. A chancre heals spontaneously in 1–2 months. Rare on the lip (upper) or intraorally – usually the tongue. *Treponema pallidum* in smear (dark-field examination). Serology is positive late in this stage. Differentiate from trauma, herpes labialis, pyogenic granuloma and carcinoma.
- *Secondary syphilis*: oral lesions include mucous patches, split papules or snail-track ulcers, which are highly infectious. Rash (coppery coloured typically on palms and soles), condylomata lata and generalized lymph node enlargement can also be present.
- *Tertiary syphilis*: this may cause glossitis (leukoplakia) and gumma (usually midline in the palate or tongue). These are non-infectious, but may be associated with cardiovascular complications (aortic aneurysm) or neurosyphilis (tabes dorsalis, general paralysis of the insane, Argyll–Robinson pupils).

Teething Teething is the name sometimes given to children who are irritable, febrile and drooling, sometimes with a rash, but tooth eruption per se may cause a little discomfort but is not associated with fever or a rash, and most examples of 'teething' are probably infections such as herpetic stomatitis, pharyngitis or tonsillitis. Paracetamol is of value and the most important measure is to ensure hydration. Teething gels containing lidocaine, tannic acid, glycerol or essential oils (e.g. menthol, thymol) may be of some benefit but those containing salicylates or alcohol are best avoided.

Temporomandibular joint dislocation Occurs if the condyle moves too far forwards and over the articular eminence. The jaw locks in an open position with intense pain. The liability is increased in people with hypermobility syndromes. The dislocation must be reduced, under sedation or GA.

Thyroglossal cyst Arises from remnants of the thyroglossal duct and is midline at any point between the tongue and thyroid gland, and moves up on protrusion of the tongue. The cyst may cause dysphagia or become infected. It should be surgically removed.

Tobacco Use can cause a range of oral conditions from staining, to malodour, candidosis, dry mouth, taste disturbances, dry socket, implant failure, ANUG, periodontitis, keratosis, leukoplakia, to oral cancer.

Tooth root resorption Can arise because of:

- chronic infection
- chronic trauma
- impactions
- cysts and tumours
- tooth subluxation, luxation or radiotherapy
- systemic disease (Paget disease; hypo or hyper-parathyroidism; Turner syndrome; Gaucher disease or calcinosis: see Ch. 56).

Tooth surface loss Tooth surface loss includes attrition (**Fig. 57.9**), abrasion and erosion (and possibly abfraction).

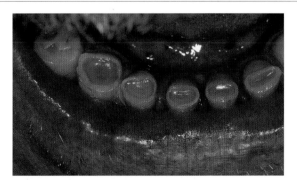

Fig. 57.9 Attrition, showing exposure of dentine and formation of secondary dentine

TORCH syndrome or complex Foetal anomalies involving the heart, skin, eye, and CNS, caused by perinatal infections with toxoplasmosis; other infections (hepatitis B, Coxsackie, syphilis, VZV, HIV, parvovirus B19) rubella; cytomegalovirus; or herpes simplex virus.

Toxic epidermal necrolysis (TEN; Lyell disease: Ch. 56) A rare clinicopathological entity, with a high mortality, characterized by extensive detachment of full-thickness epithelium. The distinction from erythema multiforme is unclear, but most cases of TEN are drug-induced and the lesions are extremely widespread. Drugs appear to trigger what appears to be an immunologically related reaction with sub- and intraepithelial vesiculation. Recently, an increased number of cases in HIV/AIDS patients has been recorded. TEN presents with a cough, sore throat, burning eyes, malaise and low fever, followed after about 1–2 days by skin and mucous membrane lesions. The entire skin surface and oral mucosa may be involved, with up to 100% sloughing off. Oral mucosae are involved in almost all cases. Gingival lesions are common and clinically are inflamed, with blister formation leading to painful widespread erosions.

Sheet-like loss of the epithelium and a positive Nikolsky sign (Ch. 56) are characteristic. Biopsy of perilesional tissue, with histological and immunostaining examination are essential to the diagnosis. Histopathological examination is characteristic, showing necrosis of the whole epithelium detached from the lamina propria. Patients with TEN must be admitted to a hospital intensive care unit as soon as possible for management.

Toxoplasmosis Infection by the parasite *Toxoplasma gondii*, which infests members of the cat family who excrete it in faeces. *T. gondii* survives in soil for up to 1 year, and infection is generally by ingestion of cysts or oocysts, which are present in up to 10% of lamb and 25% of pork used for human consumption. In normal healthy patients symptomatic toxoplasmosis manifests as:

- glandular fever syndrome, with a negative Paul–Bunell test (Ch. 56)
- ocular toxoplasmosis with chorioretinitis.

Transplacental transmission may result in foetal defects. In immunocompromised patients such as those with HIV/AIDS, *T. gondii* may produce CNS involvement.

Toxoplasmosis is diagnosed by detection of serum antibodies by the Sabin–Feldmann dye test, indirect haemagglutination or IgM fluorescent antibody tests, and isolation of *T. gondii* or histological demonstration of trophozoites. Toxoplasmosis is treated with pyrimethamine and sulfadiazine.

Trichodento-osseous syndrome Autosomal dominant; kinky hair, amelogenesis imperfecta; taurodont molars and brittle nails.

Tuberculosis Infection with mycobacteria, usually *Mycobacterium tuberculosis*, but rarely atypical mycobacteria, e.g. *M. avium-intracellulare*, *M. scrofulaceum* and *M. kansasii*, especially in HIV infection. Uncommon, tuberculosis is usually pulmonary and seen mainly in alcoholics, diabetics, patients with immune defects (including HIV infection), and certain racial groups (e.g. Asian). Clinical features may include a single chronic ulcer on the dorsum of tongue associated with (postprimary) pulmonary infection. Diagnosis is confirmed by biopsy, sputum culture, tuberculin testing and chest radiography. Management is with combination chemotherapy. Treatment is started with three drugs in combination in order to minimize the emergence of bacterial resistance, and is then continued with two or more antibiotics, usually from the following: rifampicin, isoniazid, ethambutol or streptomycin. Chemotherapy is usually effective treatment, but must be given for prolonged periods and, if chemotherapy is less than adequate, bacterial resistance readily develops. Multi-drug resistance (MDR) and highly resistant strains (X DR-TB) are increasing in HIV/AIDS.

TUGSE (traumatic ulcerative granuloma with stromal eosinophilia) Also known as traumatic granuloma, eosinophilic ulcer and eosinophilic granuloma this is not related to eosinophilic granuloma of bone as in Langerhans cell histiocytosis. TUGSE may affect patients of all ages, including neonates, when it is known as Riga-Fede disease. TUGSE is a reactive condition seen most commonly on the dorsal and lateral tongue, followed by the lips and buccal mucosa as a deep, rolled bordered and indurated ulcer to exophytic and lobular looking like a pyogenic granuloma. It probably is initiated by trauma, resolves spontaneously slowly over many weeks and may recur. The clinical features may mimic squamous cell carcinoma (SCC). Biopsy is indicated if the ulcer persists >3 weeks, and shows eosinophils in areas of muscle damage. The treatment is surgery; intralesional corticosteroids if it recurs.

Tularaemia Infection by the coccobacillus *Francisella tularensis*. The epidemics are thought to be waterborne. Most patients are young and female. In most of the cases the disease presents itself in oropharyngeal form, with fever and tonsillopharyngitis and cervical lymphadenopathy. Streptomycin is given to most patients in combination with tetracycline, doxycycline or chloramphenicol.

Ulcerative colitis Inflammatory bowel disease, which may present with persistent diarrhoea and is frequently painless, with passage of blood and mucus in severe cases, iron deficiency anaemia, weight loss, and mucosal pustules (pyostomatitis vegetans), irregular chronic ulcers and aphthae. Diagnosis is by biopsy, full blood picture, sigmoidoscopy and barium enema. Management is with haematinics for any secondary deficiencies; topical corticosteroids may be helpful; as may sulphasalazine, or corticosteroid enemas.

White sponge naevus (Cannon disease, pachyderma oralis, white folded gingivostomatitis). Rare autosomal-dominant defect of keratin causing a benign familial disorder with lesions, typically:

- symptomless
- white
- shaggy or folded or wrinkled
- bilateral
- seen in the buccal mucosa.

Lesions are sometimes seen in other oral sites especially the tongue, the floor of the mouth, or elsewhere, or in the:

- nose and upper respiratory tract
- pharynx
- oesophagus
- genitals
- anus.

The family history and examination are usually adequate to make the diagnosis, but there may be confusion with other white lesions, when a biopsy is indicated.

Glossary

AC angular cheilitis

ACA anti-centromere antibodies

ACTH adrenocorticotrophic hormone

ALU aphthous-like ulcers

ANA antinuclear antibodies

ANCA anti-neutrophil cytoplasmic antigen

ANUG acute necrotizing ulcerative gingivitis

ART antiretroviral therapy

ATA anti-topoisomerase antibodies

BANA benzoyl-arginine-naphthyl-amide

BARK Bilateral Alveolar Ridge Keratosis

bid or bd twice a day

BMS burning mouth syndrome

BNF *British National Formulary*

BP blood pressure

BRONJ bisphosphonate related osteonecrosis

BS Behçet syndrome

CAT computed tomography

CATCH 22 cardiac defects, abnormal facies, thymic hypoplasia, cleft palate, and hypocalcaemia resulting from chromosome 22 deletions

CBCT cone beam CT

CBT cognitive behavioural therapy

CD4 cluster of differentiation 4 (a type of helper T lymphocyte)

CDC Centers for Disease Control and Prevention (USA)

CMC chronic mucocutaneous candidosis

CMV cytomegalovirus

CNS central nervous system

CO complaining of

COPD chronic obstructive pulmonary disease

CPITN community periodontal index of treatment needs

CRP C-reactive protein

CSF cerebrospinal fluid

CT computed tomography

CTR chemoradiotherapy

CTX chemotherapy

CVA cerebrovascular accident

CVE cerebrovascular event

CXR chest X-ray

DEXA dual-emission X-ray absorptiometry

DIF direct immunofluorescence

DIHS drug-induced hypersensitivity syndrome

DIGO drug-induced gingival overgrowth

DLE disseminated lupus erythematosus

DPF *Dental Practitioners Formulary*

DRESS drug rash with eosinophilia and systemic symptoms

Ds DNA double strand deoxyribonucleic acid

Dsg desmoglein

DXR radiotherapy

EB epidermolysis bullosa

EBV Epstein–Barr virus

ECG electrocardiogram

EGFR epidermal growth factor receptor

ELISA enzyme linked immunosorbent assay

EM erythema multiforme

EMA European Medicines Agency

ENA Extractable Nuclear Antigen

ENT ears, nose and throat (otorhinolaryngology)

ESR erythrocyte sedimentation rate

EUA examination under (general) anaesthetic

FBC full blood count

FBP full blood picture

FDA Food and Drug Administration (USA)

FH family history

FNA fine needle aspiration

FNAB fine needle aspiration biopsy

GA general anaesthesia

GI gastrointestinal

GDP general dental practitioner

GIT gastrointestinal tract

GMH general medical history

GMP general medical practitioner

GORD gastro-oesophageal reflux disease

G6PD glucose 6 phosphate dehydrogenase

GP general practitioner

GU genitourinary

GVHD graft-versus-host disease

HAART highly active antiretroviral therapy

HBV hepatitis B virus

HCV hepatitis C virus

HHV human herpesviruses

HIV human immunodeficiency virus(es)

HL Hodgkin lymphoma

HLA human leukocyte antigen

HPA hypothalamo-pituitary–adrenal

HPA Health Protection Agency (UK)

HPC history of the present complaint

HPV human papilloma viruses

HRQoL health related quality of life

HSCT haematopoietic stem cell transplantation

HSV herpes simplex virus

HTLV human lymphotropic virus

IFN interferon

IgG immunoglobulin G

IIF indirect immunofluorescence

IL interleukin

IRIS immune reconstitution inflammatory syndrome

KCOT keratocystic odontogenic tumour

KS Kaposi sarcoma

KSHV Kaposi sarcoma herpesvirus (HHV-8)

LA local anaesthesia

LFT liver function tests

LMS locomotor system

LP lichen planus
MALT mucosa associated lymphoid tissue
MDR-TB multidrug resistant tuberculosis
MDT multidisciplinary team
MEN multiple endocrine neoplasia
mg milligram
MMP mucous membrane pemphigoid
MRG median rhomboid glossitis
MRI magnetic resonance imaging
MRS Melkersson-Rosenthal syndrome
MRSA meticillin resistant *Staphylococcus aureus*
MS multiple (disseminated) sclerosis
NAAT nucleic acid amplification test
NHL non-Hodgkin lymphoma
NICE National Institute for Health and Clinical Excellence (UK)
NSAID nonsteroidal antiinflammatory drugs
NSM necrotizing sialometaplasia
OFG orofacial granulomatosis
OLP oral lichen planus
ORN osteoradionecrosis
OTC over-the-counter
PAS periodic acid Schiff
PCR polymerase chain reaction
PET positron emission tomography
PFAPA periodic fever, adenitis, pharyngitis, aphthae
PI protease inhibitor
PMH past medical history
POM prescription-only medicine
PPI proton pump inhibitor
PRN as necessary
PV pemphigus vulgaris; plasma viscosity
QoL quality of life
RAS recurrent aphthous stomatitis
RAST radioallergosorbent test
RF rheumatoid factor
RMH relevant medical history
ROM range-of-movement
RS respiratory system

RT radiotherapy
SACE serum angiotensin converting enzyme
SCID severe combined immune deficiency
SH social history
SJS Stevens-Johnson syndrome
SLE systemic lupus erythematosus
SLN sentinel lymph node
SNRI serotonin–norepinephrine reuptake inhibitor
SPT second primary tumour
SS Sjögren syndrome
SS-A antibodies in Sjögren syndrome
SS-B antibodies in Sjögren syndrome
SSI sexually shared infections
SSRI selective serotonin re-uptake inhibitor
STI sexually transmitted infections
SUNCT severe unilateral neuralgia with conjunctivitis and tearing
TAC trigeminal autonomic cephalgia
TB tuberculosis
TEN toxic epidermal necrolysis
TMJ temporomandibular joint
TMPD temporomandibular pain-dysfunction
TORCH toxoplasmosis; rubella; cytomegalovirus; herpes
TN trigeminal neuralgia
TNF tumour necrosis factor
TPMT thiopurine methyl transferase
TUGSE traumatic ulcerative granuloma with stromal eosinophilia
U&E urea and electrolytes
UADT upper aerodigestive tract
URTI upper respiratory tract infection
US ultrasound
UTI urinary tract infection
WBC white blood cell count
WCC white cell count
VRSA vancomycin resistant *Staphylococcus aureus*
VZV varicella zoster virus
XTR-TB extended drug resistant tuberculosis

Index

415